Gerontologic
Nursing
Wholistic Care of the Older Adult

Gerontologic Nursing
Wholistic Care of the Older Adult

Second Edition

Mary M. Burke, RN, DNSc, GNP-C
Associate Professor
Nurse Practitioner Program
George Washington University
Washington, DC

Mary B. Walsh, RN, MSN, FAAN
Associate Professor, Retired
School of Nursing
The Catholic University of America
Washington, DC

With 100 illustrations

St. Louis Baltimore Boston Carlsbad Chicago Naples New York Philadelphia Portland
London Madrid Mexico City Singapore Sydney Tokyo Toronto Wiesbaden

Publisher: Nancy Coon
Editor: Michael S. Ledbetter
Associate Developmental Editor: Cecily Barolak
Project Manager: Dana Peick
Senior Production Editor: Stavra Demetrulias
Designer: Amy Buxton
Manufacturing Supervisor: Karen Lewis

A NOTE TO THE READER:

The author and publisher have made every attempt to check dosages and nursing content for accuracy. Because the science of pharmacology is continually advancing, our knowledge base continues to expand. Therefore we recommend that the reader always check product information for changes in dosage or administration before administering any medication. This is particularly important with new or rarely used drugs.

SECOND EDITION

© 1997 by Mosby-Year Book, Inc.

Previous edition copyrighted 1992.

Printed in the United States of America
Composition by Carlisle Communications, Ltd.
Lithography/color film by Color Dot Graphics, Inc.
Printing/binding by R.R. Donnelley and Sons, Inc.

Mosby-Year Book, Inc.
11830 Westline Industrial Drive
St. Louis, Missouri 63146

International Standard Book Number
0-8151-1331-5

96 97 98 99 00 / 9 8 7 6 5 4 3 2 1

CONTRIBUTORS

to Second Edition

Mary Beth Bigley, MSN, ANP-C
Assistant Professor of Health Care
  Science
George Washington University
Washington, DC

Francis J. Burke, JD
Attorney
Washington, DC

**Mary M. (Mickie) Burke,
  RN, DNSc, GNP-C**
Associate Professor
Nurse Practitioner Program
George Washington University
Washington, DC

**Caroline Bagley Burnett,
  RN, ScD**
Clinical Associate Professor
  of Nursing
Georgetown University
Division of Cancer Prevention
  and Control
Lombardi Cancer Center
School of Nursing
Washington, DC

Charles A. Cefalu, MD, MS
Director of Geriatrics and
  Associate Professor
Department of Family Medicine
Georgetown University School of
  Medicine/Providence Hospital
Washington, DC

Helene M. Clark, RN, PhD
Assistant Professor
School of Nursing
The Catholic University of America
Washington, DC

Sister Maureen Duffy, MS, RD
Clinical Dietician
Providence Hospital
Washington, DC

Theresa Ferlotti, RN, MSN, GNP
Staff Nurse/Clinician II
Georgetown University Medical
  Center
Washington, DC

Barbara Galen, MSN, CANP
Rockville, MD

Myrtle R. McCulloch, EdD, RD
Assistant Professor of Nursing
Georgetown University School
  of Nursing
Washington, DC

**B. Joan McDowell, PhD,
  CRNP, FAAN**
Associate Professor of Nursing
University of Pittsburgh
Pittsburgh, Pennsylvania

Karen Ehlke Reilly, ScD
Project Director
Allied Technology Group, Inc.
Rockville, Maryland

Helen T. Roach, RN, MSN
Critical Care Clinical Educator
Georgetown University Medical
  Center
Washington, DC

**Sister Maria Salerno, OSF, DNSc,
  RNCS, NP**
Associate Professor
Director Primary Care
  ANP Program
Codirector FNP Program
School of Nursing
The Catholic University of America
Washington, DC

Susan E. Sherman, RN, MA
President
Independence Foundation
Philadelphia, PA

Sheila M. Sparks, RN, DNSc, CS
Assistant Professor
School of Nursing
Georgetown University
Washington, DC

Patricia Stockton, M. PHIL
Research Associate
Department of Psychiatry, Division
  of Psychosocial Research
Georgetown Medical Center
Washington, DC

Catherine A. Swanson, RN, MSN
Case Manager
Lung Cancer
Lombardi Cancer Center
Georgetown University Medical
  Center
Washington, DC

**Sister Carol Taylor, RN, CSFN,
  PhD Candidate, MSN**
Assistant Professor, Humanities
Clinical Ethicist
Health Care Ethicist
Holy Family College
Philadelphia, Pennsylvania

**Mary B. Walsh, RN, MSN,
  FAAN**
Associate Professor, Retired
School of Nursing
The Catholic University of America
Washington, DC

CONTRIBUTORS

to First Edition

Kathleen Adams, RN, MSN, CANP
Adjunct Assistant Professor
Nurse Practitioner Program
George Washington University
Washington, DC

Mary Beth Bigley, RN, MSN, CANP
Cardiovascular Nurse Specialist
Arlington Hospital
Arlington, Virginia

Kathryn L. Burgio, PhD
Research Assistant Professor
of Medicine
Assistant Professor of Nursing
University of Pittsburgh–
Falk Clinic
Pittsburgh, Pennsylvania

Mary M. Burke, RN, DNSc, CRNP
Assistant Professor
School of Nursing
Georgetown University
Washington, DC

Helene M. Clark, PhD, RNC
Assistant Professor
School of Nursing
The Catholic University
of America
Washington, DC

Janice C. Hallal, RN, DNSc
Associate Professor
School of Nursing
The Catholic University
of America
Washington, DC

M. Anne Hart, MSG, MPA
District of Columbia Long Term
Care Ombudsman
Legal Counsel for the Elderly
Washington, DC

Jean Johnson, RN, MSN, NPC
Associate Professor
Department of Health Care
Sciences
George Washington University
Washington, DC

Carol N. Knowlton, RN, MSN
Assistant Dean for Student Affairs
School of Nursing
The Catholic University
of America
Washington, DC

B. Joan McDowell, CRNP, PhD, RNC
Research Assistant Professor
of Medicine
Assistant Professor of Nursing
University of Pittsburgh
Pittsburgh, Pennsylvania

Mary Eletta Morse, RN, MSN, GNPC
Geriatric Clinical Nurse Specialist
Alexandria Hospital
Alexandria, Virginia

Helen T. Roach, RN, MSN
Clinical Educator
Nursing Education and Research
Georgetown University Hospital
Washington, DC

Claudia Schlosberg, JD
Dixon Implementation
Monitoring Committee
Mental Health Law Project
Washington, DC

Sandra C. Sewell, RN, MSN
Program Manager,
Care Management
Gerontological Center
Suburban Hospital
Bethesda, Maryland

Sheila Sparks, RN, DNSc
Assistant Professor
School of Nursing
Georgetown University
Washington, DC

Patricia Stockton, BSc, MCSP
Research Associate
Department of Psychiatry
and Center on Aging
Georgetown University
Washington, DC

Catherine A. Swanson, RN, MSN, NPC
Clinical Educator
Nursing Education and Research
Georgetown University Hospital
Washington, DC

Kyriake Valassi, PhD
Professor of Nutritional
Biochemistry
School of Nursing
The Catholic University
of America
Washington, DC

Mary B. Walsh, RN, MSN, FAAN
Associate Professor, Retired
School of Nursing
The Catholic University
of America
Washington, DC

Sister Paul Gabriel Wilhere, RN, MEd
Nursing Home Consultant,
Long Term Care
Pittsburgh, Pennsylvania

To Frank and Paul,
spouses extraordinaire,
who provided patience, humor, and support
throughout the two editions of this text

PREFACE

When the authors/editors prepared the first edition of this text, the recognition of increased numbers of older adults was more true then than it is now. The difference is, there are so many more older adults in the population now (see Chapter 1), and their needs are greater in number today and are wider in variety than they were upon publication of the first edition. In view of the changes in the population today, the authors/editors felt it necessary to update the data that were presented at that time, as well as to incorporate new data that are now available about older adults.

The subtitle of the original text has been adjusted to exclude "care of the frail elderly"; however, the content of this text will continue to address the needs of the frail elderly, while not making them the sole or primary focus. The new subtitle, "Wholistic Care of the Older Adult," highlights a change in focus to include all older adults who may be healthy *or* ill; their needs will be considered throughout the text. The nurse's role in assisting older persons to prevent illness for as long as possible, and to remain as independent as possible, despite alterations in health in whatever form they appear, will also be incorporated into the text. The basic assumption throughout the text will be that of health and independence, while maintaining a realistic tone. Utilization of all of one's talents and abilities will be the thrust, with the hope that the achievements of the older persons will far exceed those predicted or projected by others.

The focus of this text is on the gerontologic knowledge that is needed by those health care professionals who are responsible for promoting and maintaining the health of older adults. Primarily, the intent is to provide information for the student of nursing that will increase the student's ability to provide quality care for the older person. While the idea of "student" places the emphasis on the beginning learner, this can have various connotations. It is possible that the beginning student will be the high school graduate who has just entered a baccalaureate nursing program; or, this beginning student may be one of several types of students who has transferred to a nursing major from an educational program with various types of preparation. The ultimate goal of such a learner is to become a health caregiver for the older person whose concern is to maintain or restore health and/or to ameliorate illness. While this is the primary focus for the development of content for this text, it is quite possible that other persons can benefit from the knowledge presentation; that is, graduate students in nursing programs, or nurses who are employed in various settings as they care for older patients.

■ Organization

Each of the chapters that addresses clinical content does so with a selection of content that the authors/editors believe is crucial to the care of gerontologic patients/persons. The contributors for these chapters have been selected according to their professional expertise in the appropriate area.

The nursing process framework is the structure for each of the clinical chapters. Elements of the nursing process are considered to be: assessing, diagnosing, planning and identifying outcomes, implementing, and evaluating.

In view of the locations where gerontologic patients or older persons live, the settings for the care of the older person include:

the acute care setting
the nursing home setting
the community or personal home.

The second edition has updated all existing chapters; furthermore, in response to readers' comments and the changing health care system, five new chapters have been added: The Transition Years, Drug Therapy in Older Adults, Bowel Elimination, Cancer in the Older Adult, and Ethical Perspectives. The scope of the book has been adapted to accommodate the emphasis on the early years of aging and the enhancement of the health of the older adult.

The first five chapters address the demography of the older population today, critical elements of gerontologic nursing, the theories about aging that guide the care of older adults, the psychosocial components of the transitional years, and the pharmacodynamics of the care of older adults.

Fourteen clinical chapters deal with the predominant issues and problems that are presently faced by older persons. These include an update of the following topics that were presented in the first edition: sexuality, sensation, integument, regulation, cardiovascular, respiration, mobility, urinary incontinence, nutrition, sleep, cognition, and safety. In addition to these twelve topics, there are two additional chapters about cancer and bowel elimination.

Finally, the last four chapters are presented as a cluster of content dealing with the topics of grief, legal issues, ethics, and some dreams and fears about the future for older adults.

Clusters of topics are similar to the groups of data that were presented in the first edition. The content under each chapter heading has been updated according to the experiences of the authors, and according to the reports of progress and change as defined in the literature. Research reports are included as they have been reported in the extant literature. The progress of health care may appear to proceed too slowly as we live out the changes and improvements that are swirling around us as we function in the care of older adults. However, in retrospect, examining the past five years is quite revealing and surprising. It is encouraging to note the number of studies that have been initiated and completed in the area of gerontologic nursing. It is heartening to see a rise in interested and well-prepared health personnel to care for the older citizen. It gives one a true boost in spirits to become aware of the improved stature that gerontology and gerontologic nursing have acquired in a relatively brief time. This is also to say that much more needs to be done by all who now function in this critical specialty, but this is to say that much has been done and much is underway.

■ Features

Various features throughout the text, both new and included from the first edition, are utilized to enhance content and serve as useful teaching tools. **Learning Objectives** at the beginning of each chapter identify key areas to be discussed. **Aging Alerts,** integrated throughout the text, highlight important aging considerations. Assessment criteria, age-related changes, pharmacology, lab and diagnostic testing, pathology, and risk factors are included in numerous **tables and boxes.**

To incorporate the wholistic approach of this edition, two new features have been added: **Health Promotion boxes** in the clinical chapters include suggestions for the nurse to encourage healthy behaviors in older adults; and *Healthy People 2000 Objectives* highlight goals for health promotion and disease prevention.

■ Instructor's Resource Manual

The **Instructor's Resource Manual** has been created in response to great demand for such an ancillary. This IRM follows the text chapter by chapter and includes chapter outlines and overviews; Teaching Suggestions for Classroom and Practice Applications and Critical Thinking Exercises to aid students in applying what they have learned; Chapter Review Questions/Activities; and a Test Bank.

■ Acknowledgments

To accept the challenge of editing a textbook on Gerontologic Nursing is quite adequate to show any person(s) how inadequate each of us is to function alone. The greater the information about the subject matter, the greater is our dependence on our peers and colleagues. There are wonderful and impressive people in the health care profession who are anxious to share with others the information gained through experience. Sharing this information with peers and colleagues is quite beneficial to the knowledge base of all of us. We are truly indebted to our co-workers, to our students, and to our patients. A special word of thanks to Sister Paul Gabriel, who has been our mentor and model for many years. They have all contributed to increasing our knowledge base about gerontologic nursing—and for this we are grateful. For all those persons who have pursued research studies, large and small, we thank you for reporting the results of your efforts so that all of us will gain from your experiences. Keep up the good work!

Accessibility to the published data about gerontologic nursing is essential for those who are involved with the care of older adults. Several persons are outstanding in this respect for this edition. Nellie Lee Powell, at the School of Nursing Library at The Catholic University of America, continues to be supportive and valuable to the production of printed data; we could not have proceeded without her. Amy Holloway at George Washington University was a great help in the development of computer illustrations and the reference librarians at the George Washington Himmelfarb library were extremely helpful. We would also like to acknowledge Debbie Drake, Mary Reuther Herring, and Cora Zembrzuski for their helpful suggestions for revising the manuscript. We thank you all.

This book may be written by authors/editors and their names appear on the cover and chapters, but the people behind the scenes are the ones who deserve the kudos. We were most fortunate with our experience with the Mosby staff. We would like to continue to thank Linda Duncan, our editor on the first edition. Our current editor, Michael Ledbetter, provides us with encouragement, understanding, and always graciousness. We couldn't have had a better editor. But the best is saved for last: Cecily Barolak, Associate Development Editor, was always there when we needed anything. What to do? Where to send it? How to say it? Who will do it? The list goes on and on, but Cecily, with her calm and friendly way, was never rushed, always available, and able to listen.

Our families are still with us, quite a feat through two editions. We love them all and thank them for their patience, and are grateful for their encouragement.

Mary M. Burke
Mary B. Walsh

CONTENTS

Gerontologic
Nursing
Wholistic Care of the Older Adult

Grow old along with me!
The best is yet to be,
The last of life, for which the first was made.

ROBERT BROWNING

The Older Adult Population

■ Learning Objectives

On completion of this chapter, the reader will be able to do the following:

1. Define the older adult population, recognizing stereotypes applied to this population.
2. Recognize the complexity of factors that influence the lives of older adults—including health maintenance, available care during illness or disability, and current health care financing and services—and the significance of environmental factors that include geographic location and features of the individual's community and home.
3. Describe sociologic, economic, and educational trends among older adults.
4. Recognize current demographic trends among older adults in the United States, identifying present and predictive trends.

■ Background

A statement of a 5-year-old kindergartner in Silver Spring, Maryland: "My teacher [26] is really old, like you, Mom [41]." A statement of a 73-year-old man in Milwaukee, Wisconsin: "I certainly am looking forward to my wedding next month! No, I'm not old yet." These two statements illustrate how varied and relative is the concept of age. When speaking of age, every person has a subjective view of the term *old*. The multitude of differences among older adults makes it both difficult and unwise to generalize traits as applicable to all older adults. In the conceptualizing and speaking of old age and older adults, terms and specific individuals or groups must be defined

clearly. Vague labels, such as "old," "elderly," or "senior citizen," suggest stereotypes that are misleading and inappropriate when applied to individuals within the labeled populations.

In the United States, further misinterpretation results from linking the concept of retirement to specific ages or age groups. Stereotypes regarding retirement may have been somewhat justifiable in the mid-1800s, when Bismarck announced the first nationwide pension plan for the German people. He decided that retirement would be mandated at age 65 and that a pension plan would be available to all retirees. Bismarck's action actually affected few Germans (Mitchell, 1971) because in the mid–nineteenth century

1

few people ever reached age 65. Today quite the opposite is true. Not only are there greater numbers of people living to age 65 and beyond, but the social contributions of those in their 60s, 70s, and 80s are quite significant. For example, one in five of those over 75 help their children or grandchildren in daily living activities (Commonwealth Fund, 1992). As life expectancy continues to increase, employers are revising their ideas and policies about retirement and even soliciting the expertise of older adults. The chronologic age for retirement now varies widely. Although early retirement may be unavoidable for people in some occupations, such as dancers or pilots, retirement age remains virtually undefined for people in less physical occupations, such as writers, artists, or accountants. Fullerton (1993) projected that the labor force made up of those 55 years old and older would increase by more than 38% between 1992 and 2005.

Many view older adults as frail or feeble, with limited capacity for making contributions society would view as beneficial. Unfortunately, the common perception of aging and older adults often differs sharply from the reality of aging. A Commonwealth Fund study (1992), *The Nation's Great Overlooked Resource: The Contributions of Americans 55+,* found that almost 38 million Americans over age 55 contribute to American society; their contributions are estimated to equal those of 20 million full-time employees. One in 5 contribute a sizable portion to their children's or grandchildren's income; only 1 in 20 receive a sizable portion from their children or grandchildren. Impressions and interpretations about older adults can vary widely, depending on one's beliefs, knowledge, experience, orientation, and age. The astute and objective observer will view each aging person according to individual talents, abilities, and state of health, thereby minimizing or avoiding misconceptions about aging.

Although the astute observer looks past aging generalities and focuses on the unique individual, there are times when it is useful to view older adults as a group or special population. The special population can be defined in terms of common characteristics and social situations. For example, the health care planner must make generalizations about the older adult population when defining health care financing or health care delivery alternatives for those over 65. Decisions regarding allocation of social goods are often based on population groups and their needs. An understanding of some common group characteristics of those 65 and older is useful in decision making and understanding human needs. Three alternative social structures, aimed at describing human needs, will be discussed here.

Human life processes continue throughout the life span. Individuals of any age experience a spectrum of human needs. For example, anyone, regardless of age, experiences fundamental physiologic needs, as well as needs for safety and security, love and belonging, self-esteem, and self-actualization (Maslow, 1970). The relative significance of each need and the hierarchic relationships among these needs are shown in Maslow's hierarchy (Figure 1-1). (Extensive illustration and discussion of Maslow's interpretation of human needs is presented in Ebersole & Hess, 1994.) The most basic needs are physiologic; life

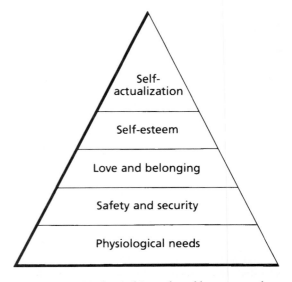

FIGURE 1-1 Maslow's hierarchy of human needs.

cannot continue without these needs being met. The psychosocial need of self-actualization is at the top of Maslow's pyramid.

Galtung (1980) suggests a second approach to the identification and analysis of human needs. Basic human needs are differentiated, according to two pairs of interrelated factors, as material versus nonmaterial needs and as actor-dependent versus structure-dependent needs. The first pair of factors concerns the needs of an individual's body versus those of the mind. There is a clear delineation between material and nonmaterial needs. For example, a material need might be housing, whereas freedom might be a nonmaterial need. The second pair of factors is related to the means by which needs are satisfied, or source of satisfaction. This involves the social context of human needs. Human need satisfaction depends on either the actor or the structure of the need situation. Actor-dependent needs depend on the motivation and capacity of some *one* person to satisfy those needs. Structure-dependent needs are met by satisfiers built into the social structure itself, without being dependent on particular persons. Table 1-1 illustrates the typology of human needs suggested by Galtung.

A third approach in describing human needs is one that arranges human needs in specific clusters. Yura and Walsh (1988) arranged a selected group of human needs according to three clusters, adapting the work of Galtung and others. They classify human needs as follows:

TABLE 1-1 Galtung's typology of human needs

Source of satisfaction	Material needs	Nonmaterial needs
Actor dependent	Security needs	Freedom needs
Structure dependent	Welfare needs	Identity needs

Adapted from Galtung, J. (1980). The basic human needs approach. In K. Lederer (Ed.), *Human needs*. Cambridge, MA: Oelgeschlager, Gunn, and Hain.

Survival needs
Closeness needs
Freedom needs

These are particularly useful ways of grouping and labeling human needs when dealing with the family and with the community (Table 1-2).

Human needs continue to exist throughout the life of each person, with multiple variables affecting the intensity of these needs as a person grows older. Because health is perceived as a major factor in realizing a satisfactory, high-quality life, most older adults devote a reasonable amount of energy to achieving the highest level of health possible. Being over 65 years old does not by any means prohibit participation in a variety of activities that promote and encourage healthy living. The range and variety of activities continue to exist, with perhaps the intensity of the activity adjusted according to individual endurance.

This text makes some generalizations about older adults, yet readers are encouraged to avoid overgeneralizing about all older people. Instead, readers are urged to meet each older person as an individual, to treat each person in a wholistic manner, and to consider each as a unique person with particular needs, desires, talents, and interests. This approach recognizes the challenge, the excitement, and the satisfaction of living and working with older adults.

■ Definition of Older Adults

For purposes of this text, *older adults* are people 65 years old or older. In 1993 older adults made up almost 13% of the U.S. population, numbering almost 33 million (American Association of Retired Persons [AARP], 1994). By the year 2000 older adults are projected to make up approximately 20% of the U.S. population, with a greater racial diversity. The term *65 and older* describes individuals with a broad spectrum of ages, health statuses, and general capacities. Not only does the term *older adult* apply to the married, employed 68-year-old; it also applies to the single, 92-year-old nursing home resident. Age subcategories are sometimes useful in further describing

TABLE 1-2 Human needs

Survival needs	Closeness needs	Freedom needs
Activity	Acceptance	Autonomy
Adaption	Appreciation	Beauty
Air	Belonging	Challenge
Elimination	Confidence	Conceptualization
Fluids intake	Humor	Freedom from pain
Gas interchange	Love, being loved	Self-control
Nutrition	Personal recognition	Self-fulfillment
Protection from fear	Sexual integrity	Spiritual experience
Perception of reality	Tenderness	Territoriality
Rest, leisure	Wholesome body image	Value system
Safety		
Sensory integrity		
Skin integrity		
Sleep		

Adapted from Yura, H., & Walsh, M. B. (1988). *The nursing process.* E. Norwalk, CT: Appleton and Lange.

the population known as *older adults* and are presented accordingly in this text.

As a normal process of aging, changes occur that slow nerve impulses, lengthen healing time, and reduce the body's ability to fend off disease (Schaie and Willis, 1986). Although physical, mental, and sensory impairments do increase with age, severe and disabling limitations are still relatively rare among older people. The fear of disability is greater than the incidence of disability, and if unchecked, this fear can handicap the lifestyle of a person. Anxiety and fear about health problems become greater as people get older. These concerns should not be ignored, but neither should they be magnified. The best antidote for such fears is to provide accurate information, education, and reassurance regarding the health problems—many of them treatable—and to focus on the most active and fullest life possible. Emphasis should be on the positive ways to maintain health. Neglect of problems can quickly lead to loss of function, and older adults can rapidly become unnecessarily dependent as a result of such neglect. On the other hand, a focus on healthy aging enables older adults to maximize their human potential and enjoy the "golden years."

■ Myths and Stereotypes

Myths and stereotypes perpetuate erroneous ideas regarding aging, as shown in Box 1-1. Reaching age 65 does not provide automatic entry into inactive frailty. In fact, the onset of aging is a gradual, subtle process, varying in rate and intensity by individual. Aging is not an abrupt change, nor is it a sure and steady retrogression from good health to poor health (Abdellah, 1989). Rather, it is a developmental stage of life, with challenges and opportunities that may vary by issue but that are similar in principle to those of other developmental stages.

Although the number of chronic ailments does increase as people grow older, these ailments do not necessarily inhibit or impair every older person. Some people do become more frail as they get older, but many do not. For example, George Burns was 95 years old in 1991, and he had already scheduled a personal performance for his one-hundredth birthday. Another celebrated oldster, similarly visible to the general public, is actor Bob Hope, 92 years old in 1995, continuing his Christmas tradition of performing for U.S. troops by traveling to the Persian Gulf.

BOX 1-1 NATIONAL INSTITUTE ON AGING: WHAT IS YOUR AGING IQ?

TRUE OR FALSE?

1. Baby boomers are the fastest growing segment of the population.
2. Families don't bother with their older relatives.
3. Everyone becomes confused or forgetful if they live long enough.
4. You can be too old to exercise.
5. Heart disease is a much bigger problem for older men than for older women.
6. The older you get, the less you sleep.
7. People should watch their weight as they age.
8. Most older people are depressed. Why shouldn't they be?
9. Older people should not have screening tests for cancer. Why bother?
10. Older people take more medications than younger people.
11. People begin to lose interest in sex around age 55.
12. If your parents had Alzheimer's disease, you will inevitably get it.
13. Diet and exercise reduce the risk of osteoporosis.
14. As your body changes with age, so does your personality.
15. Older people might as well accept urinary accidents as a fact of life.
16. Suicide is mainly a problem for teenagers.
17. Falls and injuries "just happen" to older people.
18. Everybody gets cataracts.
19. Extremes of heat and cold can be especially dangerous for older people.
20. "You can't teach an old dog new tricks."

ANSWERS

1. **False.** There are more than 3 million Americans over the age of 85. That number is expected to quadruple by the year 2040, when there will be more than 12 million people in that age group. The population age 85 and older is the fastest growing age group in the United States.
2. **False.** Most older people live close to their children and see them often. Many live with their spouses. An estimated 80% of men and 60% of women live in family settings. Only 5% of the older population live in nursing homes.
3. **False.** Confusion and serious forgetfulness in old age can be caused by Alzheimer's disease or other conditions that result in irreversible damage to the brain. But at least 100 other problems can bring on the same symptoms. A minor head injury, high fever, poor nutrition, adverse drug reactions, and depression also can lead to confusion. These conditions are treatable, however, and the confusion they cause can be eliminated.
4. **False.** Exercise at any age can help strengthen the heart and lungs and lower blood pressure. It also can improve muscle strength and, if carefully chosen, lessen bone loss with age. See a physician before beginning a new exercise program.
5. **False.** The risk of heart disease increases dramatically for women after menopause. By age 65 both men and women have a one-in-three chance of showing symptoms. But risks can be significantly reduced by following a healthy diet and exercising.
6. **False.** In later life it's the quality of sleep that declines, not total sleep time. Researchers have found that sleep tends to become more fragmented as people age. A number of reports suggest that older people are less likely than younger people to stay awake throughout the day and that older people tend to take more naps than younger people.

Continued

BOX 1-1 NATIONAL INSTITUTE ON AGING: WHAT IS YOUR AGING IQ?—cont'd

7. **True.** Most people gain weight as they age. Because of changes in the body and decreasing physical activity, older people usually need fewer calories. Still, a balanced diet is important. Older people require essential nutrients just like younger adults. You should be concerned about your weight if there has been an involuntary gain or loss of 10 pounds in the past 6 months.

8. **False.** Most older people are not depressed. When it does occur, depression is treatable throughout the life cycle using a variety of approaches such as family support, psychotherapy, or antidepressant medications. A physician can determine whether the depression is caused by medication an older person might be taking, by physical illness, by stress, or by other factors.

9. **False.** Many older people can beat cancer, especially if it's found early. Over half of all cancers occur in people 65 and older, which means that screening for cancer in this age group is especially important.

10. **True.** Older people often have a combination of conditions that require drugs. They consume 25% of all medications and can have many more problems with adverse reactions. Check with your doctor to make sure all drugs and dosages are appropriate.

11. **False.** Most older people can lead an active, satisfying sex life.

12. **False.** The overwhelming majority of people with Alzheimer's disease have not inherited the disorder. In a few families, scientists have seen an extremely high incidence of the disease and have identified genes in these families that they think may be responsible.

13. **True.** Women are at particular risk for osteoporosis. They can help prevent bone loss by eating foods rich in calcium and exercising regularly throughout life. Foods such as milk and other dairy products, dark green leafy vegetables, salmon, sardines, and tofu promote new bone growth. Activities such as walking, biking, and simple exercises to strengthen the upper body also can be effective.

14. **False.** Research has found that, except for the changes that can result from Alzheimer's disease and other forms of dementia, personality is one of the few constants of life. That is, you are likely to age much as you've lived.

15. **False.** Urinary incontinence is a symptom, not a disease. Usually it is caused by specific changes in body function that can result from infection, diseases, pregnancy, or the use of certain medications. A variety of treatment options is available for people who seek medical attention.

16. **False.** Suicide is most prevalent among people age 65 and older. An older person's concern with suicide should be taken very seriously, and professional help should be sought quickly.

17. **False.** Falls are the most common cause of injuries among people over age 65. But many of these injuries, which result in broken bones, can be avoided. Regular vision and hearing tests and good safety habits can help prevent accidents. Knowing whether your medications affect balance and coordination also is a good idea.

18. **False.** Not everyone gets cataracts, although a great many older people do. Some 18% of people between the ages of 65 and 74 have cataracts, and more than 40% of those between 75 and 85 have the problem. Cataracts can be treated very successfully with surgery; more than 90% of people say they can see better after the procedure.

19. **True.** The body's thermostat tends to function less efficiently with age, making the older person's body less able to adapt to heat or cold.

20. **False.** People at any age can learn new information and skills. Research indicates that older people can obtain new skills and improve old ones, including learning how to use a computer.

From U.S. Department of Health and Human Services, Public Health Service, National Institutes of Health (1991).

Julia Child, at the age of 82, continues with public appearances and book publishing. At the age of 85, Jacques Cousteau will set sail next year to explore and film the rivers and coast of China.

■ Complex Factors in the Lives of Older Adults

HEALTH AND ILLNESS

Health can be defined in various ways. The World Health Organization defines health as "a state of complete physical, mental, and social well-being and not merely the absence of disease and infirmity" (Brockington, 1975, p. 5). Pender (1982) defines *wholistic health* as the "actualization of human potential through purposeful, self-initiated behavior, satisfying relationships with others, and competent personal care." The National Council on Aging (1994) talks of organizational, political, and economic instruments affecting behavior and environment geared to preventing, delaying, or minimizing disease or disability while promoting independence. Many other definitions of health can be found in the literature, and each definition reflects the purpose and orientation of the author. Some view health as it relates to illness or disease rather than emphasizing the positive dimensions of health. Other authors view health positively, identifying it as a normal, expected state in people of any age. They view coping with illness or disease as an associated state, but not the dominant state of existence.

Healthy aging programs, an increased understanding of the aging process, and advances in health care technology all have contributed to increased longevity. The life expectancy of someone born in 1992 was 28 years longer than that of someone born in 1900 (AARP, 1994). Centenarians, those who reach the age of 100 years, have more than doubled during the 1980s (Taeuber, 1993). Many more older adults are living healthier lives. Conversely, as a result of modern medicine's ability to arrest disease stages, many older adults are living with various types of chronic ailments and illnesses. For impaired older adults, a focus on their strengths often assists them in achieving goals once conceptualized as unattainable. Most people are familiar with the negative cycle associated with the inability to perform an activity. The lack of accomplishment is followed by discouragement and depression, which is then followed by increased inability to perform activities, and finally by complete withdrawal from the activity. A positive cycle works in the same way. Goal achievement in activities leads to encouragement and a positive self-image, which, in turn, enhances identification and achievement of future goals.

Facilitating a positive cycle becomes increasingly important as older adults live longer (Table 1-3). In 1990 there were over 3 million Americans 85 years old and older. By the year 2050 the U.S. Bureau of the Census has projected that the number of Americans 85 years old and older will have increased to over 17 million. Furthermore, in 1985 25,000 Americans were 100 years old or older. By the year 2050 the number of Americans 100 years old and older is expected to be over 1 million ("**The Facts of Life,**" 1987) (Figure 1-2). These life expectancy figures underscore the importance of highlighting the health, abilities, and strengths of people moving into the seventh, eighth, and even ninth decades of life. The importance of enhancing the quality of life cannot be overemphasized.

Maintaining a positive attitude may be particularly difficult as older adults adapt to changes in health that accompany the aging process. There is little risk of people in their 20s and 30s suffering a chronic disease such as arthritis or osteoporosis. From the age of 40 on, however, the risk doubles exponentially about every 5 years (Table 1-4). By the time a person reaches age 85, there is also a one-in-three chance that that person will have dementia, immobility, incontinence, or other age-related disabilities.

To enhance a positive attitude among older adults by minimizing disabilities related to older

TABLE 1-3 Actual and projected growth of the older population: 1900 to 2050[*]

Year	Total population all ages	55 to 64 years Number[†]	%	65 to 74 years Number[†]	%	75 to 84 years Number[†]	%	85 years and over Number[†]	%	65 years and over Number[†]	%
1900	76,303	4,009	5.3	2,189	2.9	772	1.0	123	0.2	3,084	4.0
1910	91,972	5,054	5.5	2,793	3.0	989	1.1	167	0.2	3,950	4.3
1920	105,711	6,532	6.2	3,464	3.3	1,259	1.2	210	0.2	4,933	4.7
1930	122,775	8,397	6.8	4,721	3.8	1,641	1.3	272	0.2	6,634	5.4
1940	131,669	10,572	8.0	6,375	4.8	2,278	1.7	365	0.3	9,019	6.8
1950	150,967	13,295	8.8	8,415	5.6	3,278	2.2	577	0.4	12,270	8.1
1960	179,323	15,572	8.7	10,997	6.1	4,633	2.6	929	0.5	16,560	9.2
1970	203,302	18,608	9.2	12,447	6.1	6,124	3.0	1,409	0.7	19,980	9.8
1980	226,505	21,700	9.6	15,578	6.9	7,727	3.4	2,240	1.0	25,544	11.3
1990	249,657	21,051	8.4	18,035	7.2	10,349	4.1	3,313	1.3	31,697	12.7
2000	274,815	23,988	8.7	18,258	6.6	12,339	4.5	4,289	1.6	34,886	12.7
2010	298,109	34,378	11.5	21,235	7.1	12,767	4.3	5,702	1.9	39,705	13.1
2020	322,602	41,959	13.0	31,680	9.8	15,467	4.8	6,480	2.0	53,627	16.6
2030	344,951	36,866	10.7	37,865	11.0	23,592	6.8	8,381	2.4	69,839	20.2
2040	364,349	38,079	10.5	33,683	9.2	28,689	7.9	13,221	3.6	75,588	20.7
2050	382,674	42,620	11.1	35,217	9.2	26,008	6.8	17,652	4.6	78,876	20.6

From U.S. Bureau of the Census, Decennial Censuses of Population (for 1900-1980). U.S. Bureau of the Census, Projections of the Populations of the United States, by Age, Sex, and Race: 1983 to 2080. Current Population Reports, Series P-25, no. 1092, November 1992.
*Projections are middle series.
†Numbers in thousands.

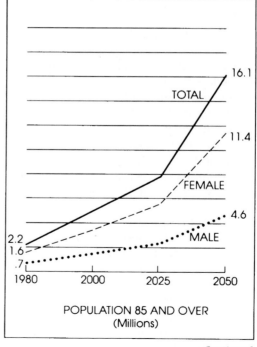

Continued

FIGURE 1-2 Projected demographic trends for the elderly, 1980-2050. (From U.S. Bureau of the Census.)

9

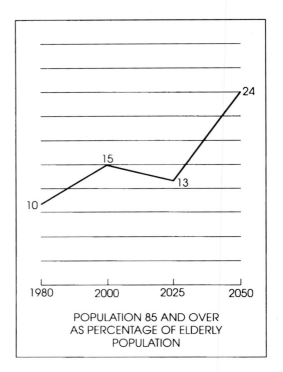

FIGURE 1-2, cont'd. For legend see p. 9.

age, Perry and Butler (1988) suggest earmarking research dollars for reducing frailty, improving health, and increasing independence among older adults. Given the common, but incorrect, belief that not much can be done to alter the aging process, coupled with the competition for research initiative dollars, aging research often loses out to other programs. Unless research dollars are directed toward minimizing older adult disabilities, recognizing the costliness of disabilities in terms of both social good and human suffering, Perry and Butler predict, for example, that Alzheimer's disease victims will increase fivefold by the middle of the next century. Unless advances are made relating to conditions associated with nursing home admissions, such as incontinence, memory loss, and immobility, there will be up to 6 million older Americans in nursing homes by the middle of the twenty-first century, as compared to 1.8 million residents in 1990. Perry and Butler plead for reducing or

eliminating "costly medical procedures, lengthy hospital stays, and financially draining long-term care."

Some research initiatives are presently underway that attempt to address these issues. For example, the Health Care Financing Administration (HCFA), within the U.S. Department of Health and Human Services, sponsors demonstrations aimed at integrating acute and long-term care benefits for older adults. The Program of All-inclusive Care for the Elderly (PACE) incorporates both acute and long-term care services for frail older adults available through Medicare and Medicaid, through a team case management approach (Vladeck et al., 1993). Another HCFA demonstration is the Social Health Maintenance Organization, which provides a wide range of support care for functionally limited Medicare recipients. HCFA's EverCare demonstration is aimed at managing the special acute care needs of the institutionalized older adult population.

TABLE 1-4 Prevalence of selected reported chronic conditions, by age, during 1987

Chronic conditions	Number of cases*	Rate per 1000 persons				
		Under 18 years	18 to 44 years	45 to 64 years	65 to 74 years	75 years and over
Heart conditions	19,656	22.2	40.7	126.1	284.7	322.2
Chronic bronchitis	12,749	62.1	40.4	56.9	86.9	58.2
Arthritis	31,438	2.8	52.8	273.3	463.6	511.9
Diabetes	6,641	2.0	11.9	56.4	98.3	98.2
Diseases of urinary system	6,769	7.3	27.8	39.6	54.8	67.7
Orthopedic impairment	27,725	35.8	135.4	155.0	154.9	182.0

From U.S. National Center for Health Statistics. (1990). *Vital and health statistics* (Series 10).
*Numbers in thousands.

Some gerontologists believe that the ability to reset the biologic clock, that is, to delay or eliminate the decline caused by aging, may be on the horizon. New information about aging is constantly being uncovered, and present-day advances in immunology and molecular aging genetics have provided valuable insights into the aging process. With reasonable, perhaps only modest, extensions of technology, there may be early resolution of problems associated with immobility, osteoporosis, and incontinence. Doubling the present monetary allotment for osteoporosis research could conceivably eliminate this major health problem, which now afflicts approximately 90% of women over the age of 75. Postponement of health deficits associated with aging has a threefold benefit: (1) the individual's health status improves, thus increasing the quality of life; (2) society's health care costs decrease; and (3) older adults' contributions to society increase, resulting in an increase in total social good. An increase in an older adult's health expectancy through reductions in chronic and disabling conditions is closely associated with an increase in enjoying the later years in life (Perry and Butler, 1988). Though one may tire of frequent references to *the improvement or maintenance of a high quality of life,* continued discussion of this term and its meaning to older adults is appropriate—even essential. As health care

providers continue to strive to increase life expectancy, of equal concern is adding quality of life to later years.

Mortality data both answer longevity questions and raise related concerns among health care delivery personnel and health policy researchers. Projections for future health care delivery and categoric financial allocation depend on data generated from current experiences and events. Various studies and reports address these concerns. One such study was prepared by K. G. Manton (1986) to determine (1) whether people are living past age 85 because better medical care and new treatments are helping those with chronic health problems to live longer and (2) whether people who live to age 85 and beyond are, on average, healthier.

One of Manton's observations was the large gain in life expectancy for those at age 85. Between 1960 and 1980, 85-year-old white men gained almost 1 year in life expectancy and 85-year-old white women gained almost 2 years in life expectancy (Tables 1-5 and 1-6). The health policy and social implications of this sizable increase are considered to be enormous. For example, this suggests a significant increase in the population who will be entitled to receive Social Security benefits. In fact, in 1995 the Social Security Administration was made an independent federal agency to increase administrative efficiency

TABLE 1-5 Expectation of life at birth, 1960 to 1988, and projections, 1990 to 2010*

Year	Total			White			Black and other			Black		
	Total	Male	Female	Total	Male	Female	Total	Male	Female	Total	Male	Female
1960	69.7	66.6	73.1	70.6	67.4	74.1	63.6	61.1	66.3	—	—	—
1970	70.8	67.1	74.7	71.7	68.0	75.6	65.3	61.3	69.4	64.1	60.0	68.3
1975	72.6	68.8	76.6	73.4	69.5	77.3	68.0	63.7	72.4	66.8	62.4	71.3
1976	72.9	69.1	76.8	73.6	69.9	77.5	68.4	64.2	72.7	67.2	62.9	71.6
1977	73.3	69.5	77.2	74.0	70.2	77.9	68.9	64.7	73.2	67.7	63.4	72.0
1978	73.5	69.6	77.3	74.1	70.4	78.0	69.3	65.0	73.5	68.1	63.7	72.4
1979	73.9	70.0	77.8	74.6	70.8	78.4	69.8	65.4	74.1	68.5	64.0	72.9
1980	73.7	70.0	77.4	74.4	70.7	78.1	69.5	65.3	73.6	68.1	63.8	72.5
1981	74.2	70.4	77.8	74.8	71.1	78.4	70.3	66.1	74.4	68.9	64.5	73.2
1982	74.5	70.9	78.1	75.1	71.5	78.7	71.0	66.8	75.0	69.4	65.1	73.7
1983	74.6	71.0	78.1	75.2	71.7	78.7	71.1	67.2	74.9	69.6	65.4	73.6
1984	74.7	71.2	78.2	75.3	71.8	78.7	71.3	67.4	75.0	69.7	65.6	73.7
1985	74.7	71.2	78.2	75.3	71.9	78.7	71.2	67.2	75.0	69.5	65.3	73.5
1986	74.8	71.3	78.3	75.4	72.0	78.8	71.2	67.2	75.1	69.4	65.2	73.5
1987	75.0	71.5	78.4	75.6	72.2	78.9	71.3	67.3	75.2	69.4	65.2	73.6
1988, preliminary	74.9	71.4	78.3	75.5	72.1	78.9	71.5	67.4	75.5	69.5	65.1	73.8
1990, projected[†]	75.4	71.8	78.8	76.1	72.7	79.4	69.1	64.5	73.6	71.2	67.0	75.2
1995, projected[†]	76.3	72.8	79.7	76.8	73.4	80.2	—	—	—	72.4	68.8	76.0
2000, projected[†]	77.0	73.5	80.4	77.5	74.0	80.9	—	—	—	73.5	69.9	77.1
2005, projected[†]	77.6	74.2	81.0	78.1	74.6	81.5	—	—	—	74.6	71.0	78.1
2010, projected[†]	77.9	74.4	81.3	78.3	74.9	81.7	—	—	—	75.0	71.4	78.5

From U.S. National Center for Health Statistics. *Vital statistics of the United States* (unpublished date).
*Data are annual, except as noted. Life expectancy is expressed in years; beginning in 1970, it excludes deaths of nonresidents of the United States, see also *Historical statistics: Colonial times to 1970* (Series B 107-115).
[†]From U.S. Bureau of the Census. *Current population reports* (Series P-25, No. 1018). Based on middle mortality assumptions.

TABLE 1-6 Life expectancy at birth and at age 65, by sex and calendar year: 1900 to 2050

Year of birth	Male life expectancy		Female life expectancy	
	At birth	At age 65	At birth	At age 65
1900	46.4	11.3	49.0	12.0
1910	50.1	11.4	53.6	12.1
1920	54.5	11.8	56.3	12.3
1930	58.0	11.8	61.3	12.9
1940	61.4	11.9	65.7	13.4
1950	65.6	12.8	71.1	15.1
1960	66.7	12.9	73.2	15.9
1970	67.1	13.1	74.9	17.1
1980	69.9	14.0	77.5	18.4
1990	71.4	14.5	78.9	19.2
2000	72.1	14.8	79.5	19.5
2010	72.4	15.0	79.8	19.8
2020	72.7	15.2	80.1	20.1
2030	73.0	15.4	80.4	20.3
2040	73.3	15.6	80.7	20.6
2050	73.6	15.8	81.0	20.8

From Social Security Administration. (1984). *Social Security area population projections, 1984* (Actuarial Study No. 92, Alternative 1).

and meet some of these increased demands. Because older adults typically consume a higher proportion of acute and long-term care services, health policy planners' work often focuses on the over-65 age group, to better forecast data and overlay potential health care delivery system costs. Total federal expenditures for the group of citizens over age 80 are expected to have increased by 67% between the years 1980 and 2000.

In 1990 heart disease was the leading cause of death among those 65 and older, accounting for 44% of deaths among those 85 years old and older (Taeuber, 1993). It is predicted that elimination of deaths from heart disease, through health promotion programs and other initiatives, will add over 5 years to life expectancy at age 65 and over 3½ years to life expectancy at age 85. Among those 65 to 74 years old, cancer, along with heart disease, accounted for approximately 33% of all deaths in 1990. Other leading causes

of death were stroke, influenza, and pneumonia. A major health problem among older adults is their susceptibility to various infections (Besdine and Rose, 1982). Infection often becomes the immediate cause of death for the very old who also have one or more chronic diseases. The number of deaths attributed to multiple causes has increased over the years. Reasons for this are an increase in age at time of death, a decrease in deaths from infectious diseases, and more accurate reporting. See the discussion under comorbidity and disability for further elaboration.

Understanding issues related to reducing mortality in advanced age is important for three reasons: (1) It would allow forecasters to more accurately predict life expectancy trends. (2) Health care researchers could assess the impact and cost effectiveness of interventions for further reducing the mortality rate. (3) Health care planners and clinicians could improve the health status of older people and assess how such improvements would affect various types of health services and the demand for those services.

COMORBIDITY AND DISABILITY

Although the occurrence of various illnesses and ailments may not be synonymous with aging, there is evidence that the incidence of health problems usually increases with a person's years of life (Figure 1-3). In addition, an older adult may experience more than one ailment or health problem at a time. This is referred to as *comorbidity*. Caregivers of older adults have witnessed and reported a special burden experienced by older

people with more than one health problem. Comorbidity affects the overall health status and functional ability of aging people to a greater extent than do the simpler difficulties of dealing with one disease. Despite these reported observations, there is a paucity of systematic studies describing the prevalence, specific patterns, and impact of comorbidity among noninstitutionalized older adults.

U.S. mortality statistics were reviewed to determine the prevalency of comorbidity at the time of death. In 1979 73% of all death certificates listed more than one cause of death; 33% listed two causes, 25% listed three causes, and 16% listed four or more causes (Table 1-7). A

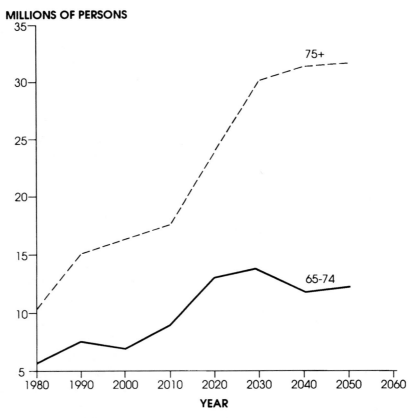

FIGURE 1-3 Limitation in activity due to actual and projected chronic conditions, 1980-2060. (Based on 1980 Health Interview Surveys, National Center for Health Statistics, and U.S. Bureau of the Census [1982], Projections of the U.S.: 1982-2050 [Current Population Reports, Series P-25, No. 922], Washington, DC: U.S. Government Printing Office.)

TABLE 1-7 Prevalence of comorbidity recorded on death certificates in 1979

Causes of death	Death certificates (%)
1+	73
2	33
3	25
4 or more	16

From Guralnik, J. M., LaCroix, A. Z., Everett, D. F., & Kovar, M. G. (1989, May 26). *Aging in the '80s: The prevalence of comorbidity and its association with disability* (Advance data from Vital and Health Statistics of the National Center for Health Statistics, No. 170). Washington, DC: U. S. Department of Health and Human Services, Public Health Service, Centers for Disease Control.

TABLE 1-8 Number of deaths due to more than one cause

Year	Deaths due to multiple causes (%)
1917	35
1955	50
1979	73

From Guralnik, J. M., LaCroix, A. Z., Everett, D. F., & Kovar, M. G. (1989, May 26). *Aging in the '80s: The prevalence of comorbidity and its association with disability* (Advance data from Vital and Health Statistics of the National Center for Health Statistics, No. 170). Washington, DC: U.S. Department of Health and Human Services, Public Health Service, Centers for Disease Control.

review of other data reveals an increase during the twentieth century in the proportion of deaths attributable to more than one cause. For example, more than one cause of death was reported in 35% of deaths in 1917, in 50% in 1955, and in 73% in 1979 (Table 1-8).

The increase probably can be attributed to several factors: (1) an increase in the average age of death; (2) fewer deaths resulting from acute, infectious diseases; and (3) more complete and accurate medical diagnoses (Guralnik et al., 1989). Before the discovery of antibiotics, pneumonia was called the "old man's friend"; each winter, one fifth of the people who lived in county homes or on poor farms died of pneumonia. In a 1989 report the National Health Interview Survey (NHIS) presented information about the prevalence and coprevalence of nine common chronic conditions in a national sample of people 60 years of age and older. It also estimated the prevalence of disability that affected participation in activities of daily living (ADLs), according to the number of conditions present (Guralnik, et al., 1989).

Approximately 42,000 households are interviewed each year by U.S. Bureau of the Census personnel who are trained to conduct surveys. Response rates are usually about 97%. In 1984 a special Supplement on Aging (SOA) was added to the survey to collect information from middle-aged and older people about chronic conditions, physical limitations, housing, retirement status, interactions with family and organizations, use of community resources, and other health-related and social information. There were 16,148 persons interviewed for the SOA, with a 95% response rate in this first year of use; 13,807 of the respondents were 60 years of age and older. Nine common chronic conditions were selected for reporting purposes: arthritis, hypertension, cataracts, heart disease, varicose veins, diabetes, cancer, osteoporosis (including hip fracture), and stroke. When these nine chronic conditions were used as a baseline, there was a measurable and significant incidence of comorbidity. High rates of comorbidity were evident for women; incidence rates were 45% for people ages 60 to 69 and 70% for people 80 years of age and older. Furthermore, as the chronologic age of people increased beyond 80 years, the number of conditions reported for those people increased. In 1985 70% of women and 53% of men had two or more of the nine chronic conditions.

A major problem among the older populations is their susceptibility to various infections (Besdine and Rose, 1982). Infections often become the immediate cause of death for older adults with chronic diseases. In addition, Manton (1986) recognized the high incidence of two or more interacting illnesses, diseases, or pathologic conditions in people of advanced age (Table 1-9,

TABLE 1-9 Functional limitations of persons 65 years old and over: 1984*

	65 years and over	Age — 65 to 74 years Total	Male	Female	75 to 84 years Total	Male	Female	85 years and over	Living — Alone	With others
Total, 65 years and over	27,537	16,987	9490	9496	8552	3251	5301	1999	8716	18,822
Percent with difficulty† in—										
Walking	18.2	13.5	12.6	14.2	23.4	17.3	27.2	35.9	21.3	16.7
Getting outside	11.7	7.0	5.7	8.0	16.9	9.2	21.6	30.1	14.0	10.7
Bathing or showering	10.0	6.3	6.0	6.5	13.9	7.8	13.8	24.8	10.7	9.7
Transferring‡	8.5	6.2	5.6	6.7	11.2	6.9	17.6	17.1	9.5	8.1
Dressing	6.0	4.2	4.5	4.0	7.3	5.2	8.6	15.1	5.2	6.3
Using toilet	4.7	2.8	2.7	2.8	6.3	3.4	8.0	14.0	5.1	4.5
Eating	1.8	1.5	1.7	1.3	1.8	1.1	2.3	4.4	1.1	2.2
Preparing meals	9.2	4.0	3.1	4.7	9.9	5.3	12.7	23.4	6.9	7.4
Shopping for personal items	12.8	7.3	5.7	8.7	18.1	10.5	22.8	36.0	15.6	11.5
Managing money	5.2	2.5	2.6	2.4	7.3	5.7	8.3	19.5	5.3	5.2
Using the telephone	5.0	3.2	3.4	3.1	5.9	6.3	5.6	16.1	3.6	5.6
Doing heavy housework	23.8	18.0	10.6	23.9	29.5	15.2	38.3	48.0	29.5	21.1
Doing light housework	8.1	4.6	3.8	5.3	11.1	6.9	13.7	24.4	7.5	8.3
Percent not performing activity—										
Preparing meals	5.2	4.6	9.8	0.5	5.5	12.0	1.6	8.9	1.1	7.1
Shopping for personal item	2.0	1.1	1.9	0.5	2.5	2.9	2.3	7.5	2.2	1.9
Managing money	1.9	1.3	1.6	1.1	2.2	2.1	2.2	5.9	0.8	2.4
Using the telephone	0.8	0.5	0.8	0.3	0.9	1.4	0.6	2.1	0.8	0.7
Doing heavy housework	9.7	8.1	12.7	4.6	11.5	16.3	8.6	15.9	7.1	11.0
Doing light housework	3.5	2.8	6.1	0.3	4.0	7.8	1.7	7.1	0.7	4.8

Percent of total receiving help§—

Walking	4.6	2.6	2.3	2.8	6.4	3.7	8.0	14.8	—
Getting outside	6.3	3.2	2.7	3.5	9.2	4.8	11.9	20.6	—
Bathing or showering	6.0	3.2	3.3	3.1	8.6	4.9	10.9	19.0	—
Transferring‡	3.2	2.1	2.3	2.0	4.0	2.3	5.0	9.4	—
Dressing	4.4	2.9	3.2	2.6	5.4	4.2	6.1	12.6	—
Using toilet	2.4	1.4	1.5	1.3	3.3	1.9	4.1	7.5	—
Eating	1.1	0.8	0.9	0.6	1.1	0.6	1.3	4.1	—
Preparing meals	6.5	3.5	2.8	4.0	8.7	5.2	10.9	22.3	—
Shopping for personal items	12.0	6.7	5.4	7.8	17.1	9.5	21.7	35.1	—
Managing money	4.9	2.1	2.4	2.0	7.1	5.7	7.9	19.2	—
Using the telephone	3.0	1.8	1.9	1.8	3.6	3.4	3.7	10.8	—
Doing heavy housework	19.1	13.7	7.9	18.2	24.2	11.4	32.0	43.1	—
Doing light housework	7.0	3.8	3.1	4.3	9.7	6.4	11.7	23.1	—

Percent of those with difficulty‡ receiving help—

Walking	24.8	20.4	21.8	19.4	24.9	20.2	26.9	38.3	11.8	31.7
Getting outside	55.8	48.0	49.4	47.3	55.7	49.4	57.5	68.0	42.0	62.4
Bathing or showering	60.9	51.9	58.4	47.9	62.6	71.6	59.1	75.1	36.5	72.5

From U.S. Department of Health and Human Services, National Center for Health Statistics. (1993, January). *National Health Interview Survey, 1986, functional limitations supplement.* And unpublished data from the Supplement on Aging to the 1984 National Health Interview Survey.

*Numbers of persons are expressed in thousands; proportions of persons expressed in percentages. Covers people 65 or more years old who were living in communities outside of nursing homes or other institutions (civilian noninstitutional population). Living arrangement figures include those not performing the activity. All other figures exclude those not performing the activity.

†Difficulty due to a health or physical problem.

‡Getting into or out of a bed or chair.

§Help received because of a health-related problem with performing the specified activity.

TABLE 1-10 Average number of chronic conditions or impairments per 1000 persons:
United States, 1985 to 1987*

Population	Ischemic heart disease	Hypertension	Diabetes	Visual impairments	Cataract	Hearing impairment	Deformity or orthopedic impairment
All 65 years and over	121.5	392.5	99.7	89.5	155.7	383.0	203.2
Male	152.6	331.1	102.5	—	—	—	—
Female	99.8	435.7	97.7	—	—	—	—
All 65 to 74 years	114.4	400.8	99.0	69.7	71.1	365.0	380.8
Male	150.7	359.3	101.9	—	—	—	—
Female	85.3	433.4	96.7	—	—	—	—
All 75 years and over	133.6	379.3	100.8	125.2	246.9	435.7	222.4
Male	156.3	276.6	103.6	—	—	—	—
Female	120.4	438.9	99.1	—	—	—	—

From U.S. Department of Health and Human Services, National Center for Health Statistics. (1993). *Vital and health statistics: Health data on older Americans: United States, 1992.*
*Rates are based on unduplicated counts. Visual impairment includes blindness in both eyes and other visual impairments. Hearing impairments include deafness in both ears, other hearing impairments, and tinnitus. Deformity or orthopedic impairment includes back, upper extremities, and lower extremities.

Table 1-10, and Figure 1-4). Incidence of comorbidity for any two of the conditions was related to the incidence of each condition. For example, high blood pressure and arthritis were the two most prevalent conditions, occurring in approximately 24% of people age 60 and over. Cataracts and arthritis occurred in over 11% of people in this age group (Figure 1-5).

From among interacting disease conditions, Manton selected three that occur among older adults, and he assumed these three to be associated with frailty or debility: septicemia, pneumonia, and hip fracture. Manton further suggested that selection of these three conditions and identification of their mortality trends might provide some markers of frailty or debilitation.

The incidence of hip fracture is high among people with osteoporosis, a long-term, noninfectious, degenerative process often seen in older women. The death rate from complications of hip fracture is very high among people who are already markedly debilitated.

Generally, Manton concluded that the proportions of deaths affected by septicemia, pneumonia, and hip fracture had declined, as reflected in increased life expectancies estimated both at birth and at or beyond age 85. However, the proportion of deaths affected by causal agents associated with debilitation did not seem to be increasing. Specifically, he concluded the following: (1) Septicemia is still a rare cause of death but is an important mortality factor at any age, not just for those who are extremely old. (2) Pneumonia is an important cause of death among the frail and debilitated, though the proportionate number of deaths resulting from pneumonia among older adults showed no marked increase over a 12-year span (1968 to 1980). (3) Hip fracture is primarily a cause of death at advanced ages. It is 3 times more prevalent in men age 85 and over than in all other age groups. It is a more important factor in female mortality than in male mortality.

FIGURE 1-4 Percentage distribution of population 60 years of age and over by number of chronic conditions, according to age group and gender; United States, 1984. (From Guralnik et al: *National Center for Health Statistics,* 1989.)

There is a clear association between the number of conditions and the proportion of people with resulting disabilities. As the number of disabilities increases, the older adult's ability to perform ADLs decreases. Furthermore, there is a graded increase in the incidence of disability with increased age (Figure 1-6). Although further studies of chronic conditions and their relationship to older adults and disabilities are needed, these comorbidity data

benchmarks indicate that these nine chronic conditions are useful measures of the burden of illness experienced by older people (Guralnik et al., 1989).

HEALTH CARE ACCESS AND DELIVERY

The health care delivery system in the United States has become increasingly complex over the years. Its complexity has become especially noticeable for several reasons: (1) The population

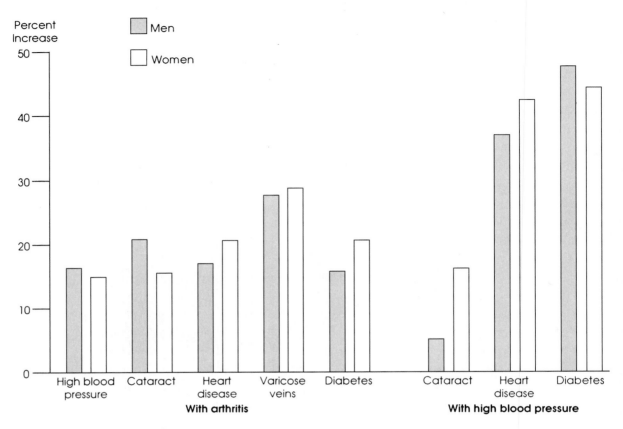

FIGURE 1-5 Percentage of increase in observed over expected frequency of most common comorbid conditions among men and women 60 years of age and over: United States, 1984. (From Guralnik et al., May 26, 1989. *Aging in the eighties. The prevalence of comorbidity and its association with disability.* Advance data from Vital and Health Statistics, No. 170, U.S. Department of Health and Human Services, Public Health Services, Centers for Disease Control.)

of the United States has increased significantly. (2) Advances in science have resulted in negating or delaying life-threatening situations of the past. (3) There have been dramatic increases in life expectancy. (4) There has been an increase in the number and types of medications and treatments. (5) There has been an emerging focus on bioethical and legal issues related to life, disease, research, and dying.

Health Care Financing

The increasing demand and competition for total U.S. dollars to be spent on health, coupled with the rising proportion of older adults, has moved health care financing to the forefront of individual concern and national policy debate in the 1990s (Gilford, 1988). The concern over issues of financing was evidenced in the vigorous health care reform debates during the first years of the Clinton

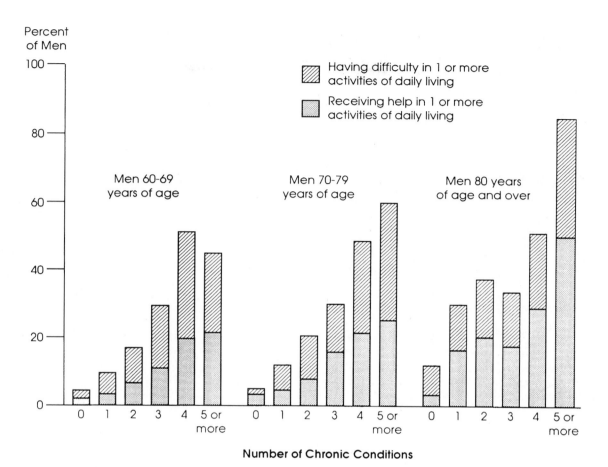

FIGURE 1-6 Prevalence of men 60 years of age and over having difficulty and receiving help in one or more activities of daily living, by number of chronic conditions and age group: United States, 1984. (From Guralnik et al., May 26, 1989. *Aging in the eighties. The prevalence of comorbidity and its association with disability.* Advance data from Vital and Health Statistics, No. 170, U.S. Department of Health and Human Services, Public Health Services, Centers for Disease Control.)

administration. In addition to increasing health care costs borne by individual older adults through personal expenditure, higher health care costs are also of paramount concern to federal and state governments. Total health care costs for health care delivery programs such as Medicare and Medicaid have risen tremendously. The Medicare program's cost has increased from under 5% of the 1960 gross national product to over 10% in 1990 (Helbing, 1992). Medicaid program expenditures have doubled between fiscal years 1987 and 1991 (Buck & Klemm, 1992). The Medicare and Medicaid programs finance a large portion of public health dollars for older adults. Though the private sector also offers some health insurance policies, many of these policies are written to enhance coverage offered by federal and state programs (Gilford, 1988) (Table 1-11).

TABLE 1-11 Medicare and Medicaid—summary, by state and other areas: 1980 and 1990[a,b]

| Region, division, and state | Medicare | | | Medicaid[c] | | |
| | Enrollment,[d] 1990 (1,000) | Payments[e] (mil. dol.) | | Recipients,[f] 1990 (1,000) | Payments (mil. dol.) | |
		1980	1990		1980	1990
Total	34,213	35,699	NA	27,967	23,311	88,378
U.S.[g]	33,499	35,561	100,894	21,628	23,213	88,212
Region						
Northeast	7,436	9,071	24,779	4,900	8,138	30,092
North Central	8,405	9,507	24,468	5,273	5,637	18,789
South	11,544	10,412	34,454	6,510	5,558	25,718
West	6,114	6,529	17,193	4,944	3,878	13,439
N. Eng.	1,890	2,238	5,833	1,069	1,781	7,910
ME	183	177	442	151	131	589
NH	136	120	349	60	72	390
VT	75	68	172	71	59	197
MA	868	1,179	2,991	651	1,009	4,574
RI	159	189	451	164	160	643
CT	469	505	1,428	272	350	1,517
Mid. Atl.	5,545	6,833	18,946	3,831	6,357	22,182
N.Y.	2,505	3,409	8,842	2,462	4,543	15,007
N.J.	1,090	1,198	3,283	614	756	3,102
PA	1,950	2,226	6,821	1,277	1,058	4,073
E. No. Cent.	5,782	6,720	17,750	3,970	4,114	13,180
OH	1,541	1,606	5,039	1,299	809	3,804
IN	755	719	2,130	415	354	1,775
IL	1,535	2,046	4,729	1,144	1,192	2,511
MI	1,239	1,620	4,079	1,113	1,072	3,359
WI	712	729	1,773	416	687	1,731
W. No. Cent.	2,624	2,787	6,718	1,303	1,523	5,609
MN	587	594	1,283	422	590	1,703
IA	456	453	1,082	261	230	791
MO	777	888	2,305	503	295	1,675
ND	99	109	251	53	47	227
SD	110	96	250	57	55	203
NE	234	234	543	134	109	401
KS	361	413	1,004	209	197	609
So. Atl.	6,169	5,555	18,078	2,980	2,512	12,609
DE	87	87	263	51	45	185
MD	546	622	2,002	363	322	1,434
DC	81	149	325	100	168	500
VA	728	614	1,985	442	360	1,259
WV	309	260	818	284	104	614
NC	894	642	2,314	667	401	2,070
SC	446	302	1,019	375	258	1,286
GA	735	601	2,240	746	462	1,974
FL	2,343	2,278	7,213	1,249	392	3,287

TABLE 1-11 Medicare and Medicaid—summary, by state and other areas: 1980 and 1990[a,b]— cont'd

Region, division, and state	Medicare Enrollment,[d] 1990 (1,000)	Medicare Payments[e] (mil. dol.) 1980	Medicare Payments[e] (mil. dol.) 1990	Medicaid[c] Recipients,[f] 1990 (1,000)	Medicaid[c] Payments (mil. dol.) 1980	Medicaid[c] Payments (mil. dol.) 1990
E. So. Cent.	2,182	1,878	6,415	1,563	1,150	5,277
KY	539	437	1,555	426	296	1,508
TN	693	594	2,867	697	380	1,896
AL	583	523	1,808	403	263	1,056
MS	367	324	985	470	211	817
W. So. Cent.	3,194	2,979	9,961	1,967	1,896	7,832
AR	392	333	1,082	285	235	732
LA	528	467	1,965	641	415	1,894
OK.	452	443	1,271	305	265	857
TX	1,822	1,736	5,643	1,729	981	4,349
Mt.	1,640	1,304	4,329	554	505	2,190
MT	117	99	294	64	62	235
ID	132	97	293	70	52	211
WY	51	44	135	37	14	93
CO	359	315	906	223	182	747
NM	179	137	450	162	70	370
AZ	498	383	1,457	(x)	(x)	
UT	161	110	382	129	80	347
NV	152	119	412	59	45	187
Pac.	4,475	5,225	12,863	4,391	3,373	11,249
WA	620	507	1,558	506	329	1,518
OR	431	385	882	263	179	660
CA	3,272	4,219	10,082	4,019	2,728	8,085
AK	25	18	82	51	28	732
HI	127	96	259	91	109	354
Outlying areas[h]	714	4	NA	1,213	99	150

[a]Modified from U.S. Health Care Financing Administration. (1984, May). *Medicare program statistics, selected state data.* And unpublished data.

[b]x = not applicable; NA = not available.

[c]For fiscal year ending September 30.

[d]Hospital and/or medical insurance enrollment as of July 1.

[e]Payments are for calendar year and represent total disbursements from federal hospital and supplementary medical insurance trust funds. Estimates of distribution by state based on interim reimbursements. 1990 figures exclude outlying areas.

[f]People receiving Medicaid at any time during the fiscal year 1991.

[g]Includes data for enrollees whose residence is unknown.

[h]Virgin Islands and Puerto Rico only.

Medicare is a federal health insurance program, enacted in 1966 under Title XVIII of the Social Security Act, for people age 65 and older and for some disabled people. Ninety-eight percent of all people age 65 and over are covered by some type of Medicare benefit (Moon, 1993). The Health Care Financing Administration of the U.S. Department of Health and Human Services (USDHHS) administers the Medicare program, which covers acute care services (USDHHS, 1993a). Medicare also covers enrollment in certain health maintenance organizations (HMOs). The Medicare program is usually divided into two parts.

Part A is the hospital insurance (HI) portion of Medicare. This component covers 90 days of inpatient hospital care per spell of illness, 100 days of skilled nursing facility care following a 3-day hospital stay, rehabilitative home health care, and hospice care for the terminally ill (USDHHS, 1993a). This part of Medicare is financed primarily through a payroll tax.

Part B is the supplementary medical insurance (SMI) portion of Medicare. This component covers 80% of reasonable charges for physician services, diagnostic tests, and home dialysis supplies; outpatient hospital services and ambulatory surgery; and durable medical equipment and prostheses (USDHHS, 1993a). It is financed through monthly premiums, paid by or on behalf of the Medicare beneficiary and from the general revenues of the federal government.

The Medicare program excludes certain mental health services, outpatient drugs, dental care, hearing aids, and eyeglasses. The primary purposes of Medicare, as it was originally designed, were to ensure access to health care for those 65 and older and to cover the major costs of acute illnesses (Moon, 1993). The Medicare program was never designed to cover long-term care services, and today coverage in this area remains very limited (Gilford, 1988).

Although the Medicare program covers 98% of all older adults with some type of health service, the state *Medicaid* program also provides health insurance coverage in some instances (USDHHS, 1993a). The Medicaid program, enacted into law under Title XIX of the Social Security Act, is an entitlement program providing health care for low-income individuals, including older adults. After Medicare, Medicaid is the secondary payer of health care expenses for older adults meeting certain eligibility requirements. The Medicaid program covers far fewer older adults than the Medicare program, covering less than 9% of older adults as opposed to Medicare's 95%. Unlike the Medicare program that is administered at the federal level, the Medicaid program is jointly administered by the state and federal governments. Although the Medicaid program receives federal assistance in addition to its own state dollars, the program is state operated and administered, with final eligibility criteria defined by the state. To qualify for Medicaid coverage, a person must first meet eligibility criteria as imposed by the individual state administering the Medicaid program.

Private insurance policies for long-term care are relatively limited, but this market is rapidly changing. The number of policies more than tripled between 1983 and 1987, with improved benefits being offered by many (Table 1-12). Nonetheless, few older adults own private insurance policies for long-term care because the premiums are often beyond the financial reach of many older adults. In the best case, it is estimated that by the year 2020 only one third of older adults will be able to afford a moderately priced insurance policy. Policyholders also express the concern that private health care insurance policies provide only limited coverage while sometimes boasting much more. For example, skilled nursing home care coverage is often not clearly defined, and in-home care (in the patient's own home) is not typically covered or is covered only in very limited instances. Despite these limitations, private health care policies continue to be written and sold, often aimed at providing "Medigap" insurance to supplement Medicare coverage. Older adults often face difficult decisions

TABLE 1-12 Health insurance coverage status, by selected characteristics: 1985 to 1987[a]

	Number (in millions)						Percentage				
		Covered by private or government health insurance				Not covered by health insurance		Covered by private or government health insurance			Not covered by health insurance
			Covered by private insurance								
	Total	Total	Total	Related to employment[c]	Medicaid		Total	Total[b]	Private insurance	Medicaid	
1985[d]	234.0	199.4	174.6	141.3	16.1	34.6	100.0	85.2	74.6	6.9	14.8
1986	236.7	202.6	177.5	144.1	16.7	34.2	100.0	85.6	75.0	7.1	14.4
1987, total persons[e]	238.8	205.9	180.9	146.6	17.6	32.9	100.0	86.2	75.8	7.4	13.8
Male	116.0	98.4	88.0	72.8	6.5	17.5	100.0	84.9	75.9	5.6	15.1
Female	122.8	107.5	92.9	73.8	11.0	15.3	100.0	87.5	75.6	9.0	12.5
White	202.8	117.2	160.2	129.5	10.7	25.6	100.0	87.4	79.0	5.3	12.6
Black	29.0	23.1	16.1	13.2	6.1	5.9	100.0	79.6	55.5	21.0	20.4
Hispanic origin[f]	18.7	13.1	9.7	8.3	3.0	5.6	100.0	69.9	52.0	15.9	30.1
Under 16 years	55.8	46.8	38.8	33.5	7.5	9.0	100.0	83.8	69.4	13.4	16.2
16 to 24 years	34.0	26.2	23.8	18.6	2.2	7.7	100.0	77.2	70.0	6.4	22.8
25 to 34 years	42.6	35.5	32.4	28.9	2.5	7.1	100.0	83.3	76.1	6.0	16.7
35 to 44 years	33.7	29.7	27.9	25.3	1.3	4.0	100.0	88.0	82.6	3.9	12.0
45 to 54 years	22.8	20.2	19.0	16.6	0.8	2.6	100.0	88.7	83.2	3.5	11.3
55 to 64 years	22.0	19.7	18.0	14.6	1.0	2.2	100.0	89.8	82.1	4.6	10.2
65 years and over	27.9	27.7	21.1	9.2	2.2	0.2	100.0	99.5	75.7	7.9	0.5

Modified from U.S. Bureau of the Census: unpublished data.

[a]Data represents monthly averages for first quarter. Government health insurance includes Medicare, Medicaid, and military plans. Based on a survey of income and program participation.

[b]Includes other government insurance, not shown separately.

[c]Related to current or prior employment of self or other family members.

[d]Revised since originally published.

[e]Includes other races, not shown separately.

[f]Hispanic persons may be of any race.

25

regarding the purchase of private health insurance coverage that allegedly supplements their Medicare coverage. Prospective purchasers are urged to be cautious in the selection of supplemental health insurance and to seek assistance and advice through their own state's insurance department or their state's agency on aging. New benefits were anticipated in 1989 under the Medicare Catastrophic Coverage Act. However, this law was repealed in December 1989. The national health insurance debates in the Clinton administration continue to rage; the future of catastrophic, extended benefits and supplemental insurance for older adults continues to evolve.

In summary, the major sources of health care financing for older adults are the federal Medicare program, the federal-state Medicaid program, and private health insurance policies. No single one of these three would typically cover completely the variety of services needed by older adults. For most older adults, Medicare provides basic protection against the high cost of health care with limitations in long-term care or assisted living coverage.

Health care services

The very nature of long-term illness among older adults demands that a variety of services be available for different periods of time. The challenge of how to provide these services is ever present, and various and new solutions are often the topic of debate. The level of care delivered is closely linked to both available health care delivery sites and the person's physical location at the time of illness or disability. In general, older adults are located in one of four settings: an acute care setting (hospital), a long-term care facility (nursing home), an assisted living community, or the person's own home. The ease of delivering the required health care services at any of these sites determines whether the person obtains care within his present living arrangement or whether the person must be moved to an alternative health care delivery site. For example, the older adult who needs daily physical therapy and who lives either at home or in an assisted living residence may be able to remain in the community if physical therapy services are available. Quite often, multiple health services covering a wide range of health needs and focusing on long-term care are required by older adults.

A 1988 task force (Catholic Health Association's Task Force on Long-Term Care Policies) reported that a continuum of care best describes the type of service required for older adults. A continuum of care includes three features: (1) a patient focus, (2) a range of services, and (3) an organizational structure containing several integrating elements (Figure 1-7). The integrating elements are the following: community-wide planning; person-centered care management; a management information system (usually a computerized system); financial planning; and an administrative structure arranged to coordinate various health care delivery services. The success or failure of the continuum of care depends on the motivations of the providers, the various community organizations, and the leadership to facilitate the realization of a truly integrated network of health care delivery services.

The following factors demonstrate the increasing need for health care providers to collaborate with other support networks and caregivers in striving toward an integrated network of health care delivery for older adults:

The fastest growing segment of the aging population is made up of those over the age of 85.

Most of the health care for older adults is provided outside the hospital and nursing care facilities. Most caregivers are family and friends whose lives may become stress filled because of the responsibilities of caring for older adults.

Because of a fragmented health care delivery system, too many older adults are not receiving appropriate health care. Often these are the older adults who have no family, friends, or financial resources.

Facilities where older adults receive health care may be set up in one of two ways: (1) as a

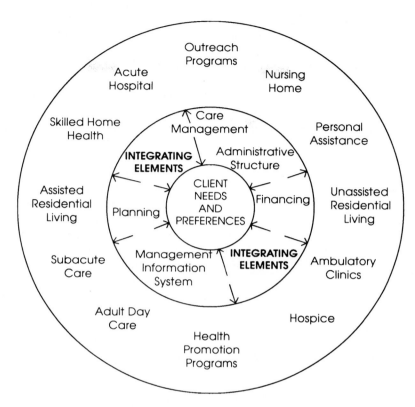

FIGURE 1-7 Example of a continuum for long-term care. (From Catholic Health Association's Task Force on Long Term Care Policy. [1988]. *A time to be old, a time to flourish—The special needs of the elderly-at-risk.* St. Louis.)

facility-focused delivery system or (2) as a patient-centered delivery system. Often the former focus is used, integrating services that focus on the facility's financial and management interests. Figure 1-8 depicts a hierarchic arrangement of integrated services in an acute care hospital. This arrangement is frequently referred to as a continuum of care, but it has little concern for individual choice. The structure requires the patient to move through all levels of care without being able to select the one or more needed services.

If the health care continuum in a health care facility is to be driven by individual need and choice, the initial step required is to perform a community assessment. The community assessment focuses on determining which services are needed by the older adult population. Once the appropriate services are identified, the next step is to ensure the availability of and access to needed services for older adults and their caregivers in the community. Figure 1-9 suggests one possible array of services that might be available to older adults. Realistically, a total patient-focused system that incorporates existing health care delivery facilities may not be financially possible, regardless of older adults' needs. The challenge of constructing a realistic patient-focused system that integrates existing health care services focuses on (1) determining community need

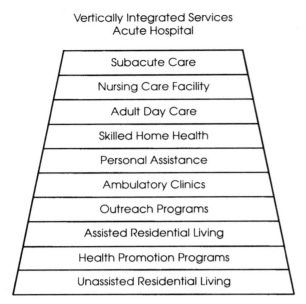

Vertically Integrated Services
Acute Hospital

Subacute Care

Nursing Care Facility

Adult Day Care

Skilled Home Health

Personal Assistance

Ambulatory Clinics

Outreach Programs

Assisted Residential Living

Health Promotion Programs

Unassisted Residential Living

FIGURE 1-8 Vertically integrated model of service acquisition. (From Catholic Health Association's Task Force on Long Term Care Policy. [1988]. *A time to be old, a time to flourish—The special needs of the elderly-at-risk.* St. Louis.)

that maximizes health benefits of older adults and (2) minimizing the financial risk to health care providers who choose to integrate, while maximizing the participants' return to ensure their continued interest. The ultimate challenge is to define and deliver "cost effective, quality of life" services.

THE ENVIRONMENT

What are the geographic location patterns of older adults? How can their physical environment be described, and what are the associated factors influencing their location choices? What are some of the housing alternatives available to older adults, especially as they age and become limited with respect to instrumental activities of daily living (IADLs)?

As people grow older, and especially as some of their functional abilities are altered, they usually seek accommodations that will be comfortable and safe. They look for homes and neighbor-

hoods that will enable them to meet their needs with as much independence as possible. Older adults consider a variety of factors that influence comfort, safety, and independence in making decisions about where, how, and with whom they will live. Table 1-13 illustrates, generally, the living arrangements experienced by selected age groups.

Older adults are less likely to change residences than members of any other age group. In 1992 only 5% of older adults had moved since the previous year, as compared to 19% of those under 65 (AARP, 1994). Older adults often prefer to remain in their own home environment, especially if it is conducive to comfortable, safe, and conveniently independent living. Within the residence, comfort may require easy access (e.g., no entry stairs), ease of movement within the residence (e.g., one level), and easy maintenance.

As it becomes more difficult for the older adult to live comfortably and independently with these arrangements, alternative living arrangements may be desirable. Assisted living communities enhance independence by providing social and physical support where necessary. For further discussion of these issues, see the section on housing.

In addition to considerations related to individual residence, the overall community also affects the older adult's choice of a living environment. Several factors affect the desirability of the community in which the residence is located—many of these factors particularly affect the relative independence of an older adult:

Safety considerations are paramount. Some older adults are unable to move about in their neighborhoods because of high crime rates. This is especially true in some urban areas.

A desire to live near family members may be the deciding factor in determining where to live.

Limited finances for moving may prohibit relocation or may mandate relocation to a less expensive residence.

Availability of transportation or easy access to community resources contributes to convenient living. Proximity to health care services, shop

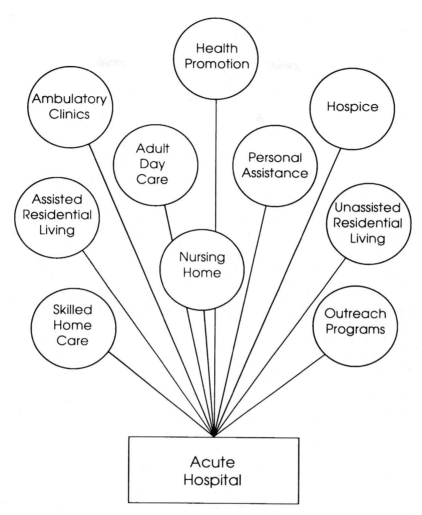

FIGURE 1-9 System development from the client's perspective. (From Catholic Health Association's Task Force on Long Term Care Policy. [1988]. *A time to be old, a time to flourish—The special needs of the elderly-at-risk.* St. Louis.)

ping, groceries, businesses, and recreational facilities greatly enhances the desirability of a community.

Geographic location

For some older adults, the warm climates of selected southern states are appealing. In 1993 over half of all older adults lived in nine states: California (over 3 million), Florida (over 2 million), New York (over 2 million), Pennsylvania (over 1 million), Texas (over 1 million), Ohio (over 1 million), Illinois (over 1 million), Michigan (over 1 million), and New Jersey (over 1 million) (AARP, 1994) (Figure 1-10). Older adults are less likely to live in central cities and more likely to live in suburbs; yet they are 3 times as

TABLE 1-13 Living arrangements of the elderly: 1990 and 1980 (In thousands. Noninstitutional populations)

Living arrangement and age	1990 Number Total	1990 Number Men	1990 Number Women	1990 Percent distribution Total	1990 Percent distribution Men	1990 Percent distribution Women	1980 Number Total	1980 Number Men	1980 Number Women	1980 Percent distribution Total	1980 Percent distribution Men	1980 Percent distribution Women
65 years and over	29,566	12,334	17,232	100.0	100.0	100.0	24,157	9,889	14,268	100.0	100.0	100.0
Living												
Alone	9,176	1,942	7,233	31.0	15.7	42.0	7,067	1,447	5,620	29.3	14.6	39.4
With spouse	16,003	9,158	6,845	54.1	74.3	39.7	12,781	7,441	5,340	52.9	75.2	37.4
With other relatives	3,734	953	2,782	12.6	7.7	16.1	3,892	832	3,060	16.1	8.4	21.4
With nonrelatives only†	653	281	372	2.2	2.3	2.2	417	169	248	1.7	1.7	1.7
65 to 74 years	17,979	8,013	9,966	100.0	100.0	100.0	15,302	6,621	8,681	100.0	100.0	100.0
Living												
Alone	4,350	1,042	3,309	24.2	13.0	33.2	3,750	797	2,953	24.5	12.0	34.0
With spouse	11,353	6,265	5,089	63.1	78.2	51.1	9,436	5,285	4,151	61.7	79.8	47.8
With other relatives	1,931	528	1,401	10.7	6.6	14.1	1,890	436	1,454	12.4	6.6	16.7
With nonrelatives only†	345	178	167	1.9	2.2	1.7	226	103	123	1.5	1.6	1.4
75 to 84 years	9,354	3,562	5,792	100.0	100.0	100.0	7,172	2,708	4,464	100.0	100.0	100.0
Living												
Alone	3,774	688	3,086	40.3	19.3	53.3	2,664	505	2,159	37.1	18.6	48.4
With spouse	4,145	2,537	1,607	44.3	71.2	27.7	2,977	1,882	1,095	41.5	69.5	24.5
With other relatives	1,237	264	974	13.2	7.4	16.8	1,394	271	1,123	19.4	10.0	25.2
With nonrelatives only†	198	73	125	2.1	2.0	2.2	137	50	87	1.9	1.8	1.9
85 years and over	2,233	758	1,475	100.0	100.0	100.0	1,683	560	1,123	100.0	100.0	100.0
Living												
Alone	1,051	213	838	47.1	28.1	56.8	653	145	508	38.8	25.9	45.2
With spouse	505	356	150	22.6	47.0	10.2	368	274	94	21.9	48.9	8.4
With other relatives	567	160	406	25.4	21.1	27.5	608	125	483	36.1	22.3	43.0
With nonrelatives only†	110	29	81	4.9	3.8	5.5	54	16	38	3.2	2.9	3.4

From Saluter, A. F., U.S. Bureau of the Census. (1991, May). *Marital status and living arrangements: March 1990* (Current Population Reports, Series P-20, No. 450). Washington, DC: U.S. Government Printing Office. Table L.
†1980 data include a small number of persons in unrelated subfamilies.

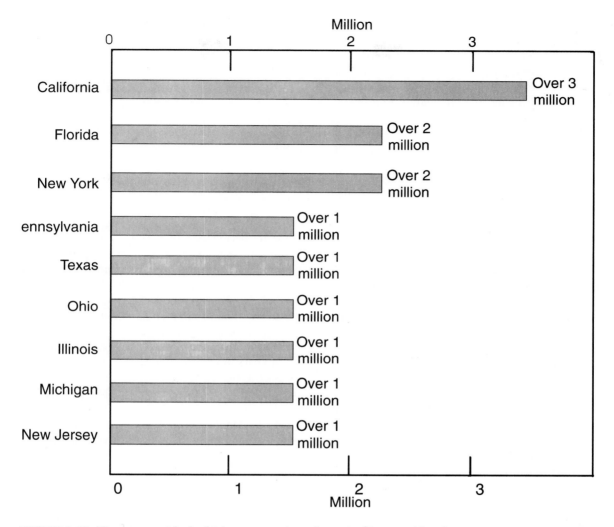

FIGURE 1-10 Nine states with the highest proportion of people 65 years old and over, 1990. States are ranked largest to smallest. (From U.S. Bureau of the Census, *Current Population Reports,* Series P-25, 1990.)

likely to live in a metropolitan area as in a nonmetropolitan area (Taeuber, 1993).

During the 1980s the greatest increase in the older adult population was in the western states and southeastern coastal states (Taeuber, 1993). By the year 2010 approximately 56% of the projected 39 million older adults will live in one of ten states—California, Florida, New York, Texas, Pennsylvania, Illinois, Ohio, New Jersey, North Carolina, or Michigan. Since the 1960s the southern and western areas of the United States have been popular areas for relocation upon retiring. This just-retired population tended to be healthy and economically secure. Since the 1970s these locations have gained popularity among the older old, a population that is typically less healthy. However, these regions may not have planned for delivering health care to a changing population.

Although older adults are less likely to change residence than are members of other age groups, some do change geographic locations for various reasons. In an AARP profile (1994), the majority of older adults (75%) who did move, moved to another location in the same state. Some older adults move their residence to be nearer other family members, especially their own children. However, one group of older adults in the profile somewhat facetiously suggested that older parents moved in order to live *further* from their children. Typically healthy and socially active, these older adults could have been illuminating their desire to avoid some of the tasks and responsibilities associated with their child's younger family, preferring to "reap the rewards" retirement years bring.

Housing

As the twenty-first century approaches, the number of older adults increases in proportion to the total U.S. population. One opportunity will be that of creatively defining alternative and accessible residence options for an adult population with a wide range of functional capabilities. Included in this population are those who require assistance with IADLs. This accounts for 45% of those who are 85 or over and who are noninstitutionalized (U.S. Bureau of the Census, 1992) and for the 1.7 million nursing home residents (Table 1-14 and Figure 1-11).

There is a wide range of living arrangements among older adults. Of the older adult, noninstitutionalized, 1990 population, 69% lived in family settings (10 million men and 9.9 million women). About 13% of people over age 65 were living with children, siblings, other relatives (excluding spouses), or nonrelatives, many of whom were under age 65. The number of older people living

TABLE 1-14 Nursing home population, by U.S. region: 1980 to 1990 percentage change*

U.S. region	1980	1990	Percentage change
Total	1,426	1,721	24.2
Northeast	327	399	22.0
Midwest	472	545	15.3
South	397	558	40.8
West	230	270	17.3

From U.S. Bureau of the Census.
*Numbers in thousands.

alone increased by 72% between 1970 and 1987, about 1½ times the growth rate for the older population in general. Approximately 9.2 million noninstitutionalized older adults lived alone in 1990, 7.2 million women and 1.9 million men. A relatively small number (1.3 million) and percentage (5%) of people age 65 or older lived in nursing homes in 1985. In 1987 1% of people 65 to 74 years old lived in nursing homes, as did 6% of people between ages 75 and 84, and 22% of people 85 years of age and over. The probability of being admitted to a nursing home increases with age. The typical nursing home resident is an older woman, with four out of five residents 75 years of age or over (Taeuber, 1993).

The American Association of Retired Persons, always at the forefront of addressing the needs of senior citizens, publishes a variety of literature aimed at facilitating exploration and decision making regarding residence options. Most older adults choose to remain in their own home environment if the specialized services they need can be made available to them. An AARP publication, *Staying at Home: A Guide to Long-Term Care and Housing,* includes data to assist people in deciding whether home care is plausible and whether specialized services can be brought to the home. For example, if an older adult needs help around the house, a potential service might be a homemaker or home health aide to help with chores or personal care. AARP

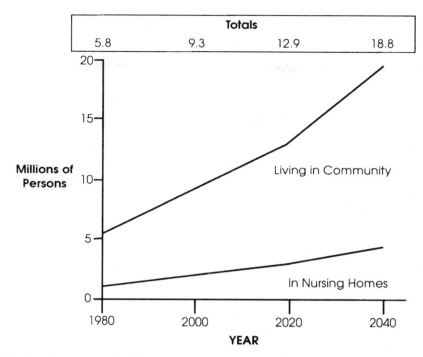

FIGURE 1-11 Older Americans in need of long-term care, 1980 to 2040. (From 1982 National Long-term Care Survey and 1977 National Nursing Home Survey and Social Security Administration Projections.)

also provides suggestions for requesting home health services and paying for long-term care, and lists specific criteria for evaluating the quality of the available services. The search for basic information might begin with a call to the Eldercare locator, a toll-free service aimed at linking older adults and their families to information about available resources (1-800-677-1116; 9 AM to 5 PM EST).

Continued residence in one's own home is only one alternative as one grows older. As the number of older adults and the need for assistance in the ADL's grow, so do the range and types of residence options. At one extreme is the continuing care retirement community (CCRC), offering a wide range of services from housekeeping to nursing care. CCRCs are one alternative for older adults needing assistance with daily living tasks. Care focuses on the older adult's needs and the desire to live in a safe and clearly—often physically—defined community environment. Another type of assisted living arrangement is the assisted living facility or board and care home. This type of arrangement offers daily assistance services for older adults, short of nursing home care. Congregate housing is another residence option. Older adults may have their own apartment, but congregate housing focuses on group living, with shared meals, planned activities, and daily housekeeping service provided. Another type of living arrangement, offering less direct support with daily living activities, is the elder cottage housing opportunity (ECHO). These are typically self-contained, barrier-free units placed in the yard of a single-family house. Home sharing is another type of living arrangement that offers little direct support with ADLs. As the name *home sharing* implies, two or more unrelated older adults share common areas of a house or apartment.

A newer concept in residence options is retirement communities constructed right on university campuses. Even in college towns where retirement communities do not exist, college campuses have been attracting increased numbers of retirees in recent years. Building a life-care community where retired faculty and alumni can reside has appeal for both retirees and property owners. One advantage for the property owner (often the university or college itself) is that people who are seeking places for retirement may offset the loss created by the shrinking pool of 18-year-olds. The retirees may feel a natural affection for returning to the environment where they spent many enjoyable days. Retirees may wish to take advantage of cultural and educational opportunities while reflecting on past memories. In addition, continuing contributions from the retirees may be both experiential and financial. Retirees can continue to teach and share their expertise and experience in a variety of ways in the educational setting, also possibly making financial contributions in the form of alumni gifts and bequests. An educational institution associated with a medical school and/or a nursing school may have an additional reason to be attracted to this arrangement. Having many retirees available close to the learning center makes for an ideal situation for geriatric-gerontology educational programs. The eventual outcome of these new ventures remains to be seen, but to many, this arrangement has a special appeal (Lewin, 1990). As the need for housing for older adults increases in the twenty-first century, it seems likely that there will be additional innovative and creative means developed for meeting this basic need.

◼ Sociologic Concerns, Economics, and Intellectual Abilities

SOCIOLOGIC CONCERNS

As older adults enter their retirement years, the majority are relatively healthy and receive retirement income from previous paid employment (Neugarten, 1978). Currently, older men retire earlier than they did 40 years ago (Taeuber, 1993). In 1950 almost 70% of men 55 years of age and over were working; in 1990 this figure decreased to under 40%. Over 45% of men 65 and older were working in 1950; in 1990 only 16% of men 65 and older were working.

Women's retirement patterns follow a similar decreasing trend. However, a policy expert panel on aging suggests that this trend may not continue (Wilson, et al., 1994). Improvements in older adults' health status, the desire to stay active, and economic constraints limiting one's choice to retire early all contribute to the likelihood of future older adults staying in the work force.

Despite these retirement projections for future older adults, the number of healthy, young retirees currently continues to grow. As a result, older adults have the opportunity to explore a wide range of activities. For example, older adults may choose to travel, attend recreational or educational events, or participate in relaxing and satisfying hobbies for which they could never find time before. They can also pursue another career, which may be similar to, or completely different from, the one from which they have just retired. Opportunities to do volunteer work abound. The expertise and experience of older adults are invaluable, making them unique contributors in countless situations.

As the pool of healthy older adults continues to grow, the social perception of hiring older workers is changing. The results are increases in new and innovative job opportunities for older adults. Concerns about older adults' productivity are proving to be unfounded, based on the experiences of companies that employ older adults. The Days Inns of America experiment in hiring older workers as reservations agents was highly successful from a cost-benefit standpoint (McNaught & Barth, 1992). Older workers remained on the job longer than younger workers; they received higher wages because they stayed on the job longer; and although they spent more time talking to callers, they were more successful in booking reservations than younger workers.

Another "do it yourself" chain experimentally staffed only older workers and found it to be very successful, with no adverse effects on profitability (Hogarth & Barth, 1991). Travelers Corporation, a large financial services company, found that older adults were the answer to maximizing the company's staffing efficiency with highly productive temporary workers (McNaught & Barth, 1991). Even the McDonald's fast-food chain developed a "McMasters' Program," which enables retired adults to fill the dearth of available employees (Beck, 1990). Often employment opportunities provide more than career enhancement or pure economic gains. The jobs also provide a means of increasing the older adult's self-esteem or satisfying the human need for social contacts.

Many companies and employers are taking innovative approaches to hiring older adults, matching the needs of their business to the expertise of older adults who wish to be employed. T. Franklin Williams suggests that this trend toward continuing employment will increase in the twenty-first century: "We're going to see more and more second and third careers" (Beck, 1990).

Depending on their state of health and underlying motivation, many retirees spend much of their time in a volunteer role. Policy experts in aging state that the growing number of healthy older adults represents an abundant volunteer resource pool (Wilson et al., 1994). On average, 25 hours per week are freed up as a result of retirement for males; 18 hours per week for females. Maintaining an active role in their community is a stimulating and attractive way of life for many older adults. For example, elementary schools recruit retirees to teach and tutor in special programs (e.g., day reading programs and evening computer classes). AARP currently funds a grant aimed at involving older adults as mentors and tutors in public elementary schools in Montgomery County, Maryland. Both children and retirees enjoy these interactions, which serve to enrich intergenerational understanding. This type of experience fosters a positive, regenera-tive cycle. The more active and involved older adults become, the healthier they are. The longer they remain healthy, the more active and involved they can remain. Most contemporary public services offer a wide range of attractive volunteer opportunities for older adults.

Another sociologic concern relates to the "sandwich generation," those older adults who bear the responsibility both for their children and for their aging parents. They are sandwiched between two dependent generations. This relatively new role for older adults is becoming increasingly common as the baby boom generation ages. It quite likely could become the norm for future older adults (Beck, 1990) (Figure 1-12). The baby boomers of today will constitute a large number of older adults tomorrow. They potentially will be more physically and financially independent and will be better educated than today's typical older adult. As a result of this, and of living longer, they will more likely be in the role of caregiver for both their children and their parents. Many American families may even see four generations living at one point in time by the year 2000. A national survey found that "sandwich generation" adults see themselves as making substantial transfers of both time and money to their frail, older parents, with women providing help in terms of time and men most likely providing financial help.

Many older adults are self-sufficient and are able to maintain healthy independence. These are the older adults who will be responsible for caring for their older parents. More older adults in their early retirement years will face the responsibility of caring for their very old, frail parents or relatives (Taeuber, 1993). As longevity increases, it is inevitable that some parents will live to see their children retire. They may even seek the assistance of their retired children for some type of support. The difficulties of these responsibilities for the older adult sandwich generation can be onerous. For example, consider the situation of an older, single adult with two grown children who also has aging parents living nearby. The adult is the only child living near the

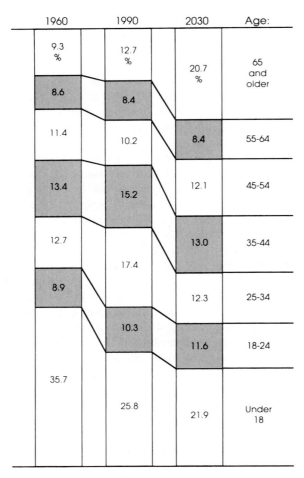

FIGURE 1-12 Age distribution of total U.S. population. (From U.S. Bureau of the Census.)

Not the least of the problems encountered in this type of situation is the psychologic task of role reversal faced when the adult child must care for dependent parents. As the dependency of the aging parent increases, the adult child increasingly assumes the caregiver role. This may set the stage for increasing psychologic dependence on the part of the parent. Role reversal may be consciously recognized and perpetuated, unconsciously recognized and perpetuated, or consciously recognized and limited. Some adult children report negative feelings, resulting in strained relationships among family members. Many adult children are able to develop significant emotional bonds with their aging parents and report, in spite of difficulties, a high level of personal satisfaction and acceptance of their filial responsibilities.

The sandwich generation problems coming to light in the 1990s will surely increase in future decades. Some statistics indicate that as of the beginning of the 1990s, about 5 million Americans were spending some of their time caring for a parent. By the year 2010 that number is likely to double.

ECONOMICS

In the past, one could perhaps make generalizations about anyone over 65 and be fairly accurate. The number of people over 65 was relatively small compared to all other age groups. Quite often there were social restrictions on older adults' roles and functions. However, as we observe increases in the proportion of older adults and changes in their health status, quality of life, social choices, and economic diversity, society's concept of those over 65 changes. Broad generalizations about anyone over 65 become very difficult to make. There is greater economic status variation among older adults than ever before. It is impossible to describe older adults in terms of a broad economic statement that might apply to every older adult.

Some view older people as being quite comfortable economically, a view supported by several reports that give evidence of financial security among a sizable number of older adults. For

parents, and the parents' health is beginning to fail. Furthermore, the adult's children still require assistance (in terms of time and money). The result is intense pressure and sometimes devastating stress on the adult, who must juggle twilight career responsibilities (which may increase because of increased financial pressures), providing assistance to the children, and filling the caretaker role for aging parents. An added challenge may involve searching for adequate resources and support services to assist in fulfilling multiple responsibilities.

example, J. B. Quinn (1990) states that members of the pre–World War II generation married in their early 20s, had children, and by age 50, finished paying for their children's college tuition. They then focused on saving for their own retirement 10 to 15 years down the road. The standard of living of pre–World War II older adults is in sharp contrast with the experiences of the baby boomer older adults. Competition for job openings and security, delays in marriage, delays in having children, increasing longevity, and caretaker responsibilities for frail parents all contribute to quite a different economic experience for retiring older adults today. Personal savings and retirement benefits amounts may be reduced in the future, putting more of an economic burden on retired older adults (Taeuber, 1993).

The professional literature and daily news stories report a concern for older baby boomers and for the responsibility they will bear in caring for parents and grandparents. Though some older baby boomers are indeed heavily burdened by the care they must provide to aging parents, one should not conclude that all older adults excessively burden their adult children. In fact, many older parents actually help their adult children by providing down payments for a home purchase or tuition assistance for their grandchildren. Many older adults may find themselves in the comfortable position of being able to reap the rewards of their diligent work and the frugality they exercised in their younger years. Contrary to concerned reports regarding the older baby boomers, others have concluded that the older generation holds unprecedented wealth. Because aging parents today are less likely than those of previous generations to need financial assistance from their children, some conclude that most older adults are wealthy.

These conflicting and extreme conclusions illustrate how stereotypes of older adults often lead to erroneous generalizations. For example, many people who write about older adults in America describe them as poor, hopeless, helpless, sick, and downtrodden—objects of pity and public charity. On the other hand, a more recent stereotype is that older adults in America are rich, greedy, self-serving, and self-centered, needing no help from their family, the U.S. government, or anyone else. Before jumping to either conclusion, it behooves the observer to be very discriminating when defining the older population (Quinn, 1990). The fact is, both kinds of older adults exist. All seek the assurance of adequate and reliable retirement income that can "spell the critical difference between dignity and despair" (AARP & Pacific Presbyterian Medical Center of San Francisco, 1989). Although many older adults can expect to be financially comfortable in their retirement years, many others live in poverty or at least near the poverty level, which seriously compromises their sense of dignity.

Income generally decreases after retirement, but the income after retirement is relatively stable because so many older adults receive Social Security payments (Taeuber, 1993). Social Security benefits represent the largest share of income for people age 85 and older (Figure 1-13). Although the primary source of income for older adults remains Social Security, there are several other income sources: property, pensions, personal savings, investments, earnings, and a variety of financial assets. Social Security income and pension benefits accounted for approximately 45% of the total household income of older adults in 1986 (Taeuber, 1993). However, not every older citizen has the benefit of all or even several of these sources. Older adults are more likely than those 25 to 64 years old to receive welfare assistance (Taeuber, 1993). Differences in income are best explained by the following factors: former occupational status, educational attainment, work history, age, sex, race, ethnicity, marital status, and living arrangements (Taeuber, 1993).

Economic facts of life for older adults in the United States during the late 1980s and early 1990s included the following:

In 1989 11.4% of people 65 and over lived in poverty. That is, their weekly income was $120

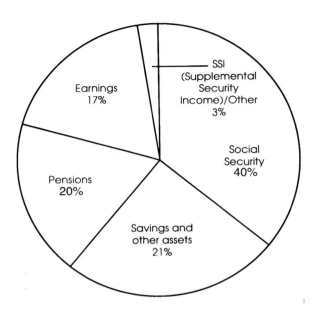

FIGURE 1-13 Sources of income for people 85 years old and older. (From U.S. Department of Health and Human Services, Social Security Administration, and Office of Research and Statistics. [1994]. *Income of the aged chartbook, 1992* [SSA Pub. No. 13-11727]. Washington, DC: U.S. Government Printing Office.)

or less for single-person households and $152 for two-person households. This was 8% lower than the poverty income figures for single-person households 15 to 64 years old and 11% lower than the poverty income figures for two-person households 15 to 64 years old (Taeuber, 1993).

Between 17% and 28% of white women 85 years of age or older in 1990 were living in poverty (Taeuber, 1993). The rate increased to between 15% and 55% for black women. Poverty levels were greater for women, minorities, older adults living alone, and the very old.

In 1990 over 27% of married-couple households of 65- to 69-year-olds received annual incomes of less than $20,000. The percentage increased to over 32% for married-couple households 70 to 74 years old and to over 40% for married-couple households 75 years old and over (Taeuber, 1993).

In 1990 the mean monthly private pension income (not including Social Security) was $652. Six out of ten older adults receiving private pension income were men. About one third of those living alone received private pension income (Taeuber, 1993).

Examination of the economic status of older adults in the United States results in a wide diversity of views. Economic and demographic statistics can support conflicting conclusions. One may find statistics supporting either the belief that older adults are very rich or that they are very poor, depending upon the statistical parameters presented and/or omitted (Table 1-15 and Figure 1-14).

In a qualitative report about "the other side of easy street," the Villers Foundation set out to separate fact from fiction and to identify what is reality for older adults versus what are myths about their economic status. At the heart of the report is a plea to eliminate the disparity between the rich and the poor, no matter their age. Goals for all ages are the elimination of poverty, providing access to health care, and creating availability of shelter (Bethell, 1987).

The Villers report examines some of the myths incorrectly describing the economics of old age. One such myth is that there is not very much poverty among older adults, as a result of their above-average income. They are believed to live better than those younger than age 65. Differences in describing who is poor and who is not would be eliminated given clear definitions and measurements of poverty. The existing poverty index has been criticized because it fails to consider poverty as a relative concept (Stone, 1989). If criteria for identifying those who are living in poverty were applied to all age groups consistently, the poverty rate among older adults would increase markedly. Because children are a large percentage of the population and there is a high rate of poverty among children, the rate of

TABLE 1-15 Persons 65 years old and over who were below poverty level, by selected characteristics: 1970 to 1987*

	Number below poverty level (in thousands)					Percentage below poverty level				
	1970	1979†	1985	1986	1987	1970	1979†	1985	1986	1987
Total, 65 years and over‡	4,793	3,682	3,456	3,477	3,491	24.6	15.2	12.6	12.4	12.2
White	4,011	2,911	2,698	2,689	2,597	22.6	13.3	11.0	10.7	10.1
Black	735	740	717	722	808	47.7	36.3	31.5	31.0	33.9
Hispanic§	—	154	219	204	247	—	26.8	23.9	22.5	27.4
In families	2,013	1,380	1,173	1,164	1,247	14.8	8.4	6.4	6.2	6.5
Householder	1,188	822	708	716	751	16.5	9.1	7.0	7.0	7.2
Male	980	629	498	520	533	15.9	8.4	6.0	6.1	6.1
Female	209	193	210	196	218	20.1	13.0	12.1	11.8	12.6
Other members	825	559	465	448	496	13.0	7.6	5.6	5.2	5.7
Unrelated individuals	2,779	2,299	2,281	2,311	2,241	47.2	29.4	25.6	25.2	24.0
Male	549	428	402	412	416	38.9	25.3	20.5	19.6	19.3
Female	2,230	1,871	1,879	1,899	1,825	49.8	30.5	27.0	26.8	25.4
Total, 60 years and over	5,977	4,753	4,677	4,547	4,657	21.3	13.9	12.3	11.7	11.8

From U.S. Bureau of the Census. *Current population reports* (Series P-60, No. 61). And unpublished data.

*Persons as of March of following year. Based on old processing procedures; therefore data will not agree with other tables.

†Population controls based on 1980 census.

‡Beginning in 1979, includes members of unrelated subfamilies not shown separately; for earlier years, unrelated subfamily members are included in the "In families" category.

§Hispanic persons may be of any race.

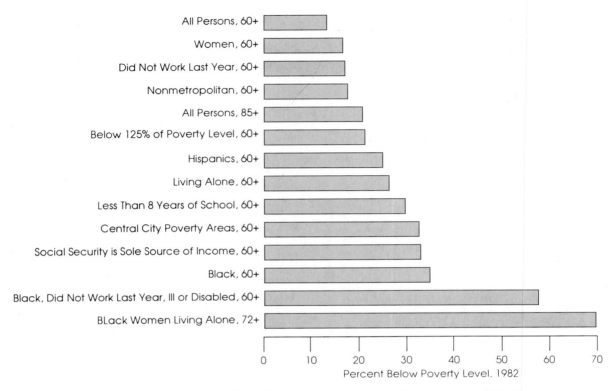

FIGURE 1-14 Percent below poverty level by selected population group. Poverty remains high for some groups. (From U.S. Bureau of the Census.)

poverty among adults who have no children is calculated as being lower than it would be if children were not considered. If only adults were considered, it could be concluded that poverty among older adults is a more serious problem than it appears to be when all age groups are considered (Bethell, 1987).

In 1989 the U.S. Bureau of the Census defined the monetary cutoff for poverty as $6240 per year for an older individual and $7904 for older couples. Some contend that this defines poverty too narrowly. A broader definition of poverty should consider availability of resources such as "basic services, decision-making power, and dignity" (Stone, 1989, p. 22). For example, the cost of health care among older adults is an

additional factor that should be considered when determining the level of poverty. Older adults spent approximately 15% of their income on health care in 1985. If the poverty level were adjusted to consider these out-of-pocket health costs, the poverty rate among older adults would rise further (Stone, 1989).

INTELLECTUAL ABILITIES AND OPPORTUNITIES IN CONTINUING EDUCATION

When considering sociologic information, one must bear in mind that what is known about a group of people may not be true of many individuals within that group. Like many other groups, the aging population defies overgeneralization. The emphasis on youth in the United States further fuels the tendency to stereotype the aging population. However, these stereotypes are being challenged as the number of older adults increases. For example, shoe advertisements depict active older adults. And it is not unusual to turn on the television and see older adults skydiving. But there remain uphill challenges to dispelling many of the myths about aging. Among the most pernicious of these is the prevailing myth that intellectual abilities automatically decline with age. Schaie (1983) has taken steps to dispel this myth by conducting a longitudinal study of about 4000 participants who have been tested throughout the study's 30 years. Schaie and the other researchers at Pennsylvania State University have concluded that "in the absence of disease, those [people] who have maintained a very high level of interaction with their environment" do not demonstrate a decline in mental skills or knowledge as they age. The "use it or lose it" principle appears to apply to the maintenance of high levels of intellectual performance, as well as to muscular strength (Keller, 1986).

Many older adults still "use it" and are far from "losing it," contradicting the stereotypes of being sick, poor, and lonely. These older adults are more concerned about seizing opportunities for learning and enjoying life than some younger people are prepared to believe. As early as 1978 Birren said the following: "I am forecasting a graying of the university where persons of all ages will be seeking knowledge about the conditions of life. They will be an informed and eager group, interested in extending their options in life as well as contemplating the meaning of their own life with a measure of maturity unique to themselves."

In the future, education systems will have to revamp their offerings, schedules, and resources to accommodate the decreasing numbers of younger people and the increasing numbers of older people. Some of the older people will be seeking skills and knowledge applicable to new and different careers. This knowledge will complement their existing experience and skills gleaned from past careers and will build new skills for new frontiers. Other older adults, rather than seeking career-related skills, will pursue further education for the sheer pleasure of learning.

Gerontologic literature contains very little information about the kind of reaction the older student can expect from the traditional university community. Without solid evidence regarding the experiences of older adult students, there was once a fear that faculty might be biased against the older person. Hays conducted a research study (supported by the Andrus Foundation) at Wichita State University in Kansas related to this issue. He found just the opposite to be true (AARP, 1989-1990). As a result of this study, the first longitudinal data base was established about older student behavior, with a focus on students ages 60 and older. Data were collected over a 6-year period. Data were obtained by encouraging older people to audit selected classes and then by interviewing the older adults auditing these classes. Findings indicated that over 75% of the faculty members whose classes were audited found that older adults were better motivated than younger students and learned just as quickly. Three out of five faculty members felt that older students contributed positively to the classes. The study also helped university officials to better understand the older student and relieved university officials' concerns regarding the cost associated with enrolling older students—the costs were found to be minimal (AARP, 1989-1990).

Older students enroll in programs for a variety of reasons—to pursue different or additional degrees, to enhance their careers, to increase their earning capabilities, or for the simple pursuit of knowledge. These various reasons for continuing education may influence which of several educational options an older adult chooses. Four options offer special advantages for many older learners:

1. Some universities open their enrollments to interested retirees who are not in degree

programs, giving open slots in selected courses. These non–degree-seeking older students register, enroll in the courses, and participate in all the same requirements and activities as the younger students.

2. The Elderhostel program exemplifies an exciting opportunity to learn. This Boston-based, nonprofit program provides an environment where older citizens are stimulated intellectually. The plan follows the tradition of hosteling as practiced in Europe. Older people live on a college or university campus and attend classes, usually for a 1-week period, to experience the life and learning of the college student. The fee for this educational experience is modest—about $250 per week for room, board, and tuition. The Elderhostel concept is based on the belief that retirement offers a time of opportunity for the older person to engage in and enjoy new experiences and new challenges.

3. The Older Adult Service and Information System (OASIS), in operation since 1982, is a partnership between governmental departments of aging, usually at a county level, and businesses, usually those located in shopping centers or shopping malls. Volunteers offer their services to provide instruction for interested older adults who learn about health care, creative writing, music appreciation, wood carving, physical fitness, dancing, and any number of creative recreational activities.

4. Full- or part-time summer programs are especially attractive to older adults who look forward to traveling and new activities in the summer months. Educators are becoming increasingly concerned that schools and classrooms may not be well utilized between the month of graduation and the beginning of a new school year. Providing opportunities for interested and motivated older adults allows the classrooms to be used constructively and enables the faculty and teachers to pursue gainful employment between academic semesters.

Whether the older student pays a full- or part-time tuition or even a reduced or discounted tuition, the gray-haired student is becoming a welcome sight on campus. The older students' interest and enthusiasm make an excellent climate for fostering teaching and learning. They stimulate and motivate younger learners and facilitate the creation of an exciting, productive, competitive atmosphere.

■ Demography of Aging in the United States

FACTORS INFLUENCING DEMOGRAPHIC TRENDS

A predictive demographic profile of older adults is paramount to a policymaker's accurate planning for the short- and long-term needs of the older adult population. Anyone involved in delivering services or care for older adults needs specific information regarding factors such as age, gender, race, living arrangements, and marital status. Articles and publications (especially from the U.S. Department of Commerce, Bureau of the Census) about aging and older adults often include these types of statistical data. In filtering through these data and assessing predictions, one must astutely gauge the accuracy of the underlying assumptions associated with predictive modeling (McFarland, 1978). Demographers often mention two factors associated with predicting trends among older adults:

1. Incidence of disease
2. Rate of aging

Reduction of the incidence of disease would lead to reduced mortality rates and an increase in the number of older adults. This projection assumes that health practices will improve, which, in turn, will contribute to the control of disease. Lifestyle changes are most directly associated with reductions in disease, typically those related to diet and exercise. Examples of lifestyle changes are the reduction or elimination of smoking and use of alcohol or drugs; increased physical activity; improved dietary habits; and annual (or more frequent) physical examinations that include health screening for early disease detection and treatment planning.

Control of the rate of aging is a bit more complex than reducing the incidence of disease. It involves first understanding the genetic and environmental factors associated with the aging process. This includes an understanding of such things as the aging body's physiologic (e.g., immune, endocrine) systems. The second step is to apply this understanding to deterring the effects of the aging process (Neugarten, 1978). The National Institute on Aging within the National Institutes of Health is responsible for conducting and supporting biomedical, social, and behavioral research and for disseminating information related to the aging process and diseases of older adults (National Institute on Aging [NIA], 1994).

CHANGING DEMOGRAPHICS AMONG OLDER ADULTS

In 1993 there were 32.8 million persons in the United States age 65 or over. This was 12.7% of the total U.S. population, or about one in eight persons. Since 1900 the number of people age 65 and over has increased more than 10 times and the percentage has tripled (AARP, 1994). The population can also be tracked by breaking out age categories for older adults. In 1990 approximately 7% of the U.S. population was between 65 and 74 (about 18 million persons). This was over 8 times the number of people in this age group in 1900. In 1990 approximately 4% of the U.S. population was between 75 and 84 years old and approximately 1.2% was 85 years old or older. These numbers were 12 times and 23 times, respectively, the numbers in 1900 (AARP & Pacific Presbyterian Medical Center, 1989; Taeuber, 1993) (Table 1-16 and Figure 1-12).

Population growth by age category is projected based on current birth and death data.

TABLE 1-16 Total population, by age: 1960 to 1991

Year	Total	65 to 74 years	75 years and over
1960	180,671	11,053	5,622
1975	215,973	13,971	8,779
1985	239,279	17,009	11,531
1988	246,329	17,897	12,470
1991	252,503	18,548	13,497

From U.S. Bureau of the Census. *Current population reports* (Series P-25, Nos. 519-917).

The U.S. Bureau of the Census provides such data and generates forecasting models that estimate future U.S. population growth. The older adult population is expected to continue to grow in the future, slowing somewhat in the 1990s because of the smaller number of births during the 1930s. However, an accelerated increase is forecast between 2010 and 2030, when the baby boom generation reaches age 65 (AARP, 1994). At that time, 77 million persons (one third of the current U.S. population) will be senior citizens (Beck, 1990). Based on current data and trends, demographers project that there will be almost 80 million older adults in the United States by the year 2030 (or over 20% of the total U.S. population). This is almost 3 times the number of older adults that were in the United States in 1980 (AARP, 1994). The age groups made up of people over 55 will be the only U.S. age groups to experience significant growth in the next century, especially if current fertility and immigration levels remain stable (AARP & Pacific Presbyterian Medical Center, 1989).

The total population of the United States is expected to rise from 249 million in 1990 to 345 million in 2030 and 383 million in 2050. Following this peak, it is predicted that a slow decline in numbers will occur until 2080, when the population will stabilize.

Other changes in population in the United States will create subtle but certain alterations in the workplace, education, and health care. Some businesses, professions, and industries will expand. For example, as the population ages, deaths will outnumber births, so the funeral business and associated industries (e.g., casket companies, cemeteries, florists, and funeral equipment suppliers) will expand. Total birth rates will drop, and there could be labor shortages in those industries in which labor supplies depend on young workers. Factors, unknown at the present, could alter these scenarios. For example, technologic breakthroughs could dramatically change the manner and shape of current business and industry practices.

In the future the health care system will be challenged to provide institutional care for those who need it. At present, this is usually the very old person with comorbidity and significant disabilities. The health care system will also be challenged to promote healthy aging directives among older adults. Those who are interested in assisting older adults in maximizing their quality of life will have to provide creative programs and novel initiatives to meet the unique needs of the increasingly complex mix of older individuals.

Gender

Women make up the majority of the expanding number of older adults and are more likely than men to live alone, to be poor, and to suffer from long-term chronic illnesses. In 1990 there were about 67 men age 65 and over for every 100 women age 65 and over. This was approximately 18.5 million older adult women and about 12.5 million older adult men. The ratio of men to women in 1990 was 81:100 for people 65 to 69 years of age; 74:100 for people 70 to 74 years of age; 64:100 for people 75 to 79 years of age; 53:100 for people 80 to 84 years of age; and 39:100 for people 85 years of age and older (Taeuber, 1993) (Figure 1-15).

Racial and ethnic groups

Studies of the racial and ethnic characteristics of older populations depict the following: In 1993 about 86% of people age 65 and over in the United States were white, non-Hispanics; 8% were African American; 3% were of Hispanic origin; 2% were Asian or Pacific Islander; and less than 1% were American Indian or Native Alaskan (AARP, 1994) (Figure 1-16). Haub (1990), of the Population Reference Bureau, predicts that the dramatically lower birth rates among whites will partially account for some dramatic changes in the United States' racial and ethnic mix in the future. By the year 2080 Haub suggests that white, non-Hispanic Americans will be on the verge of losing their majority to the current three largest minority groups: African Americans, Asian Americans, and Hispanics. This prediction suggests a change from that of a U.S. Bureau of the Census 1988 report estimating a U.S. population of 245 million in 2080, with 84.4% being white, 12.3% black, and 3.3% "other races" (Asians, Pacific Islanders, Native Americans, and Eskimos and other Alaskan Native Americans).

Marital status

In 1993 about 77% of older adult men were married, as compared to 42% of older adult women. Almost half of the older adult women were widows (48%, or 8.6 million). This was 5 times the number of older adult widowers (1.8 million). Approximately 5% of older adults were divorced (1.6 million). The number of divorced older adults has increased 3 times as fast as the entire older adult population since 1980 (AARP, 1994). This trend is quite likely to continue into the future. Approximately the same percentage of older adult men and older adult women had never married (5%) (AARP & Pacific Presbyterian Medical Center, 1989).

Education

As the baby boom generation reaches old age, it will enjoy an educational advantage over other

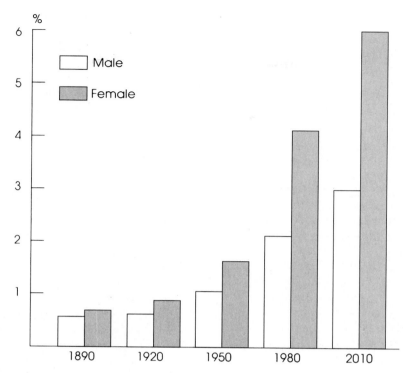

FIGURE 1-15 Percentage of total U.S. population (male and female) age 75 years and older. (From U.S. Bureau of the Census.)

older generations. The goal of parents in the early part of the twentieth century was to see their children complete high school. By midcentury the goal was to complete the first or second level of a college or university education. In 1993 approximately 12% of older adults had a bachelor's degree (AARP, 1994). This percentage varied considerably by race. In the latter years of the twentieth century the number of doctoral-prepared people has increased phenomenally. When the twenty-first century begins, older adults are predicted to be recipients of various types of education, received in a variety of settings, with multiple applications.

The education level of older adults has increased in the last 20 years. The percentage of

older adults who have completed high school increased from 28% in 1970 to 60% in 1993 (AARP, 1994).

Still greater changes are expected for the next generation of aging Americans—those students who entered first grade in 1991, with expected high school graduation in the year 2003. By 2003 a world of change is predicted. The following list highlights just a few of the facts that will confront the high school graduate, class of 2003 ("What the Class . . ." 1988):

The body of available knowledge will have doubled 4 times since 1988. They will have been exposed to more information in 18 years than their grandparents were exposed to in a lifetime.

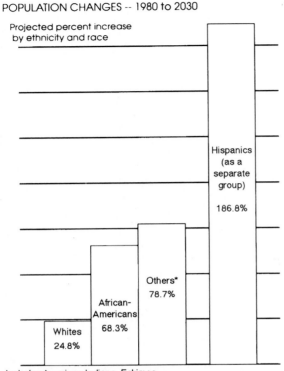

POPULATION CHANGES -- 1980 to 2030

Projected percent increase
by ethnicity and race

Hispanics
(as a
separate
group)

186.8%

Others*
78.7%

African-
Americans
68.3%

Whites
24.8%

Includes American Indians, Eskimos,
plus Aleuts, Asian, and Pacific Islanders

FIGURE 1-16 Population changes related to cultural diversity, 1980-2030.

Only 15% of jobs will require a college education but nearly all will require job-specific training.

In three families out of four, both spouses will have full-time jobs.

Salaries for women will have grown from within 70% of men's salaries in 1988 to within 90% of men's salaries.

Of the people in the United States, 118,000 will be older than 100 (in 1988 there were 26,000 centenarians).

Life expectancy

The U.S. Department of Health and Human Services reports that someone born in 1900 was expected to live to be 47 years of age. Someone born in 1988 could expect to live to an average age of 74 years or more (Figure 1-17).

The number of people age 85 and older is expected to double by the year 2010 and to triple by the year 2025. So the fastest growing segment of the population will continue to be people over 85 years of age. In 1988 1 in every 15 persons was more than 85 years old. By 2030 1 in every 10 persons will be more than 85 years old (Fisk, 1988). There are several implications to be considered as one ponders these statistics:

Most of the nursing home residents who are 85 and older require some assistance with at least one activity of daily living, and many have three or more dependencies.

These include activities such as eating, bathing, dressing, getting out of bed, and going to the bathroom.

Projected increases in the number of older adults and the very old resulting from the baby boom generation raise concerns regarding available services and personnel to care for this population.

People will be old much longer in the future, because of increasing life expectancy.

Four-generation families will be the norm by the year 2000, with some families having great-great-grandparents in their midst. This prediction has serious implications for family finances. Will money be spent on college tuition for children or on some type of eldercare for aging parents or grandparents?

Members of the sandwich generation will be faced with caring for their own children while caring for their parents as well.

Because of changing demographic statistics, some policy experts believe that in the future the United States will be run by older adults. The population cohort of younger people is shrinking. Instead of those under age 35 making up 55% of the population as they did in 1989, their percentage will drop to 41% by the year 2030. There will be more than a million people over the age of 100 by the year 2050 and nearly 3 million between 95 and 99 years old.

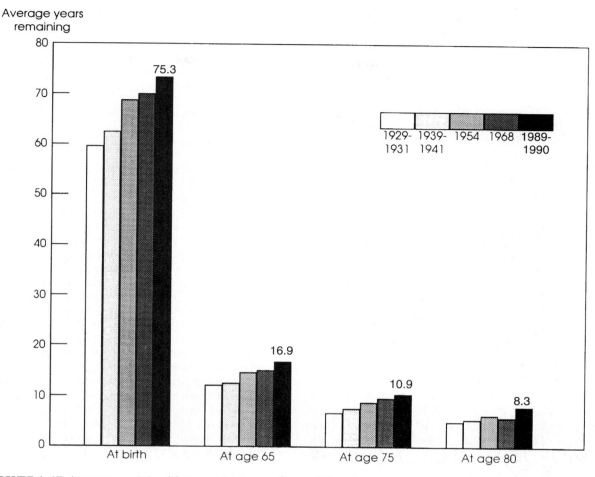

FIGURE 1-17 Average remaining lifetime at birth, age 65, age 75, and age 80; 1929-1931, 1939-1941, 1954, 1968, and 1989-1990. (From U.S. Bureau of the Census.)

■ Summarizing Major Trends Among the Older Adult Population

The following statements summarize major trends among the older adult population (Taeuber, 1993):

1. Currently there are more older adults than ever before in history.
2. Older adults are an increasing proportion of the U.S. population.

3. The increase in older adults will be steady until 2011, when the baby boomers turn 65.
4. Older adult women outnumber older adult men.
5. More people will survive to older ages in the future.
6. As more people survive to older ages, more will experience chronic disease disabilities.
7. Concern over identifying appropriate care for the older adults will increase, and the

young-old will experience new opportunities in extended careers and retirement activities.

8. The population of older adults will be more racially diverse.

9. The educational attainment of older adults will increase significantly.

10. Although currently some older adults are economically secure, there remains a sub-population of the oldest old with high rates of poverty.

Many questions remain that require continued study of older adults. Many are related to predictions in the demographics of aging. In the future, how many older adults will be young-old and how many will be old-old? How healthy will they be? Other research relates to social structure and older adults. How will the quality of their life be described? What are alternative living arrangements for the very old? Still other research is related to genetic and environmental issues. Will projections that consider disease control promote more healthful living and facilitate a healthier, more active and independent lifestyle? Will expanding knowledge of genetic and environmental factors associated with aging result in increases in years and quality of life? What alterations in diet and exercise yield the largest return in an older adult's life? Perhaps the most important research question relates to improving the quality of life as a whole, no matter when it ends.

Most policymakers now acknowledge that the wave of the future will be mightily swayed by senior power, sometimes referred to as the "gerontocracy." Though few experts agree as to the extent to which older adults will influence future trends and events, few would dispute that older adults will surely have a large and multifaceted impact on society.

REFERENCES

Abdellah, F. (1989). Foreword. In M. E. O'Brien, *Anatomy of a nursing home: A new view of resident life.* Owings Mills, MD: National Health Publishing.

American Association of Retired Persons. (1989, December-1990, January). AARP older students, quick studies. *Modern Maturity, 32*(6), 97.

American Association of Retired Persons. (1994). *A profile of older Americans* (Brochure No. PF3049 [1294]-D996). Washington, DC: Program Resources Department.

American Association of Retired Persons & Pacific Presbyterian Medical Center of San Francisco. (1989). *Aging in America.* Washington, DC: American Association of Retired Persons.

Beck, M. (1990, Winter-Spring). The geezer boom. *Newsweek,* pp. 62-68.

Besdine, R. W., & Rose, R. M. (1982). Aspects of infection in the elderly. In C. Eisdorfer (Ed.), *Annual review of gerontology and geriatrics.* New York: Springer.

Bethell, T. N. (Ed.). (1987). *On the other side of easy street: Myths and facts about the economics of old age.* Washington, DC: Villers Foundation.

Birren, J. (1978). A gerontologist's overview. In L. F. Jarvik (Ed.), *Aging into the twenty-first century: Middle-agers today.* New York: Gardner Press.

Brockington, F. (1975). *World health.* New York: Churchill Livingstone.

Buck, J., & Klemm, J. (1992). Recent trends in Medicaid expenditures. *Health Care Financing Review: Medicare and Medicaid Statistical Supplement,* 123-54. Baltimore: U.S. Department of Health and Human Services, Health Care Financing Administration, ORD.

Catholic Health Association's Task Force on Long Term Care Policy. (1988). *A time to be old, a time to flourish—The special needs of the elderly-at-risk.* St. Louis: Author.

Commonwealth Fund. (1992). *The nation's great overlooked resource: The contributions of Americans 55+.* New York: Commonwealth Fund, Americans over 55 at Work Program.

Ebersole, P., & Hess, P. (1994). *Toward healthy aging: Human needs and nursing response* (4th ed.). St. Louis: Mosby.

The facts of life in older America. (1987, October-November). *Modern Maturity, 30*(5), 13.

Fisk, C. F. (1988). Address to the surgeon general's workshop. In *Health promotion and aging.* Washington, DC: U.S. Department of Health and Human Services, Public Health Service.

Fullerton, H. N. (1993, November). Another look at the labor force. *Monthly Labor Review,* pp. 31-40.

Galtung, J. (1980). The basic needs approach. In K. Lederer (Ed.), *Human needs* (pp. 55-130). Cambridge, MA: Oelgeschlager, Gunn, and Hain.

Gilford, D. M. (Ed.). (1988). *The aging population in the twenty-first century*. Washington, DC: National Academy Press.

Guralnik, J. M., LaCroix, A. Z., Everett, D. F., & Kovar, M. G. (1989, May 26). *Aging in the '80s: The prevalence of comorbidity and its association with disability* (Advance data from Vital and Health Statistics of the National Center for Health Statistics, No. 170). Washington, DC: U.S. Department of Health and Human Services, Public Health Service, Centers for Disease Control.

Haub, C. (1990, July 8). 2050: Standing room only? *Washington Post Outposts*, p. C3.

Helbing, C. (1992). Medicare program expenditures. *Health Care Financing Review: Medicare and Medicaid Statistical Supplement*, 123-54. Baltimore: U.S. Department of Health and Human Services, Health Care Financing Administration, ORD.

Hogarth, T., & Barth, M. (1991). Costs and benefits of hiring older workers: A case study of B & Q. *International Journal of Manpower, 12*(8), 5-17. MCB University Press.

Keller, A. S. (1986, November 18). Exercising the mind. *Washington Post Health/Aging*, p. 10.

Lewin, T. (1990, February 19). Retirees return to campus in housing trend for elderly. *New York Times*, p. A1.

Manton, K. G. (1986). Cause of specific mortality patterns among the oldest old: Multiple causes of death trends 1968 to 1980. *Journal of Gerontology, 41*(2), 282-289.

Maslow, A. H. (1970). *Motivation and personality* (2nd ed.). New York: Harper and Row.

McFarland, D. D. (1978). The aged in the twenty-first century: A demographer's view. In L. F. Jarvik (Ed.), *Aging into the twenty-first century: Middle-agers today*. New York: Gardner Press.

McNaught, W., & Barth, M. (1991). *Using retirees to fill temporary labor needs: The Travelers' experience* (Background Paper Series, No. 5). New York: Commonwealth Fund, Americans over 55 at Work Program.

McNaught, W., & Barth, M. (1992, Spring). Are older workers "good buys"?—A case study of Days Inns of America. *Sloan Management Review, 33*(3), 53-63.

Mitchell, A. (1971). *Bismarck and the French nation*. New York: Pegasus.

Moon, M. (1993). *Medicare now and in the future*. Washington, DC: Urban Institute Press.

National Council on the Aging. (1994). Promotional literature regarding the Health Promotion Institute. Washington, DC: Author.

National Institute on Aging. (1994). *Aging research: Practice, promise, and priorities*. Washington, DC: National Institutes of Health.

Neugarten, B. L. (1978). The future and the young-old. In L. F. Jarvik (Ed.), *Aging into the twenty-first century: Middle-agers today*. New York: Gardner Press.

Older, slower-growing America predicted. (1989, February 1). *Washington Post*, p. B4.

Pender, N. J. (1982). *Health promotion in nursing practice*. Norwalk, CT: Appleton-Century-Crofts.

Perry, D., & Butler, R.N. (1988, December 20). Aim not just for longer life, but extended "health span." *Washington Post Health*, p. 16.

Quinn, J. B. (1990, Winter-Spring). Growing old frugally [Special issue]. *Newsweek*, pp. 102-105.

Schaie, K. W. (1983). The Seattle longitudinal study: A 21-year exploration in psychometric intelligence in adulthood. In K. W. Schaie (Ed.), *Longitudinal studies of adult psychological development*. New York: Guilford.

Schaie, K. W., & Willis, S. L. (1986). *Adult development and aging* (2nd ed.). Boston: Little, Brown.

Stone, R. I. (1989). *The feminization of poverty among the elderly*. Rockville, MD: U.S. Department of Health and Human Services, Public Health Service, National Center for Health Services Research and Health Care Technology Assessment.

Taeuber, C. (1993). *Sixty-five plus in America* (Current Population Reports, Special Studies, No. P23-178RV). Washington, DC: U.S. Department of Commerce, Economics, and Statistics Administration, Bureau of the Census.

U.S. Bureau of the Census. (1990). *Persons in institutions and other group quarters*. (1980 Census of Population, No. PC80-2-4D; 1990 Census of Population and Housing, Summary Tape File 1A). Washington, DC: Author.

U.S. Bureau of the Census. (1992a). *Population projections of the United States, by age, sex, race, and Hispanic origin: 1992 to 2050* (Current Population Reports, No. P25-1092). Washington, DC: U.S. Government Printing Office.

U.S. Bureau of the Census. (1992b). *Sixty-five plus in America* (Current Population Reports, Special Studies,

No. P23-178RV). Washington, DC: U.S. Government Printing Office.

U.S. Department of Health and Human Services. (1990). *The Medicare handbook* (DHHS Pub. No. HCFA 10050). Washington, DC: U.S. Department of Health and Human Services, Health Care Financing Administration.

U.S. Department of Health and Human Services. (1993a). *Health Care Financing Review: Medicare and Medicaid Statistical Supplement.* Washington, DC: U.S. Department of Health and Human Services, Health Care Financing Administration.

U.S. Department of Health and Human Services. (1993b). *Vital and health statistics: Health data on older Americans—United States, 1992.* (DHHS Pub. No. [PHS] 93-1411). Washington, DC: Public Health Service, Centers for Disease Control and Prevention, National Center for Health Statistics.

Vladeck, B., Miller, N., & Clauser, S. (1993). *The changing face of long-term care. Health Care Financing Review* (Vol. 14, No. 4). Baltimore.

Watson, W. (1982). *Aging and social behavior.* Monterey, CA: Wadsworth.

What the class of '00 needs to know. (1988, July 3). *Washington Post Magazine,* p. 11.

Wilson, L., Simon-Rusinowitz, L., & Marks, L. (1994). *Policy issues and trends influencing employment and volunteerism in the next generation of older Americans: Views from policy experts* (Project summary). College Park: University of Maryland, Center on Aging.

Yura, H., & Walsh, M. B. (1988). *The nursing process.* E. Norwalk, CT: Appleton and Lange.

Yurick, et al. (1984). *The aged person and the nursing process.* Norwalk, CT: Appleton-Century-Crofts.

BIBLIOGRAPHY

American Association of Retired Persons. (1986). *A home away from home.* Washington, DC: Author.

American Association of Retired Persons. (1987). *A handbook about care in the home.* Washington, DC: Author.

American Association of Retired Persons. (1988). *Tomorrow's choices.* Washington, DC: Author.

American Public Health Association. (1989). Nursing home data report is released to the public. *Nation's Health, 19*(1), 5.

Atchley, R. C. (1980). *The social forces in later life: An introduction to social gerontology* (3rd ed.). Belmont, CA: Wadsworth.

Comfort, A. (1978). A biologist laments and exhorts. In L. F. Jarvik (Ed.), *Aging into the twenty-first century: Middle-agers today.* New York: Gardner Press.

Dychtwald, K., & Flower, J. (1989). The challenges and opportunities of an aging America. In K. Dychtwald (Ed.), *Age wave.* Los Angeles: Jeremy P. Tarcher.

Jarvik, L. F. (Ed.). (1978). *Aging into the twenty-first century: Middle-agers today.* New York: Gardner Press.

LaRue, A., & Jarvik, L. F. (1978). Aging and intellectual functioning: Great expectations? In L. F. Jarvik (Ed.), *Aging into the twenty-first century: Middle-agers today.* New York: Gardner Press.

Lawrence, B. (1990, March 6). An oasis of education for seniors. *Prince George's Journal,* p. A6.

National Institute on Aging. (1993). *The health and retirement study—Preliminary findings.* Washington, DC: National Institutes of Health.

Rivlin, A. M., & Wiener, J. M. (1988). *Caring for the disabled elderly.* Washington, DC: Brookings Institution.

Rosenwaike, I. (1985). *The extreme aged in America: A portrait of an expanding population.* Westport, CT: Greenwood Press.

Rowan, T. (1989, May 11). The grim effects of loneliness. *Catholic Standard,* p. 2.

Theories of longevity—The search for the fountain of youth. (1986, February-March). *Bostonia,* pp. 29-32.

U.S. Department of Health and Human Services. (1991). *What's your aging I.Q.?* (NIH Pub. No. 1991-281-837/40019). Washington, DC: Public Health Service.

U.S. Department of Health, Education, and Welfare. (1977). *A staff report: Public policy and the frail elderly* (DHEW Pub. No. 79-2059). Washington, DC: Office of Human Development Services, Federal Council on Aging.

World Health Organization. (1946). *Constitution of the World Health Organization.* New York: Author.

If I can stop one heart from breaking, I shall not live in vain.
If I can ease one life the aching, or cool one pain,
Or help one lonely person into happiness again
I shall not live in vain.

EMILY DICKINSON

Gerontologic Nursing

■ Learning Objectives

On completion of this chapter, the reader will be able to do the following:

1. Discuss the history of gerontologic nursing.
2. Describe the current status of gerontologic nursing.
3. Identify the importance of the nursing process, including nursing diagnosis.
4. Recognize several conceptual or theoretic frameworks for nursing.
5. Describe the results of the leadership efforts of the American Nurses' Association in defining standards for gerontologic nursing, initiating and maintaining nursing certification, and defining the nature and scope of nursing.
6. Recognize the contributions of the teaching nursing homes.

■ Historical Overview of Gerontologic Nursing

The nursing profession has developed dramatically during the second half of the twentieth century, partly because of a tremendous increase in the knowledge of human physiology, biochemistry, medicine, medical technology, and pharmacology. In like manner, gerontologic nursing has undergone major changes, especially because of the changing demographics of the U.S. populations. The nursing profession and the gerontologic nursing specialty have enjoyed tremendous professional development during recent decades; many challenges have been faced and many are yet to be defined, but all are accepted as legitimate obstacles that can be overcome.

One purpose of this chapter is to consider several perspectives of gerontologic nursing. Box 2-1 highlights selected events and people in the history of nursing that have had a significant influence on the development of nursing in general, and on gerontologic nursing in particular. Because history helps us understand our present state of development, it behooves all of us occasionally to reflect on the past. Although some would have preferred that the rate of change and development of new ideas in nursing had been faster, a careful and thoughtful analysis of historic

51

BOX 2-1 EVENTS AND PEOPLE WHO HAVE INFLUENCED GERONTOLOGIC NURSING

Florence Nightingale (1820–1910)—Nursing gained stature as a profession with professional goals:

- To care for the patient as a person
- To approach patient care wholistically, emphasizing the patient's physical, psychologic, and spiritual needs
- To promote wellness, as well as to provide care during illness
- To provide care according to a plan based on scientific principles and practices

Early twentieth century (1900-1940)

- Nursing was task oriented.
- Nurses followed hospital regulations and physicians' orders.
- There was little autonomy in nursing.
- Nurse actions were reactive rather than proactive.
- Gerontologic nursing was minimal; older adults were not as numerous in the population as they are today.
- Care of ill patients was the primary focus.
- Little or no attention was given to health maintenance.
- Older adults were cared for in hospitals or in nursing homes, and no deliberate plans were made for the older person to return home.
- Little attention was given to rehabilitation.

Housing for older adults (before 1930)—Few facilities existed for the older adults who were destitute or without family; many older adults lived on "poor farms."

Social Security Act (1935)—This welcome legislation made funds available to older adults who were needy or who had limited financial resources.

World War II and postwar years (1940-1960)

- The population of older adults began to gradually increase.
- While emphasis on care during illness continued, nurses increasingly gave attention to wellness activities such as exercise, nutrition, ambulation, and rehabilitation for patients of all ages.
- Nursing education programs moved into institutions of higher education.
- Educational grants and funding for professional nurses became available.

Latter twentieth century (1960-1995)

- Theories of nursing evolved.
- Critical care nurses entered the health care system.
- Cardiac surgery, recovery rooms, and critical care units became integral parts of acute care systems.
- Technology advances included ventilators, cardiac and hemodynamic monitoring, and computerized documentation.
- Medicare and Medicaid payment and regulations and diagnosis-related groups (DRGs) were introduced.
- Nurse practitioners entered the health care system.
- Master's and doctoral education in nursing increased.
- Cycles of oversupply and shortages of nurses were recognized.

BOX 2-2 POINTS OF VIEW ABOUT GERONTOLOGIC NURSING

- An opportunity to exercise professional skills, to apply clinical knowledge in practice, and to use clinical decision-making skills
- An opportunity to be creative and to use initiative in providing patient care
- An opportunity to care for older adults in various settings, such as community clinics, the patient's own home, the nursing home, and the acute care hospital
- An opportunity to collaborate with other health care disciplines in the planning and implementation of care for older adults
- An opportunity to teach and to support older adults in performing activities of daily living and in maintaining their independence
- An opportunity to appreciate the wisdom of older adults and to be enriched as they share memories of their life experiences
- A specialty that has a poor image among many professional nurses
- Often equated with employment and nursing practice exclusively in nursing homes, which is frequently viewed negatively
- Often, lower wages than those received by nurses in nongerontologic specialties
- Indirect reimbursement for nursing services
- Limited opportunities for career advancement
- Limited opportunities for collaborating with peers because of fewer colleagues in this specialty than in others
- Limited assignment of nursing students to gerontologic nursing as part of their educational practice

events suggests that nursing has progressed at a reasonable pace when compared with other professions. What is most important, advances in nursing are still continuing.

In addition to significant strides in the development of the nursing profession generally, gerontologic nursing in particular has become an important and legitimate specialty in professional nursing. The development of this specialty can be more fully understood by comparing pros and cons of gerontologic nursing. On the one hand, gerontologic nursing offers a variety of challenging opportunities for professional development. On the other hand, nurses who choose to care for older adults are just beginning to receive the professional recognition and rewards they deserve. Elaboration on the perceptions of this specialty are presented in Box 2-2.

While fully recognizing that the professional nurse continues to face many uphill challenges as

the care of older adults becomes more complex, this chapter examines recent progress in nursing. Specific benchmarks of progress are identified, as are relationships between nursing generally and the specialty of gerontologic nursing. In the future, nurses will be able to rely on the foundation of professional gerontologic nursing that is currently being established and to build on this foundation so that care of older adults will be less frustrating in the future than it has been in the past.

Since midcentury, several events in nursing stand out as important turning points in the profession:

In the 1960s

- The nursing process was defined.
- Theoretic-conceptual frameworks of nursing were developed.

In the 1970s

- Nursing diagnoses were identified.
- Nursing certification was established and nursing standards were defined.

In the 1980s

- Nursing was defined in a social policy statement.
- Teaching nursing homes were developed as models for care.

In the 1990s (to date)

- A White House Conference on Aging was held, the first since 1981.
- The Biennial Nurse Theorist Conference was held in 1993.
- Revisions of the social policy statement for nursing were published, as was a statement of the standards and scope of gerontologic nursing.

These events have established nursing as a respected profession among the health care disciplines and have moved nursing into roles that are both respected by health care colleagues and peers and appreciated by patients and families who seek and receive the services provided by nurses. The remainder of this chapter describes these key events of the 1960s, the 1970s, the 1980s, and the first half of the 1990s.

■ In the 1960s

During the 1960s two important developments occurred that continue to have an impact on nursing:

1. The nursing process was defined.
2. Theoretic-conceptual frameworks for nursing were enunciated.

DEFINITION OF THE NURSING PROCESS

During the 1960s, nursing was defined as a scientifically based problem-solving process. Many nurses welcomed this defining statement about how nurses perform patient care. The nursing process was defined clearly and specifically so that colleagues in the health care profession could understand it; this helped to establish clearer lines of communication among nurses and colleagues than had existed previously.

Two mid-1960s publications were instrumental in spelling out the nursing process as the base on which nursing has continued to build. One report was issued by the Western Interstate Commission of Higher Education (WICHE), in which the nursing process was defined as "that which goes on between the patient and the nurse in a given setting" (Lewis et al., 1967, p. 6). It identified components of the process as being perception, communication, interpretation (assessment), intervention (nursing action), and evaluation.

The second publication was a report of an 8-week continuing education program that defined and discussed *The Nursing Process: Assessing, Planning, Implementing, Evaluating* (Yura & Walsh, 1967). These two history-making publications set the stage for defining the essence of nursing as being a process "central to all nursing actions . . . applicable in any setting." It is flexible and adaptable, and it provides "a base from which all systematic nursing actions can proceed" (Yura & Walsh, 1983, p. 1). All nursing specialists, including gerontologic nurses, rely on the framework of the nursing process. Nurses adapt specific components of the process according to the needs and the traits of the population for whom they are caring in each nursing situation.

For purposes of this text the nursing process is made up of the following steps: (1) collecting data about the patient to identify real or potential problems (assessment), (2) on the basis of the data collected, arriving at a conclusion about the patient's needs (diagnosis), (3) specifying the goals toward which patient care will be directed (outcome identification), (4) developing plans to prevent or to solve the patient problems that have been identified (planning), (5) putting the plans into action (implementation), and (6) determining to what extent the plans and actions were effective in preventing or resolving the identified problems and diagnoses (evaluation).

Over the past 30 years different authors have used various labels to present, discuss, and apply the nursing process. Despite differences in labeling, all recognize the process as scientific, orderly, and systematic. The crucial common feature of all descriptions of the process is that all the aforementioned activities are included in the process, whatever the terminology being used. The present text does not explicate the various differences among the numerous descriptions of this process. Interested readers who would like a more comprehensive description of the many perspectives on this problem-solving process are urged to obtain a text that addresses the nursing process in detail.

The following pages describe each component of the nursing process in terms of the nurse's role and responsibility in using the nursing process to assess, diagnose, identify outcomes, plan, implement, and evaluate the care of the older person.

Characteristics of the nursing process

The logical problem-solving process of nursing requires nurses to collect and analyze data about the patient. Having reached conclusions about the patient's health status, the nurse informs the patient and the caregivers about the patient's health-related needs, desires, concerns, and problems. Based upon the data gathered about the patient, the nurse determines the goals to be achieved, sets priorities regarding these goals, plans and carries out appropriate strategies and interventions, and then reexamines the situation to ensure that the patient's problems will be resolved.

Nurses possess three kinds of qualifications for satisfactorily applying the nursing process: knowledge, technical skills, and interpersonal skills. An extensive repertoire of sound *knowledge* provides a solid foundation from which all aspects of the process can proceed. *Technical skills* enable the nurse to carry out the activities that constitute the craft of nursing. The nurse's *interpersonal skills* allow the establishment of good relationships between the nurse and the older person. To achieve this goal, there needs to be clear communication, trust, and mutual respect in the intimate and vital situations of nursing care. With full understanding of their responsibility for care of older adults in any setting, professional nurses establish and maintain the following:

1. Honest, clear communications with the patient, caregivers, and family members
2. A sense of mutual trust between the patient and the nurse
3. The patient's confidence in the ability of nursing personnel to meet needs and to help with problem prevention and solution

Preparation for initiating the nursing process

To facilitate communication between the nurse and the patient, the nurse should arrange seating and body positioning that optimize eye-to-eye contact with the patient. If the patient is sitting in a chair, the nurse should arrange a chair to sit nearby. It may be necessary to adjust furniture to facilitate comfortable eye contact if the patient is lying down or sitting in a low seat. A nurse who stands or sits above the eye level of the patient may intimidate the patient or otherwise hinder the nurse-to-patient communication.

Seating arrangements should allow the nurse to face the patient. This enables communication via facial expressions and gestures, clear reception of verbal inquiries and messages, and observation of the facial features and moving lips of the speaker. This is especially important for the older person who may have some hearing impairment or some difficulty in speaking audibly and distinctly. Though neither communicator may be proficient in lipreading, the communication will be enhanced by these visual cues.

Regarding the placement of light fixtures, the nurse should be positioned so that the light falls on the nurse's face. Again, this aids the patient in observing facial expressions and interpreting the messages being communicated by the nurse.

One of the major goals of this preparation is to establish a sense of trust between the nurse and the patient. Through the adept use of interpersonal skills, mutual respect can be established, which can set the stage for a trusting, comfortable relationship. This kind of nurse-patient relationship can be critical to maintaining a high quality of life for older patients who may be experiencing numerous insults and difficulties.

In addition to physically preparing the setting for the nursing process, the nurse mentally prepares for interactions with patients. A hurried, anxious nurse may neglect subtle signs being given by the patient or may overwhelm the patient with more information than the patient can absorb. The pace of communication and data collection must be appropriate for the particular nurse-patient interaction. It is important for the patients that the nurse speak clearly and slowly so that patients can grasp what is being said. Adequate time should be allowed for the patients to respond to questions. The nurse communicates, by words and actions, that the patients are important and that the information being given is important. When initiating the nursing process, the nurse must foster the patient's comfort and trust that the patient's strengths will be recognized and fostered to prevent problems from developing and to solve any identified health problems. Once rapport is established, the patient and nurse can smoothly begin the assessment data-collecting activities.

Assessment

The nurse reviews the older patient's situation for the purpose of collecting data about the patient, particularly to identify the strengths and limitations (actual and potential) of the individual. These data that are gathered by the nurse lead to the nursing diagnoses that will guide the patient's care.

The nurse gathers data based on an overall plan for the assessment. The nurse selects an appropriate assessment form or some other organizational plan, which has been developed by the nurse or by the gerontologic nursing team, to guide data collection. This plan uses a theoretic framework to guide nursing practice in the applicable setting. The nurse's values and philosophy about life and about nursing are inherent in this framework.

During the assessment the nurse guides the dialogue and directs questions and comments to the patient to collect the information necessary for determining the patient's needs. Throughout this process the nurse acknowledges each older person as a unique individual, subject to the same environmental insults experienced by younger people, and possibly even more sensitive to these insults than are younger people. Therefore the nurse should allow time for the patient to communicate, both in replying to the nurse's questions and in asking questions of the nurse. An effective assessment is a dialogue, not a monologue. As in any communication experience, the participants *take time to listen* to each other.

If family members are available and are knowledgeable about the patient's needs and interests, they should be included in the assessment discussion, given the full consent and approval of the patient. Family involvement can produce positive results for the patient, the family, and the nurse. This type of exchange provides insight about the family's perspective and allows the nurse to observe and assess the kinds of relationships that exist within the patient's family. For example, does a family member interrupt a cognitively alert patient's responses, providing answers before the patient has had an opportunity to do so?

Some older patients may have lived alone for many years and may have had limited social activities. If this is the case, the patient may relish the presence of the nurse as an interested person who is asking about the patient's needs and desires; this may stimulate an interest in more communication than was anticipated. When this occurs, the nurse will be challenged to use creative interpersonal skills in directing the patient's verbalizations to those areas of assessment that will provide the kinds of data

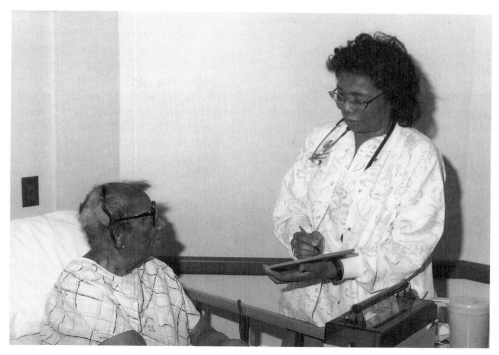

Nurse gathering assessment data. *Courtesy Loy Ledbetter, St. Louis.*

needed for nursing diagnosis. The nurse should also include the observation of this perceived social need in the assessment data; it will be significant information to use in planning the care of this person, because the opportunity to converse with an interested person may well be therapeutic in itself.

Nursing diagnosis

Nursing diagnosis is a clinical judgment about individual, family, or community responses to actual or potential health problems or life processes. Nursing diagnoses provide the basis for selection of nursing interventions to achieve outcomes for which the nurse is accountable (Gordon, 1994).

Following the collection of data during assessment, the nurse analyzes and logically clusters the data. When the data have been organized, the nurse determines the strengths and the needs of the patient to determine the nursing diagnoses.

The three major components of the nursing diagnosis are (1) the problem, (2) the etiology of the problem, and (3) the signs or symptoms of the problem, referred to collectively as *PES* (Gordon, 1994). The problem (P) occurs in the health state of the older person. This can be an actual problem or a potential problem. The nurse identifies potential problems as a result of inquiry and observation about the patient's habits, practices, and nutrition, and other factors that contribute to or detract from health.

The etiology (E) comprises those influences in the patient's environment that contribute to the person's identified health problems. The signs or symptoms (S), or defining characteristics of the problem, are those objective and subjective clues that the nurse observes and detects and that lead the nurse to the nursing diagnosis.

Some of these defining characteristics are based on group consensus about probable associations rather than on hard data about known links; intensive research remains to be done in this area. The developing of research-based diagnoses for each PES based on accurate clinical data depends on the nurse's prudent judgment. Clinical judgment and decision making facilitate the development of accurate nursing diagnoses. These skills are especially significant for gerontologic nurses, who find a limited number of research publications to guide the development of these very important dimensions of nursing.

Outcome identification

To influence health outcomes, the nurse and the health care team derive the expected outcomes of care from the nursing diagnoses. It is the patient's care that is being planned, and the patient's choices and decisions must be given primary consideration. If the patient is unable to participate in defining the goals to be achieved, the family members (as appropriate) may speak for the patient.

The group should specify both short-range ("proximate") goals and long-range ("ultimate") goals, including general time lines within which to meet these goals. For example, if the older patient is in an acute care setting, an immediate goal may be to orient the patient to the new surroundings. A long-range goal may be to enable the patient to walk around in the hospital unit without getting lost. The health care team may decide that this should be accomplished by the end of 24 hours of hospitalization. Identification of these goals, stated in measurable terms and including a reasonable time estimate, will be important for moving the patient toward wellness. The goals also are consistent with the diagnosis-related group, or DRG, criteria that influence the length of time available for the patient, depending on the patient's diagnosis and progress.

In addition to defining expected outcomes, the nurse and the health care team will also set priorities to determine which of the identified problems to address first. Assuming that more than one nursing diagnosis is specified, it usually is not possible to resolve all diagnoses simultaneously. To assist with priority setting, the patient should indicate which problem is most troublesome and should be resolved first. With input from the patient and the family, the nurse considers which of the problems is most important from a health care standpoint. For example, if a nursing home patient is dehydrated, resolution of this deficit will assume a higher priority than will the resolution of a problem related to inadequate socialization.

Planning

The purpose of planning is to determine what can be done to help the patient achieve optimal wellness; it involves reviewing the goals, setting priorities, and designing methods to resolve the problems that were identified by the nursing diagnoses. The nurse leads these care-planning activities. In addition, the patient, family members, and other health care personnel who play a role in the patient's health maintenance may be involved in the planning.

Once the goals are determined and the priorities are set, the planning team designs the means by which to resolve the problems (diagnoses). If the patient has a problem with constipation, for example, the planning team will discuss the foods that will encourage elimination and the activities in which the older person can engage to stimulate intestinal peristalsis.

Throughout the planning discussions, the patient's perceptions must be considered. The other members of the planning team may identify a problem and a plan for resolution quite differently than would the patient. The final plan is more likely to be implemented and to succeed when the team considers the patient's views and reactions to the other team members' ideas, suggestions, and proposals.

Careful, deliberate planning, based on the assessment data and valid nursing diagnoses, is critical to the successful outcome of patient care activities. Through astute perception, knowledgeable observation, and effective communication, the nurse and the other team members can prescribe a plan that will meet the needs of the older patient. In the past, nurses have largely used intuition to guide their plans and decisions about patient care, but nurses now use patient data, scientific processes, and their own intellectual skills to determine the direction of that care. This is very important with all patients, but especially significant in the care of the older person whose age may play an important role.

Implementation

Implementation involves the initiation and completion of the actions necessary for accomplishing the goals that were defined in the planning sessions. By definition, this is the action phase of the nursing process: someone *does* something to address the problems that the older adults are experiencing. The people who perform the activity may be the patients themselves, family members, nurses, or other designated members of the health team. The team will determine who is responsible for the action before initiating the implementation phase. Throughout the activity of caring for the older person, important concepts to bear in mind include health promotion, illness prevention, health maintenance, rehabilitation, and palliation. All of the knowledge and interpersonal and technical skills that can be mustered will be employed to make the implementation successful. As the challenges of resolving the older patients' problems become more complex, the skills of the nurse become more essential.

The acute care setting In the acute care setting, the older patient usually depends on the actions of the nursing personnel. Among these people is a registered professional nurse who is responsible for carrying out the agreed-on plans of action. Associated with the nurse are other levels of nursing personnel who assist in the caregiving activities. The nurse assigns these caregiving activities among the associated personnel; to make appropriate assignments, the nurse considers each person's level of preparation, as well as the personality traits and strengths of the multiple caregivers. Matching these traits to the needs of the older patient challenges the intellectual skills of the most able professionals: Will the nurse aide respect the frailty of an older patient? How will the patient react to the nurse aide? Many factors are considered by gerontologic nurses in hospital settings.

The nursing home setting In the nursing home the older resident is usually more familiar with the routines of care than in the acute care setting. Most residents spend a longer period of time in nursing homes than patients spend in hospitals. However, this does not reduce the challenge of matching caregiver traits to the patient, the diagnoses, and the situation. When the nurse delegates activities to other personnel, the nurse is responsible for ensuring that the goals are understood and that all activities are directed toward achieving these goals. The nurse encourages reassurance that the patient's needs are being considered and that the choices and participation of the older patient and family members are constantly being reviewed. Although the assessment and planning activities begin before implementation is initiated, assessment and planning continue during the implementation phase. New data, as they become available, are used for revising the plan; as the plan is revised, the implementation actions are reconsidered and redefined. In other words, the nurse constantly rethinks, reviews, and revises the action plan, using intellectual and interpersonal skills to ensure that the needs of the older patient are foremost in the minds of the caregivers. This is especially true in the nursing home setting.

The patient's private home setting In the patient's own home in the community, professional nurses rely on the data they obtain during assessment, the nursing diagnoses they define, the outcomes they identify, and the plans they develop, for meeting the health needs of the patient. The variable that directs the activities of the nurse is the nurse's ability to function on the patient's turf, always aware of being in the patient's environs and territory. Professionals respect the patient's privacy in all settings, but it is imperative to do so when functioning in the patient's private home.

It is crucial to establish rapport with older adults to identify expected outcomes, define plans, and determine the necessary activities that the older person, the family members, or the significant others will carry out. Although the same data are sought in this setting as in all other settings, it is important here to define the patient's needs so that care can be continued in the absence of the professional person. The teaching role of the nurse assumes major significance in the patient's private home. Mutual understanding of the expected outcomes and the goals of care, and agreement about the projected care activities are critical to achieving comfort and health for older people in their own homes.

Evaluation

Evaluation appraises the changes experienced by the patient as a result of the actions conducted during the nursing process. That is, it asks how effectively the identified outcomes were achieved. To what extent were the defined goals realized?

To initiate evaluation, the nurse reexamines the blueprint for action that was designed in the early phase of the nursing process. The patient is included in this activity to be certain that the patient's perspective is respected. If the patient believes that the goals were not achieved, this sends a clear message to the nurse, whether or not the nurse believes that the goals were met. The focus of the evaluation phase is the viewpoint of the patient and the patient's response to care. If the patient is not satisfied, and if the nursing team identifies deficits in the expected outcomes of care, the evaluation process directs the team members to reassess, replan, reimplement, and reevaluate the care as many times as

necessary until the goals are achieved. That is, the patient's needs are assessed and diagnoses are defined again, outcomes are reidentified, and a revised plan is made in terms of this reappraisal. The appropriate people implement the new plan of care, and the team then evaluates the patient's satisfaction with—and the health outcomes of—the revised care. Each of the steps is repeated in this cycle of activity as many times as necessary until satisfactory results are achieved.

Conclusion

These phases of the nursing process—assessing, diagnosing, identifying outcomes, planning, implementing, and evaluating—provide the basis of nursing care for all older adults who require a nurse's expertise in a health-related situation. To care for older adults, the nursing caregivers tailor these phases to meet the unique needs of each older person, recognizing that the care of older adults differs from the care of one who is younger.

FRAMEWORKS FOR NURSING

In addition to the elucidation of the nursing process, a second development in the 1960s was the enunciation of several theoretic frameworks for care. The writings of Florence Nightingale (published in 1859 and 1946), Hildegarde Peplau (1952), and Virginia Henderson (1966) provided valuable pronouncements about nursing and clear explanations of the goals and purposes of many professional nursing functions. Ideas such as these were being referred to as "nursing concepts" and later were called "nursing theories." These early writings stimulated discussions about professional nursing responsibilities that have continued for the past 3½ decades.

A number of these ideas have been presented in the literature and have been labeled as theories, although most of the ideas have not been validated by sufficient research. Nonetheless, many nurses are cautiously referring to these ideas as theories that aid in exploring intellectually stimulating concepts that guide nursing practice. As continuing research increasingly validates many of these nurses' ideas, the label of theory is gradually becoming justified. Meanwhile, whether labeled as theories or as ideas about nursing, these frameworks for nursing are critical to the structural formulation of what nursing is, how nurses help patients in need, and why nurses perform the activities that are called "nursing." To date, an insufficient number of research efforts have included the older population as subjects for study. This is a fertile area for exploration, offering myriad opportunities for systematic and scientific study.

Nightingale, Peplau, and Henderson had the temerity to present previously unpublished aspects of nursing, thereby stimulating others to formulate ideas that have guided major intellectual developments in nursing. For example, in the 1960s Ida Jean Orlando (1961), Ernestine Wiedenbach (1964), Myra Levine (1969), and Dorothy Johnson (1961) published their ideas about nursing. In the 1970s Martha Rogers (1970), Dorothea Orem (1971), Imogene King (1971), Joyce Travelbee (1971), Sister Callista Roy (1976), and Josephine Paterson and Loretta Zderad (1976) presented their concepts about nursing. In the 1980s Betty Neuman (1980), Jean Watson (1985), and the team of Helen Yura and Mary Walsh (1988) announced their views to their colleagues in nursing. In addition, nurses began to emphasize the applicability of these ideas to nursing practice. Thus began a greater thrust toward wholistic nursing and an emphasis on the use of frameworks to guide nursing practice.

Building on consensus developed in the 1980s regarding the "domain concepts" of nursing—person, environment, health, and nursing—nurse theorists of the 1990s remain focused on the tenor and interrelation of these concepts (Fawcett, 1984). Additionally, literature reveals continued debate regarding the type of science nursing represents—basic, applied, or practical—as well as the necessity for a practice theory separate from scientific and ethical theory (Beckstrand, 1992; Collins & Fielder, 1992; Johnson, 1991).

Despite and because of ongoing controversy regarding some basic tenets of the development and investigation of nursing knowledge, the current decade holds great promise for refinement of the scientific discipline of nursing. The wonder of the possibilities is reflected in the frameworks of contemporary nursing theorists and their application to nursing practice. Specifically, Patricia Benner, Rosemarie Parse, and Margaret Newman hold promise for further theory development, application of theory to practice, and the differentiation of nurses in their roles as health care providers.

So far, the development of theories and concepts about nursing has given little attention to the structure that can best guide the care of older adults. However, among the several frameworks for nursing that have been enunciated, the following have particular appeal for and potential applicability to the care of older people: frameworks suggested by Imogene King, Betty Neuman, Dorothea Orem, Martha Rogers, Sister Callista Roy, Jean Watson, and the team of Helen Yura and Mary Walsh. These frameworks seem to be the most constructive for guiding the care of older adults. Further research to validate these ideas in the gerontologic setting will be very important.

Gerontologic nurses are encouraged to select from the framework or frameworks with which they are most comfortable. Because some elements of several ideas may be appropriate for the care of older adults, nurses are encouraged to consider the use of an eclectic approach, which integrates the most appropriate ideas from several of the authors.

Interaction theory (Imogene King) focuses on the ways in which older adults interact both with their environment and with the nurse to set and achieve goals of health care. King defines nursing as a process of action, reaction, interaction, and transaction. She highlights the establishment of the nurse-patient relationship as the means to help the patient maintain health and to support the patient in making changes and adapting to the changes in order to improve health. The older person is perceived by King as an open system that consists of social systems (society), interpersonal systems (groups), and personal systems (individuals).

The health care systems model (Betty Neuman) views the older person as a total person who experiences stress and adversity that can affect the individual's functioning. The nurse's role in this health care systems model is to help the older person, as well as the person's family if necessary, to achieve a maximum level of wellness through purposeful interventions. Two assumptions proposed by Neuman are appropriate to the care of older adults: (1) Each person is unique and is exposed to a variety of stressors that can disturb the equilibrium of the individual. (2) Reactions to these stressors can vary, depending upon the status of each person's inherent lines of defense.

The self-care deficit theory (Dorothea Orem) encourages, supports, and empowers older adults in meeting their own needs to the extent that they are able. Orem suggests that the nurse is responsible for identifying what the person needs and then providing and managing the resources that will enable the patient to engage in self-care; assuming that these activities are continual, the outcome of these nursing endeavors will be to help the older person to sustain life and health, to recover from disease or injury, and to cope with the effects of disease or injury. The essence of Orem's ideas are the constructs of self-care, self-care deficits, and nursing systems.

Unitary man concepts (Martha Rogers) emphasize the interaction between older adults and the environment, with the goal of achieving maximal health. Rogers's beliefs that apply to the care of older adults include the concepts that each person is unique, that each human and the environment are involved in a continuous interactive process, and that all human beings are more than and different from the sum of their parts. Rogers stresses the importance of nursing

practice in multiple settings and identifies the nurse's role as helping people to prevent disease and to achieve optimal health.

Adaptation theory (Sister Callista Roy) points to the need for older people to adapt to the changes they may be experiencing. Four modes of adaptation are defined: physiologic needs, self-concept, role function, and interdependence. These constitute the framework that the nurse can use to determine how effectively older people are adapting to their life and health status. Three types of stimuli are defined in this theory: focal, contextual, and residual. These can be adjusted and/or manipulated to promote and to ensure adaptation; the patients may be the ones to manipulate these stimuli with the assistance and support of the nurse.

An interpersonal concept (Jean Watson) directs the focus of nursing to meeting the needs of the older person through a caring interpersonal relationship. The focus is a philosophy and science of caring to guide the action of the nurse. Caring is viewed as an interpersonal process that promotes health; accepts patients wherever they may be in terms of their health, their health awareness, and their health activity; and creates an environment that enables the patients to exercise choice as they consider what will be best for them. Watson views decision making as being the responsibility of the older patient. Nursing intervention is perceived as a legitimate activity that is based on a scientific-humanistic approach, using caring as a framework to direct activity. Nurses are encouraged to approach older adults in a positive manner with a wholistic outlook, liberally using faith and hope. Watson believes that without these concepts, it would not be possible to establish an interpersonal relationship. Through a positive relationship, both nurse and patient can realize teaching and learning, help and trust, and the acceptance of feelings.

Human need theory (Helen Yura and Mary Walsh) views the older person as an integrated, organized whole whose goal-directed behavior leads the person to satisfy human needs. As the nurse supports and encourages the older adults' attempts to satisfy their needs, wholistic care is practiced and the integrity of the older person is recognized. With guidance and direction from the health care professional who respects the patient's ability, it is reasonable to expect that the individual person will achieve those goals that satisfy the person's unique human needs.

A framework of *pragmatic phenomenology* is described by *Patricia Benner* and serves as a bridge between the nursing theorists of the 1980s and those of the 1990s. Her model embraces the basic domain concepts of person, environment, health, and nursing. The framework is pragmatic in that nursing is characterized as a caring association. The nurse is viewed as facilitating a relationship with the patient in which help is given and received (Benner & Wrubel, 1989). The framework is phenomenologic in that Benner's views of health, person, and situation (environment) are grounded in the works of existential phenomenologists Heidegger and Merleau-Ponty. Existential phenomenology is difficult to define; however, all existential philosophers stress individual existence, subjectivity, individual freedom, and choice. Knowing this will serve as a good basis for discerning Benner's wholistic view of nursing practice relative to the interrelationships of health, person, situation, and nursing.

Health is described as a dialectic, "the lived experience of being healthy and being ill" (Benner & Wrubel, 1989, p. 7). Benner views health as being capable of assessment and as being more than the absence of disease and illness. She further makes the distinction between illness and disease. Benner posits that people may not see themselves as ill because illness is interpreted as a "loss or dysfunction." In other words, an aging person may not recognize symptoms of congestive heart failure if those symptoms do not translate into a loss of function from the person's perspective.

Person is described as "embodied" or capable of responding to meaningful situations. "A person is a self-interpreting being" (Benner & Wrubel, 1989, p. 41), defined throughout the course of living life. Consistent with her grounding in existential phenomenology, Benner clearly views the person as being interactive with the world, a summation of mind and body, evolving over time.

Environment is described by Benner within a phenomenologic framework. Situation, rather than environment, is described in the model to emphasize meaningfulness in a full social context. This creates a comprehensive context for the concept of environment. Benner states that the unique perspectives, habits, and assigned meanings of a person enter into each situation with the person.

Benner views nursing practice as the application and study of the lived experiences of health, illness, and disease and their interrelationships framed within the caring paradigm of nursing practice. The concept of how a "person is in the situation sets up different possibilities" (Benner & Wrubel, 1989, p. 63), both for the person and for the nurse involved in the care of that person. Benner purports that "a nurse's clinical knowledge is relevant to the extent to which its manifestation in nursing skills makes a difference in patient care and patient outcomes" (Benner & Wrubel, 1989, p. 63). A thorough accounting of Benner's concepts regarding skill acquisition and nursing can be studied in her work *From Novice to Expert*. Benner resides well within the caring paradigm of nursing. Although caring is clearly a component of the application of her work with Wrubel in *Primace of Caring,* her offering is specifically related to the philosophy of caring. What remains to be articulated is the relevance and function of caring in nursing (Radsma, 1994).

Rosemarie Parse has developed a theory firmly entrenched in the domain concepts central to nursing. Although never expressly stated, this focus is understood in the process orientation of the original title of her theory: man-living-health. She further made this explicit in the coining of the term *simultaneity paradigm* to describe alternative views of the domain concepts relative to the Rogers and Parse conceptual frameworks (Parse, 1981). It is critical to point out that the language requires some work from the reader. Parse has been criticized for her difficult terminology. Holmes (1990) states the following:

Unfortunately, [Parse's] efforts have not had the impact on nursing that might have been hoped. Their accessibility is undermined by an obscure style, a penchant for the utterly novel use of familiar words, and a large crop of ill-explained neologisms. These problems are exacerbated if the reader is not familiar with esoteric language and idiosyncratic conceptual tools of existential phenomenologists (p. 193).

That said, the reader is challenged to take up the study of this theory for all it offers.

The human becoming theory of Parse evolves from Martha Rogers's holistic interactive framework of nursing and major tenets from existential-phenomenologic works of Heidegger, Sarte, Merleau-Pongy, and Marcel (Parse, 1981). The outcome is theory rooted in the human sciences intended to guide nursing by serving as the theoretic basis of a practice and research methodology unique to nursing. The central theme is the interrelationship of the elements of the human-universe-health process described as *human becoming* (Parse, 1992). Three main principles emerge from the three central themes of meaning, rhythmicity, and cotranscendence. The three principles are as follows (Parse, 1981):

1. Structuring meaning multidimensionally is cocreating reality through the *languaging* of *valuing* and *imaging.*
2. Cocreating rhythmic patterns of relating is living the paradoxic unity of *revealing-concealing* and *enabling-limiting,* while *connecting-separating.*

3. Cotranscending with the possibles is *powering* unique ways of *originating* in the process of *transforming.*

Each principle contains three major concepts central to the understanding of Parse's theory of human becoming (as highlighted with italics).

Languaging is the communication of personal experiences through verbal and nonverbal means. Valuing is the process of living cherished beliefs while assimilating the new into a personal world view. It emerges in the human-universe process and is the human being's confirming of cherished beliefs. Imaging is the creation of perceptions of one's experiences. "What is real for each individual is structured by that individual." Revealing-concealing is the process of choosing what is to be known of one's self while simultaneously hiding other things. Connecting-separating represents the rhythm of the patterns created by making choices throughout one's life. Choosing to move toward something or someone is a simultaneous decision to move away from another. Enabling-limiting describes the paradoxic patterns that emerge when one chooses a particular path in life. Each path represents limitations, as well as possibilities. Powering is the force of human existence. It is self-affirmation in light of the possibility of nonbeing. Originating is self-differentiation through personal choices within given situations, despite uncertainty of the outcome. Transforming is defined as the changing of change. Changing unfolds as the familiar is seen in a different light, thus shifting the view and illuminating new possibilities.

Parse (1990) describes health as "a process of becoming, experienced by the person" (p. 137), whereas most others view health as a value. Parse states that "health is an unfolding that cannot be prescribed or described by societal norms, only by the person living the health. It is just the way the human is!" (Parse, 1992). She further states the following:

Health as personal commitment, then, means that health is one's own unfolding in interconnectedness with the world. It does not imply that one's health is an entity, lived in a vacuum without connectedness with others and environment. The belief is that one cocreates health with others and the world in mutual interrelationship and that cocreation of health is the set of choices the person with the world makes from all levels of the universe, not just from the explicit level. The person is responsible for the outcomes of choices in that the choices themselves incarnate the person's unique was, is, and will be (Parse, 1990, p. 137).

People, or human beings, are conceptualized through the simultaneity paradigm. They are thought to be a "living unity" free to choose meaning, create patterns of relating and being, assume responsibility for choices made, and move beyond the present en route to changing in the future. Consistent with these views of the human being is the broader view of human nature that depicts the human as a "creative author." This view posits that "the human creates a personal world with spirit, compassion, and honor. This view of the human shuns the idea of control, fixing, and manipulation" (Parse, 1981, 1990).

Parse refers to environment and the universe interchangeably. Her concept of environment is most clearly seen within principle #2: Cocreating rhythmic patterns of relating is living the paradoxic unity of revealing-concealing and enabling-limiting, while connecting-separating. The interrelation of man and environment is reflected in this principle. *Cocreating* meaning together, man and the environment are partners in the origination of the other (Parse, 1981).

The goal of nursing is to enhance the quality of life as perceived by the person and family. The nurse who is guided by Parse's theory in practice "seeks to participate with persons in enhancing their quality of life through being with them in true presence as they explore the meaning of personal situations and choose ways of becoming" (Cody & Mitchell, 1992). This requires a different approach to nursing. Nurses do not

assume the positions of authority. They trust the individuals' commitment to the process of health and remain present with the individuals as they align their realities with those of their current or future situation. To this end Parse created a practice methodology capable of application in any given environment or nurse-client relationship (Cody & Mitchell, 1992). Dimensions and processes of this methodology are advocated: illuminating through *explication,* synchronizing rhythms through *dwelling with,* and mobilizing transcendence processes, imagine a person being allowed to explore the meaning of smoking cessation and relate it to the quality of that person's life. One way of moving beyond the current reality to future realities is to assist people in viewing their past, present, and future health with and without smoking with no imposition of the "shoulds" of a different value structure. This allows the individuals to review the meanings they have placed on smoking, its role in their lives, and possibly how those meanings have changed or will change. The first step to changing health, then, is within the context of one's own values and preferences (Parse, 1990).

The basis of *Margaret Newman's* theory of nursing is *health as expanding consciousness.* This concept describes the patterns of time, space, and movement as directly corresponding to evolving consciousness. The roots of her theory were derived from several varied disciplines: nursing, philosophy, physics, psychology, and chemistry. Flowing from the influences of Hegel's dialectic process and Rogers's model of nursing, Newman's theory concentrates on wholeness, person-environment, pattern organization, life process, and the capacity for advanced, complex process of the mind (Newman, 1979, 1986). Her major assumptions are as follows:

- Health encompasses conditions heretofore described as illness, or in medical terms, pathologic conditions.

- These "pathologic" conditions can be considered a manifestation of the total pattern of the individual.
- The pattern of the individual that eventually manifests itself as a pathologic condition is primary and exists before structural or functional changes.
- Removal of the pathologic condition in itself will not change the pattern of the individual.
- If an individual's pattern can manifest itself only through the individual's becoming "ill," then that is health for that person.

The theory of expanding consciousness is posited along a continuum from potential consciousness (freedom) to the ideal of absolute consciousness (real freedom). The continuum of consciousness is related to the dimensions of time and space. Described is a process of interrelationships among time, space, movement, and consciousness. It begins with the person coming into being in a state of potential consciousness, circumscribed in time, defined in space, and propelled toward absolute consciousness by choices made within patterns of life (movement) (Newman, 1979).

The domain concepts universal to nursing, much as in the case of Parse's theory, are not directly discussed within the theory of expanding consciousness. However, they can be inferred through examining several conceptual definitions.

Health is the focus of Newman's theory of expanding consciousness. Health is viewed as being composed of both disease and nondisease. It follows that health is "the pattern of the whole of a person"—the "undivided wholeness of the person in interaction with the environment." Newman further states that the recognition of patterns is the essence of health, thus concluding that health and evolving consciousness are one and the same (Newman, 1986, 1990).

People are defined as extensions of consciousness. They are identified and differentiated by their individual patterns. Newman describes both implicit and explicit order in her concept of pattern and states that pattern is somehow intimately involved in energy exchange and transformation (Newman, 1986).

Newman (1986) postulates that "consciousness is coextensive in the universe and resides in all matter" (p. 33). It is through movement that one is able to control one's environment. Incorporating the concept of pattern, Newman describes the pattern of consciousness of a person as interacting with the collective consciousness of the family and/or community at large (Newman, 1986).

Newman views nursing as facilitating a relationship with the patient within the process of expanding consciousness. The nurse is capable of developing this relationship when the person is at the point of choice or movement. The task for nursing is to recognize the patterns of a person and to understand them as a unified entity, thus enabling the nurse to facilitate health within the context of person-environment (Newman, 1986).

Conclusion

A few theoretic frameworks have been summarized in this chapter. Several publications present far more comprehensive overviews of these theoreticians who have fostered a sophisticated level of intellectualization in the discussion of the practice of nursing. Readers of this text are advised to review these publications, which present the various authors' ideas in considerable detail, and which provide guidance regarding the use and value of specific frameworks in clinical practice. Students and practitioners are encouraged to consider each author's views about nursing, about people, and about how to apply these ideas in practice.

A more recent group of publications provides the scholar of theories with presentations and analyses that enable deeper thoughts about the proposed theories of nursing. A variety of nurses have accepted the challenge of describing conceptual frameworks and theories. Each monograph presents a biographic sketch of the theorist, the origin of the theory, assumptions, concepts, propositions, examples for application to practice and research, a glossary of terms, and a bibliography of classic works, critiques, and research. These monographs have been published by the National League for Nursing Press, in 1993 and 1994, under the following titles:

1. Martha Rogers: The Science of Unitary Human Beings
2. Imogene King: A Conceptual Framework for Nursing (by Christina L. Sieloff Evans)
3. Callista Roy: An Adaptation Model
4. Dorothea Orem: Self-Care Deficit Theory (by Donna L. Hartweg)
5. Rosemarie Parse: Theory of Human Becoming (by Sheila Bunting)
6. Margaret Newman: Health as Expanding Consciousness (by Joanne Marchione)
7. Jo Patterson and L. Zderad: Health as Expanding Consciousness (by Nancy O'Conor)
8. Florence Nightingale: An Environmental Adaptation Theory (by Louise C. Selanders)
9. Hildegarde E. Peplau: Interpersonal Nursing Theory (by Cheryl Forchuk)
10. Betty Neuman: The Neuman Systems Model (by Karen S. Reed)
11. Ida Jean Orlando: A Nursing Process Theory (by Norma Jean Schmieding)

■ In the 1970s

IDENTIFICATION OF NURSING DIAGNOSES

In 1973 the fledgling North American Nursing Diagnosis Association (NANDA) got off to an optimistic start. Kristine Gebbie and Mary Ann Lavin initiated the first national conference on the classification of nursing diagnoses held in 1975 at St. Louis University. The ultimate goal of this group of forward thinkers was to "identify, standardize, and classify health problems treated by nurses" (Gordon, 1982, p. xi). Four assumptions formed the underpinnings of the discussion

among the first group of 95 conference participants and 24 group leaders:

1. Nursing diagnosis is an integral part of the nursing process.
2. Nursing diagnoses are not made without substantiating clinical data.
3. Understanding of the diagnostic process facilitates the development of clinical reasoning and diagnostic judgment.
4. Professional nurse graduates and students will assume the professional responsibility for defining nursing diagnoses.

Also, concern was expressed that nurses must not only define and understand the *process* of nursing diagnosis but also understand the *clinical judgment* that is used to arrive at this diagnosis.

The first eight conferences on nursing diagnoses were hosted in St. Louis; the ninth conference was held in Orlando, Florida. The definition of nursing diagnosis was accepted at the ninth biennial conference of the North American Nursing Diagnosis Association in Orlando in March 1990, which represented the culmination of 17 years of deliberating and discussing the development of nursing diagnoses. Nonetheless, the definition is considered to be a working definition; nurses are encouraged to use this definition, critique its content, and contribute to its evaluation for future endeavors in research, education, and practice.

Before 1982 the conferences were open to invitees only. The 1982 conference saw the initiation of several changes: (1) All interested nurses were invited to the conferences; (2) the North American Nursing Diagnosis Association was formally organized; (3) formal bylaws of the association were accepted; and (4) a taxonomy committee was established to develop the classification scheme for nursing diagnosis. The present charge to the taxonomy committee is to develop the taxonomy in such a way that it will meet the criteria for inclusion in the tenth revision of the International Classification of Diseases

(ICD-10) of the World Health Organization (WHO) (Fitzpatrick et al., 1989). The currently approved NANDA nursing diagnoses appear in Box 2-3.

NURSING CERTIFICATION

Among the indications of professional achievement is the certification (credentialing) of nurses. The development of certification within the profession enables gerontologic nurses to demonstrate the level of expertise that they have attained. It is a means of identifying those nurses who have demonstrated capability in using expert clinical judgment and high-level skills in managing patient care. In addition to proving to oneself that these distinctive levels of knowledge and practice have been achieved, certification demonstrates to colleagues and to peers that a level of expertise has been reached that is worthy of recognition.

In 1973 the American Nurses' Association (ANA) established the ANA certification program. The primary purpose of certification is to recognize the professional achievement of nurses in a defined clinical area or in one of the functional areas of nursing (ANA, 1995b).

The American Nurses' Credentialing Center (ANCC) was established as a separately incorporated center as a result of the 1989 recommendation from the ANA Commission on Organized Assessment and Renewal. The credentialing programs of the ANCC are based on standards set by the ANA Congress for Nursing Practice. Each test development committee from each of the ten boards on certification of the ANCC develops examinations that cover knowledge, understanding, and application of nursing theory and practice. The committees define the content areas that are to be covered in the tests, what the relative emphases are to be, and what is the nature of professional skills and abilities to be measured. The examinations assess both knowledge of and skills in professional nursing practice. Seeking certification as a specialist or an advanced practitioner in nursing is a voluntary pursuit on the part of the individual nurse.

The certification examination is available for an increasing number of specialties in nursing. Interested nurses can obtain, on request, from the ANA, an appropriate handbook that contains the necessary information regarding the existing specialty certification boards, as well as the requirements that must be met to apply for the certification examination. A wide range of nurses have satisfactorily completed the certification examinations, and the numbers are continuing to increase. To date, approximately 400 nurses are certified as clinical specialists in gerontologic nursing, and approximately 1500 nurses have satisfied the requirements for certification as gerontologic nurse practitioners.

STANDARDS OF GERONTOLOGIC NURSING

As the official organization of professional nursing, the ANA has defined the standards and scope of gerontologic nursing practice, which are shown in Box 2-4. The ANA recognizes the complexity of caring for the illness needs and of promoting the health of older people who live in the technology-oriented society of today. Nurses need continual updating of knowledge about the demographics of the older population, the services available to older adults to help them meet their needs, and the services that they may be unable to obtain unless nursing support is provided, as well as the social and political factors that impinge on the health and illness of older adults.

The ANA standards were defined to cite a level of quality care that is beyond the care required by minimal regulatory standards. These professional standards are models toward which gerontologic nursing can strive in practice, whatever the setting in which care is given. They may also be used in quality assurance programs, as a guide for evaluating care, as a resource for assessment tools, as a model for plans of care, and as a form of guidance for peer review and performance appraisal (ANA, 1995c).

The roles of generalist and specialist in gerontologic nursing practice are described in the statement of the scope of gerontologic practice

BOX 2-3 NANDA-APPROVED NURSING DIAGNOSES

This list represents the NANDA-approved nursing diagnoses for clinical use and testing (1994).

PATTERN 1: EXCHANGING

Altered Nutrition: More than Body Requirements
Altered Nutrition: Less than Body Requirements
Altered Nutrition: Risk for More than Body
  Requirements
Risk for Infection
Risk for Altered Body Temperature
Hypothermia
Hyperthermia
Ineffective Thermoregulation
Dysreflexia
Perceived Constipation
Colonic Constipation
Diarrhea
Bowel Incontinence
Altered Urinary Elimination
Stress Incontinence
Reflex Incontinence
Urge Incontinence
Functional Incontinence
Total Incontinence
Urinary Retention
Altered (Specify Type) Tissue Perfusion (Renal,
  Cerebral, Cardiopulmonary, Gastrointestinal,
  Peripheral)
Decreased Coronary Tissue Perfusion
Fluid Volume Excess
Fluid Volume Deficit
Risk for Fluid Volume Deficit
Decreased Cardiac Output
Impaired Gas Exchange
Ineffective Airway Clearance
Ineffective Breathing Pattern
Inability to Sustain Spontaneous Ventilation
Dysfunctional Ventilatory Weaning Response
Risk for Injury
Risk for Suffocation
Risk for Poisoning
Risk for Trauma
Risk for Aspiration
Risk for Disuse Syndrome

Altered Protection
Impaired Tissue Integrity
Altered Oral Mucous Membranes
Impaired Skin Integrity
Risk for Impaired Skin Integrity
Decreased Adaptive Capacity: Intracranial
Energy Field Disturbance

PATTERN 2: COMMUNICATING

Impaired Verbal Communication

PATTERN 3: RELATING

Impaired Social Interaction
Social Isolation
Risk for Loneliness
Altered Role Performance
Altered Parenting
Risk for Altered Parenting
Risk for Altered Parent/Infant/Child Attachment
Sexual Dysfunction
Altered Family Processes
Caregiver Role Strain
Risk for Caregiver Role Strain
Altered Family Process: Alcoholism
Parental Role Conflict
Altered Sexuality Patterns

PATTERN 4: VALUING

Spiritual Distress (Distress of the Human Spirit)
Potential for Enhanced Spiritual Well-Being

PATTERN 5: CHOOSING

Ineffective Individual Coping
Impaired Adjustment
Defensive Coping
Ineffective Denial
Ineffective Family Coping: Disabling
Ineffective Family Coping: Compromised
Family Coping: Potential for Growth
Potential for Enhanced Community Coping
Ineffective Community Coping

Continued

BOX 2-3 NANDA-APPROVED NURSING DIAGNOSES—cont'd

Ineffective Management of Therapeutic Regimen
  (Individuals)
Noncompliance (Specify)
Ineffective Management of Therapeutic Regimen:
  Families
Ineffective Management of Therapeutic Regimen:
  Community
Ineffective Management of Therapeutic Regimen:
  Individual
Decisional Conflict (Specify)
Health Seeking Behaviors (Specify)

PATTERN 6: MOVING

Impaired Physical Mobility
Risk for Peripheral Neurovascular Dysfunction
Risk for Perioperative Positioning Injury
Activity Intolerance
Fatigue
Risk for Activity Intolerance
Sleep Pattern Disturbance
Diversional Activity Deficit
Impaired Home Maintenance Management
Altered Health Maintenance
Feeding Self-Care Deficit
Impaired Swallowing
Ineffective Breastfeeding
Interrupted Breastfeeding
Effective Breastfeeding
Ineffective Infant Feeding Pattern
Bathing/Hygiene Self-Care Deficit
Dressing/Grooming Self-Care Deficit
Toileting Self-Care Deficit
Altered Growth and Development
Relocation Stress Syndrome
Risk for Disorganized Infant Behavior
Disorganized Infant Behavior
Potential for Enhanced Organized Infant Behavior

PATTERN 7: PERCEIVING

Body Image Disturbance
Self-Esteem Disturbance
Chronic Low Self-Esteem
Situational Low Self-Esteem
Personal Identity Disturbance
Sensory/Perceptual Alterations (Specify)
  (Visual, Auditory, Kinesthetic, Gustatory, Tactile,
  Olfactory)
Unilateral Neglect
Hopelessness
Powerlessness

PATTERN 8: KNOWING

Knowledge Deficit (Specify)
Impaired Environmental Interpretation Syndrome
Acute Confusion
Chronic Confusion
Altered Thought Processes
Impaired Memory

PATTERN 9: FEELING

Pain
Chronic Pain
Dysfunctional Grieving
Anticipatory Grieving
Risk for Violence: Self-Directed or Directed
  at Others
Risk for Self-Mutilation
Post-Trauma Response
Rape-Trauma Syndrome
Rape-Trauma Syndrome: Compound Reaction
Rape-Trauma Syndrome: Silent Reaction
Anxiety
Fear

From: *NANDA nursing diagnoses: Definitions and classification 1997-1998.* (1997). Philadelphia: North American Nursing Diagnosis Association.

BOX 2-4 STANDARDS OF GERONTOLOGIC NURSING PRACTICE

The nursing process encompasses all significant actions taken by gerontologic nurses in providing care to patients and forms the foundation of clinical decision making (McFarland & McFarlane, 1996).

STANDARD I. ASSESSMENT
The gerontologic nurse collects patient health data.

STANDARD II. DIAGNOSIS
The gerontologic nurse analyzes the assessment data in determining diagnoses.

STANDARD III. OUTCOME IDENTIFICATION
The gerontologic nurse identifies expected outcomes individualized to the patient.

STANDARD IV. PLANNING
The gerontologic nurse develops a plan of care that prescribes interventions to attain expected outcomes.

STANDARD V. IMPLEMENTATION
The gerontologic nurse implements the interventions identified in the care plan.

STANDARD VI. EVALUATION
The gerontologic nurse evaluates the aging person's progress toward attainment of expected outcomes.

From American Nurses' Association (1995). *Scope and standards of gerontological nursing practice.* Washington, DC: Author.

(ANA, 1995c). The nurse generalist is perceived as the one who provides care primarily to older individuals and their families and who participates in the planning, implementation, and evaluation of care for older adults. The generalist draws on the expertise of the specialist and may assume some aspect of the specialist role if such a person is not present, but the generalist is urged to seek and use the expertise of a consultant when a specialist is not available.

The nurse specialist is prepared to perform all of the functions of the generalist, in addition to performing in those areas requiring special-ization—namely in those areas that require preparation in terms of extensive clinical experience with older individuals, their families, and groups of people; expertise in the formulation of health and social policy; and proficiency in planning, implementing, and evaluating health programs for older adults. Changes will be made in the ANA standards and in the ANA scope statements as the gerontologic nursing specialty indicates the need for revision. Professional nurses are urged to continue contributing ideas and data to the ongoing refinement and revision of these foundation blocks of the profession.

■ In the 1980s

THE ANA DEFINITION OF NURSING

For many years professional nurses focused on specifying the essence of nursing, pursuing questions such as the following: What is nursing? What makes nursing different from the other health care professions? Is there a profile, a plan, a pattern that can distinguish nursing from other caregiving services? These and other questions were posed in a variety of settings and with various groups of nurses, including nursing educators, practitioners, administrators, and researchers. These questions stimulated much discussion and debate regarding how to clearly define nursing. The challenge was to define the activities of the professional nurse so that nurses could agree with the definition of nursing and could accept an unambiguous statement of the defined practices of nursing. Such a definition would help colleagues in associated disciplines to understand and appreciate what nurses do that is specific to the nursing profession. In other words, it was necessary to define the essence of nursing in a way that was sufficiently narrow to distinguish it from other health care disciplines, yet sufficiently broad to encompass all the common elements of nursing practice in its various settings.

The American Nurses' Association, which is the professional organization of nursing in the United States, assumed leadership in defining a social policy statement that would articulate, strengthen, and maintain the social contract between nursing and society (ANA, 1980). The statement included the identification of the following:

- The social context of nursing
- The nature and scope of nursing practice
- Specialization in nursing, to differentiate levels of practice

Despite a variety of statements about nursing that had been proposed, one consistent theme had been identified in all statements: nurses are responsible for promoting the well-being of people and for caring for and nurturing the sick and the well. To maintain the historical orientation of nursing and to reflect the influence of nursing theory, the following definition of nursing was accepted: "nursing is the diagnosis and treatment of human responses to actual or potential health problems" (ANA, 1980, p. 9). This landmark document provided the profession of nursing with the first description of its social responsibility and defined for all to read what roles nursing played in the American health care system. Because society's health needs have changed since this definition was accepted, and because clinical nursing practice has changed since 1980, a task force was appointed in 1992 to update and revise the social policy statement. Hundreds of nurses contributed to the final statement that was published by the ANA near the end of 1995. Discussions in the published statement include the following:

- Definition of nursing
- Knowledge base for nursing practice
- Scope of nursing practice
- Regulation of nursing practice

In the statement that includes the definition of nursing, four areas are highlighted:

- Attention to the full range of human experiences and responses to health and illness without restriction to a problem-focused orientation
- Integration of objective data with knowledge gained from an understanding of the patient's or group's subjective experience
- Application of scientific knowledge to the processes of diagnosis and treatment
- Provision of a caring relationship that facilitates health and healing

This document is valuable to nurses in teaching, practice, research, or administration; each nurse should possess and study the policy statement to be intimately familiar with the ideas contained therein (ANA, 1995a).

TEACHING NURSING HOMES

During the 1980s various teaching nursing home models were planned, established, maintained, and evaluated. This came about because members of both the medical and the nursing professions were equally concerned about the predicted challenge to provide for the existing and future health care needs of the older age groups, especially older adults who generally seek the assistance of nursing homes. The fastest growing age group in America comprises the people 85 years old or older, and predictions suggest that their numbers may triple in the next 50 years. Although health clinicians and researchers certainly seek to prevent the disorders that disable older adults, they also realistically recognize that as acute illnesses are prevented and successfully treated and chronic diseases are more adequately controlled, longevity will increase, which will certainly lead to an increasing need for long-term care for older adults.

The quality of care in the nursing home has become a critical health care policy issue for several reasons: (1) the number of older adults has increased, (2) the number of nursing homes has increased, and (3) the total U.S. nursing home costs have grown rapidly. *Nursing home reform* was a catchphrase of the 1980s. In an effort to exercise regulatory control over the care of nursing home residents, the Omnibus Budget Reconciliation Act (OBRA) of 1987 (Public Law [PL] 100-203) was formulated and implemented in October 1990. From a nursing perspective, all reports suggest a greater shortage of nursing home nurses than of hospital nurses. There are a number of reasons for fewer professional nurses being employed in nursing homes:

1. Nurses who work in nursing homes often work in isolation.
2. Legislation in some states supports unrealistically low staffing patterns in the nursing home.
3. Many people do not understand or appreciate the role of the professional nurse in the nursing home.

4. Nursing home nurses often receive low salaries and unattractive fringe benefit packages.
5. Nurses are able to exercise only limited if any control over nursing practice. Professional autonomy is often nonexistent.

In an effort to address and improve the quality of patient care in the nursing home, a 5-year demonstration program, with nursing as the focus, was implemented in 1982 in which an affiliation was established between 11 schools of nursing and 12 nursing homes. Funding for the program was provided by the Robert Wood Johnson Foundation, with cosponsorship by the American Academy of Nurses (Mezey et al., 1985). Each of the program participants took part in determining the objectives of the joint endeavor. The nursing home and the nursing school had equal responsibility in identifying and achieving these objectives. Some objectives were more readily developed and achieved than others; however, efforts to achieve all of the objectives were stimulated and invigorated by the opportunity to participate in the creative project (Small & Walsh, 1988).

Evaluation of the program was reported by the University of Colorado Health Science Center, which identified a number of encouraging conclusions (Shaughnessy et al., 1990):

1. Active participation of nurse clinicians in patient care assessment and planning was a significant factor in the success of the program.
2. Involvement of nurses with advanced educational preparation was identified as a "catalyst" for positively influencing the behavior of the nursing staff, especially the nurse aides.
3. Quality assurance through education appears to be quite possible.
4. Reduced hospitalization can be realized through nursing home programs that are designed to maximize the physical and cognitive functioning of residents, to enhance incontinence care, and to regularly review the use of psychotropic drugs.

It was concluded by the evaluators that teaching nursing homes should be established in multiple sites, by using various means of funding and by defining specific objectives that would improve the quality of life for nursing home residents.

THE COMMUNITY COLLEGE–NURSING HOME PARTNERSHIP PROJECT

An ongoing project was initiated in 1987 to link six associate degree nursing programs with selected long-term care facilities. Funding for the project was provided by the W.K. Kellogg Foundation. Established goals were the following:

* To develop nursing potential in long-term care through in-service education
* To influence associate degree nursing education to include active preparation for nursing roles in the long-term care setting.

Creativity and diversity were hallmarks of the project. The positive outcomes of the project and the project's contributions to nursing education and to long-term care are being carefully described and tracked as the project continues (The Community College, 1990).

■ In the 1990s

Five nurse theorists met at the Biennial Nurse Theorist Conference in 1993, namely, Imogene King, Madeleine Leininger, Rosemarie Parse, Hildegarde Peplau, and Martha Rogers. They discussed the following:

* Caring as an essence of nursing
* The value of continuing to develop nursing theory
* What constitutes nursing research
* The role of advanced practice nurses

Although no conclusions were reached by this group, the stage was set for further collaboration and discussion among the scholars of nursing.

■ The World of Tomorrow

Prognostications for nursing and the direction in which it will go in the future are yet to be determined. However, based on the positive directions that have been observed to date, and based on the discussions among leaders in nursing, one can speculate about some exciting possibilities for the future of nursing in a variety of settings. In the future the settings for older adults will probably be creatively diverse.

Acute care facilities will still exist, and the level of illness of older adults in acute care settings will be more serious and critical. Nonetheless, the length of stay in hospitals will be further reduced. Increasingly, economics will dictate where older people can be cared for and for what period of time they may stay in one setting.

Nursing homes will still exist, and those older people who enter long-term care facilities will be much more frail than the current residents of such facilities. Economics will drive the existence of such facilities, as well as defining the services available in them.

Residing in one's own home will continue to be preferred by the older people in our society. With innovative and increased community services, this may more often be possible in the coming years. Support services that can be made available to older adults in their homes will expand, will increase the number and types of services, and will be open to innovative and creative ideas to help the older person. Present accessibility of grocery shopping via telephone, home delivery of food and pharmaceutical supplies, a wide variety and availability of homemaker services, and gerontologic nurse specialists who provide care in the community via clinics, home visits, and other convenient means will be commonplace among multiple delivery systems.

REFERENCES

American Nurses' Association. (1980). *Nursing: A social policy statement* (p. 32). Kansas City, MO: Author.

American Nurses' Association. (1995a). *Nursing's social policy statement* (p. 21). Washington, DC: Author.

American Nurses' Association. (1995b). *Professional certification: 1995 certification catalog.* Washington, DC: Author.

American Nurses' Association. (1995c). *Scope and standards of gerontological clinical nursing practice.* Washington, DC: Author.

Beckstrand, J. (1992). The notion of a practice theory and the relationship of scientific and ethical knowledge to practice. In L. H. Nicoll (Ed.), *Perspectives on nursing theory* (2nd ed., pp. 529-537). Philadelphia: Lippincott.

Benner, P., & Wrubel, J. (1989). *The primace of caring: Stress and coping in health and illness.* Menlo Park, CA: Addison-Wesley.

Cody, W. K., & Mitchell, G. J. (1992). Parse's theory as a model for practice: The cutting edge. *Advances in Nursing Science, 15* (2), 52-65.

Collins, R., & Felder, J. (1992). Beckstrand's concept of practice theory: A critique. In L. H. Nicoll (Ed.), *Perspectives on nursing theory* (2nd ed., pp. 556-561). Philadelphia: Lippincott.

The community college–nursing home partnership. (1990, Spring). *Newslink.* Fremont, CA: Ohlone College.

Fawcett, J. (1984). The metaparadigm of nursing: Present status and future refinements. *Image, 16* (3), 84-87.

Fitzpatrick, J. J., et al. (1989). Nursing diagnosis: Translating nursing diagnosis into ICD code. *American Journal of Nursing, 89* (4), 493-495.

Gordon, M. (1982). *Nursing diagnosis: Process and application.* New York: McGraw-Hill.

Gordon, M. (1994). *Nursing diagnosis: Process and application* (3rd ed.). New York: McGraw-Hill.

Holmes, C. A. (1990). Alternatives to natural science foundations for nursing. *International Journal of Nursing Studies, 27,* 187-198.

Johnson, J. (1991). Nursing science: Basic, applied or practical? *Advances in Nursing Science, 14* (1), 7-16.

Lewis, L., et al. (1967). *Defining clinical content, graduate nursing programs, medical-surgical nursing.* Boulder, CO: Western Interstate Commission for Higher Education.

McFarland, G. K., & McFarlane, E. A. (1996). *Nursing diagnosis and intervention—Planning for patient care.* St. Louis: Mosby.

Mezey, M. D., Lynaugh, J. E., & Aiken, L. H. (1985). The Robert Wood Johnson Foundation. In E. L. Schneider (Ed.), *The teaching nursing home.* New York: Raven Press.

Newman, M. A. (1979). *Theory development in nursing.* Philadelphia: F. A. Davis.

Newman, M. A. (1986). *Health as expanding consciousness.* St. Louis: Mosby.

Newman, M. A. (1990). Newman's theory of health as praxis. *Nursing Science Quarterly, 3,* 37-41.

Parse, R. R. (1981). *Man-living-health: A theory of nursing.* New York: John Wiley and Sons.

Parse, R. R. (1990). Health: A personal commitment. *Nursing Science Quarterly, 3*(3), 136-140.

Parse, R. R. (1992). Human becoming: Parse's theory of nursing. *Nursing Science Quarterly, 5*(1), 35-42.

Radsma, J. (1994). Caring and nursing: A dilemma. *Journal of Advanced Nursing, 20,* 444-449.

Shaughnessy, P. W., Kramer, A. M., & Hittle, D. F. (1990). *The teaching nursing home experiment: Its effects and implications.* Denver: University of Colorado Health Sciences Center.

Small, N. R., & Walsh, M. B. (Eds.). (1988). *Teaching nursing homes—The nursing perspective.* Owings Mills, MD: National Health Publishing.

Yura, H., & Walsh, M. B. (1967). *The nursing process—Assessing, planning, implementing, evaluating.* Washington, DC: The Catholic University of America Press.

Yura, H., & Walsh, M. B. (1983). *The nursing process—Assessing, planning, implementing, evaluating* (4th ed.). Norwalk, CT: Appleton-Century-Crofts.

BIBLIOGRAPHY

Gebbie, K. M., & Lavin, M. A. (Eds.). (1975). *Classification of nursing diagnoses: Proceedings of the first national conference on classification of nursing diagnoses.* St. Louis: Mosby.

Henderson, V. (1966). *The nature of nursing: A definition and its implications—Practice, research, and education.* New York: Macmillan.

Johnson, D. (1961, November). The significance of nursing care. *American Journal of Nursing, 61,* 63-66.

King, I. M. (1971). *Toward a theory for nursing.* New York: John Wiley and Sons.

Levine, M. (1969). *Introduction to clinical nursing.* Philadelphia: F. A. Davis.

Neuman, B. (1980). The Betty Neuman health care systems model: A total person approach to patient problems. In J. P. Riehl & C. Roy (Eds.), *Conceptual models for nursing practice* (2nd ed., pp. 119-134). New York: Appleton-Century-Crofts.

Nightingale, F. (1946). *Notes on nursing: What it is and what it is not* [Facsimile of 1859 edition]. Philadelphia: Lippincott. (Original work published 1859)

North American Nursing Diagnosis Association. (1990). *Taxonomy I revised, with official nursing diagnoses.* St. Louis: Author.

Orem, D. E. (1971). *Nursing: Concepts of practice.* New York: McGraw-Hill.

Orlando, I. J. (1961). *The dynamic nurse-patient relationship.* New York: Putnam.

Paterson, J. G., & Zderad, L. T. (1976). *Humanistic nursing.* New York: John Wiley and Sons.

Peplau, H. (1952). *Interpersonal relations in nursing.* New York: Putnam.

Rogers, M. E. (1970). *An introduction to the theoretical basis of nursing.* Philadelphia: Davis.

Roy, C. (1976). *Introduction to nursing: An adaptation model.* Englewood Cliffs, NJ: Prentice Hall.

Travelbee, J. (1971). *Interpersonal aspects of nursing* (2nd ed.). Philadelphia: Davis.

Watson, J. (1985). *Nursing, human science, and human care: A theory of nursing.* New York: National League for Nursing.

Wiedenbach, E. (1964). *Clinical nursing: A helping art.* New York: Springer.

Yura, H., & Walsh, M. B. (1988). *The nursing process—Assessing, planning, implementing, evaluating* (5th ed.). Norwalk, CT: Appleton and Lange.

C H A P T E R 3

*A theory is a cluster
of conclusions in
search of a premise.*

NR HANSON

Theories of Aging

■ Learning Objectives

On completion of this chapter, the reader will be able to do the following:

1. Identify what is known about the causes of aging.
2. Recognize that overlap and duplication exist among the aging theories that have been reported to date.
3. Discuss selected biologic and psychosocial theories about aging.
4. Understand that application of theories about aging can enhance the nursing care of older adults.

"Aging defies easy definition, at least in biological terms. Aging is not merely the passage of time. It is the manifestation of biological events that occur over a span of time. There is no perfect definition of aging but, as with love and beauty, most of us know it when we experience it or see it" (Hayflick, 1994).

Some scholars tend to identify one cause or offer one explanation for aging. It is reasonable to consider the possibility that "mortality among living things might have a universal cause" (Brookbank, 1990). However, among the many theories about aging that are being reported in the current literature, each has a number of advocates who offer convincing arguments and favorable evidence. Unfortunately, many of these apparently valid perspectives conflict, and each theory may be said to have dissenters and antago-

nists, as well as proponents and advocates. These disputing proponents and opponents are all armed with research data that appear to prove their contradictory points. These diverse arguments and appeals for one theory or another only serve to emphasize the fact that many people continue to search for answers to the following questions: What is aging? Why do humans age? What causes aging? What factors influence aging? Can a change in these factors alter or change the aging process?

Humans have long shown great curiosity and limitless zeal in seeking profound answers about the nature of life and death; this striving continues to intensify as humans experience ever-increasing longevity. Several questions then arise: What is the alternative to growing old? Is there an alternative to dying? What is the price of increased longevity? What are investigators from various disciplines finding out about the aging process? How much interdisciplinary communication about aging is being conveyed among the various scientists? For example, are sociologists and biologists talking with each other, to maximize collaboration and minimize competition and duplication of effort?

Some gerontologists are exploring the quality of human life in later years: What defines *quality of life?* Can or should it be better than it is now? In what way? How can this be achieved? Though this term is widely used, those who use it quite freely are seldom challenged to define its meaning. If longevity is extended, will there be a meaningful place in society for those people who benefit from such extension? "There must be work, pleasure, medical care, and a role to play for life to be worth" the extension that is realized (Brookbank, 1990).

The identification of theories about aging and the explanation of the underlying causes of aging will be very important to scientists as they continue to accumulate knowledge about aging. The justification for using theory is that it provides anchors for thinking and guidelines for examining data. The development of theory will assist in the integration of what is already known about aging and will help to point out directions for future research in this field (Birren & Bengtson, 1988).

As the work goes forward in this area of growing interest and potential, there will be increased literature available to report the findings and work of the scholars and scientists in various disciplines. The report prepared by Birren and Bengtson (1988) was the result of their wish to address the "data-rich but theory-poor" state of research on aging and to encourage an interchange of communication among the various disciplines that study and work with the aging. According to these two experts, there is so much activity being initiated and carried out in this area of study that small "islands of knowledge" (Birren & Bengtson, 1988) have been created, and there is little communication among them.

A consequence of this interdisciplinary isolation is that most aging theories are described and labeled uniquely by individual scientists and scholars; few studies use identical labeling to describe similar phenomena across the various studies. Though the broad areas of biologic, psychologic, social, or psychosocial theories may use some consistent labels, the subclassifications of theories within these disciplines are often labeled quite differently. Interested readers may seek more detail regarding the theories presented in this chapter by using various references and seeking other resources as published materials become increasingly available. This chapter provides an overview of a selected few of the major theories that are most frequently found in the literature. Specific authors are identified as each theory is mentioned, to enable the student to associate a specific author's name with a specific theory. It is hoped that this will facilitate further exploration of any one or several of the theorists and/or theories.

While the reader is studying the theories of aging, it will become obvious that these are not discrete ideas; there is a great deal of overlap and relationship among the ideas. As with many areas of human functioning, interdependence among data may sometimes offer comfort, but it may also seem baffling. The challenge is to explore and investigate all avenues in order to clarify the ideas that are being promoted about aging.

Biogerontology has assumed an important role among scientists in recent years, and it is now recognized as a respected science. Understanding of the aging phenomenon has advanced a great deal. The scientific study of the biology of aging has created greater interest among scholars and researchers than ever before. The student of aging recognizes that gerontology is the scientific study of the aging process, whereas geriatrics is concerned with the medical problems of older adults (Hayflick, 1994).

The focus of gerontology experts is on determining answers about the normal aging process rather than the diseases of old age. There has been a concerted effort during these recent years to address the changes that occur in every human cell as a person ages; hence, the emergence of biogerontology. This is a science with a vast subject area for those who are courageous enough to explore it (Hayflick, 1994).

Biogerontologists generally agree that there is enough observational data available about aging to test a number of theories about aging. Theories that are presently accepted are continuously changing as new research reports become available. The recent increase in theories about the causes of age changes can cause confusion about the validity of the multiple theories.

Strehler (1977) suggested a group of criteria that must be met before any theory is accepted. According to Strehler, the theory must explain why

1. The losses in physiologic function occur (deleterious)
2. The losses are gradual (progressive)
3. The losses cannot be corrected (intrinsic)
4. The losses occur in all members of a species (universal)

Application of these criteria allows a more precise definition of biologic aging, setting aside, for example, the effect of disease on the human cell (Strehler, 1977).

The major challenge for nurses is to determine just what areas of knowledge are important for providing the best care for older adults. The more nurses understand about the process of aging, the better they will be able to meet the needs of older people. This knowledge provides a better basis for decision making about measures to control and cope with the major problems of aging, such as incontinence, cognitive impairment, susceptibility to infection, lack of or difficulty with mobility, loneliness, changes in human needs, and a host of other difficulties that continue to grow in number and complexity as people age.

■ Psychosociologic Theories

Psychologic aging is characterized primarily by behavioral changes. Closely associated with the psychologic and biologic sciences are the sociologic changes that relate to the environmental influences that contribute to and affect aging people.

As research about aging increases, "there appears to be an openness to accept contributions from . . . adjacent sciences," as well as pressure to establish a theoretic structural framework for reporting the results of scientific study (Birren & Birren, 1990, p. 14). Each of the three disciplines (psychology, sociology, and biology) is increasingly aware of the need for research to explain the aging process, and a multidisciplinary approach is being strongly advocated.

Potential for the growth of knowledge within each discipline is phenomenal. Witness the growth in the psychologic gerontologic literature alone. Until 1945, only about 500 publications could be found in this area. In each 10-year period since 1945 the literature has doubled. The reports about research and aging in each discipline have continued to increase exponentially. Similar pronouncements can be made about the biologic and sociologic literature, which indicates the potential significance and value of the literature in guiding the study of gerontology.

Explanation for psychosocial (i.e., psychosociologic) aging are complex. Psychologists and sociologists show a marked desire to arrive at a single cause or explanation for aging. As the population of older adults increases, the complexity of this issue also grows. Each older person is an individual, and each life experience and each change in a person's environment has an effect on that person. Explaining these events and experiences, tracing the origin of each change, and describing the resulting influences on the person leads the scholar down a very convoluted trail. By isolating one experience at a time and discretely analyzing the data related to

---

BOX 3-1 PSYCHOSOCIOLOGIC THEORIES OF AGING

- Disengagement theory
- Activity theory
- Life-course theories
- Continuity theory

---

the particular experience across a variety of individuals, one can reach logical conclusions about the experience. If this process is implemented for a variety of experiences, the various conclusions about each experience can be clustered and arranged in some order that will allow inspection and application to future groups of people.

A few psychosocial theories, listed in Box 3-1, are presented in the following pages. Experts are also discussing many other valid and intriguing theories. Readers are advised to consider the theories presented here to be only a sampling among the many that will be developed in the future. Readers should critically analyze each of the theories they encounter, whether presented here or elsewhere. The developments in the theories of aging are emerging so rapidly that while new reports are being written, still-newer information is being discovered. The diligent and conscientious reader is challenged to maintain an open and inquiring mind while carefully monitoring the exciting emergence of information in this rapidly developing field.

PSYCHOSOCIAL PERSPECTIVES ON AGING

Aging is defined as the transformation of the human organism after the age of physical maturity so that the probability of survival constantly decreases, and it is accompanied by regular transformations in appearance, behavior, experience, and social roles (Birren, 1988). The underlying assumption on which all scholars of aging theory operate is that whatever is observed or described will change in some way, given time, experience, and exposure to the environment. Growth, development, and aging are characterized by change; stagnation is not a characteristic of life.

Psychosocial aging can be described as a result of the disuse of previously acquired skills; a consequence of random wear and tear; a change in adaptive capacity because of environmental variables; a loss of various internal and external resources; a result of genetic influences over the life span, which cause changes in an individual's psychosocial characteristics; and/or a consequence of the choices made by an individual and the creation of new solutions that have never been used before.

Social scientists generally agree that genetics—that is, heredity—is a major factor in determining the length of human life, although environment plays an important role in modifying the expected life span. Within the limits of heredity and despite the environmental factors that influence life, scientists recognize that genetically controlled characteristics interact with the biologic characteristics of individuals and their knowledge and attitudes about life; the resulting characteristics become known as "culture." Culture can be considered the "DNA of society"—that is, the collection of roles, beliefs, and behaviors that are handed down from one generation to another (Birren, 1988).

The psychosocial literature of gerontology contains many closely related yet different views of aging. These various perspectives agree that as people grow older, their behavior changes, their social interactions change, and the activities in which they engage change. At this point, the common views diverge into a great variety of theories, two of which focus on either the individual's social interactions (disengagement theory) or the individual's activities (activity theory—originally called implicit theory).

DISENGAGEMENT THEORY

Cumming and Henry (1961), of the University of Chicago, reported the empiric study that prompted their development of disengagement theory and activity theory. These two scholars investigated various aspects of the aging process and reported the results of their work in publications that others have relied on for more than the past 35 years. Data were gathered by observing and interviewing a sample of older people to "construct inductively a theory of aging" (Cumming & Henry, 1961). Cumming and Henry acknowledged the work of colleagues who had identified and described "outcomes of the aging process," or the end point of the aging process. However, their colleagues had not identified the actual *process* of aging. Unanswered questions were, How did the older person reach the end point? What stages were experienced by the individual in reaching the end point? Stimulated by the desire to describe what happens between adulthood and old age, these researchers observed a panel of aging people over a period of time to identify what occurs to healthy, economically stable Americans as they experience the process of aging. Based on the resulting data, they enunciated two theories of aging. Talcott Parsons presciently predicted, in the foreword to the report of their findings, that this study would serve as a focus of discussion for some time to come, and indeed it has proven to be just that.

As a result of this investigation, the disengagement theory of aging was developed. This was perceived as a commonsense theory. *Disengagement* was viewed as "an inevitable process in which many of the relationships between a person and other members of society are severed, and those remaining are altered in quality" (Cumming & Henry, 1961, p. 14). The process may be initiated by aging people themselves, or it may be initiated by others in society. When the withdrawal takes place, it may be partial or total; that is, the aging people need not withdraw from everyone around them. They might selectively withdraw from some groups of people and not from others.

The research plan was based on a social-psychologic theory, and it was suggested that the theory was a bridge between personality theory and social theory. A wide variety of hereditary and environmental factors were known to influence human behavior, and all of these factors were to be considered when studying human behavior. Cumming and Henry went on to acknowledge that development follows a pattern in which each phase of development is influenced by the phase that has preceded it. For example, older people are influenced by the experiences they have had in adulthood, which in turn have been influenced by experiences during adolescence and, still earlier, by occurrences in childhood. The major emphasis of the researchers, however, was on the experiences of old age and adulthood, with little attention given to childhood experiences. Given these assumptions, the goal of the study was to develop a theory of aging through the use of the *inductive process* (i.e., the process of deriving general ideas from a lot of specific information).

It was observed that older people are less involved with life than they were as younger adults. This is a statement of fact; no value judgments were made regarding whether older people should or should not behave in this way. It was noted that during middle age, adults usually establish an equilibrium between themselves and society; as they age, this state of equilibrium is altered and a new equilibrium is established, in which the older people experience a greater distance from society, and they develop a new kind of relationship with society. In America there is evidence that society forces withdrawal on the older people whether or not they wish it.

Although this theory has had staunch supporters over the years, it has also had strong opponents. Some suggest that this theory does not consider the large number of older people who do not withdraw from society. The rebuttal to this criticism is that the theory still holds and that those older people who do keep in touch with society are "unsuccessful adjusters to old age," or "off time" disengagers, or members of a "biological or psychological elite." Although disengagement theory has been roundly criticized and its limitations are acknowledged, even those who argue against it admit that it has stimulated important discussion and investigation and has had a lasting effect on theory development in social gerontology. It is recognized as the first formal theory that attempted to explain the process of growing older.

ACTIVITY THEORY

Disengagement theory is not the only common-sense theory that describes the psychosocial aging process. The implicit theory of aging, more recently called the activity theory of aging, looks at and considers the phenomenon of aging quite differently than does disengagement theory. Missing from the literature and from research reports were data that could provide a basis for an *explicit* theory of aging. Many assumptions about aging gave credence to an implicit theory of the aging process. The following were among the assumptions that supported the implicit theory:

- There is an abrupt beginning of old age after a specified period of time in middle age.
- The process of aging leaves the older person alone or cut off from the usual acquaintances and friends.
- People should be encouraged to remain active and to develop friendships with other people in their own age group.
- Standards and expectations of middle-aged people should be projected onto the behavior of the older person. Being successful in the aging process depends on being like a middle-aged person as much as possible.
- The aging person should be encouraged to expand and to be involved, because the more active older adult is more satisfied with life.

Activity theory emphasizes the importance of ongoing social activity; as a result of this activity, older adults develop a positive concept of self. Those who adhere to this theory suggest that a person's self-concept is related to the roles held by that person; for example, retiring from an occupational role may not be so harmful to self-concept if the person actively maintains other roles, such as familial roles, recreational roles, and volunteer and community roles. As one ages, it is expected that roles will change, but to maintain a positive sense of self, the activity theory assumes that one must substitute new roles for those roles that are lost because of age; hence well-being in later life depends on activity in newly acquired roles.

A basic assumption that underlies activity theory is that social activity, in and of itself, is beneficial for older adults and that it contributes to the achievement of life satisfaction for older adults. Also, it is assumed that older adults need and desire high levels of social activity and that older adults interpret different types of activity in exactly the same way that younger people do. Studies have reported that the relationship between activity and well-being among older adults depends on the type of activity in which they are engaged. A further component of this theory considers the preferences of the older people and their choices regarding the extent to which they wish to be active; setting aside time for quiet reflection may be as important as more active pursuits for some older people.

LIFE-COURSE THEORIES

Various scholars have placed marked emphasis on the developmental features of aging. The life span theories of the 1950s and 1960s made valuable contributions to the psychosocial literature. Their views about human development from infancy through adulthood have been a stimulus to further inquiry.

E.H. Erikson (1963) approached maturity as a process. He perceived each person as developing as a biologic organism and a social being. To illustrate this development, he defined eight distinct stages and proposed that each person progresses through these stages, from birth through maturity. Within each stage, he identified features of complete development and of incomplete development. This model cites crises that involve dilemmas that confront people as they develop. Erikson contends that each crisis can be resolved by moving forward to another stage of development or by remaining fixed at a level of incomplete development. Those who disagree with Erikson's theory acknowledge that there may be some substance to his ideas, especially regarding the early and middle years of life. However, it is felt that the model neither incorporates nor adequately defines the maturity of old age. Though the model does provide some sound ideas on which study of maturity and development can be based, the theory does not adequately address the dilemmas and crises through which older adults proceed.

Havighurst (1972) also suggested some development-related ideas and suggested that if older people (age 60 and older) are to experience satisfaction in later life, they should successfully complete the following tasks:

1. Adjustment to declining health and decreasing physical strength
2. Adjustment to the life of retirement, as well as to reduced income
3. Adjustment to the death of a spouse, of family members, and of significant others
4. Adjustment to living arrangements that differ from those to which they have been accustomed
5. Adjustment to the pleasures that accompany aging, such as increased leisure time and playing with grandchildren

In the more recent past (the 1970s and 1980s), scholars have addressed the life-course perspective, which is a conceptual development within social and behavioral analysis of aging (Passuth & Bengtson, 1988). This perspective is perceived as a "conceptual framework for conducting research and interpreting data" rather than as an exact theory. Key elements of this framework are the following assumptions:

- Aging occurs from birth to death.
- Aging involves biologic, psychologic, and sociologic processes.
- Experiences during aging are shaped by historical factors.

Some who share this perspective express concern that loosely using the term *life course* in social gerontology may dilute and reduce the significance of the life-course perspective.

CONTINUITY THEORY

The central premise of continuity theory is that older adults try to preserve and maintain internal and external structures by using strategies that maintain continuity; that is, the older people may seek to use familiar strategies in familiar arenas of life. Continuity is a subjective perception, and each person must uniquely adjust to changes by forming personal links to tie the new experiences to the person's previous experiences in life (Cohler, 1982). Continuity is very much *person oriented*—that is, oriented to the individual person. Only the older person can assess the here and now because the basis for assessing is the result of the person's retrospection—the recollection of the person's remembered past. In later life, adults tend to use continuity as an adaptive strategy to deal with changes that occur during normal aging. Continuity theory has excellent potential for explaining how people adapt to their own aging. It is supported by individual preference and social approval (Atchley, 1989).

A fundamental assumption of this theory is that evolution occurs as people age and that change can be integrated into a person's historical context without causing major upheaval or disequilibrium. Change comes about as a result of the aging person's reflecting upon past experience and setting goals for the future. The aging people exercise choice over their experiences and recognize that some of the changes are occurring because of normal aging, which they may not have chosen for themselves.

Atchley (1989) defines *continuity* as "coherence or consistency of patterns over time." He refers to this as a dynamic concept of continuity and applies it to the issue of adaptation to normal aging. Change is ever present and may be perceived as such against the backdrop of the person's past, especially the person's perceived past. Thus continuity may be a general cognitive construct within which many specific changes can occur.

Continuity may be viewed more readily over a long life span than over a short one. Thus the changes that occur in human development in later life appear to be more subtle than the changes that occur earlier (Fry, 1992).

■ Biologic Theories

Theories of cellular aging have been classified as genetic and nongenetic by Brookbank (1990), with the suggestion that genetic theories seem to be the most promising in terms of arriving at answers through research. Genetic theories include those involving deoxyribonucleic acid (DNA), error and fidelity, somatic mutation, and glycation. Nongenetic theories include those involving "wear and tear," nutrient deprivation, and aging pigment accumulation, as shown in Box 3-2.

GENETIC THEORIES
Theories of molecular aging

Error and fidelity theory The error theory of aging has been extensively studied, yet it is difficult to determine exactly where an identified error might have occurred in the molecular development of the cell. The error may have occurred at the level of DNA or at the level of transcription, translation, or posttranslation. *Fidelity* is defined as the faithful reproduction of the correct proteins from the point of gene transcription and translation of the messenger ribonucleic acid (RNA) into the proteins that become components of cellular structure. As the

BOX 3-2 GENETIC AND NONGENETIC THEORIES OF AGING

Genetic theories
  Theories of molecular aging
    Error and fidelity
    Somatic mutation
    Glycation
  Theories of cellular aging
    Programmed cellular aging
    Aging pacemaker
  Theories of the organ system
    Autoimmunity
    Neuroendocrine control
Nongenetic theories
  Effects of temperature
  Nutrient deprivation
  Lipofuscin

fidelity of transcription or translation is decreased, an error occurs that results in the insertion of improper amino acids into the sequence of a particular protein. As a result of the identification of these data in scientific experiments, further studies were done to determine the relationship of this information to aging. Despite the demonstrated existence of altered proteins in aging cells, there is little evidence to support the theory of error and fidelity as a cause of aging (Brookbank, 1990).

According to Cristofalo (1988), the theory of error is an example of a *stochastic theory*—that is, a theory describing random events that occur in the organism or in the environment that may have a cumulative and predictable effect. The core of this theory recognizes that the normal process of faithfully replicating that is carried out by normal molecules of protein occasionally—at random—goes awry. The error occurs when an incorrectly replicated or synthesized protein is faithfully (fidelity) replicated over and over, which produces numerous faulty molecules in the genetic apparatus. Over a lifetime these random changes lead to a continually increasing production of erroneous protein molecules, which eventually leads to an "error catastrophe" that causes the death of the person.

Somatic mutation theory A very similar example of a stochastic theory is the somatic mutation theory. *Mutations* are those inheritable changes that occur in the cellular DNA. If there is extensive damage to DNA and it is not repaired, then there will probably be an alteration in a genetic sequence. The suggestion is that random genetic mutations caused by background radiation of various types, as well as other factors, gradually produce failure in various body systems that eventually causes death (Cristofalo, 1988). The frequency of spontaneous somatic mutation is low, and the possibility of linking the aging process to these genetic changes is not very likely. Although x-rays do increase the rate of mutation, the lesions of aging and of radiation damage differ. Radiation primarily affects the cells of the skin, of the intestinal lining, and of the bone marrow. Age effects, however, are noted primarily on the nerve and muscle cells. Scientists advise that much more research and study will be necessary before a direct link can be established between radiation-related or other mutations and aging (Brookbank, 1990).

Glycation theory Glycation theory suggests that glucose acts as a mediator of aging. *Glycation* is the nonenzymic reaction between glucose and tissue protein. Cellular studies of the effect of glycation suggest that glycated proteins show less enzyme activity, less degradation of abnormal proteins, and inappropriate *cross-linking* (i.e., they do not form appropriately parallel connections with other proteins). A number of studies conclude that glycation may have a profound cumulative effect during a person's life. The negative effects of this process on proteins may be a major contributor to age changes. In addition, the effects of this process appear to parallel the elevated glucose levels and shorter life span of diabetic patients (Masoro, et

al., 1989). However, no definitive relationship between diabetes and aging has been shown, and it has not been clearly determined that glycation effects either cause aging or are caused by aging-related changes that occur in other body processes (Brookbank, 1990).

Theories of cellular aging

Programmed cellular aging theory The theory of programmed cellular aging, sometimes termed *program restriction,* suggests that aging may be the result of an impairment of the cell in translating necessary RNAs as a result of increased turnoffs of DNA. Some scientists speculate that though the essential messages may be transcribed at all ages, the translation of these messages into functional proteins may be restricted in older people. They suggest that the cell may stop exchanging genetic information, and without genetic guidance, the cell may undergo senescence.

The significance of this theory is being debated. It has been established that either some segments of DNA become depleted with advancing age, or selected cellular structures seem to change with age so that DNA transcription is restricted. However, if aging were attributable to this alteration in the program of cellular development, a more regular and more predictable sequence of organ system failures might be expected than occurs at present (Brookbank, 1990).

Aging pacemaker theory The aging pacemaker theory proposes that one cell, or one type of tissue, interferes with cell proliferation, thereby initiating the process of senescence throughout the body. Some authors have attempted to explain this process by studying the thymus as the pacemaker, or "biologic clock," that is responsible for activating and maintaining this aging activity in humans. This theory has not been definitively and universally accepted.

Conclusion Cellular aging remains a fascinating area of study. Though various authorities agree that cells have finite limits of reproduction, they continue to debate exactly what these limits are. Some doubt that the finite limit is ever reached by cells living in the body. The body cells lose their functional abilities well before they lose their ability to reproduce; hence signs of aging cannot be attributed to cell death alone.

Theories of the organ system

Autoimmune theory Many of the health problems that older people encounter can be explained by some degree of immune system dysfunction, including diseases such as cancer, mature-onset diabetes, senile dementia, and some vascular diseases. The immune system is closely linked to the neuroendocrine system, and each body system can react to changes in the other systems. It is also known that the immune system is less able to deal with foreign organisms as the body ages, and the immune system also increasingly makes mistakes by erroneously identifying autologous tissues as being foreign. The altered ability of the body to deal with alien organisms and the increase in identification errors by the immune system increase the susceptibility to disease and to abnormalities that result from autoimmune responses (Brookbank, 1990); many known causes of death relate to these problems of the immune system.

Neuroendocrine control theory The neurologic and endocrine systems are major controllers of body activity. The loss of cells from both of these systems is documented by scientists who study the brain. During the human life span there is a 10% decrease in the weight of the brain, which is accounted for by both a loss of cells and a loss of fluids in the cerebrum. Some investigators suggest that the documented age-related changes in response to hormones may be the result of changes in the receptors for hormones rather than changes in the activity of the endocrines themselves.

Conclusion General acceptance of the neuroendocrine control theory is just as elusive as is general acceptance of the autoimmune theory. As with many scientifically correlated events, it is difficult to know which one may be causing the other or whether still other factors may be causing both events. Thus the changes in the body that are ascribed to the processes described by either of these theories may simply reflect what is happening to the systems of the body as a result of the aging process (Brookbank, 1990).

NONGENETIC THEORIES
Effects-of-temperature theory

The life span of warm-blooded species is inversely proportional to their metabolic rate; observations confirm that mammals with high metabolic rates tend to be the smaller, shorter-lived species. However, this cannot explain why members of the same species die at different ages despite a similar metabolic rate. Aging among those species with a higher metabolic rate is usually explained in terms of the cells wearing out; the rationale for this is that chemical reactions in living systems are slower at lower temperatures and are accelerated at higher temperatures. Humans might live at a much slower pace if their body temperatures were just 5 degrees lower than the usual 98.6 degrees Fahrenheit. If such a reduction were attained, humans could expect to live about 20% longer than they live at present (Brookbank, 1990).

Nutrient deprivation theory

Nutrient deprivation is another perplexing correlational theory: thus far, scientists do not know whether deprivation of cellular nutrients causes aging or is caused by aging, or even whether both may be caused by some other factor. Some theorists propose that oxygen deprivation leads to senescence of deprived cells, but the pattern of such deprivation does not approximate that of normal aging, in which cells randomly disappear from tissues (Brookbank, 1990).

Lipofuscin theory

As people age, pigment accumulates, and this accumulation becomes apparent in the skin of older people. These "age spots" have been referred to as "biochemical debris" by biochemists, and it is theorized that these waste products of the metabolic processes of the cells accumulate until they reach a critical point, when they begin to interfere with cellular functioning. This is referred to by some people as the "wear and tear" theory. However, there has been no demonstrable association between the existence of these age spots and alterations in cellular function. Scientists have concluded that this pigmentation is a result of aging rather than a cause of it (Brookbank, 1990).

CURRENT THINKING AND OLD IDEAS

In the present situation of defining theories of aging, most biogerontologists believe that several mechanisms are operating simultaneously to cause aging; there probably is not one single cause of aging, but many causes. Until there is definitive data about the causes of aging, a number of ideas and efforts will be studied, read, and reported. Those presented by Brookbank are stimulating and give cause for thought and study. In the following section, equally valid ideas are presented from the studies and work done by Hayflick.

According to Hayflick (1994), current thinking about aging is influenced by some old ideas. Three of these ideas are the following:

1. The "vital substance" theory
2. The genetic mutation theory
3. The reproductive exhaustion theory

Vital substance theory

Each person is born with a specific amount of some vital substance. Aging occurs as this vital substance is consumed, or exhausted, and the person dies. Variations in individual life expectations are the result of differences in the amount of vital substance that each person has at birth. To date, there has been no evidence to support this theory.

Genetic mutation theory

Mutations are changes that occur in genes, and several kinds of changes are known to occur.

Some are harmful and some are beneficial. Because of their essential role in the diversity of life and the adaptation of animals to their environment, mutations are serious contenders for the locus of aging and longevity phenomena. Although this idea has been intriguing to scientists, there is no experimental evidence to support it as a sound theory.

Reproductive exhaustion theory

The reproductive exhaustion theory has few followers. The central idea in this theory is that there is an initial burst of reproductive activity, then a period of rapid aging followed by death. It was concluded that this does not meet the criteria for being an acceptable theory.

■ Theories Presuming a Preexisting Master Plan

Theories of aging that are worthy of consideration at present can be classified into two broad groups: those that presume a preexisting master plan and those that are based on random events.

The chief theory in the first group suggests the presence of a *biologic clock* governed by a series of chemical events. Especially significant in this idea is the secretion of hormones by the hypothalamus or the pituitary gland in the brain.

Biologists generally accept the phenomenon of *programmed cell death*. Hayflick, however, questions the relationship of massive cell death to aging. The complex molecular changes that precede cell death might cause age changes and eventual death of the person long before the cells die. The current beliefs about programmed aging make it an unpopular theory today.

The release of hormones into the human blood creates many kinds of activity in the body. Hormones can accelerate some aging processes and can slow down other processes. Modern gerontologic endocrinologists are especially concerned with hormones as possible causes of age changes rather than looking to the hormones as a means of rejuvenation. The role of the *neuroendocrine system* is significant in reproduction and in the presence and function of biologic clocks. However, despite various research efforts to define the relationship of the endocrines to aging, conclusions can only point to the fact that the neuroendocrine system has an effect on our bodies—there is no conclusive evidence that it is the origin of age changes.

Biogerontologists cannot agree about whether or not we lose nerve cells as we age. They do agree that profound changes occur in the brain as humans age, but the effect of these changes on the life of other cells in the body is not clear. At one time it was thought that the brain produced a "death hormone," allegedly made by the pituitary. The studies have not been confirmed, and researchers are not pursuing this area of research at present. Despite the tendency to rely on the neuroendocrine theory to account for age-associated deficits, there seems to be no more compelling reason to "blame" the neuroendocrine system for age changes than to select any other body system as being responsible for these changes.

■ Theories Based on Random Events

The *wear and tear theory* has been on record for many years. The idea that supports this theory is that a body tissue, as it becomes worn from use, cannot continuously renew itself. It is generally agreed that normal cells cannot divide or function forever, but this admission does not explain *why* age changes occur. In fact, this recognition may have nothing at all to do with aging causes. Although biogerontologists may be admired for their ingenuity in developing such a theory, it will not be possible to test this theory scientifically until some type of experiment is devised to determine whether the wear and tear on body parts can account for aging.

The *rate-of-living theory* is based on the premise that animals and humans are born with a limited amount of potential or physiologic capacity that is expended at various rates. Rapid expenditure of energy precipitates early aging; slow expenditure results in slower aging. This is often referred to as the "live fast, die young" theory. Life in the fast lane is also referred to as "burning the candle at both ends"; maintaining a slower lifestyle is referred to as "being laid back." Proponents of the rate-of-living theory, and of the wear and tear theory, would assume that one who lives a laid-back life will age more slowly and will live longer. Appealing as this may sound to some, there has not been any scientific evidence generated to support this idea.

The *waste product accumulation theory* suggests that a kind of cellular constipation results if cells accumulate more waste than can be disposed of efficiently. Over time, such cells will accumulate toxins that could hamper normal cell function and the cell will slowly die. Among some scientists this is called the lipofuscin theory. The most evident sign of this process is the brownish pigment that becomes apparent in the skin of people as they age. One writer calls these age pigments "the ashes of our dwindling metabolic fires." However, this theory does not meet the criterion of universality, and there is no proven evidence that the presence of age pigmentation interferes with cell functioning. Some merchants promote the use of centrophenoxine, which in laboratory animals seems to reduce the pipovuscin content of cells. When studied in humans, the drug does reduce blood sugar levels and increase oxygen consumption; however, there is no sound evidence that this pigmentation—or the centrophenoxine—plays any role in aging.

The *cross-linking theory* of aging contends that, with age, some body proteins become cross-linked and may impede metabolic processes. Advocates of this theory contend that as errors accumulate in various molecules, age changes can occur. Belief that cross-linking of molecules in the human body causes age changes is not based on experimental evidence. Even if cross-linking of the human collagen molecules does occur, there is no good evidence that it actually interferes with the metabolic processes. Perhaps this is only one of the many biochemical changes that occur over time and contribute to aspects of aging. More systematic study is needed to arrive at conclusive evidence about the significance of this phenomenon.

■ Conclusion

There are other theories about aging, and there is a great deal of speculation about what may cause this reality of life. None of the theories that have been proposed can claim sufficient evidence to account for the aging effects that are witnessed and experienced in humans. Any one of the proposals can be pursued and studied with great interest and enthusiasm. The basic truth about the explanation of the cause or causes of aging is this: we do not know why we age. Some biogerontologists believe that aging has many causes that probably include aspects of all of the extant theories. Other scientists adhere to one or a few theories and discount all the other proposals. Because gerontology is such a young science, there is not sufficient knowledge to explain why aging occurs. For the first time in the history of biology, however, there is hope that available knowledge will be made known soon because of the increase in the number of dedicated scientists who are working in the field of aging. Hayflick suggests that our thinking about aging can be reordered by rearranging the format of the question we ask; in other words, instead of asking, Why do we age? the question should be, Why do we live as long as we do? By reformulating the question, we may conclude that the body has changed over a period of time as evidenced by the fact that longevity has increased and by the possibility that the aging process has slowed. The studies of biogerontology could prove to be very exciting and revealing in the future.

The theories of aging presented in the preceding pages share one common denominator, or central theme: change. As molecules, cells, and organ systems continue to live, they change. An interesting observation about change: When considered at the beginning of life, change is referred to and talked about as *development.* Later in life, when change is considered, it is referred to as *aging.* This idea offers an interesting basis for discussion.

The following summarizes several characteristics of the complex process of aging (Cristofalo, 1988):

- There is increased mortality with increasing age.
- Changes in the chemical composition of the body occur during the aging process.
- A broad spectrum of progressive deteriorative changes occurs with aging.
- The reduced ability of the older person to adapt to environmental change is probably a major factor in aging.
- People who are aging are increasingly vulnerable to disease.

Examination of and reflection on the theories of aging are stimulating and intellectually invigorating experiences. Witness the ever-increasing research and number of publications in the biologic, psychologic, and sociologic specialties of gerontology; with these before them, scholars cannot help but wax enthusiastic and feel very positive about the future of gerontologic knowledge. On the other hand, several improvements are sorely needed:

- Experts must communicate more, building on the strengths of existing interdisciplinary collaboration and communication.
- Researchers must develop and use a more uniform, shared language, both within each discipline and across the disciplines, to enhance communication.
- Nurses must intensively analyze existing theories to develop more specific ideas and to reduce the complexity and overlap among the defined theories.
- Nurses must maintain, and increase, the emphasis on the quality of life of older adults.
- Society must develop a positive view of older adults and their potential for contributing to

society, yet at the same time, realistically recognize when their strengths may be temporarily reduced.

- Nurses must incorporate the concept of the individuality of each older person, respecting the uniqueness of the individual whose life holds valuable experiences and recollections that should be utilized.
- Nurses must recognize the physical, psychologic, and social losses experienced by all older people.
- Society must change or eliminate the existing stereotypes about older adults.

As studies about older adults continue, it is encouraging to note that there is room for many ideas and a multitude of systematic studies.

Specialists in aging predict an "endless agenda for empirical research on the social aspects of aging" (Streib & Binstock, 1990). They advocate the development of theories and models so that acquired knowledge and discoveries about aging can be organized in such a way that the interested scholars can build on data already identified (Birren & Bengtson, 1988).

The task of defining theories of aging is complex. Biology uses genetics and evolution (commonly termed *nature*) as concepts for organizing data, whereas the social sciences use concepts of culture, social structure, and socialization (commonly termed *nurture*). Each human being is a product of both domains; hence the theories that can be called "psychologic theories" will have dimensions of genetics (nature), as well as social dimensions (nurture). To develop a theory in the behavioral sciences, multiple factors must be considered, and each must be specified carefully as the theorist struggles to meet the challenge of defining the process of aging.

During the 1950s, 1960s, and 1970s older adults in the developed nations were examined and studied as a disadvantaged group with low socioeconomic status, as compared to younger people in society (Streib & Binstock, 1990). This stereotype of older people changed in the 1980s, probably because of society's awareness of their increased numbers and the fear of their becoming an economic burden; indeed, the stereotype became the reverse as U.S. society came to believe that all older adults were "prosperous, hedonistic and selfish" (Streib & Binstock, 1990). As a result of the change in society's view of older adults, which showed a fear of the influence that older adults will wield on the nation's economy, groups of advocates for the aging have been established. It is predicted this trend will continue throughout the remaining years of the twentieth century. These issues will probably be studied by analyzing the socioeconomic status of older adults, as well as by further developing the proposed theories about aging.

There is general agreement among the gerontologic scientists that the research efforts of many scholars will be needed to adequately explore the various theories of aging. It will take a great deal of time to explore, refine, and elaborate upon the many ideas that are being proposed as explanations of the aging process. It will be important for many to participate, especially those who work with older adults in community settings, in long-term care facilities, and in acute care settings. There are rich sources of data available to the gerontologic researcher; the availability of many hands to assist in the data collection and analysis will surely be appreciated by all older adults of today and tomorrow, as well as by their families and caregivers.

REFERENCES

Atchley, R.C. (1989, April). A continuity theory of normal aging. *Gerontologist, 29*(2), 183-190.

Birren, J.E. (1988). A contribution to the theory of the psychology of aging: As a counterpart of development. In J.E. Birren & V.L. Bengtson (Eds.), *Emergent theories of aging.* New York: Springer.

Birren, J.E., & Bengtson, V.L. (Eds.). (1988). *Emergent theories of aging.* New York: Springer.

Birren, J.E., & Birren, B.A. (1990). The concepts, models, and history of the psychology of aging. In J.E. Birren &

K.W. Schaie (Eds.), *Handbook of the psychology of aging*. New York: Academic Press.

Brookbank, J.W. (1990). *The biology of aging*. New York: Harper and Row.

Cohler, B.J. (1982). Personal narrative and life course. In P.B. Baltes & O.G. Brim (Eds.), *Life-span development and behavior* (Vol. 4). New York: Academic Press.

Cristofalo, V.J. (1988). An overview of the theories of biological aging. In J.E. Birren & V.L. Bengston (Eds.), *Emergent theories of aging*. New York: Springer.

Cumming, E., & Henry, W.E. (1961). *Growing old: The process of disengagement*. New York: Basic Books.

Erikson, E.H. (1963). *Childhood and society* (2nd ed.). New York: W.W. Norton.

Fry, P.S. (1992, April). Major social theories of aging and their implications for counseling concepts and practice. *Counseling Psychologist, 30*(2), 246-329.

Havighurst, R. (1972). *Developmental tasks and education*. New York: David McKay.

Hayflick, L. (1994). *How and why we age*. New York: Ballantine Books.

Masoro, E.J., Katz, M.S., & McMahan, C.A. (1989). Evidence for the glycation hypothesis of aging from the food-restricted rodent model. *Journal of Gerontology, 44*, B20.

Passuth, P.M., & Bengtson, V.L. (1988). Sociological theories of aging: Current perspectives and future directions. In J.E. Birren & V.L. Bengtson (Eds.), *Emergent theories of aging*. New York: Springer.

Strehler, B.L. (1977). *Time, cells and aging* (2nd ed.). New York: Academic Press.

Streib, G.F., & Binstock, R.H. (1990). Aging and the social sciences: Changes in the field. In R.H. Binstock & L.K. George (Eds.), *Handbook of aging and the social sciences* (3rd ed.). New York: Academic Press.

CHAPTER 4

If I should live to a ripe old age
May I possess some bit of
individuality, charm and wit
that I may not be discarded
when I am withered, worn, and weak
But sought after and cherished
like a fine antique.

ANONYMOUS

The Transition Years

■ Learning Objectives

On completion of this chapter, the reader will be able to do the following:

1. Describe social role changes experienced by older adults in the United States.
2. Describe changing family roles experienced by older adults in the United States.
3. Discuss the patterns of late-life marriages.
4. Examine the positive and negative consequences of retirement for older adults.

Most people do not experience aging by waking each morning saying, "Well, today I am much older than yesterday." Rather, for many people the song "Sunrise, Sunset" from the musical *Fiddler on the Roof* captures their experience of growing older. Tevye, a traditional father, suddenly notices that his oldest daughter is a beautiful woman and his young neighbor has grown into a man who dearly loves her. He reveals his sense of aging by singing, "I don't remember growing older; when did they?"

Perhaps that is the way most people come to the realization of their own aging—watching their children reach adulthood, losing their parents, and realizing that they now are the oldest generation in their families.

Middle age is said to begin when a person starts to think of time in terms of the amount left to accomplish life's tasks; there is an awareness of one's mortality different from the younger person's sense of unlimited time and immortality. Taking stock of one's life is another aspect of middle age. Furthermore, as people move into their late 50s and early 60s, there is a sense, for some, of coming to terms with their own passage into the older age group. What this actually means to people is not clearly understood, especially in our youth-oriented culture.

The ambiguity surrounding the perception of growing older in the United States in the last part of the twentieth century is suggested in an interesting sociologic study. Goldstein and Heiens (1992) examined self-perceptions of aging. They asked subjects to evaluate, when compared to members of a given age group, how they looked, how they felt, and how their interests compared. The results demonstrated that older subjects overwhelmingly perceived themselves as being within younger age groups rather than within their own chronologic age boundaries, leading the investigators to conclude that perceived subjective age is less than chronologic age (Goldstein & Heiens, 1992). There is a sense of the ageless self, an identity that maintains continuity over time, that draws meaning from the past and provides courage for the future (Kaufman, 1993).

There is a creative tension in the lives of many older people as they strive to meet new role expectations, to continue to develop their gifts and talents, and to realize their ambitions and dreams for their retirement years. The tension comes from being older and living in a society that values youth, speed, productivity in terms of work, and individual independence. These attributes are difficult for older people to generate and exacting for them to maintain.

What then are the psychosocial challenges and the realities that face an older person? How does society respond to the needs of older adults? And lastly, what are the gifts, talents, and dreams of older people that have the potential to enrich the community and society while providing a sense of satisfaction and fulfillment for the older adult? While trying to address these questions, this chapter will provide a view of family and social roles available to the older person and will discuss the effects of retirement, successful aging, and the involvement of older people in overall society.

■ Social Challenges of Aging

As a result of extensive studies of today's older population, a great deal is known about the older people of today. Significant for nursing is the realization of the wide diversity of the older population and the important differences in health care needs. Because of the wide diversity, it is most difficult to generalize about appropriate health care for the individual older adult. The diversity is seen in ethnic origin, language, health, family relationships, intelligence, lifestyle, educational background, and socioeconomic status (Silverstone, 1996). The need for individualized health care is of vital importance and should be uppermost in the nurse's mind when the nurse approaches the care of older adults. The need for nursing care soars as people age because of increases in disabling illness, the occurrence of which rises sharply in the older age groups. There is an opportunity for nurses to focus on the functional level of the older person rather than on the disease or illness state. The understanding of diversity among older people will assist the nurse in bringing a realistic but wholistic perspective to the delivery of services to older people.

The social roles available to older adults are in a way reflections of their lives. Family roles many times are a result of investments made over years of being a family member. Traditions handed down through generations—celebrations of holidays, family events, celebration of family members' accomplishments, traditional gifts, vacations—are part of the glue that binds generations together through both good and bad times. There is a reciprocity in life, a mutuality of sharing, celebrating, laughing, and crying together. To live fully is to give of oneself for the joy of life's journeys. Not always, but most of the time, people make a place for the older person as they journey through life.

Today many older people are challenged to embrace the leisure time they have forfeited along their life's journey. The rewards of an older age should not be dismissed. The freedom from the competitive struggle so often typical of the workplace, the time to pursue creative talents, and the time to travel to faraway and exotic places are a few of the pleasures that are afforded to many of today's older adults.

FAMILY ROLES

Significant changes in family composition—such as declining family size with fewer children, changes caused by increasing divorce and second-marriage rates, and expanding numbers of women in the work force with dual workers, single parents, and single-person households—will lead to adjustments in the lives of older adults. Although these changes may seem overwhelming, it is appropriate to pause and realize that older adults in their 70s, 80s, and beyond have survived and adapted to depression, war, countercultures, and phenomenal changes in the use of information processes, from listening to radios on crystal sets to working with computers and the Internet. As society responds to the cultural changes, it may be that the older and wiser people will provide the continuity that will support growth and stability for family life.

The family roles depend on the composition of the family and the availability of different members to augment whatever roles are played by the older person. Family life provides many roles for older people. The connections in three-, four-, and even five-generation families lead to multiple roles. Many older people have roles that stretch from being a caregiver for a frail 80-plus-year-old parent to being a great-grandparent. Over 50% of people over 65 years of age are members of four-generation families, and 20% of women over 80 who died were great-great-grandmothers, the matriarchs of five generations (Silverstone & Hyman, 1992). Longevity and early childbearing create multiple roles for older members.

The following two situations emphasize factors that influence role attainment for an older adult:

Charles and Maria have been married for 45 years. Charles, who is 67 years old, has his 86-year-old mother living with his family; he shares expenses for her care with his two brothers. Maria's father, who has severe dementia, lives in a nursing home close to their home. Charles's eldest son, Harold, who is 45, is a new grandfather; his 22-year-old daughter, Emily, has just given birth to her first child. Charles's roles in this family include husband, son, son-in-law, brother, father, father-in-law, grandfather, and great-grandfather. Charles has made a lifetime investment in his family roles. He enjoys close relationships with his wife, his children, his siblings, his mother, his father-in-law, and his grandchildren.

Bryan is 62 years old and has been divorced once and has remarried. He was 35 years old when he first married, and his marriage lasted for 14 years. He had two sons by this marriage; they are 13 and 19 years old. Bryan remarried when he was 52. He is an only child and his parents are both deceased. He has a poor relationship with his sons and does not see them more than twice a year. His second wife's parents are also deceased. She has a sister who lives close to them and is often a visitor at their home. Bryan's family roles are husband, father, and brother-in-law. His strained relationship with his sons will probably limit his future enjoyment of not only the father role, but also the grandparent role. At present he is very satisfied with his life, but the structure of the family system may limit his ability to fulfill all available family roles.

GRANDPARENTING

Age is not an accurate predictor of family roles, although grandparenting is always projected to be the special role reserved for older adults. A favorite saying regarding grandchildren is the classic "If I had known grandchildren were such fun, I would have had them first"; or consider another statement, overheard from a retired money manager: "The children are the investment, the grandchildren the dividends."

How older adults assume the role of grandparenting varies, with interactions ranging from fun loving and game playing to a distant, formal type of interaction. One role of grandparenting that has become too common is that of caregiver or protector of grandchildren. As the scourge of drug abuse ravages some young adults, their parents are stepping in to take care of their grandchildren. Many times grandparents have gone to court to protect the grandchildren from abuse or neglect and have won custody of their grandchildren (Minkler et al., 1992).

Most grandparents are not faced with such a heavy responsibility, but enjoy the role of grandparent with a sense of continuity of family and a sense of fulfillment. The old idea of the grandparents' being aged, doddering, fragile, and dependent has been changed. Grandparents are now often hale, hearty, active, healthy, and quite independent. As the younger, middle-aged, and older generations consider grandparents of today, they think of quite a different group of people than existed a few years ago.

Because people are living longer, healthier lives, the role of the grandparent has taken on a very different style. This is the age when grandparents celebrate life and love; they love and are involved with grandchildren very intimately, quite a bit more freely than they interacted with their own brood. They celebrate their life with their spouse in a more romantic way than when they were burdened with the responsibilities of child rearing, mortgage paying, grocery shopping, meal preparing, and all the other daily tasks of working families. The grandparent couple can spend time with the grandchildren in a relaxed, fun-loving way; they can involve themselves and the children in games and activities, depending on the ages of all. They can reflect and comment on the strengths of their grandchildren, appreciate the talents and potential they observe in the children, and introduce and use humor to appreciate and talk about the mistakes and shenanigans that are experienced in the course of the days when they are together. The ease with which the children and the grandparents experience being together, for whatever purpose and period, is certainly one of the potential gifts available to the older adult.

This relationship with grandchildren affords an opportunity for the older person's own children, now parents themselves, to view their older parents in a special way. The bonds between generations may become stronger as the young parents come to appreciate not only the

Strong intergenerational bonds are important.
Courtesy Loy Ledbetter, St. Louis.

present grandparenting, but also the parenting they received when they were young. They may now come to an increased understanding of all the trials and tribulations that are part of childrearing experiences. There is great opportunity for intergenerational reflection and expression of love and affection through the act of active grandparenting.

■ Late-Life Marriage

The role of spouse or the role of being part of a couple is available to those who choose marriage as part of their life's journey. Silverstone and Hyman (1992) suggest that couples who grow old together live out their later years in several different patterns. With great respect for the diversity in relationships and the difficulty in categorizing people, it is helpful for nurses to look at the different patterns late-life marriage may take.

How individual partners in a marriage respond to aging influences the life of the married couple. Certainly health and illness are key factors in the couple's ability to maintain the relationship over time. Nonetheless, taking these factors into consideration, there are six patterns that typify late-life marriage: the inseparables, the collaborators, the quiet despairers, the not-so-quiet despairers, the parallel pairs, and the tie breakers (Silverstone & Hyman, 1992).

THE INSEPARABLES

The inseparable couple is a poet's dream—love forever, together forever. The partners in these couples talk for each other, always referring to themselves as "us," and their entangled identity leaves no room for individual differences. They like the same sports, vacations, movies, people, and other elements in their lives. Whether or not this type of marriage pattern makes for a healthy relationship for individuals is not for anyone to judge. The important thing for nurses to recognize with this pattern is that the partners need one another, and illness in one has the potential to leave the other incapacitated.

THE COLLABORATORS

The collaborators have developed, over time, the ability to respect individual differences, but they are emotionally connected, with mutual appreciation for each other's talents and gifts. Problem solving is their mode of operation, and this continues into their later life. They work efficiently together; at times there are disagreements and arguments, but solutions are their goals. One example of a late-life problem could be the simultaneous retirement of both members of a professional working couple. Collaborators will spend time working toward an equitable solution, which may entail different times for individual retirement. The problem-solving focus of this couple will need to be recognized and valued by any health professional who will be providing the spouses' health care.

THE QUIET DESPAIRERS

Marriage is viewed as a trap by the quiet despairers. Many spouses have gone through long years of not experiencing intimacy, support, or personal recognition for their talents or gifts. Many lead lives of quiet desperation. They stay together for a myriad of reasons that others may find incomprehensible: for the good of the children, for financial security, because of religious or social beliefs, or out of fear of being alone. These are some of the reasons health professionals may hear as individuals explain their lives together, although most suffer in silence. In fact, many times these couples go unrecognized; they seem contented and perhaps even comfortable in their relationship. The nurse, however, should always be aware that there may be despair below the surface of silent contentment.

THE NOT-SO-QUIET DESPAIRERS

For the not-so-quiet despairers, fighting is a way of life, and the partners have spent years bickering, carping, and even physically abusing one another. In fact, later years may see an increase rather than a decrease in the fighting. One or both individuals may have difficulty in accepting changes brought about by the aging process. These feelings of frustration may lead to venting of unrecognized rage that increases hostility and results in more fighting within the marriage. Because these spouses do not endear themselves to many, they become more dependent on each other as their children and their friends maintain a distance from the constant discomfort of watching or participating in the pattern of fighting.

THE PARALLEL PAIR

The parallel pair long ago decided, for reasons similar to those of the quiet despairers, that marriage was essential but not necessarily an emotional or loving involvement. Many times, either one or both of the partners have found intimacy outside of the marriage. There is either open or tacit acknowledgment of the arrangement, and these spouses live compatible but separate lives. Later years may find that this pattern does not continue, and disruption may bring forth resentment if in fact there was not mutual acceptance of extramarital behavior.

THE TIE BREAKERS

Some spouses find that the late-life transition is not one they want to share, and they realize that their goal is to escape the relationship. Late-life divorce and separation are still uncommon, but they are on the rise. Although infrequent, divorce among older couples has become such a major concern that the American Association of Retired Persons has published a guide entitled "Getting Divorced after 50" (Silverstone & Hyman, 1992).

CONCLUSION

How older adults relate to each other through their marriage is a reflection of their history together. Most marriages maintain or actually escalate their pattern of relationship. It is important for the nurse to be aware of the diversity of marriage patterns and the possible impact these relationships will have on the health of the individual partner.

■ Widowhood

Even though older couples know that they will be separated by the death of one member, most older adults experience great difficulties in adjusting to the reality. The adjustment includes coping with loss and acceptance of the role of widow or widower. Following the death of their husbands, older women are most economically vulnerable because of a loss of income and benefits.

For many older adults, widowhood is accompanied by adverse health. It is difficult to appreciate all the stresses that impinge on an older person who has suffered a severe loss such as the loss of a long-term spouse. Whether or not this type of stress is related to or a cause of illness is a moot question. The reality is that the recent widow may be at risk because of a combination of factors, such as increased age, self-neglect, stress response, and genetic makeup. The nurse must consider where the person is in the life cycle and incorporate this knowledge in the assessment process when managing the care of older adults.

On the other hand, the new role of widowhood may in time bring unforeseen joys as many older adults are able to find new companionship with new marriage partners. The gender distribution in the older population, of three women for every man over the age of 65 years, favors the remarriage of older men over that of older women (White House Conference on Aging, 1995).

■ Retirement

Retirement is defined as the withdrawal from the labor force, either voluntary or involuntary, coupled with the earned right to pension income. This is a recent sociologic development, which may not survive in its current form for future older generations. Actually, the practice of setting retirement age at 65 years was started in Germany in 1889 by Chancellor Bismarck. He arrived at the age of 65 by adding 20 years to the average life expectancy, which at that time was 45 years. Bismarck ensured that few, if any, pension benefits would be paid to workers. Even though life expectancy has increased, the age of 65 has remained the marker for retirement in Western countries.

Two historical events have influenced the American retirement process: (1) in 1908 Great Britain adopted 70 as the age of retirement, and (2) in 1935 the United States established the first nationalized pension system for adults 65 years of age. In 1967 age discrimination in places of employment was made illegal in the United States, ending a long history of age discrimination in the workplace. In 1986 the Age Discrimination in Employment Act made involuntary retirement at either 65 or 70 a thing of the past. As of then, involuntary retirement predicated on age alone was to be considered an act of discrimination and therefore illegal.

In 1900 an average man spent about 3% of his life in retirement; men and women in the late 1990s will spend from 20 to 35 years in retirement. Therefore retirement is to be considered a normative event in the third age of life, and for most people it is a welcome and widely anticipated stage of life: a time to reap the rewards of work and family life and to have an abundance of free time to pursue forestalled pleasures.

Retirement can have a major impact on the financial condition of the retiree. The economic status of older Americans has improved significantly since the 1950s, with poverty rates declining from 35% in 1959 to 12% in 1986 (McLaughlin & Jensen, 1993). Income in older age is linked to multiple interacting past and present variables such as past and current labor force participation, marital status, gender, age, educational attainment, and living arrangements. Factors that increase the possibility of a comfortable income stream during later life are high wages during the work years, higher educational attainment, being male and married, and living in an urban area.

Professional and self-employed older adults have personal investments and continued employment opportunities and are more apt to retire later rather than earlier. However, more people are retiring earlier, and the trend is thought to be accelerating because of the restructuring of the American business community. Younger retirees have lower projected Social Security benefits, fewer private pensions, and longer life expectancy. This does not bode well for their future economic well-being. (Table 4-1.)

A Canadian longitudinal study of men over the age of 65 indicated that men with higher earnings in midlife had significantly lower mortality at older ages and that mortality was associated with early retirement (Wolfson et al., 1993).

TABLE 4-1 U.S. labor force participation

Year	Age	Men (%)	Women (%)
1950	55-64	87.0	27
	65+	45.8	10
1980	55-64	72.0	42
	65+	19.0	8

From Social Security Administration (1995). *Social Security Handbook* (12 ed.). Washington D.C.: Government Printing Office.

On the other hand, many studies show a continuity of involvement and well-being among most retirees as they make the transition to retirement. A study of the short-term effects of retirement on a group of 60- to 66-year-old health maintenance organization (HMO) participants indicated no negative effects. Retired men reported less stress and were more apt to exercise regularly than those who were still working (Midanik et al., 1994). The mixed results of retirement studies demonstrate the diversity of experiences and characteristics of older adults. Retirement is a personal experience and a shared family experience.

There are large ethnic inequalities in the income of older U.S. citizens, with black and Hispanic Americans having much less in assets and private pensions than white citizens. Median income of white older men is almost twice that of black and Hispanic older men. Retirement patterns are sensitive to differences in mortality rates and to the occurrence of disability over the life course. Black men spend more time working, experience more disability, die younger than white men, and therefore spend less time in retirement (Hayward et al., 1996).

Women make up one half of the population, but they compose 75% of the poverty group of older adults. Median income of single older men is substantially higher than that of single older women. Poverty in retirement for women is a result of past discrimination in the workplace coupled with lifetime low salaries. Eighty percent of all working women can be found in 20 of the 420 jobs listed by the Department of Labor. Women are most frequently found in clerical and sales and service jobs. They occupy a limited number of professional jobs including teacher, nurse, librarian, and dental assistant—certainly not the highest-paying jobs in America. Poverty of postretirement women affects social, psychologic, and physical well-being (Perkins, 1993). Noncash factors that benefit all older adults are tax treatment, reduced family size, Medicare, and Medicaid.

The inequality in the distribution of wealth is mitigated, though not resolved, in the United States through our social program known as

BOX 4-1 POTENTIAL RETIREMENT ISSUES

LOSSES
Psychologic

1. Loss of valued self-identity
2. Loss of prestige

3. Loss of companionship
4. Loss of satisfaction

Social

1. Loss of income
2. Loss of valued role

3. Loss of benefits

Physical

1. Loss of physical routine
2. Loss of health

GAINS

1. Gain in companionship of family members
2. Increase in involvement in community affairs as volunteer
3. Increase in control of own time

1. Acceptance of new roles
2. Increase in value to family for grandparenting skills

1. Increase in time to exercise
2. Increase in attention to health behaviors
3. Decrease in stress

Social Security. Thirty-five percent of income for older persons comes from the Social Security system, and nine out of ten people over 65 receive benefits (Social Security Administration 1995). Interesting is the fact that after a lifetime of work, only 29% of Americans over 65 years of age receive a private pension.

Issues that surround retirement reflect the complexity of the human condition, which becomes more extreme as people age. When assessing a person's response to retirement, the nurse should consider that that response may have psychologic, social, and physical aspects (Box 4-1).

How retired people spend their time is of interest to the nurse because social interaction is considered a fundamental element of a healthy lifestyle. However, it must be remembered that individuals differ greatly in their approach to life. Furthermore, the diversity of the older population is a major premise of this chapter, and it calls for great respect for the patterns of social interaction that older adults have chosen for their third age. It is of interest to note that 22.6 million people over the age of 55 provide direct help for their children or grandchildren. Seventy percent report membership in churches or synagogues, and 60% attend religious activities once a week. Another important aspect of life for people who have retired from the work force is volunteerism. Over 6 million older Americans volunteer through organizations and add their contributions to maintaining community structures. The services of older volunteers influence the nation's political system and support much of the country's system of social programs. For a summary of leisure activities of older adults, see Table 4-2 (White House Conference on Aging, 1995).

In spite of the potential losses associated with retirement, there are certainly significant gains for many retired people, including more leisure time, relief from monotonous work patterns, more control over daily living patterns, ability to pursue interests, time to renew relationships, and time to travel. Retirement has become

TABLE 4-2 Leisure activities of older adults

Activity	Percentage participating
Travel	50
Handcrafts	43
Photography	30
Playing musical instruments	18
Singing in choir	18
Painting	15
Writing	12

Tennis anyone? *Courtesy Loy Ledbetter, St. Louis.*

an acceptable and anticipated role in modern society. Studies have shown that men and women look forward to retirement and suffer few if any adverse effects that can be attributed solely to retirement from the organized work force.

The nurse must be cognizant of the social roles that older adults carry out in their daily lives. The older person's response to social roles of later life and to retirement may fall anywhere within a wide range—the changes may result in almost no difference in daily life, or they may constitute the best or worst event that the couple or individual has had to face. The event may be a life crisis or the reason for unending joy. But the nurse will always consider social roles and response to retirement—both psychosocial and economic aspects—when doing any assessment of an older adult.

REFERENCES

Goldstein, R., & Heiens, R. (1992). Subjective age: A test of five hypotheses. *Gerontologist, 32*(3), 312-317.

Hayward, M., Friedman, S., & Chen, H. (1996). Race inequities in men's retirement. *Journal of Gerontology, 51B*(1), S1-S10.

Kaufman, S. (1993). Reflections on the "ageless self." *Generations, 17*(2), 13-16.

McLaughlin, D., & Jensen, L. (1993). Poverty among older Americans: The plight of the nonmetropolitan elders. *Journal of Gerontology, 48*(2), S44-S54.

Midanik, et al. (1994). Retirement and health behaviors. *Journal of Gerontology: Social Sciences, 50*(1), S59-S61.

Minkler, M., Roe, K., & Price, M. (1992). The physical and emotional health of grandmothers raising grandchildren in the crack cocaine epidemic. *Gerontologist, 32*(6), 752-762.

Perkins, K. (1993). Recycling poverty: From the workplace to retirement. *Journal of Women and Aging, 5*(1), 5-23.

Silverstone, B. (1996). Older people of tomorrow: A psychosocial profile. *Gerontologist, 36*(1), 27-32.

Silverstone & Hyman. (1992). *Growing older together.* New York: Pantheon Books.

Social Security Administration. (1995). *Social Security handbook* (12th ed.). Washington, DC: U.S. Government Printing Office.

White House Conference on Aging. (1995, May). Background papers. Meeting held in Washington, DC.

Wolfson, M., et al. (1993). Career earnings and death: A longitudinal analysis of older Canadian men. *Journal of Gerontology: Social Sciences, 48*(4), S167-S179.

C H A P T E R 5

In spite of illness, in spite even of the archenemy sorrow, one can *remain alive long past the usual date of disintegration if one is unafraid of change, insatiable in intellectual curiosity, interested in big things, and happy in small ways.*

EDITH WHARTON

Drug Therapy in Older Adults

■ Learning Objectives

On completion of this chapter, the reader will be able to do the following:

1. Discuss physiologic-age-related changes that affect the pharmacologic dynamics of the older person.
2. Identify signs and symptoms of adverse drug reactions common in older adults.
3. Recognize high-risk drugs and their potential for harm and benefit to older adults.
4. Identify drug-drug interactions in older adults.
5. Recognize the risks and benefits of the use of over-the-counter (OTC) drugs in older adults.
6. Discuss methods to increase older adults' ability to understand and to follow medication prescriptions.

Appropriate drug prescribing in older adults is an important component of both the day-to-day primary care evaluation and comprehensive assessment of an older patient. The basic concepts of appropriate drug prescribing in older adults differ significantly from those used in other age groups because the effects of a drug on an older patient may be magnified by certain changes that occur during the aging process. This may be secondary to either an alteration of absorption, metabolism, or excretion of the drug; structural and physiologic changes of aging organ systems; or blunting of immune defenses (Hazzard et al., 1994).

Because of these changes and because older patients in general have significantly more ill-nesses, they take more prescription and over-the-counter-drugs, and in many instances, inappropriately, than do members of other age groups. This syndrome, referred to as polypharmacy, is defined as the use or administration of many medications; it differs according to subgroup within the older population. The average older American takes 4.5 prescription and 3.5 over-the-counter medications at any given time. That same individual may refill about 15 prescriptions per year. As would be expected, the highest incidence of polypharmacy occurs in the nursing home population burdened with advanced age and chronic disease, averaging eight medications per patient. The least incidence occurs in the

101

community-dwelling older adult population (Beck, 1991-1992).

Older adults are at greater risk for and experience the greatest severity of adverse drug reactions (ADRs). An adverse drug reaction is "the development of unwanted symptoms, signs, changes in laboratory values, or death directly related to the use of a medication" (Beck, 1991-1992). In addition to those instances secondary to alterations in drug absorption, metabolism, or elimination, ADRs may also occur in the form of drug-drug or drug-disease interactions (Gurwitz & Avorn, 1991; Lesage, 1991; Lindley et al., 1992). This increased risk is not independently related to age, however.

Older adults are also at greater risk for both polypharmacy and adverse drug reactions because they tend to be referred to or to visit more specialist physicians. Therefore they may visit more pharmacies, both in frequency and in numbers of sites, possibly because their regular pharmacy may not have the drug "in stock" and they perceive an urgent need to take the drug as soon as possible. Also, various family members serving as caregivers for an older loved one may use their own respective pharmacies, when refilling the drug, adding to the confusion and the number of "pill" bottles. Older patients may not be aware that they are taking several different forms of aspirin or acetaminophen because they are not aware of some of the basic ingredients of OTC drugs.

■ Physiologic-Age-Related Changes

Older adults, especially the advanced elderly (those over 85 years of age), have blunted immune defense systems to fight infection, leading to a greater risk of pneumonia and influenza, and less chance of recovery because of inadequate antibody production (Hazzard et al., 1994). Manifestations of this blunted response may be seen in the gastrointestinal system (at the junction of the esophagus and the stomach-cardiac sphincter of the stomach) and genitourinary system (at the junction of the urinary sphincter and urethra), in which bacteria may have a tendency to reflux

beyond otherwise "sterile" areas close to these sphincters, leading to a greater risk of aspiration pneumonia or bladder infection in the presence of disease (Beck, 1991-1992). Therefore these patients lose the "margin of reserve" that allows the human body to fight off stresses, whether physiologic, psychologic, or physical. In the presence of various disease processes, this loss of reserve plays a significant role. An example is precipitation of congestive heart failure (CHF) in a patient with angina and cardiomegaly when the system is challenged with intake of a "few" grams of extra dietary salt, failure to take a morning dose of fluid medication or digoxin, a mild upper respiratory tract infection, or slight excesses of physical exertion (Beck, 1991-1992).

Normal changes of aging include reduction in total body water and muscle mass, and increase in total body fat (Beck, 1991-1992). These changes may translate into a greater risk of adverse drug reactions. Water-soluble drugs, such as digoxin and theophylline, and alcohol are distributed in a smaller compartment in older adults and may accumulate at toxic levels at the same dose that would be safe in other age groups. Fat-soluble, long-acting benzodiazepine minor tranquilizers accumulate in body fat to a greater extent, leading to excess sedation, lethargy, and risk of falls, whereas these problems do not tend to occur in younger patients with less body fat (Calkins et al., 1992). Reduction in muscle mass with "normal" aging translates into reductions in renal clearance, especially in the advanced elderly and for drugs dependent on renal clearance, including digoxin, H_2 blocking agents, fluoroquinolones, penicillins, and aminoglycosides (Calkins et al., 1992).

The normal aging process is accompanied by a reduction of the total number of receptors in the nervous system. In some older adults there is a reduction in the number of functioning receptors in the pancreas; in the responsiveness to stimuli of organ-specific receptors and specific organ systems; in blood supply to the liver; and in the size of organs such as the kidneys, liver, and brain (Beck, 1991-1992; Calkins et al., 1992). Examples of reduction of responsiveness of a specific organ (central nervous system) to stimuli are increased refractory time between responses and inability to learn new material with advancing age. An example of reduction of organ-specific receptors' responsiveness to a stimulus is reduced maximum heart rate, or "blunted" heart rate increase, initiated by the carotid baroreceptors, sensing an acute change in blood pressure when the patient is standing or sitting from a supine position. Normally the expected increase in heart rate would neutralize the negative effects of any transient reduction in blood pressure and prevent any symptoms of "dizziness" or lightheadedness. The blunted process may precipitate postural hypotension in an otherwise normal older patient in 10% to 15% of instances. Postural hypotension is a reduction in systolic blood pressure of 15 mm Hg or more when the patient stands or sits from the supine position (Calkins et al., 1992). The presence of various disease processes and drugs may potentiate these responses. Examples of drug-induced exaggeration of normal aging responses include development of cognitive dysfunction secondary to usage of alcohol and other drugs, including centrally acting antihypertensive agents; psychotropics in high doses or with high anticholinergic activity; long-acting minor tranquilizers; anticholinergic agents; high doses of certain antibiotics—aminoglycosides, fluoroquinolones, and penicillins; high doses of H_2 blocking agents; and nonsteroidal anti-inflammatory drugs (NSAIDs). These agents might cause reduction in responsiveness to stimuli, leading to confusion, sedation, or lethargy. An example of drug-induced exaggeration of reduced responsiveness of an organ-specific receptor to a stimulus is the heart block that might be caused by the use of cardiovascular agents—including digoxin, antiarrhythmic drugs, and calcium channel blocker drugs—at high doses in older adults.

"*Five body systems*" deserve mention in a discussion of the absorption, metabolism, and excretion of drugs in older adults and the development of adverse drug reactions. The least important system is the "*integumentary system.*" In the outer layers of the skin, 7-dehydrocholesterol is converted by ultraviolet light of the sun to vitamin D_3 (Hazzard et al., 1994). Though the sun is not the only source of vitamin D production, institutionalized older patients with chronic renal or liver failure who do not get regular exercise may develop vitamin D deficiency, leading to the development of osteomalacia, because the metabolically active form of vitamin D requires metabolism in the liver and the kidney (Hazzard et al., 1994). (See Table 5-1 for a summary of the effects of drugs on body systems.)

The "*central nervous system*" plays an important role in the development of adverse drug reactions in older adults primarily because of normal structural and physiologic changes; in addition, Alzheimer's and related diseases may cause the patient to be more susceptible to acute confusion (delirium) and chronic confusion (cognitive dysfunction). The development of confusion syndromes is thought to be related to an anticholinergic hypothesis (Hazzard et al., 1994; Mach et al., 1995). Use of drugs with significant anticholinergic or muscarinic activity (e.g., antihistamines, antispasmodics, tricyclic antidepressants, phenothiazines, and narcotics) should be minimized or avoided in older patients.

The second least important system involves the "*gastrointestinal tract.*" In the normal older adult, physiologic changes include a reduction in acid secretion and motility, an increase in transit time, and a greater tendency for constipation (Hazzard et al., 1994). These changes do not usually translate into clinically significant disease. Certain drugs dependent on an acid medium in the stomach may be absorbed to a greater or lesser degree (Calkins et al., 1992). Albumin decreases slightly with normal aging, which is of no clinical significance. However, in the presence of gastrointestinal tract disease (previous gastrectomy, Crohn's disease, ulcerative colitis, or sprue), older patients may develop malabsorption syndromes leading to hypoproteinemia and hypoalbuminemia. Albumin and total protein levels may also decrease in older adults secondary to one or a combination of three other possible

TABLE 5-1 Classes of drugs associated with frequent adverse drug reactions by mechanism and body system

Body system	Drug class	Mechanism of ADR	ADR
Cardiovascular system	Diuretics	Fluid contraction, hypokalemia, hyponatremia	Lethargy; inappropriate antidiuretic syndrome; postural hypotension, falls, hip and other fracture
	Alpha-blocker drugs	Arterial vasodilation	Presyncopal lightheadedness and falls, especially with high doses
	Beta-blocker drugs	Nonselective blockade of beta-receptors	Precipitation or exaggeration of congestive heart failure, masking of hypoglycemia, postural hypotension, masking of symptoms of endocrine disease, reduction in exercise capacity, exacerbation of chronic lung disease or bronchospasm, memory loss, depression, arthropathy
Central nervous system	Anticholinergic agents (antihistamines, antispasmodics, phenothiazine and tricyclic antidepressants)	Stimulation of parasympathetic nervous system, central anticholinergic disruption	Sedation, cognitive dysfunction, lethargy, acute confusion; postural hypotension, falls, hip fracture; constipation, fecal impaction; worsening of glaucoma; urinary retention; dry mouth
	Benzodiazepine tranquilizers, barbiturates, hypnotics	Depression of central nervous system	Sedation, cognitive dysfunction, lethargy, acute confusion; postural hypotension, falls, hip and other fracture
	Centrally acting antihypertensive agents (methyldopa, reserpine, clonidine)	Depression of central nervous system	Sedation, cognitive dysfunction, lethargy, acute confusion; postural hypotension
	Nonsteroidal anti-inflammatory drugs	—	Sedation, cognitive dysfunction, lethargy, acute confusion

TABLE 5-1 Classes of drugs associated with frequent adverse drug reactions by mechanism and body system—cont'd

Body system	Drug class	Mechanism of ADR	ADR
Gastrointestinal system	H₂ blocking agents, sucralfate	Reduction in acid secretion leading to achlorhydria	Increased risk of aspiration pneumonia in the presence of swallowing dysfunction in bed-bound patients
	Nonsteroidal anti-inflammatory drugs	Direct irritation of gastric and duodenal mucosa (inhibition of surface prostaglandin)	Gastrointestinal bleeding
	Antacids, iron preparations, tetracyclines	Binding between agents	Diarrhea or constipation; malabsorption
Liver	Anticoagulant (warfarin) and antiseizure medications (carbamazepine [Tegretol], phenytoin [Dilantin], barbiturates, meperidine)	Increased bleeding time (warfarin); sedation, lethargy, acute confusion, cognitive dysfunction (phenytoin, carbamazepine, barbiturates, meperidine); ataxia and incoordination (phenytoin)	—
	Barbiturates, meperidine, diphenhydramine, lidocaine, theophylline, ibuprofen, tolbutamide, salicylates, long-acting benzodiazepine tranquilizers (diazepam, chlordiazepoxide, flurazepam)	Increased risk of gastrointestinal or other bleeding (salicylates, ibuprofen)	Sedation, lethargy, acute confusion, cognitive dysfunction, postural hypotension, falls, hip fracture
Kidney	H₂ blocker drugs, antibiotics (penicillins, aminoglycosides, fluoroquinolones)	Reduction in creatinine clearance	Confusion, irritability, drowsiness, lethargy, dizziness
	Digoxin	Reduction in creatinine clearance	Anorexia, decreased appetite, nausea, cardiac conduction problems, confusion, irritability, anxiety
	Nonsteroidal anti-inflammatory drugs	Inhibition of prostaglandin-mediated renal vasodilation	Fluid retention, worsening hypertension, aggravation of CHF
Integumentary system	Tetracyclines	Photosensitivity	Dermatitis

mechanisms: decreased metabolism secondary to liver diseases such as cirrhosis; increased catabolism secondary to malignancy; or decreased intake secondary to socioeconomic issues or the anorexia associated with dementia or depression. Certain drugs are highly bound to protein or albumin in the inactive (ineffective) state. A reduction in total protein or albumin level may lead to a greater fraction of free drug that is bioavailable, leading to toxicity. Examples include phenytoin, meperidine, digoxin, and warfarin (Calkins et al., 1992). Reduction of the dosage of these drugs may be necessary to prevent confusion and ataxia secondary to the use of phenytoin; lethargy, drowsiness, falls, or cognitive dysfunction secondary to the use of meperidine; confusion, anorexia, and nausea secondary to the use of digoxin; and bleeding secondary to the use of warfarin. Specific formulas are available that allow dose-specific adjustments according to protein and albumin levels (Winter, 1988). The use of anticholinergic drugs or sucralfate may predispose the older patient to constipation or gastric reflux (by relaxation of the sphincter of the stomach) and aspiration risk. In addition, the use of H_2 blocking drugs to reduce acid secretion in the stomach of an older patient with peptic ulcer disease or hiatal hernia theoretically might seem a logical step in the treatment process; however, the use of such drugs could lead to further reduction in acid secretion and a neutral or basic medium that would be an appropriate environment for bacteria refluxing from the stomach cavity to the lower esophagus. The problem is compounded when the patient develops swallowing problems from a stroke, Parkinson's disease, or other esophageal disorder and becomes bed bound, becoming further predisposed to aspiration risk (Beck, 1991-1992; Cook et al., 1994).

The second most important system regarding the development of adverse drug reactions in older adults is the "*liver*." The liver is the most important organ system for metabolism of various drugs. This metabolism involves two processes. The first one, phase I metabolism, undergoes significant reduction in activity with age. Drugs metabolized in this phase are either oxidized, reduced, or hydrolyzed, and their half-lives are prolonged because of this phase. This includes drugs such as diazepam, chlordiazepoxide, flurazepam, barbiturates, meperidine, phenytoin, propranolol, quinidine, warfarin, theophylline, tolbutamide, salicylates, nortriptyline, diphenhydramine, lidocaine, and ibuprofen. Phase II metabolism, conjugation or deactivation, is not altered with age. Drugs metabolized by phase II include the short-acting benzodiazepines (lorazepam, oxazepam, temazepam, and triazolam) with relatively short half-lives (Calkins et al., 1992). This correlation of metabolism phase to half-life is reflected clinically by studies indicating a difference in hip fracture risk between patients using long-acting and short-acting benzodiazepines, with the long-acting drugs causing a greater risk (Berggren et al., 1987; Cummings et al., 1995).

The most important organ system involved in the elimination of drugs dependent on renal blood flow is the "*kidney*," because kidneys are dependent on creatinine clearance, which decreases with advancing age even in the presence of normal blood urea nitrogen and serum creatinine levels. Examples of these drugs are digoxin, penicillins, aminoglycosides, H_2 blocking agents, and fluoroquinolones (Calkins et al., 1992). Significant reduction in the dose of these drugs is necessary with reduced creatinine clearance to avoid adverse drug reactions, which may manifest themselves with acute changes in mental status, cognitive dysfunction, dizziness, falls, or syncope. A formula useful for estimating creatinine clearance is as follows: creatinine clearance (CrCl) equals 140 minus the age of the patient times the weight of the patient in kilograms divided by the serum creatinine value (values less than 1 rounded to 1) times 72. In the case of women, the creatinine clearance should be multiplied by 0.85 (Calkins et al., 1992). A useful rule of thumb to remember is that if the serum blood urea nitrogen or serum creatinine is elevated above the normal range, the creatinine clearance will be below at least 50 ml/min and the dosage of these drugs should be reduced by one half.

■ High-Risk Drugs

Certain categories of drugs that present high risk of adverse drug reactions to the older patient warrant special consideration and discussion. This list includes the nonsteroidal anti-inflammatory drugs, H_2 blocking drugs, beta-blocking drugs, diuretics, psychotropics, centrally acting alpha-blocker drugs, ganglionic antihypertensive drugs, anticholinergic drugs, antibiotics, antiarrhythmic drugs, drugs for dementia, and other miscellaneous drugs.

Recent studies show a correlation between advancing age, peptic ulcer disease, and the presence of helicobacter pylori, a gram-negative bacterium that colonizes the lining of the stomach, especially in the presence of chronic disease (Graham et al., 1991). Excluding alcoholic and nonsteroidal anti-inflammatory drug–induced causes, one study of 49 older patients with gastritis showed a high correlation with helicobacter pylori (O'Riordan et al., 1991). In such cases, "H_2 blocker drugs" have been shown to be inadequate for healing stomach and duodenal ulcers, with a greater chance of recurrence than with a combination of 2 weeks of antibiotics, metronidazole, and milk of bismuth (Graham et al., 1992; Hentschel et al., 1993). Because of this increasingly popular concept about the etiology of gastrointestinal disease, this regimen appears to be gaining momentum as an ideal alternative in the presence of a positive helicobacter stomach biopsy, urea breath test, or serum antibody level (Culter et al., 1995; Peura, 1995). Both H_2 blocker drugs and sucralfate have been used nonspecifically as prophylaxes to prevent stomach ulceration—in older patients with or without a history of gastrointestinal disease and in patients placed on salicylates or nonsteroidal anti-inflammatory drugs to prevent ulceration. This regimen is not an accepted indication for use of these drugs (*Physicians Desk Reference,*

1995). A study of over 700 nursing home patients revealed that 41% were taking H_2 blocker drugs per indications that had not been substantiated by clinical studies (Gurwitz et al., 1992). Another common protocol is for critically ill patients in the intensive care unit setting to receive one of these agents to prevent stress-related gastrointestinal bleeding. Another study, however, indicated only two conditions that warranted use of these agents in this setting to prevent this complication: respiratory failure or coagulopathy (Cook et al., 1994).

Omeprazole and lansoprazole are proton pump inhibitors, a new class of drugs useful for the treatment of duodenal ulcer and gastroesophageal reflux disease. They have been shown to be more effective than conventional therapy with H_2 blocker drugs in the short-term (2- to 4-week) healing of duodenal ulcer disease. They should not be used for longer than 8 weeks because they may produce achlorhydria and hypergastrinemia; prolonged use has been associated with a dose-related increase in the production of gastric carcinoid tumors in rats (*Physicians Desk Reference,* 1995). These drugs should be reserved for treating intractable symptoms after conventional therapy has failed or for severe disease.

Metoclopramide and cisapride are drugs commonly used to increase gastric emptying and cause contraction of the lower esophageal (cardiac) sphincter. Indications for metoclopramide use are for the treatment of gastroesophageal reflux, diabetic gastroparesis, prevention of nausea and vomiting secondary to chemotherapy and postoperatively, and before implementation procedures. Common side effects include restlessness, drowsiness, confusion, fatigue, extrapyramidal symptoms, and diarrhea. Because cisapride has less affinity for crossing the blood-brain barrier than does metoclopramide, central nervous system symptoms are negligible. Cisapride is the preferred agent for treating gastroesophageal reflux in older adults but is not currently indicated for the other conditions. Both drugs are frequently used nonspecifically to increase gastric emptying in older patients with feeding tubes to prevent aspiration. However, they are not approved for this use (*Physicians Desk Reference,* 1995).

In addition to their effects on cognitive status, other common side effects of *anticholinergic drugs* include dry mouth, constipation, dry eyes, difficulty with urination, blurred vision, drying of bronchial secretions, and prevention of sweating. Medical diseases such as glaucoma, benign prostatic hyperplasia, Sjögren's syndrome (dry eyes and dry mouth), constipation, chronic bronchitis, and peripheral vascular disease may be aggravated by these drugs, predisposing the older patient to the development of fecal impaction, worsening glaucoma, urinary retention, hypothermia and hyperthermia, and exacerbation of chronic bronchitis secondary to mucous plugging (Beck, 1991-1992; Cahill et al., 1994; *Physicians Desk Reference,* 1995).

Nonsteroidal anti-inflammatory drugs, known as NSAIDs, are a particularly hazardous category of drugs that should be avoided in older adults, if at all possible, because of their potential for causing adverse drug reactions by three different mechanisms: precipitating confusion, gastrointestinal bleeding, and renal insufficiency or failure. In one study, NSAID use was found to have caused or exacerbated medical conditions in 86% of the 500 emergency admissions to a general hospital ward (Jones et al., 1992). In high doses, all of these drugs may cause acute or cognitive dysfunction. Indomethacin, because of its high affinity for penetrating the blood-brain barrier, causes the greatest risk of central nervous system side effects such as confusion, dizziness, lethargy, restlessness, and depression (*Physicians Desk Reference,* 1995), and thus is inappropriate for use in older adults (Willcox et al., 1994). NSAIDs also cause direct irritation of the gastric and duodenal mucosa leading to gastritis, peptic ulcer, and esophagitis after first-time or sustained use. Often, a patient may develop bleeding from an undiagnosed, asymptomatic hiatal hernia or reflux that was precipitated by the use of these drugs. Several studies indicate that all NSAIDs, in high enough doses, may cause gastrointestinal bleeding, with the least risk being from low doses of ibuprofen (200 to 400 mg) (Griffin et al., 1991; Langman et al., 1994).

The third mechanism by which NSAIDs cause adverse drug reactions in older adults is by prostaglandin-mediated renal vasodilation leading to fluid retention and subsequent renal injury via several mechanisms, renal failure, and glomerulopathy (Shankel et al., 1992). By causing fluid retention, NSAIDs may be responsible for worsening of hypertension or inability to control existing hypertension adequately, or for precipitating or aggravating existing congestive heart failure. Discontinuance of NSAIDs in an older patient with hypertension may result in a statistically significant reduction in mean blood pressure (Gottlief et al., 1992; Gurwitz et al., 1994).

The use of NSAIDs also is associated with acute liver injury and a hepatitis-like syndrome (Garcia Rodriquez et al., 1992). A recent study comparing acetaminophen (4000 mg) to high (2400 mg/day) and low doses of ibuprofen (1200 mg/day) for osteoarthritis of the knee indicated no difference in relief of symptoms (Bradley et al., 1991). However, for acute flare-ups of inflammation (swollen, warm, tender joints), for which a nonsteroidal agent may be beneficial, some practical guidelines include the following: (1) using the agent as needed, alternating it with acetaminophen; (2) using the agent in the lowest possible dose; and (3) using the agent for 5 to 7 days and then discontinuing use. Occasionally, persistent patients will demand that they be prescribed an NSAID for continuous use. In such cases, patients should be advised of the potential side effects and should agree to routine monitoring of the blood urea nitrogen for early signs of renal insufficiency, and a hemogram to monitor for early gastrointestinal bleeding. In these cases, misoprostol, a cytoprotective agent given 4 times daily, may provide some protection of the mucosa from gastrointestinal problems (Levine, 1995). Disadvantages of the drug include high cost, the need to be administered 4 times daily, and the common side effect of diarrhea. NSAIDs should not be used concomitantly with aspirin or warfarin because of the higher risk of causing bleeding complications (*The Complete Drug Reference*, 1992).

"*Beta-blocker drugs*" should be used with caution in older adults, particularly propranolol, which is often an inappropriate drug because of its side effects. These include the precipitation or exacerbation of congestive heart failure, masking of hypoglycemia, development of postural hypotension, masking of symptoms of endocrine disease such as hypothyroidism, reduction in exercise capacity, exacerbation of chronic lung disease or bronchospasm, depression, memory loss, and production of arthropathy (Cahill et al., 1994; Newbern, 1991; Thiessen et al., 1990). However, some studies indicate that propranolol may be beneficial for the treatment of anxiety in demented patients and tremor disorders in older adults (Colenda, 1991). The drug was also used to prove efficacy of treatment of systolic hypertension (systolic blood pressure greater than 160) for the prevention of stroke and death (Systolic Hypertension in the Elderly Program [SHEP] Cooperative Research Group, 1991). Use of the drug should be based on a risk-benefit ratio for the particular patient, including an evaluation of the patient's medical conditions.

Beta-blocker drugs may also produce adverse effects on lipid metabolism (*Physicians Desk Reference*, 1995). Pragmatically, the use of beta-blocker drugs in older adults would seem illogical because of the low incidence of high-renin, high-aldosterone hypertension in this group and because renin and aldosterone levels decrease with normal aging (Beck, 1991-1992). However, beta-blocker drugs may be used as first-line agents for the older hypertensive patient with a history of angina or myocardial infarction because they can reduce overall mortality by as much as 76% in this population (Park et al., 1995). Beta selective blocking drugs such as atenolol or metoprolol have fewer side effects and also have the advantage of once- or twice-daily dosing and therefore increased compliance. They also may be particularly appropriate for the older patient for treatment of dual conditions of atrial arrhythmias and hypertension. Beta-blocker drugs used selectively in patients with good left ventricular function have been shown to decrease the risk of congestive heart failure and death over a 2-year period (Lichstein et al., 1990).

"*Diuretics*" constitute another class of high-risk drugs that should be used with caution in older adults because of the reduction in total body water with normal aging and other factors. Side effects include hypokalemia, possibly linked to sudden death; worsening renal function, left ventricular hypertrophy; and increase in total cholesterol and triglycerides. Diuretics also may cause a contraction alkalosis. In addition, they may precipitate an exaggerated postural hypotensive response leading to lightheadedness, falling, and further morbidity or death from a hip or other fracture (Beck, 1991-1992; *Physicians Desk Reference*, 1995; Weinberger, 1992). Extreme caution is advised in administering thiazides to older patients with dementia or depression because of the tendency of these patients to drink less or even to forget to drink fluids because of the associated memory loss. Frail older adults and those over 85 years of age are also at high risk because of their greater tendency to develop postural hypotension. Older patients taking diuretics should be advised to drink lots of isotonic fluids during the summer months, especially during times of exercise and sweating. Diuretics may actually be harmful in hypertensive diabetic patients. A recent study indicated that such patients treated with diuretics had higher cardiovascular and total mortality than untreated patients (Warram et al., 1991).

Thiazides are generally not effective in the presence of renal insufficiency. Loop diuretics (metolazone, furosemide, bumetanide) are popular drugs used to treat dependent leg edema in older adults but also have the potential of exaggerating the postural hypotension caused by chronic venous insufficiency and stasis, further increasing the risk of inducing lightheadedness, dizziness, falls, and fracture or other morbidity (Beck, 1991-1992). These agents should be reserved for severe edema that is refractory to leg elevation, stockings, and exercise, or for patients with renal insufficiency or congestive heart failure, to mobilize fluid and promote brisk diuresis. By causing calciuria, they may serve a useful purpose in the initial treatment of hypercalcemia (Beck, 1991-1992). Both loop and thiazide diuretics may be a significant cause of urinary incontinence. Removing or minimizing the dose or changing the time of day for administration from the afternoon to midmorning may alleviate the problem in many cases (Beck, 1991-1992).

Advantages of using thiazide diuretics in older adults for treating mild hypertension include low cost and once-per-day dosing. The systolic hypertension in the elderly program, or SHEP, trial, using a first-line drug of chlorthalidone, a long-acting diuretic, showed that reduction in systolic blood pressure below 160 mm Hg reduced significantly the incidence of stroke and cardiovascular disease and, to a lesser extent, cardiovascular deaths and total mortality (SHEP Cooperative Research Group, 1991). Recent case control studies indicate that older women with hypertension using thiazides as compared to those not using thiazides have a significantly lower risk of hip fracture, possibly secondary to reduced excretion of calcium in the urine and resulting retardation of osteoporosis (Heidrich et al., 1991). Doses of more than 50 mg are generally not effective in achieving blood pressure control. African-American patients seem to benefit more from thiazides than do Caucasian patients. For stepwise treatment of hypertension, diuretics used in combination with other agents may potentiate the effect of other drugs but also have the disadvantage of being more expensive.

Centrally acting and "*alpha-blocker antihypertensives*" represent another group of high-risk drugs. Centrally acting drugs such as clonidine, reserpine, and methyldopa can cause significant central nervous system side effects in older adults, including headache, irritability, sedation, cognitive dysfunction, and depressive symptoms (*Physicians Desk Reference,* 1995). Alphamethyldopa is an old drug that must be given 4 times per day because of its short half-life. It may also cause drug-induced lupus syndrome, a rare hemolytic anemia, and hepatitis syndrome in a small percentage of cases (*Physicians Desk Reference,* 1995). Reserpine offers the advantage of once-per-day dosing and is inexpensive, but may produce other bothersome side effects including postural hypotension, dry mouth, constipation, bradycardia, bronchospasm, and hypersecretion of the digestive tract. It causes a hypertensive crisis when used in conjunction with food and drugs containing MAO inhibitor. Thus the use of methyldopa and reserpine is inappropriate in older adults (Willcox et al., 1994). Alpha-blocker drugs such as prazosin, terazosin, and doxazosin reduce blood pressure by causing vasodilation (*Physicians Desk Reference,* 1995). They have become popular because of their recent promotion as first-line agents for treating hypertension in the older patient with benign prostatic hyperplasia with associated signs and symptoms of urgency, frequency, or hesitancy. They have the added advantage of once- or twice-daily dosing. However, to achieve the dual effect of blood pressure and prostatic symptom control, dosages of 7 to 10 mg are often necessary, which also increase the risk of postural hypotension. This risk can be minimized by giving the drug before bedtime (Guthrie, 1994).

Apresoline is an old drug that has traditionally been used for treating hypertension. Its mechanism of action involves vasodilation, especially of the renal arteries. Side effects of the drug include negative effects on the cardiac muscle and increase in heart rate, which subsequently increase the work load of the heart and, in some cases, contribute to the development of congestive heart failure, especially in patients with impaired left ventricular function (*Physicians Desk Reference,* 1995). Disadvantages of the drug include short half-life and 4-times-per-day dosage. The drug can also cause a lupus-like syndrome. The dual-acting alpha- and beta-blocking drugs are newer agents that combine the advantages of beta-blockers with the vasodilating effects of alpha-blockers without increasing heart rate; they can be used for treating heart failure (Lessem & Weber, 1993). However, these combination drugs tend to be more expensive than other classes of drugs in general. Other classes of drugs appropriate for the treatment of hypertension in older adults include the angiotensin-converting enzyme (ACE) inhibitor and calcium channel blocker drugs.

The *angiotensin-converting enzyme, or ACE inhibitors* are a popular group of drugs used to treat hypertension. They have been shown in numerous studies to improve cardiac function in cases of acute congestive heart failure secondary to diastolic dysfunction and to increase survival in patients with chronic severe congestive heart failure, with one study showing a reduction in mortality in cases of mild to moderate congestive heart failure at 41 months using enalapril (Braunwald, 1991; Cohn et al., 1991). Captopril, the first of these agents, has been shown to reverse the reduction in renal blood flow that occurs with normal aging in healthy normotensive older adults by causing significant renal vasodilation (Hollenberg & Moore, 1994). It also has been shown to limit myocardial infarction expansion if given within 24 hours (Oldroyd et al., 1991), and to limit short-term mortality at 5 weeks (ISIS-4 Collaborative Group, 1995). This drug may also slow the progression of renal disease, reduce mortality, and alleviate the need for transplantation or dialysis as opposed to placebo when followed for 3 years (Lewis et al., 1993). Enalapril has also been shown to slow the progression of renal disease, proteinuria, and albuminuria when taken for hypertension, as compared to the effects of using metoprolol, when followed for 3 years (Bjorck et al., 1992). Furthermore, use of enalapril, as compared to beta-blocker drugs,

resulted in a significant reduction in proteinuria at 6 months and significant reduction in end-stage renal failure when followed for 3 years in patients with nondiabetic renal insufficiency (Hannedouche et al., 1994). Other positive effects of ACE inhibitor drugs include slower rates of renal function decline and significant reductions in albuminuria using lisinopril, as opposed to using furosemide and atenolol, in hypertensive patients with moderate diabetic renal insufficiency when followed for 18 months (Slataper et al., 1993). In most cases, ACE inhibitor drugs offer the added advantage of once- or twice-daily dosing. ACE inhibitor drugs are contraindicated in the presence of renal artery stenosis. Frequent side effects of these drugs include cough and angioedema (*Physicians Desk Reference,* 1995). Potassium levels should be monitored in patients given ACE inhibitors because of the tendency for these patients to develop hyperkalemia.

Calcium channel blocker drugs are another popular group of drugs used to treat older hypertensive patients by producing vasodilation and promoting loss of sodium and water. Side effects include flushing, headache, dependent edema, and constipation, depending on the specific drug. Calcium channel blocker drugs also offer the advantage of once- or twice-daily dosing, although they are more expensive than diuretics or beta-blocker drugs (Weinberger, 1992). However, a recent case control study suggests increased mortality in hypertensive patients treated with these agents, with the risk increasing with increasing dose, particularly of short-acting agents. Because of the possible limitations and criticisms of the study, a clinical trial is ongoing to prove or disprove these findings, but the results are not expected until 2002. Because these findings relate mostly to the short-acting agents, until there are further findings, long-acting agents are the preferred agents for treating hypertension according to recommendations of the National Heart, Lung, and Blood Institute (Buring et al., 1995; Furberg et al., 1995; Pinkowish, 1995).

PSYCHOTROPIC DRUGS

Another group of high-risk drugs is the *psychotropic drugs* that include minor tranquilizers, major tranquilizers, antidepressants, barbiturates, and hypnotics. Adverse effects of these drugs in general include cognitive dysfunction, sedation, drowsiness, lethargy, and functional decline. In inappropriately high doses for the older patient, they may produce or exaggerate postural hypotension leading to lightheadedness on standing or sitting from a supine position, leading to falls, fracture, and other morbidity (Beck, 1991-1992; Cummings et al., 1995; Grisso et al., 1991; Ray et al., 1991). Because of their side effect profile and their traditional overuse in institutional settings for such nonspecific conditions as insomnia, general agitation, anxiety, and dementia syndromes, OBRA 1987, a federal law, limits use of psychotropics in these settings to specific indications only and in a time-limited fashion. Proper documentation in the medical record is also required. Major and minor tranquilizers are only indicated for psychotic behavior, for hallucinations or delusions that are potentially harmful to the patient or to his or her surroundings, or for the prevention of aggressive, hostile, or combative behavior. Antidepressants should only be used for depressive symptoms. Antianxiety drugs should only be used to alleviate these symptoms in a patient with anxiety that is potentially harmful to the patient's medical or social condition. Barbiturates should only be used for prevention of specific seizures. Hypnotics should only be used for occasional inducing of sleep and not on a daily basis. The first component of the law involving the use of major tranquilizers was implemented in 1994. As a result, the use of these agents has decreased significantly (Rovner et al., 1990).

The *"major tranquilizers,"* commonly known as the phenothiazines, can also cause a drug-induced Parkinsonian syndrome consisting of bradykinesia, resting tremor, and cogwheel rigidity of the extremities (Beck, 1991-1992). It has been traditional that they be prescribed prophy-lactically with an anticholinergic drug (diphenhydramine, benztropine, trihexyphenidyl) to prevent these side effects. However, the older patient with this syndrome may not have the associated tremor, alleviating the need for these agents, especially with their additional troublesome side effects mentioned previously. In many cases, older patients are inappropriately treated for presumed Parkinson's disease instead of having their dose of phenothiazine eliminated or lowered (Kalish et al., 1995). The phenothiazines have a particularly disturbing and, in many cases, nonreversible side effect of tardive dyskinesia, characterized by abnormal, involuntary, repetitious muscle movements. Increasing the drug dosage may temporarily suppress the involuntary movements with subsequent "breakthrough" and worsening of the involuntary movements. Discontinuance of the drug may help to alleviate the movement disorder, but there is no predictable pattern to the syndrome. Anticholinergic drugs used to treat the parkinsonian side effects of phenothiazine major tranquilizers usually are of no benefit for this condition. The antipsychotic clozapine may be effective in treating severe cases, but can cause agranulocytosis in 1% of cases. Patients treated with this drug should have a hemogram performed monthly to monitor for this side effect. The risk of tardive dyskinesia in older adults may be as high as 6 times that for younger patients using the phenothiazine drugs (Saltz, 1992; Saltz et al., 1991; Yassa & Nair, 1992). The newest agent available for the treatment of psychotic disorders in older adults is risperidone, a serotonin and dopamine antagonist. Because it is not a phenothiazine derivative, it has a safer side effect profile, especially as related to dyskinesia (*Physicians Desk Reference,* 1995).

The choice of a major tranquilizer (phenothiazine) used in the older patient depends on the side effect of the agent and the patient's signs and symptoms. All of the phenothiazine major tranquilizers cause tardive dyskinesia, postural hypotension, anticholinergic side effects, and sedation, and have differing potency. For instance, an older patient with sleep-wake cycle problems secondary to sundowning from Alzheimer's disease may benefit from the sedative properties of chlorpromazine (10 to 25 mg) or thioridazine (25 mg at bedtime) to produce sleep; a dose sufficient to induce postural hypotension or cause significant anticholinergic disruption, leading to the development of delirium, worsening cognitive dysfunction, or other anticholinergic or parkinsonian side effects, is not warranted. On the other hand, haloperidol in a dose of 0.5 to 1 mg may be an ideal drug to treat aggressive, hostile, combative, or psychotic behavior in an agitated demented patient during the day because it is the least sedating, is the least hypotensive, and has the least anticholinergic side effects of these agents, yet is the most potent. However, the use of haloperidol at night for sleep would be counterproductive. The use of these agents, especially in high doses, may reduce the older demented patient's self-care activities, as a result of cognitive dysfunction secondary to the drug. This may lead to the development of functional decline manifested by reduction in independent mobility, bathing, feeding, dressing, eating, and toileting, leading to fecal and urinary incontinence and subsequent hygiene problems (Beck, 1991-1992).

The *"tricyclic antidepressants"* should be used with caution because of their side effect profile, similar to that of the phenothiazines, including postural hypotension, anticholinergic side effects (dry mouth, blurred vision, tachycardia, constipation, urinary retention), sedation, and cognitive dysfunction, and because of their differing potency (Beck, 1991-1992; Calkins et al., 1992; *Physicians Desk Reference,* 1995; Sheikh, 1995). They nonselectively block the reuptake of various neurotransmitters, including norepinephrine, serotonin, and dopamine. In low doses these agents promote a "quieting" or quinidine-like effect on the myocardium, and they produce an arrhythmogenic effect when used in high doses. These drugs can cause significant risk to older adults because of their high rate of successful suicide. Suicide risk related to anti-

depressants in general is not related to the specific class, but rather to the dose used, with higher doses associated with increased risk (Jick et al., 1995). Tricyclic drugs with the least anticholinergic properties should be used over those with high-anticholinergic side effects to limit the risk of precipitating acute confusion or precipitating or worsening cognitive dysfunction, especially at high doses. Desipramine and nortriptyline should be given during the morning because of their nonsedating properties. They also offer the safest profile, whereas imipramine and amitriptyline offer the worst. The latter, considered an inappropriate drug for older adults in a majority of cases (Willcox et al., 1994), should not be given during the day because of the associated high risk of sedation and postural hypotension, and it should be avoided in doses exceeding 25 mg. Few current indications exist for its use, except to treat chronic pain syndromes associated with depressed mood, or depression associated with both insomnia and anorexia, because of its ability to stimulate appetite. It should be used with caution in patients with Alzheimer's disease.

The newest and most popular class of agents useful for the treatment of depression in older adults includes the *"serotonin selective reuptake inhibitors (SSRIs)."* These have the same efficacy as the tricyclic agents, but may be tolerated better because of their selectivity (Sheikh, 1995). Recent studies indicate that depression may be caused primarily by a deficiency of serotonin, among other chemical agents in the brain. These agents offer an advantage over the traditional tricyclic antidepressants because of their lack of significant anticholinergic side effects. Theoretically, their use in patients with Alzheimer's disease would seem appropriate to avoid worsening the anticholinergic disruption that typically occurs in these patients structurally as the disease process worsens (Hazzard et al., 1994; Mach et al., 1995). This is an especially important concept because Alzheimer's disease accounts for 93% of cases of dementia, either in the pure form

(51%) or combined with vascular causes (42%) (Calkins et al., 1992). However, side effects of SSRIs include insomnia, agitation, decreased appetite, and nausea (Sheikh, 1995). Fluoxetine, the first of these agents, has a half-life of several days and is less selective in its side effect profile. Other, newer agents such as sertraline and paroxytyline, with half-lives approximating 24 hours and more selectivity for serotonin receptors, are more appropriate for the older patient (*Physicians Desk Reference,* 1995). The SSRIs are strong inhibitors of the cytochrome P-450 system, which is involved in the metabolism of many medications. When used with other agents such as the tricyclic agents, antihistamines, theophylline, erythromycin, benzodiazepines, and steroids, they can double or triple the levels of these agents, leading to a greater risk of adverse drug reactions (Sheikh, 1995). Fluoxetine has been shown to be an independent factor related to higher suicide risk, probably because of its multiple antidepressant use (Jick et al., 1995). Caution should be exercised when using SSRIs to treat depressive symptoms with or without dementia and in the malnourished patient, because the drug may magnify the symptoms of weight loss, nausea, and anorexia related to the disease process itself. This class of drugs also has the advantages of once-daily dosing and rapid onset of action—in 2 to 4 weeks, as compared to the tricyclic antidepressants, which require 6 to 8 weeks. These drugs should be administered in the morning because of their side effect profile. Because of its direct serotonergic effects, trazodone, in an initial dose of 25 to 50 mg at bedtime, provides an excellent option for the dual purpose of treating dementia and/or depression along with insomnia or sundowning. Side effects include postural hypotension and—rarely, if the drug is given in much higher doses than normally used in older adults (150 to 300 mg)—priapism (Beck, 1991-1992). The SSRIs are also used in combination with trazodone for treating depression. Patients given such a combination should be monitored for signs and symptoms of the so-called serotonin syndrome, associated with restlessness and increased anxiety (Hazzard et al., 1994).

Atypical antidepressants include venlafaxine and bupropion. Venlafaxine has a broader spectrum of neurotransmitter reuptake in addition to that of serotonin, but it does not inhibit the cytochrome P-450 system, which results in less risk of adverse drug reactions when it is used in combination with other drugs (Sheikh, 1995). Bupropion is a relatively safe drug with low anticholinergic and antiadrenergic side effects used for the treatment of depression. However, it should be used with caution in patients with a history of seizure disorder because it lowers the seizure threshold (Beck, 1991-1992).

Lithium is a drug used to treat bipolar (manic depressive) disorder. Regular monitoring of serum levels is recommended because of the frequency of adverse side effects associated with this drug, especially when used with other agents. Because the drug is distributed in the total body water content, excretion is dependent on adequate renal function. Dosages should be reduced for renal insufficiency. Levels of the drug may be increased in patients taking ACE inhibitor and nonsteroidal anti-inflammatory drugs. Other agents such as acetazolamide, urea, xanthine preparations (theophylline), and alkalinizing agents may decrease serum levels. Lithium may interfere with blood monitoring for thyroid disease. Use with calcium channel blocker drugs can increase the risk of nervous system toxicity. Use of lithium with diuretics or in patients with restricted sodium diets for treatment of congestive heart failure or hypertension decreases sodium reabsorption by the renal tubules, leading to an increased risk of hyponatremia and lithium toxicity (*Physicians Desk Reference,* 1995). Other agents that may interfere with lithium metabolism include antipsychotics and medications containing iodine. Early symptoms of toxicity include diarrhea, drowsiness, loss of appetite, muscle weakness, nausea or vomiting, slurred speech, and trembling. Late symptoms include confusion, unsteadiness or blurred vision, convulsions, dizziness, and increased urination. Less common side effects include postural hypotension, weight gain, bradycardia, cardiac arrhythmias, and heart block (*The Complete Drug Reference,* 1992).

The *"benzodiazepine minor tranquilizers"* are useful agents for the treatment of agitation, anxiety, and insomnia in older adults. In this category, short-acting drugs such as lorazepam (0.5 to 1 mg) and oxazepam (15 mg) are the drugs of choice to prevent worrisome side effects encountered with the long-acting agents (Beck, 1991-1992; *Physicians Desk Reference,* 1995). Flurazepam, chlordiazepoxide, and diazepam are inappropriate for use in older adults (Willcox et al., 1994). Although requiring metabolism by the liver, alprazolam, a short-acting benzodiazepine, has minor antidepressant effects in addition to its antianxiety effect if used in a low dose (0.25 mg) 2 or 3 times daily (*Physicians Desk Reference,* 1995). Other relatively short-acting benzodiazepines (triazolam and temazepam) serve a useful purpose for the occasional treatment of insomnia. Triazolam, having a half-life of 4 to 6 hours, is useful for inducing sleep, whereas temazepam will maintain sleep. Triazolam, in doses higher than 0.125 mg and when used on a regular basis, has been implicated as a cause of delayed recall of tasks in older patients. For this reason it should be used in a dose of 0.125 mg only on an occasional basis (Bixler et al., 1991; Greenblatt et al., 1991). The benzodiazepines in general are known to cause short-term memory impairment, although the long-term effect is unknown (Rummans et al., 1993). Meprobamate is an older drug used for the treatment of anxiety. However, its use in older adults is inappropriate because of its risk of causing sedation, confusion, and lethargy (*The Complete Drug Reference,* 1992; Willcox et al., 1994). Buspirone is a useful agent for the treatment of chronic anxiety, but must be given on a regular basis to be effective. Because onset of action requires 7 to 10 days, use of a short-acting benzodiazepine for this period may be necessary (*Physicians Desk Reference,* 1995).

Zolpidem tartrate is a new, short-acting non-benzodiazepine hypnotic with a chemical structure unrelated to the benzodiazepines, barbiturates, or other hypnotic drugs. Because it interacts with GABA receptor sites, it shares some of the properties of the benzodiazepines, including the potential to depress the central nervous system and impair motor and cognitive performance in older adults. It also has been associated with signs and symptoms of other central nervous system depressant drugs with abrupt withdrawal. It is indicated for the occasional treatment of insomnia, but because it is a new drug, experience in older adults is limited (*Physicians Desk Reference,* 1995).

Agents useful in the treatment of agitation and anxiety associated with dementia syndromes include trazodone and buspirone (Colenda, 1991). Carbamazepine has also recently become a popular agent for the treatment of agitation and aggressive, hostile, and combative behavior in such cases—in lower doses traditionally used to treat seizure disorder (100 to 200 mg twice daily). It offers a safer side effect profile than the traditional psychotropic agents, with little toxicity (Tariot et al., 1994, 1995).

"Drug therapy for dementia" has shown little to no progress in ameliorating the symptomatology of the disease. Various agents have been recommended in the past for the treatment of Alzheimer's disease, because of the recognition that lecithin deficiency and acetylcholine deficiency may play a role in its development. These various agents include lecithin-containing health foods and megadoses of other vitamins. Even though popularly used, clinical trials do not prove their efficacy. Hydergine, an old drug, has been used in the past for the treatment of dementia but has shown no clinically significant effects (Beck, 1991-1992). Cerebral vasodilators were once a popular group of drugs for the treatment of organic brain syndrome, Alzheimer's disease, or vascular dementia. The theory

behind the use of these agents was that vascular and oxygen supply to the brain should be increased. These drugs are contraindicated because of their risk of causing postural hypotension, falls, fracture, and other morbidity (Willcox et al., 1994). Pentoxifylline, a drug approved for use in treating peripheral vascular insufficiency, has been shown to slow the cognitive deterioration in patients with multiinfarct dementia, but with little effect on memory (Black et al., 1992).

Tacrine, an acetylcholinesterase inhibitor, is the first of a new class of drugs approved for Alzheimer's disease. Studies prove its effectiveness for mild cases of the disease and only for short-term benefit (up to 30 weeks); long-term studies are not available. In addition to cost, disadvantages include the need for regular blood monitoring because the drug causes asymptomatic elevation of the liver function tests. This toxicity is usually associated with higher doses of the drug, and discontinuance of the drug will usually resolve the problem. Another disadvantage is a high frequency of other side effects, including diarrhea and nausea, occurring in up to 74% of patients, with 59% of patients stopping the drug (Knapp et al., 1994; Maltby et al., 1994).

ANTIBIOTICS

Because of their risk of causing confusion, sedation, and lethargy, classes of antibiotics for which the dosage should be reduced in older adults consistent with creatinine clearance (as mentioned earlier) include the orally and parenterally administered penicillins and fluoroquinolones (Beck, 1991-1992; Calkins et al., 1992). Aminoglycosides, used in high doses, may cause hearing loss. In addition, appropriate use of antibiotics in older adults is important to prevent the development of resistant strains of bacteria, which appears to be an increasing and alarming concern among health care providers and public health officials. Appropriate general indications for the use of antibiotics include a productive-colored sputum, evidence of bacteria and leukocytes in the urine, evidence of cellulitis or sus-

pected osteomyelitis or bacterial meningitis, and abscess formation. The indiscriminate use of these agents can lead to diarrhea secondary to *clostridium difficile*, and related morbidity and death from pseudomembranous colitis, if not treated appropriately (Beck, 1991-1992). Mild cases should be treated with oral metronidazole (250 mg 3 times daily for 10 days), whereas moderate to severe cases with systemic symptoms of fever and leukocytosis should be treated with intravenous vancomycin (Beck, 1991-1992; *The Complete Drug Reference,* 1992). The fluoroquinolone group of antibiotics should be given 4 hours before or 2 hours after administration of antacids or sucralfate, because these agents may interfere with antacid's effectiveness (*The Complete Drug Reference,* 1992).

A frequent misperception among health care professionals is that the presence of bacteria or leukocytes in the urine of a patient with an indwelling urinary catheter or the presence of foul-smelling or pustular drainage from a pressure ulcer requires antibiotic administration. Patients with indwelling catheters and pressure ulcers will commonly develop colonization of the urinary tract or ulcer site, respectively. The use of oral antibiotics in such cases is not only ineffective, but will also promote resistance. Indications for the administration of parenteral antibiotics are the presence of fever greater than 102° as determined rectally, elevation of the serum leukocyte count above 15,000 with a shift to granulocytosis, and/or other signs of systemic sepsis including hypotension, change in mental status, central pallor, peripheral cyanosis, diaphoresis, and/or tachycardia (Beck, 1991-1992).

Acyclovir is an antiviral agent used for the treatment of herpes zoster (shingles). Initially approved for the treatment of herpes type II infections, this agent should be given for zoster at a much higher dose of 800 mg every 4 hours 5 times per day for 7 to 10 days. If given within 48 hours of infection, it has been shown to reduce the duration and severity of symptoms. The dosage and/or frequency of administration of the drug should be lowered in patients with creatinine clearance below 25 ml/min to prevent neurologic side effects from high doses, including confusion, dizziness, hallucinations, paresthesia, and lethargy (*Physicians Desk Reference,* 1995). Other side effects include skin rash, itching, myalgia, diarrhea, nausea, fever, headache, peripheral edema, lymphadenopathy, and leukopenia. When acyclovir is taken concomitantly with cobenemid, levels may become elevated. The drug can be administered intravenously in severe cases of infection associated with systemic involvement (ocular) or when infection is associated with immune deficiency states (*Physicians Desk Reference,* 1995). Famciclovir is a newer antiviral agent for acute zoster infection with the advantage of less frequent dosing (3 times per day) and a safer side effect profile. Dosage should be reduced for renal insufficiency (*Physicians Desk Reference,* 1995).

AGENTS FOR DIZZINESS

It is common practice among practitioners to prescribe meclizine for a patient who complains of dizziness, especially in a hurried office visit. Older patients with such a complaint may be exhibiting one or a combination of three different syndromes: "true" dizziness, presyncopal lightheadedness, or disequilibrium. True dizziness implies a vertical or horizontal spinning of the surroundings, which may or may not be associated with sensory or neurologic signs or symptoms. It can be secondary to a multitude of causes related to the inner ear or the central nervous system. Disequilibrium usually implies unsteadiness on the feet, usually on walking or turning. Disequilibrium may be secondary to a host of other disease processes as well. Presyncopal lightheadedness implies a "feeling of being faint," usually on standing or sitting from the supine position, and lasting 1 to 2 minutes in most cases. Various disease states and drugs previously mentioned in other sections may cause this syndrome. Appropriate evaluation of the type of dizziness, as well as the associated signs

and symptoms, time frame, and circumstance, is necessary before prescribing meclizine, because the treatments for these three syndromes are different. In addition, meclizine is an anticholinergic drug and should be used in as low a dose as possible, preferably 12.5 mg, to prevent side effects (Baloh, 1992).

CARDIAC DRUGS

There are only a few current indications for the use of digoxin—for systolic dysfunction of the myocardium and for the treatment of atrial arrhythmias. This drug should be avoided if possible in older adults because it is excreted 90% unchanged in the urine and is highly dependent on renal clearance, which in the absence of disease declines steadily with age. Inappropriately high doses of digoxin may cause confusion, agitation, anxiety, nausea, vomiting, heart block, arrhythmias, and the visual perception of yellow or green colors. An early sign of digitalis toxicity is usually anorexia. When used concomitantly with other cardiac drugs such as quinidine, verapamil, or amiodarone, the dosage of digoxin should be monitored closely and reduced accordingly because of the potentiating effects of these drugs. Digoxin is contraindicated in certain cardiac disease states such as incomplete heart block, pericarditis, aortic stenosis, and hypertrophic cardiomyopathy. The drug may also worsen myocardial ischemia with acute pulmonary edema (Luchi et al., 1991).

Quinidine is an old drug traditionally used to treat ventricular and atrial arrhythmias including atrial fibrillation. A recent meta-analysis of controlled trials using quinidine to control normal heart rhythm after conversion indicates that use increases mortality rate (Coplen et al., 1990). Common side effects of quinidine include ringing in the ears, diarrhea, flushing of the skin, bitter taste, nausea, stomach pain or cramping, headache, dizziness, lightheadedness, blurred vision, skin rash, and wheezing. Rare side effects include confusion, fatigue, increased bleeding, and hemolytic anemia (*The Complete Drug Reference,*

1992). Other more recent and more potent anti-arrhythmic agents such as flecainide and encain-ide have also been shown to increase mortality in patients with ventricular arrhythmias after acute myocardial infarction, with age being an indepen-dent risk factor (Akiyama et al., 1992). Amio-darone is an agent used for treatment and prophy-laxis of frequently occurring (refractory) ventricular fibrillation and unstable ventricular ta-chycardia. Hypotension is a major side effect. Procainamide has been shown to decrease short-term survival after cardiac arrest and resuscitation outside the hospital (Hallstrom et al., 1991). Side effects include diarrhea and, less commonly, fever, chills, joint pains, skin rash, confusion, depres-sion, dizziness, and lightheadedness (*The Com-plete Drug Reference,* 1992). Procainamide can also cause a lupus syndrome. Because of the lim-ited benefit-to-risk ratio for these drugs, they should be prescribed only under the close super-vision and monitoring of a cardiologist. Nitroglyc-erin preparations (nitrates), both administered orally and applied to the skin for treatment of ischemic heart disease and angina, may predis-pose the older patient to the development of lightheadedness, postural hypotension, syncope, and falls, especially when used in increasing doses. Other common side effects include head-ache, faint or rapid heartbeat, nausea, and vomit-ing. Rare side effects include blurred vision, dry mouth, skin rash occurring at the site of admin-istration for topical preparations, and—with very high doses—seizures (*The Complete Drug Refer-ence,* 1992). Patients using patch preparations should remove the patch for 4 to 6 hours per day to prevent the development of tolerance to the drug.

■ Hypolipidemic Agents

Hypocholesterolemic agents should be used with discretion in older adults because a recent meta-analysis of 35 randomized trials of cholesterol-lowering treatments questions the value of inten-sive treatment of hypercholesterolemia; this treatment is likely to benefit only people with significant risk factors for coronary heart disease, including the presence of smoking, hyperten-sion, sedentary activity, previous stroke or myo-cardial infarction, and/or family history of risk factors (Smith et al., 1993). Two recent studies indicate that serum lipid levels (elevated levels of cholesterol and low levels of high-density lipo-protein [HDL] cholesterol) are poor predictors of coronary risk (for coronary heart disease mortal-ity or hospitalization for myocardial infarction or unstable angina) and all cause death in *older adults* between the ages of 60 and 79 years and after age 70, respectively (Grover et al., 1994; Krumholz et al., 1994). A recent meta-analysis of clinical trials involving cholesterol reduction has also failed to show any correlation with stroke risk (Hebert et al., 1995). In fact, since serum cholesterol screening in healthy postmenopausal women has not been shown to change serum cholesterol levels significantly over the long term (7 to 10 years), a serum cholesterol performed every 5 to 10 years in older women without cardiovascular risk factors is sufficient (Hteland et al., 1992). Lastly, cholesterol-lowering agents used for patients with a total cholesterol level of over 309 mg/100 ml in the general population have not been shown to be cost-effective, costing $190,000 per extra year of life saved as opposed to population-based promotion of better eating habits at a cost of $20 per extra year of life saved (Kristiansen et al., 1991).

Normal aging is accompanied by dulling of taste and smell sensations (Beck, 1991-1992). Certain older patients are predisposed to the development of malnutritional states, including patients with anorexia secondary to dementia, depression, or malignancy; patients with visual or oral sensory deficits; and patients living alone, with low income and lack of transportation, or living in an institutional setting (Beck, 1991-1992). Inappropriate dietary cholesterol restric-tion in these patients is unnecessary because it may worsen the process, leading to further anorexia, weight loss, and death. Liberalization of salt, carbohydrate, protein, and cholesterol restrictions in these patients may be one of the few quality-of-life measures that may make life worth living. Hypocholesterolemia (4 mmol/L) has been linked to increased mortality in older adults, probably secondary to chronic inflammatory processes producing a catabolic state (Verdery & Goldberg, 1991). Restricted diets found in a majority of malnourished nursing home patients can contribute to the situation (Buckler, et al., 1994).

For those patients with cardiovascular risk factors and a higher-than-normal low-density lipoprotein (LDL) cholesterol level, the statin (HMG-CoA reductase inhibitor) drugs are very effective in lowering the LDL and total cholesterol, with the disadvantage of higher cost and need for regular monitoring of liver function tests because of the development of rare hepatitis (*The Complete Drug Reference,* 1992; Verdery & Goldberg, 1991). These agents should not be used in combination with cyclosporine, gemfibrozil, or niacin, because renal failure may result (*The Complete Drug Reference,* 1992). Nicotinic acid lowers total cholesterol to some extent but significantly elevates the HDL cholesterol (Vega & Grundy, 1994). Gemfibrozil reduces total cholesterol and elevates HDL cholesterol to a lesser extent than do nicotinic acid and the statin drugs (Vega & Grundy, 1994). Niacin and gemfibrozil also reduce serum triglyceride levels. When used to treat serum triglyceride levels, niacin and gemfibrozil should be used after an adequate trial of diet has failed, and for levels between 1000 and 2000 mg/100 ml, and for patients who have a history of pancreatitis or of recurrent abdominal pain resembling pancreatitis (*Physicians Desk Reference,* 1995). Frequent bothersome side effects of niacin include pruritus, flushing, tingling, headache, and diarrhea, especially when given in high doses of several grams per day (*The Complete Drug Reference,* 1992). Concomitant administration with aspirin can prevent cutaneous side effects (Whelan et al., 1992). Common side effects of gemfibrozil include stomach pain, gas, and heartburn. Less frequent side effects include diarrhea, low back pain, cough, fever or chills, nausea or vomiting, and muscle pain. This agent should not be used concomitantly with anticoagulants because it may increase the risk of bleeding. Use of the drug may increase the severity of gallstones and, in the presence of liver disease, may increase levels of the drug, subsequently increasing chances of side effects (*The Complete Drug Reference,* 1992).

Probucol is a drug used to lower LDL cholesterol and, to a lesser extent, triglycerides. Probucol is not the preferred agent for use in older adults because, in addition to causing gastrointestinal side effects, it carries the risk of worsening cardiac conduction problems, as evidenced in many instances by prolongation of the QT interval on the electrocardiogram (*The Complete Drug Reference,* 1992; *Physicians Desk Reference,* 1995). Clofibrate is a drug that causes modest reduction in cholesterol with a somewhat greater reduction in triglyceride level. The use of this drug is associated with potentially bothersome gastrointestinal side effects including diarrhea and nausea. It is relatively weak as compared to other agents. It may potentiate the effect of anticoagulants when used concomitantly with them. It also has been shown to increase the incidence of cholelithiasis and subsequent morbidity and death from surgery (*Complete Drug Reference,* 1992; *Physicians Desk Reference,* 1995). Regular isotonic exercise (walking, running, swimming, bicycling) for 20 to 30 minutes 3 times per week is a very effective way of raising the high-density cholesterol and can be effective in causing slow, progressive weight loss (Schuler et al., 1992). Moderate alcohol intake (one or more drinks per day) has been shown to be effective in elevating HDL cholesterol, and in achieving a reduction in the subsequent risk of stroke, myocardial infarction, and total cardiovascular mortality (Scherr et al., 1992).

The most potent cholesterol-lowering agent is estrogen, which increases HDL, reduces LDL, and lowers total cholesterol (Scherr et al., 1992;

Stampfer et al., 1991). Recent studies indicate that it improves word recall, increases quality of life, retards osteoporosis, and reduces fracture risk at all bone sites (Daly et al., 1993; Fogelman, 1991; Robinson et al., 1994). Other positive effects of estrogen include reduced risk for myocardial infarction, less intimal thickening of the carotid arteries, and reduced stroke risk in postmenopausal women as seen in a follow-up of less than 2 years (Finucane et al., 1993; Manolio et al., 1993; Psaty et al., 1994). In the older woman who has had a hysterectomy, in the presence of cardiovascular risk factors and an elevated total cholesterol level, low HDL component, and high LDL component, estrogen may offer a substantial advantage over the conventional cholesterol-lowering agents. In the nonhysterectomized patient, estrogen should be used sequentially or in combination with progesterone to reduce the risk of endometrial cancer caused by taking unopposed estrogen (Voight et al., 1991). New formulations that combine estrogen and progesterone are currently under review by the Food and Drug Administration. Relative contraindications to the use of estrogen include fibrocystic disease and a history of migraine headaches. Absolute contraindications include a history or family history of breast cancer and previous pelvic cancer (Colditz et al., 1995; *Physicians Desk Reference,* 1995). There is also a slight risk of breast cancer with consecutive use of estrogen (Colditz et al., 1995). Progesterone has also recently been shown to reduce the risk of osteoporosis (Prince, 1991). The effect of estrogen in regard to osteoporosis can be enhanced by the concomitant use of calcium (in a dose of at least 1000 mg daily) and Vitamin D (400 IU) (Hazzard et al., 1994).

■ Drugs for the Prevention of Osteoporosis

The question of whether to use hormone replacement therapy (estrogen and progesterone) in a woman involves the presence or absence of four factors: older age, osteoporosis risk factors,

cardiovascular risk factors, and status of the uterus and ovaries. The effect of estrogen for the prevention of osteoporosis is thought to be dependent on a "window of opportunity" during which maximum effect can be achieved. The sooner hormone replacement therapy is started after surgical or natural menopause, the greater the effect, with maximum effect achieved from therapy initiated within 3 to 5 years afterward. The usefulness of hormone replacement therapy after age 62 solely for prevention of osteoporosis is thought to be minimal, though specifics are unknown and studies are ongoing (Hazzard et al., 1994). The presence of osteoporosis risk factors after menopause may strengthen the argument for use of hormone replacement therapy for osteoporosis, although this therapy by itself will have little impact for an older woman unless cardiovascular risk factors are present, because the benefit for the latter has been shown to be short-term. The use of hormone replacement therapy for prevention of cardiovascular risk is beneficial at any age. For the older woman with osteoporosis risk factors and no cardiovascular risk factors, modification of osteoporosis risk factors may be all that is necessary, including cessation of smoking and drinking, consumption of extra calcium and vitamin D, and regular exercise. The presence of a uterus when hormone replacement therapy is used necessitates an understanding of the risk of endometrial cancer; the need for follow-up if prolonged, unexpected, or heavier than usual bleeding occurs; and the fact that the patient may have a regular period.

Other drugs that may be beneficial in the treatment of osteoporosis for the patient who has relative or absolute contraindications to hormone replacement therapy include calcitonin, sodium fluoride, and biphosphonates (Beck, 1991-1992; Hazzard et al., 1994). Calcitonin has to be given parenterally (subcutaneously) 3 times per week, and has the added disadvantage of being expensive. Sodium fluoride, considered an experimental agent, has been shown to increase bone formation, but with increased risk of fracture because the bone that is formed is more brittle. Etidronate, a biphosphonate, has been shown to be effective for the prevention of recurrent vertebral compression fractures in older women with osteoporosis when used cyclically in combination with calcium (*The Complete Drug Reference,* 1992). Disadvantages include cost and side effects, including, most commonly, diarrhea and nausea (*The Complete Drug Reference,* 1992). Sodium alendronate has recently been approved for primary prevention of postmenopausal osteoporosis. It has been shown to significantly decrease the risk of vertebral and other fractures when used over a 3-year period. Common side effects include abdominal and musculoskeletal pain, acid reflux, dyspepsia, esophageal ulcer, vomiting, abdominal distention, and gastritis in 1% to 3% of patients.

■ Drugs That Cause Anorexia

In the evaluation of causes of anorexia in older adults, review of the patient's drug list with prompt removal of the suspected offending agent is a simple but expedient method of resolving the problem before instituting a potentially unnecessary extensive workup to rule out organic causes such as malignancy, dementia, and depression. Drugs known to cause anorexia include digoxin, procainamide, thyroxin, theophylline, nitrofurantoin, and the selective serotonin reuptake inhibitors (Thompson & Morris, 1991).

Inappropriately high doses of thyroxin may also cause agitation, insomnia, unexpected weight loss, tachycardia, arrhythmias, and premature osteoporosis (*The Complete Drug Reference,* 1992; *Physicians Desk Reference,* 1995). Theophylline may also precipitate anxiety, arrhythmias, postural hypotension, nausea, insomnia, and even seizures (*The Complete Drug Reference,* 1992; Hazzard et al., 1994). Because of these side effects, higher incidence of comorbid disease, and concomitant use of other drugs, theophylline is more difficult to use in older patients. The use of theophylline and fluoroqui-

nolones together can cause a severe adverse drug reaction that includes seizures, agitation, confusion, nausea, and vomiting, because of possible doubling of the theophylline concentration (Grasela & Dreis, 1992). For these reasons, if theophylline is to be used at all, a dose in the lower therapeutic range is appropriate (Hazzard et al., 1994). It is also prudent to use theophylline for selected instances of wheezing and for the treatment of asthma; the beta-agonist drugs, oral or inhaled, are the first line of treatment for chronic lung disease (Hazzard et al., 1994).

Drugs such as cotrimoxazole, tetracyclines, and nitrofurantoin should be avoided in the advanced elderly and in patients with renal dysfunction, and used with caution in older patients in general because of these drugs' dependence on renal excretion (Sanderson, 1990). Long-term administration of tetracyclines may cause staining of the teeth and skin, photosensitivity of the skin, diarrhea, or stomach cramping. Tetracyclines also will chelate with other drugs taken orally—including antacids, iron preparations, laxatives, and calcium supplements—preventing absorption (*The Complete Drug Reference,* 1992).

■ Drugs for Health Maintenance, Disease Prevention, and General Prophylaxis, Minerals, Vitamins, and Antioxidants

Because of the greater risk of malnutrition secondary to multiple diseases, limited income, social isolation, or dental problems, patients 62 years of age or older should be prescribed a general multiple vitamin. Recent advertisements on television, on the radio, and in newspapers and periodicals encourage megadoses of specific vitamins—A, C, and E—to prevent premature aging, especially with case control studies indicating that vitamins A and C may reduce the incidence of heart disease and stroke (Gale et al., 1995; Riemersma et al., 1991). A popular theory of aging involves the production of free ionizing and chemical radical formation, which causes damage to the DNA and RNA responsible for the production of proteins and enzymes and for cell function (Kristal & Yu, 1992). These vitamins may function as scavengers against free radicals, or antioxidants, preventing the aging process, and have been shown to increase cell-mediated immunity in older adults (Penn et al., 1991). Although popular among older adults, the use of specific vitamin and health food supplements should be discouraged until the results of clinical trials prove their effectiveness. Rather than a deficiency of vitamins, a more common problem among community-dwelling older adults is hypervitaminosis (Beck, 1991-1992). The fat-soluble vitamins, A, D, E, and K, accumulate in fat tissue with continued use, leading to vague and nonspecific but toxic symptoms that may be difficult to recognize. Specifically, megadoses of vitamin C can cause gastrointestinal irritability, a false negative result on fecal occult testing, renal stones, and rebound scurvy. Megadoses of vitamin A can cause malaise, liver dysfunction, headache, hypercalcemia, and leukopenia (Beck, 1991-1992). Specific indications include the following: vitamin B_{12} for dementia, pernicious anemia, or malabsorption syndromes; vitamin C for pressure ulcers and for skin healing from incisions; vitamin D and calcium for osteomalacia and osteoporosis; vitamin K for bleeding problems; thiamine for chronic alcohol abuse; and folic acid supplementation for patients on phenytoin (phenytoin inhibits the production of folic acid) (Hazzard et al., 1994; Yao et al., 1992).

The need for supplemental iron therapy in older patients for nonspecific chronic anemia should be thoroughly investigated before use. Older adults, in general, tend to have a greater frequency of normal or increased tissue iron stores because of the high frequency of chronic diseases that cause iron-deficient erythropoiesis (Beck, 1991-1992). Side effects of oral iron therapy include constipation, black stools, hemosiderosis, and browning of the skin and teeth (*The Complete Drug Reference*, 1992). The diagnosis of a microcytic hypochromic anemia re-lated to iron deficiency in older adults should always be distinguished from the diagnosis of this anemia related to other common causes such as malignancies and acute or chronic inflammatory diseases, both of which also manifest themselves with a microcytic hypochromic anemia. Blood studies such as those measuring serum iron, ferritin level, transferrin level, and total iron binding capacity can easily distinguish between anemia secondary to iron deficiency and that secondary to other disease states (Damon, 1992).

Erythropoietin is one of the first of the new biotechnology drugs being used to treat anemias secondary to chronic disease. By stimulating the production of erythropoietin, the drug has been shown to increase mean hemoglobin levels and improve quality of life. It is indicated in patients with chronic renal failure and for rheumatoid arthritis; it also has been used to treat patients with chronic anemia secondary to human immunodeficiency virus (HIV) disease. It is a relatively safe drug, with little associated risk of anaphylactic reactions. There are no contraindications to its use in older adults. Because of its tendency to cause volume expansion, and to worsen blood control, it should be monitored in patients with high blood pressure or chronic renal insufficiency (Damon, 1992). When the drug is used, an adequate substrate of iron supplementation should be given for the production of red blood cells.

Aspirin in a dose of 75 mg has been shown to be effective in significantly reducing the incidence of cerebral infarction, fatal myocardial infarction, subsequent risk of stroke, subsequent transient ischemic attack, and death in older patients (average age 66) during a follow-up period of 32 months. These results occurred with an associated nonsignificant increase in hemorrhagic stroke in older patients with a history of transient ischemia attacks, as compared to those given a placebo (Swedish Aspirin Low-Dose Trial [SALT] Collaborative Group, 1991). Aspirin also has been shown to reduce significantly the risk of severe angina, myocardial infarction, and death at 6 and 12 months in older patients (younger than age 70) with non–Q-wave myocardial infarction or unstable angina (Wallentin et al., 1991). Because of its relative safety, a baby aspirin should be a part of every older patient's medication regimen unless contraindicated by active gastrointestinal bleeding, a history of bleeding diathesis or other blood disorder, or a history of allergy to aspirin. Higher doses of aspirin (325 mg) have been shown to be as effective as warfarin in preventing stroke in patients younger than 75 years of age with a history of nonrheumatic atrial fibrillation, except in patients with risk factors such as a history of hypertension, thromboembolism, or heart failure (Stroke Prevention in Atrial Fibrillation Investigators, 1994). Aspirin has also been shown in a case control study to reduce the risk of colon cancer (Thun et al., 1991).

Heparin, in a low dosage (5000 units twice daily), may be more effective than aspirin in preventing deep venous thrombosis and subsequent fetal or nonfetal pulmonary embolus and death in older patients who are temporarily immobile for an acute illness, for a history of deep venous thrombosis or pulmonary embolus, for obesity, for a history of congestive heart failure, or for chronic venous insufficiency (Beck, 1991-1992). This regimen is also recommended for general postoperative prophylaxis other than for patients undergoing surgery for malignancies, repair of femoral or hip fracture, or lower extremity joint replacement. In these instances, a regimen of subcutaneous heparin 3 times daily or, preferably, low-dose warfarin (coumadin) starting on the day of surgery and continuing for up to 10 weeks postoperatively is recommended, because these patients are at greater risk for deep venous thrombosis and embolization. However, to prevent significant bleeding, the prothrombin bleeding time (INR) should be adjusted to between 1.2 and 1.5. A newer regimen using enoxaparin, a low–molecular weight heparin, twice daily in a dose of 5000 units is equally effective for the prevention of deep vein thrombosis after hip replacement (*Physicians Desk Reference,* 1995).

Whether to use warfarin or aspirin in an older patient is often a difficult question. Issues that should be factored into decision making include compliance, risk of falling, associated medical conditions, economic issues, and cognitive dysfunction, weighing overall risk against benefit to the individual patient. A patient with significant cognitive dysfunction may not be an ideal candidate for warfarin because the patient may ultimately take too much in a single dose, which might lead to either increased risk of bleeding or insufficient amount in a subsequent dose to achieve a desired effect. The availability of a willing and able caregiver or interested party to administer the medication on a regular basis can resolve this issue. Pill administration vehicles may also be of benefit. In addition, communication and understanding of the need for regular monitoring of the bleeding time, physician and laboratory costs involved, availability of transportation, and distance of the patient from the medical facility are essential components in the decision. The wrong value for any of these factors will make the use of warfarin impractical. Associated medical conditions such as liver disease, malabsorption syndrome, cognitive dysfunction, and malignancy may predispose the patient to a greater risk of adverse drug (disease-drug) reactions when using warfarin because of its protein-binding properties. The presence of other chronic medical conditions necessitating the use of other medications may increase the risk of drug-drug reactions. Finally, a patient at increased risk for falls secondary to mobility problems, arthritis, neurologic disease, or specific drug therapy may be a less than optimal candidate for warfarin because of the increased risk of bleeding secondary to trauma.

Ticlopidine is a platelet aggregation inhibitor. It is indicated for the prevention of thrombotic stroke in patients with a history of transient ischemic attack who have not responded to aspirin therapy or who are intolerant to aspirin (allergy or previous bleeding). In patients with reductions in creatinine clearance (50 to 80 ml/min), there has been no significant difference in clinical effects of the drug. The drug has the potential for causing neutropenia, which is usually reversible but can be life threatening in severe cases, in less than 2% of patients. Because of this, patients who are candidates for ticlopidine therapy should have a neutrophil count taken before starting treatment, and every 2 weeks for the first 3 months of therapy. Ticlopidine becomes 50% effective within 4 days of starting treatment and 60% to 70% effective in 10 to 11 days. It is contraindicated in patients who are hypersensitive to it, or in patients with a history of hematopoietic disorders, severe liver impairment, or active intracranial or peptic ulcer (*Physicians Desk Reference,* 1995).

Influenza vaccine should be given yearly, usually between October and December, to all older adults except for those with a history of egg allergy, because 90% of deaths caused by influenza epidemics occur in patients over the age of 64. If influenza develops in a long-term care institution, patients who have not been vaccinated or those allergic to the vaccine may be prophylactically treated with amantadine in a dose of 100 mg per day until the infection resolves. When the vaccine is given in high doses, common side effects include confusion, irritability, headache, rash, lethargy, nausea, and fluid retention; rare side effects include seizures (*The Complete Drug Reference,* 1992). The drug can shorten the duration and lessen the severity of influenza type A if started early in the course of the infection, but is not effective against influenza type B (Beck, 1991-1992). Pneumonia vaccine should be administered to all older patients at least once, and some geriatricians advocate a repeat vaccination after 6 years for those at high risk for pneumococcal pneumonia, such as asplenic patients (Beck, 1991-1992). Patients who have received the older 18 polyvalent strain do not need a repeat injection. Even though older patients have the greatest need for these vaccinations, studies indicate that they often develop an inadequate antibody response to these agents because of their blunted immune responses. Diphtheria tetanus prophylaxis is often ignored in older adults, but recent studies indicate that only about 20% of older adults have adequate antibody levels. Patients especially at risk include diabetic patients with chronic foot ulcers and nursing home or homebound older adults with chronic pressure ulcers. Many older adults were not exposed to childhood tetanus vaccinations because this program had not yet been initiated in their youth. Any older patient who has not had a vaccination should receive three separate injections of diphtheria tetanus vaccination—initially, at 6 weeks, and then at 1 year from the time of the initial vaccine (Beck, 1991-1992; Gergen et al., 1995; Holt, 1992).

Older patients with a recent conversion to positive tuberculin skin testing should be treated with isoniazid—300 mg per day for 6 months—because studies of the drug indicate that it provides a high degree of protection (69%) against conversion from tuberculous infection to disease. Patients with a history of positive skin testing of unknown duration should not be treated with this drug because of the risk of morbidity and subsequent death in older patients who develop isoniazid-induced hepatitis. Patients taking the drug should have liver function tests performed monthly to monitor for the development of this adverse reaction (*Core Curriculum on Tuberculosis,* 1994). The drug should be administered with vitamin B_6 (pyridoxine), because the drug interferes with the metabolism of this vitamin.

STEROIDS

Oral corticosteroid use in the older patient population should be a last resort for specific indications and after conventional therapy has failed, because of the side effects that occur after prolonged use. These include dependence, weight gain, masking of infection, fluid retention, worsening or precipitation of hypertension, diabetes, cataracts, and osteoporosis. Steroids serve no purpose for the treatment of uncomplicated osteoarthritis and should be reserved for severe cases of rheumatoid arthritis. Steroids may be very beneficial for the treatment of asthma resistant to conventional therapy, and for initial treatment of certain dermatoses, polymyalgia rheumatica, and temporal arteritis (Beck, 1991-1992). Inhaled steroids are as effective as oral steroids for the treatment of chronic lung conditions without producing the systemic side effects seen with oral administration (Beck, 1991-1992).

LAXATIVES

The long-term use of stimulant laxatives (cascara, bisacodyl, senna) should be discouraged in older adults because of these drugs' tendency to produce a chemical deinnervation of the autonomic nerves as they detach from the mucosa of the large colon after many years of frequent use (Cefalu & Pike, 1981). This may subsequently lead to the development of a chronic, nondilating megacolon syndrome, resulting in worsening constipation and even fecal impaction when the patient becomes immobile. Non–systemically acting and bulk laxative agents (stool softener, psyllium) are the preferred agents for the treatment of constipation (*The Complete Drug Reference,* 1992). Prune juice serves an excellent purpose as a natural mild cathartic without long-term sequelae. Additional measures that should be used in conjunction with these agents include regular exercise, added fiber in the diet in the form of bran, fruits, and vegetables, and extra fluid intake (Beck, 1991-1992). An excellent laxative regimen for the patient with gastrointestinal symptoms of hyperacidity could include an inexpensive antacid containing liquid magnesium. Because these agents tend to cause diarrhea, patients should be advised that the frequency of bowel movements depends on a variety of factors, including associated medical conditions.

What may be "abnormal" for one patient may be "normal" for another. In addition to discouraging frequent laxative use, drugs known to cause constipation, including narcotics, anticholinergic agents, antispasmodics, antihistamines, and major tranquilizers, should be identified and discontinued if possible (Cefalu & Pike, 1981).

MISCELLANEOUS DRUGS

Certain groups of drugs deserve special mention as being inappropriate and in some instances having no specific indications. Dipyridamole is an old drug that has been popular for the treatment of vascular problems by decreasing platelet "stickiness" and preventing stroke or myocardial infarction. It has not been shown to be superior to aspirin alone for the treatment of cerebral or coronary artery disease, nor in maintaining the patency of autologous grafts. It is an inappropriate drug for use in older adults (Willcox et al., 1994).

Muscle relaxers can cause sedation, lethargy, confusion, and cognitive dysfunction and should be avoided in older adults if possible (Willcox et al., 1994). The need for a "short-acting" muscle relaxer can best be served by the use of a short-acting benzodiazepine such as lorazepam, administered in a dosage of 0.5 to 1 mg every 8 hours, and used in a time-limited fashion.

Chlorpropamide, a long-acting agent used for treatment of type II diabetes, is very potent and has been popular in the past. However, this agent has a half-life of 48 to 72 hours in some cases, and carries a high risk of causing prolonged hypoglycemia, especially in patients with reduced appetite or cognitive dysfunction. It is generally considered an inappropriate drug for use in older adults and should be reserved for cases of diabetes complicated with diabetes insipidus (Willcox et al., 1994).

Oxybutin, an older drug with smooth muscle and anticholinergic properties, has traditionally been used to treat detrusa hyperreflexia associated with temporary or chronic urge incontinence in older patients. A recent study, however, indicates that it is only effective in selected patients who have not responded to prompted voiding (Ouslander et al., 1995). Phenazopyridine is an old drug that may be useful for treating the uncomfortable symptoms of urinary tract infection initially (48 to 72 hours), until the antibiotic can become effective. It stains the urine a dark orange (*The Complete Drug Reference,* 1992).

Quinine is another old drug that has been used traditionally for the treatment of nonspecific, nocturnal leg cramps. A recent meta-analysis of five clinical trials using doses from 200 to 500 mg indicated that quinine reduces the frequency but not the severity or duration of leg cramps (Man-Sons-Hing & Wells, 1995).

Older patients may have intractable anorexia and weight loss, especially in association with a worsening dementia process or cancer. Cyproheptadine is a serotonin- and histamine-blocking agent that may be effective in these patients by stimulating central appetite centers (Beck, 1991-1992).

■ "Cold" and OTC Pain Medications

Older patients frequently seek advice about prescription and over-the-counter cold and cough medications. These agents will usually have an antihistamine and/or decongestant component. In general they should be avoided, especially in the presence of any medical illness that might contraindicate their use. Decongestants relieve nasal stuffiness, whereas antihistamines "dry up" bothersome watery secretions. Decongestants should be avoided for conditions such as anxiety and panic disorder, arrhythmias, and congestive heart failure. Recent studies indicate, however, that these agents do not interfere with blood pressure control in patients with hypertension (Coates et al., 1995). In addition, though studies in older patients are lacking, the use of OTC decongestant-antihistamine preparations has not been shown to improve symptoms in children (Hutton et al., 1991). Patients with chronic nasal or allergic rhinitis or stuffiness should be in-

structed to use simple, normal saline nasal spray 3 to 4 times daily to loosen secretions. If this remedy is insufficient, and if infection has been treated, topical steroid sprays combined with normal saltwater sprays are available by prescription to relieve symptoms, as a safer alternative to decongestants or antihistamines.

Many older patients take over-the-counter analgesics for pain relief. These drugs often contain caffeine, which may be responsible for chronic symptoms of insomnia, especially if the drug is taken before bedtime (Brown et al., 1995).

■ Chronic Pain Control

Chronic pain is often the rule rather than the exception in older patients burdened by multiple chronic diseases, especially secondary to arthritis and malignancy. For these patients, the intensity and chronicity of perceived pain may produce or aggravate depressive symptoms. The latter can be a common symptom complex in older patients because of the loss of independence that occurs secondary to mobility problems; multiple sensory deficits in hearing, vision, taste, and smell; social isolation; institutionalization; and other losses including family, friends, money, and personal possessions (Parmelee et al., 1991).

Relieving chronic pain for an older patient in a pharmacologically safe and effective manner requires that certain principles be followed. These include (1) avoiding high-risk drug administration that may increase the risk of adverse drug reactions and side effects; (2) avoiding use of "as needed" medications for pain relief; (3) using the oral route of administration and reserving parenteral treatment for patients with alimentary dysfunction; (4) remembering that dependence should not be a concern and tolerance is a minimal problem; (5) starting with the simplest and safest drug available and switching to other categories as necessary; (6) always providing support for the patient in the form of counseling, both informally from family, friends, and clergy, and formally from social workers and psychologists as necessary; (7) never abandoning the patient so that he or she feels alone or isolated; and (8) providing pharmacologic support for symptoms of depression (Patt, 1992; Rhymes, 1991).

Regarding specific drug therapy: Acetaminophen given around the clock starting in a dose of 5 to 10 grains every 4 to 6 hours is often effective initially in providing pain relief secondary to arthritis. Patients with chronic pain and associated depressive symptoms will often have associated insomnia and anorexia (Parmelee et al., 1991). In these cases, 25 to 50 mg of amitriptyline may be effective because of its sedating side effects and appetite stimulation properties. Trazodone, starting in a dose of 25 to 50 mg at bedtime, is an alternative antidepressant for the patient with Alzheimer's dementia that avoids the anticholinergic side effects of amitriptyline. If acetaminophen is not effective, propoxyphene and acetaminophen (*The Complete Drug Reference*, 1992), a narcotic antagonist, may be more effective without the side effect profile of nonsteroidal anti-inflammatory drugs or narcotics.

For patients with the chronic pain of bone metastasis from a terminal malignancy, nonsteroidal anti-inflammatory drugs are particularly useful, but increasing the dose creates a "ceiling effect" after which the patient gets no further relief from pain (Rhymes, 1991). Steroids may also be effective for the relief of this type of pain (Rhymes, 1991). The around-the-clock use of a narcotic such as codeine, with judicial use of laxatives, stool softeners, and phenothiazines to alleviate the side effects and potentiate the effect of the narcotic, including relief of nausea, is the next step in relieving this type of pain. If this regimen is not effective, fentanyl patches with half-lives of 72 hours or morphine infusion pumps delivering a constant infusion with steady serum levels provide better relief (Patt, 1992; Rhymes, 1991). Meperidine and meperidine-like preparations, given orally or parenterally, with their short half-lives, have the disadvantage of causing breakthrough pain and provide no added benefit over the use of morphine derivatives (*The Complete Drug Reference,* 1992). If meperidine is used for acute pain, a dose of no more than 25 mg, used in combination with an equal dose of a phenothiazine antiemetic (promethazine), may be effective. Higher doses may induce anticholinergic delirium.

■ Drug Compliance

Compliance with drug regimens is a significant problem in older adults, more so than in other age groups, because of a host of factors including the following: (1) multiplicity of disease requiring multiple medications, often obtained through multiple pharmacies, all of which may cause confusion for the patient; (2) cognitive dysfunction with associated memory loss and subsequent failure to take medication appropriately, leading to exacerbation of disease (too low a dose) or to excessive medication in some instances (too high a dose), leading to toxicity; (3) restricted income and inability to pay for medication, leading to exacerbation of disease; (4) difficulty with complying with office or hospital visits or with obtaining medication from the pharmacist promptly—or at all, in some cases—because of mobility problems or transportation problems for the patient; (5) visual problems that may increase the frequency of inappropriate medication or dosing, leading to adverse drug reactions; and (6) medical diseases—such as stroke, Parkinson's disease, cervical stenosis, dementia, and arthritis—that may interfere with fine and gross coordination of the upper extremities necessary for medication administration.

For the older patient, the nurse can enhance drug compliance in the following general ways: (1) educating the patient and/or family about the purpose of the medication and potential side effects; (2) educating the patient and/or family about the disease process and signs or symptoms of worsening disease; (3) asking the patient and/or family to bring all prescription and over-the-counter medications for each clinic or hospital visit for reevaluation; (4) assigning key family members or friends to assist the patient in securing needed medication from the pharmacy and clinic in a timely fashion; (5) asking family or friends, when available, to assist in or monitor medication administration for the older patient with visual, coordination, or cognitive problems; (6) using pill administration boxes that can be refilled weekly by the patient, family, or friends; and (7) referring the patient and/or family to social service agencies, home health agencies, senior citizen centers, and volunteer agencies for securing financial and transportation assistance.

■ Conclusion

Appropriate drug prescribing in older adults requires an understanding of normal changes that occur during the aging process, including reduction of immune defenses, blunting and reduction of receptor sites, loss of physiologic reserve, and physiologic and structural changes in organ systems. These systems include the integumentary system, gastrointestinal system, liver, kidney, and central nervous system. Advancing age is associated with the development of chronic disease, in many cases in multiple fashion, with the need to take more over-the-counter and prescription medications. All of these factors increase the risk of adverse drug reactions. The high incidence of sensory deficits, cognitive dysfunction, mobility problems, transportation difficulty, socioeconomic concerns, and arthritis necessitates extreme caution, and attention to compliance issues as well. All of these points make the topic of drug therapy in older adults much different from that of drug therapy in the general adult population. Table 5-2 summarizes the effects of drug therapy on older adults.

TABLE 5-2 Appropriate and inappropriate drug therapy in older adults

Drug	Appropriate use	Inappropriate use	Special consideration
Antiarrhythmic agents (quinidine, procainamide, flecainide, encainide)	For treatment of complicated arrhythmias	For treatment of routine arrhythmias	Use recommended for complicated cases under cardiologist supervision only
Antibiotics	For systemic symptoms of infected pressure ulcer or indwelling urinary catheter; fever; leukocytosis; hypotension; cellulitis; osteomyelitis; colored sputum	For surface exudate of pressure ulcers; bacteruria and pyuria associated with indwelling urinary catheter; uncomplicated upper respiratory tract infection (viral)	May cause pseudomembranous colitis or promote resistance to antibiotics; adjust doses of penicillins, aminoglycosides, and fluoroquinolones to be consistent with creatinine clearance
Anticholinergic agents (antihistamines, tricyclic antidepressants, phenothiazine tranquilizers, narcotics)	—	—	Minimize or avoid use in patients with benign prostatic hyperplasia, glaucoma, chronic constipation, peripheral vascular disease, chronic bronchitis, or Alzheimer's dementia, or in advanced elderly
Antidizziness agents (meclizine)	For true dizziness	For disequilibrium or presyncopal lightheadedness	Use in low doses; anticholinergic effects may cause or worsen cognitive dysfunction
ANTIHYPERTENSIVE AGENTS			
Alpha-blocker drugs	For hypertension	High doses—may cause postural hypotension or syncope	Dual indication for hypertension and benign prostatic hyperplasia
Beta-blocker drugs	Shorter-acting selective agents—atenolol or metoprolol	Propranolol	For dual indications—angina and high blood pressure or atrial arrhythmias; after myocardial infarction or angina to reduce cardiovascular mortality

Continued

TABLE 5-2 Appropriate and inappropriate drug therapy in older adults—cont'd

Drug	Appropriate use	Inappropriate use	Special consideration
CENTRALLY ACTING DRUGS			
Cold and OTC analgesic agents	See Antihistamines and Decongestants	See Antihistamines and Decongestants	Antihistamine-decongestant combination agents not found to be clinically effective in children
Antihistamines	For drying of excessive secretions	For Alzheimer's patients	See Anticholinergic Agents
Decongestants	For relief of nasal stuffiness	For patients with congestive heart failure, arrhythmias, anxiety disorders	Not found to significantly affect mean blood pressure control in patients with hypertension
Analgesic agents	For pain relief	For patients with anxiety disorders or insomnia	Caffeine a frequent ingredient
DEMENTIA DRUGS			
Hydergine	—	—	Not significantly effective
Tacrine	For mild impairment (Alzheimer's type) for up to 30 weeks	For moderate to severe Alzheimer's disease	Monitor liver function tests monthly while patient is taking drug because of potential liver toxicity
Pentoxifylline	For multi-infarct dementia?	—	Slows cognitive deterioration but not memory loss
Vasodilators	—	Not effective	May cause postural hypotension
DIGOXIN	For congestive heart failure secondary to systolic dysfunction, atrial arrhythmias	Nonspecifically for other cardiac conditions	May cause anorexia, nausea, agitation, confusion; reduce dose according to creatinine clearance

TABLE 5-2 Appropriate and inappropriate drug therapy in older adults—cont'd

Drug	Appropriate use	Inappropriate use	Special consideration
DIURETICS			
Loop diuretics	For treatment of fluid retention secondary to congestive heart failure or renal insufficiency; refractory and severe leg edema secondary to venous stasis or chronic venous insufficiency	For routine treatment of dependent edema or venous stasis secondary to chronic venous insufficiency; for treatment of hypercalcemia; to be used with caution in advanced elderly or older patients with dementia or depression; for treatment of uncomplicated hypertension	May cause contraction alkalosis, postural hypotension, hypokalemia, arrhythmias, increased mortality; causes hypercalciuria
Thiazides	For treatment of mild hypertension alone or in combination with other agents	For routine treatment of dependent edema or venous stasis secondary to chronic venous insufficiency; to be used with caution in advanced elderly or older patients with dementia or depression; doses greater than 50 mg ineffective for hypertension	May cause contraction alkalosis, postural hypotension, hypokalemia, arrhythmias, increased mortality; prevents loss of calcium in urine; may have secondary benefit in retarding osteoporosis
GASTROINTESTINAL AGENTS			
H₂ blocker drugs	For treatment or prevention of peptic ulcer disease or gastroesophageal reflux	Prophylactically to prevent NSAID-induced gastric or duodenal bleeding; as prophylaxis to prevent bleeding secondary to stress-induced gastritis in intensive care unit patients	Increases risk of aspiration pneumonia in bed-bound patients with swallowing abnormalities; indicated for prophylaxis against stress-induced gastritis for intensive care unit patients with a history of respiratory failure or bleeding disorders
Proton pump inhibitors (omeprazole, lansoprazole)	For severe or intractable gastrointestinal reflux disease	For treatment of uncomplicated peptic ulcer disease	Expensive; approved for short-term (4- to 8-week) use only

Continued

TABLE 5-2 Appropriate and inappropriate drug therapy in older adults—cont'd

Drug	Appropriate use	Inappropriate use	Special consideration
Smooth muscle relaxers (metoclopramide, cisapride)	For gastrointestinal reflux disease—for diabetic gastroparesis, prevention of nausea and vomiting postoperatively or secondary to chemotherapy, and (metoclopramide only) implementation procedures	For gastric emptying for gastrostomy patients	Less central nervous system sedation with cisapride
Sucralfate	For treatment or prevention of peptic ulcer disease	Prophylactically to prevent NSAID-induced gastric or duodenal bleeding; as prophylaxis to prevent bleeding secondary to stress-induced gastritis in intensive care unit patients	Increases risk of aspiration pneumonia in bed-bound patients with swallowing abnormalities, indicated for prophylaxis against stress-induced gastritis for intensive care unit patients with a history of respiratory failure or bleeding disorders
HYPOLIPIDEMIC AGENTS			
Hypocholesterolemic drugs	For patients with significant history of heart disease or cardiovascular risk factors	For population-based treatment of hypercholesterolemia to prevent cardiovascular mortality	HMG-CoA reductase agents used with niacin, gemfibrozil, or cyclosporine may cause rhabdomyolysis and renal failure; need to monitor liver function tests when using HMG-CoA reductase (statin) agents; HMG-CoA agents more expensive; probucol can worsen cardiac conduction abnormalities; clofibrate may increase the incidence of cholelithiasis, subsequent morbidity, and death from surgery; gemfibrozil and clofibrate may increase risk of bleeding when used with anticoagulants

TABLE 5-2 Appropriate and inappropriate drug therapy in older adults—cont'd

Drug	Appropriate use	Inappropriate use	Special consideration
Hypotriglyceridemic drugs	For patients in whom diet has failed; triglyceride levels between 1000 and 2000 mg/100 ml; pancreatitis, recurrent abdominal pain resembling pancreatitis	—	See Hypocholesterolemic Drugs
MISCELLANEOUS DRUGS			
Chlorpropamide	—	Long-acting (half-life 48 to 72 hours), potent chlorpropamide	Use only in patients with diabetes mellitus and diabetes insipidus
Dipyridamole	—	—	Not shown to be superior to aspirin for vascular disease or for autologous grafts
Meperidine	For acute pain—in low doses (25 mg)	For chronic pain	Short half-life
Muscle relaxers	—	—	May cause sedation, lethargy, cognitive dysfunction, postural hypotension, falls
Oxybutin	—	—	Only effective in selected patients who have not responded to prompted voiding
Quinine	For leg cramps—meta-analysis indicates it reduces the frequency but not the duration or severity	—	—

Continued

TABLE 5-2 Appropriate and inappropriate drug therapy in older adults—cont'd

Drug	Appropriate use	Inappropriate use	Special consideration
Nonsteroidal anti-inflammatory drugs	As needed, in lowest possible dose, for acute "flare-ups of arthritis" for 5 to 7 days	Indomethacin; frequent use of NSAIDs; for active bleeding	May cause or worsen hypertension, congestive heart failure, renal insufficiency, hepatitis; high doses associated with acute confusion and cognitive dysfunction, especially indomethacin; monitor hemogram and renal function with frequent use; acetaminophen as effective for osteoarthritis
PSYCHOTROPIC DRUGS			
Antidepressants	For treatment of depressive symptoms	For nonspecific treatment of insomnia or agitation; amitriptyline, in most cases	SSRIs can worsen appetite, insomnia, anxiety, and weight loss in frail older patients or patients with dementia or depression; high doses of tricyclic agents can cause or worsen cognitive dysfunction, precipitate postural hypotension and falls; properly document need for drug; reduce dose of drug when possible
Hypnotics	Occasional use for sleep	Regular use for sleep	Can cause sedation, cognitive dysfunction, falls
Major (phenothiazine) tranquilizers	For psychotic behavior; hallucinations or delusions that are troublesome for patient; aggressive, hostile, combative behavior in dementia patients	For nonspecific diagnosis of dementia	May cause or worsen cognitive dysfunction, functional decline, postural hypotension, falls; parkinsonian side effects and risk of tardive dyskinesia; reduce dose and discontinue drug when possible; properly document need for drug

TABLE 5-2 Appropriate and inappropriate drug therapy in older adults—cont'd

Drug	Appropriate use	Inappropriate use	Special consideration
Minor (benzodiazepine) tranquilizers	For anxiety that is troublesome for patients	Nonspecific use for sleep	Reduce dose and discontinue when possible; avoid as-needed use; properly document need for drug
Barbiturates	For seizure disorder	For nonspecific treatment of insomnia or anxiety	Monitor drug levels; properly document need for drug; may cause or worsen cognitive dysfunction, postural hypotension, falls
Theophylline	For acute wheezing or a diagnosis of asthma	For routine treatment of chronic obstructive lung disease	Can cause postural hypotension, nausea, anorexia, weight loss, arrhythmias, anxiety, insomnia
VITAMINS AND PROPHYLACTIC AGENTS			
Aspirin (75 mg)	Daily for all patients older than 62 years	For active gastrointestinal bleeding or history of bleeding diathesis or other blood disorders, allergy to aspirin	—
Aspirin (325 mg)	For patients with a history of stroke	For active gastrointestinal bleeding or history of bleeding diathesis or other blood disorders, allergy to aspirin	—
Iron supplements	For proven iron deficiency	For nonspecific treatment of microcytic hypochromic anemia	—
Vitamins (antioxidant)	For deficiency states only	For prophylaxis against premature aging	—
Vitamins (multiple)	For all patients older than 62 years		—

135

REFERENCES

Akiyama, T., et al. (1992). Effects of advancing age on the efficacy and side-effects of antiarrhythmic drugs in post-myocardial infarction patients with ventricular arrhythmias. *Journal of the American Geriatrics Society, 40,* 666-672.

Baloh, R.W. (1992). Dizziness in older people. *Journal of the American Geriatrics Society, 40,* 713-721.

Beck, J.C. (1991-1992). *Geriatric review syllabus—A core curriculum in geriatric medicine.* New York: American Geriatrics Society.

Berggren, D., et al. (1987). Postoperative confusion after anesthesia in elderly patients with femoral neck fractures. *Anesthesia and Analgesia, 66,* 497.

Bixler, E.O., et al. (1991). Next-day memory impairment with triazolam use. *Lancet, 337,* 827-831.

Bjorck, S., et al. (1992). Renal protective effect of enalapril in diabetic nephropathy. *British Medical Journal, 304,* 339-343.

Black, R.S., et al. (1992). Pentoxifylline in cerebrovascular dementia. *Journal of the American Geriatrics Society, 40,* 237-244.

Bradley, J.D., et al. (1991). Comparison of an anti-inflammatory dose of ibuprofen, an analgesic dose of ibuprofen, and acetaminophen in the treatment of patients with osteoarthritis of the knee. *New England Journal of Medicine, 325,* 87-91.

Braunwald, E. (1991). Ace inhibitors—A cornerstone of the treatment of heart failure. *New England Journal of Medicine, 325,* 351-353.

Brown, et al. (1995). Occult caffeine as a source of sleep problems in an older population. *Journal of the American Geriatrics Society, 43,* 860-864.

Buckler, D.A., Kelber, S.T., & Goodwin, J.S. (1994). The use of dietary restrictions in malnourished nursing home patients. *Journal of the American Geriatrics Society, 42,* 1100-1102.

Buring, J.E., et al. (1995). Calcium channel blockers and myocardial infarction: A hypothesis formulated but not yet tested. *Journal of the American Medical Association, 274,* 654-655.

Cahill, L., et al. (1994). Beta-adrenergic activation and memory for emotional events. *Nature, 371,* 702-704.

Calkins, E., Ford, A.B., & Katz, P.R. (1992). *Practice of geriatrics* (2nd ed.). Philadelphia: W.B. Saunders.

Cefalu, C.A., & Pike, J. (1981, May). Fecal impaction—A practical approach to the problem. *Geriatrics,* 143-145.

Coates, M.L., et al. (1995). Does pseudoephedrine increase blood pressure in patients with controlled hypertension? *Journal of Family Practice, 40,* 22-26.

Cohn, J.N., et al. (1991). A comparison of enalapril with hydralazine-isosorbide dinitrate in the treatment of chronic congestive heart failure. *New England Journal of Medicine, 325,* 303-310.

Colditz, G.A., et al. (1995). The use of estrogens and progestins and the risk of breast cancer in postmenopausal women. *New England Journal of Medicine, 332,* 1589-1593.

Colenda, C.C. (1991). Drug treatment of behavior problems in elderly patients with dementia: Part I. *Drug Therapy,* 15-20.

The Complete Drug Reference, (1992). New York: United States Pharmacopeia.

Cook, D.J., et al. (1994). Risk factors for gastrointestinal bleeding in critically ill patients. *New England Journal of Medicine, 10*(330), 377-381.

Coplen, et al. (1990). Efficacy and safety of quinidine therapy for maintenance of sinus rhythm after cardioversion. *Circulation, 82,* 1106-1116.

Core curriculum on tuberculosis—What the clinician should know (3rd ed.). (1994). U.S. Department of Health and Human Services.

Culter, A.F., et al. (1995). Accuracy of invasive and non-invasive tests to diagnose helicobacter pylori infection. *Gastroenterology, 109,* 136-141.

Cummings, S.R., et al. (1995). Risk factors for hip fracture in white women. *New England Journal of Medicine, 23* (332), 767-773.

Daly, E., et al. (1993). Measuring the impact of menopausal symptoms on quality of life. *British Medical Journal, 307,* 836-840.

Damon, L.E. (1992). Anemias of chronic disease in the aged: Diagnosis and treatment. *Geriatrics, 47,* 47-57.

Finucane, F.F., et al. (1993). Decreased risk of stroke among postmenopausal hormone users: Results from a national cohort. *Archives of Internal Medicine, 153,* 73-79.

Fogelman, L. (1991). Viewpoint: Oestrogen, the prevention of bone loss and osteoporosis. *British Journal of Rheumatology, 30,* 276-281.

Furberg, C.D., et al. (1995). Nifedipine: Dose-related increase in mortality in patients with coronary heart disease. *Circulation, 92,* 1326-1331.

Gale, C.R., et al. (1995). Vitamin C and risk of death from stroke and coronary heart disease in cohort of elderly people. *British Medical Journal, 310,* 1563-1566.

Garcia Rodriquez, et al. (1992). The role of non-steroidal anti-inflammatory drugs in acute liver injury. *British Medical Journal, 305,* 865-868.

Gergen, P.J., et al. (1995). A population-based serologic survey of immunity to tetanus in the United States. *New England Journal of Medicine, 332,* 761-766.

Gottlief, S.S., et al. (1992). Renal response to indomethacin in congestive heart failure secondary to ischemic or idiopathic dilated cardiomyopathy. *American Journal of Cardiology, 70,* 890-893.

Graham, D.Y., et al. (1991). Epidemiology of helicobacter pylori in an asymptomatic population in the United States: Effects of age, race, and socio-economic status. *Gastroenterology, 100,* 1495-1501.

Graham, D.Y., et al. (1992). Effect of treatment of helicobacter pylori infection on the long-term recurrence rate of gastric or duodenal ulcer. *Annals of Internal Medicine, 116,* 705-708.

Grasela, T.H., & Dreis, M.W. (1992). An evaluation of the quinolone-theophylline interaction using the Food and Drug Administration spontaneous reporting system. *Archives of Internal Medicine, 152,* 617-621.

Greenblatt, D.J., et al. (1991). Sensitivity to triazolam in the elderly. *New England Journal of Medicine, 324,* 1691-1698.

Griffin, M.R., et al. (1991). Nonsteroidal anti-inflammatory drug use and the increased risk for peptic ulcer disease in elderly persons. *Annals of Internal Medicine, 114,* 257-262.

Grisso, J.A., et al. (1991). Risk factors for falls as a cause of hip fracture in women. *New England Journal of Medicine, 324,* 1326-1331.

Grover, S.A., et al. (1994). Serum lipid screening to identify high-risk individuals for coronary death. *Archives of Internal Medicine, 154,* 679-684.

Gurwitz, J.H., & Avorn, J. (1991, June). The ambiguous relation between aging and adverse reactions. *Annals of Internal Medicine, 114,* 956-966.

Gurwitz, J.H., et al. (1992). Reducing the use of H_2-receptor antagonists in the long-term-care setting. *Journal of the American Geriatrics Society, 40,* 359-364.

Gurwitz, J.H., et al. (1994). Initiation of antihypertensive treatment during non-steroidal anti-inflammatory drug therapy. *Journal of the American Medical Association, 272,* 781-786.

Guthrie, R. (1994). Terazosin in the treatment of hypertension and symptomatic benign prostatic hyperplasia: A primary care trial. *Journal of Family Practice, 39,* 129-133.

Hallstrom, A.P., et al. (1991). An antiarrhythmic drug experience in 941 patients resuscitated from an initial cardiac arrest between 1970 and 1985. *American Journal of Cardiology, 68,* 1025-1031.

Hannedouche, T., et al. (1994). Randomized controlled trial of enalapril and B blockers in non-diabetic chronic renal failure. *British Medical Journal, 309,* 833-837.

Hazzard, W.R., et al. (1994). *Principles of geriatric medicine and gerontology* (3rd ed.). New York: McGraw-Hill.

Hebert, P.R., et al. (1995). An overview of trials of cholesterol lowering and risk of stroke. *Archives of Internal Medicine, 155,* 50-55.

Heidrich, F.E., et al. (1991). Diuretic drug use and the risk for hip fracture. *Annals of Internal Medicine, 115,* 1-6.

Hentschel, E., et al. (1993). Effect of ranitidine and amoxicillin plus metronidazole on the eradication of helicobacter pylori and the recurrence of duodenal ulcer. *New England Journal of Medicine, 328,* 308-312.

Hollenberg, N.K., & Moore, T.J. (1994). Age and the renal blood supply: Renal vascular responses to angiotensin converting enzyme inhibition in healthy humans. *Journal of the American Geriatrics Society, 42,* 805-808.

Holt, D.M. (1992). Recommendations, usage and efficacy of immunizations for the elderly. *Nurse Practitioner, 17,* 51-59.

Hteland, M.L., et al. (1992). One measurement of serum total cholesterol is enough to predict future levels in healthy postmenopausal women. *American Journal of Medicine, 92,* 25-28.

Hutton, N., et al. (1991). Effectiveness of an antihistamine-decongestant combination for young children with the common cold: A randomized, controlled clinical trial. *Journal of Pediatrics, 118,* 125-130.

ISIS-4 Collaborative Group. (1995). ISIS-4: A randomized factorial trial assessing early oral captopril, oral mononitrate, and intravenous magnesium sulphate in 58, 050 patients with suspected acute myocardial infarction. *Lancet, 345,* 669-685.

Jick, S.S., et al. (1995). Antidepressants and suicide. *British Medical Journal, 310,* 215-218.

Jones, A.C., Berman, P., & Doherty, M. (1992). Nonsteroidal anti-inflammatory drug usage and requirement in elderly acute hospital admissions. *British Journal of Rheumatology, 31,* 45-48.

Kalish, S.C., et al. (1995). Antipsychotic prescribing patterns and the treatment of extrapyramidal symptoms in older people. *Journal of the American Geriatrics Society, 43,* 967-973.

Knapp, M.J., et al. (1994). A 30-week randomized controlled trial of high-dose tacrine in patients with Alzheimer's disease. *Journal of the American Medical Association, 271,* 992-998.

Kristal, B.S., & Yu, B.P. (1992). An emerging hypothesis: Synergistic induction of aging by free radical and maillard reactions. *Journal of Gerontology: Biological Science, 47,* B107-B114.

Kristiansen, I.S., et al. (1991). Cost-effectiveness of incremental programmes for lowering serum cholesterol concentration: Is individual intervention worth while? *British Medical Journal, 302,* 1119-1122.

Krumholz, H.M., et al. (1994). Lack of association between cholesterol and coronary heart disease mortality and morbidity and all-cause mortality in persons older than 70 years. *Journal of the American Medical Association, 272,* 1335-1340.

Langman, M.J.S., et al. (1994). Risks of bleeding peptic ulcer associated with individual non-steroidal anti-inflammatory drugs. *Lancet, 343,* 1075-1078.

Lesage, J. (1991, June). Polypharmacy in geriatric patients. *Nursing Clinics of North America, 26,* 273-289.

Lessem, J.N., & Weber, M.A. (1993). Antihypertensive treatment with a dual-acting beta-blocker in the elderly. *Journal of Hypertension, 11,* S29-S36.

Levine, J.S. (1995). Misoprostol and non-steroidal anti-inflammatory drugs: A tale of effects, outcomes, and costs. *Annals of Internal Medicine, 123,* 309-310.

Lewis, E.J., et al. (1993). The effect of angiotensin-converting-enzyme inhibition on diabetic nephropathy. *New England Journal of Medicine, 329,* 1456-1462.

Lichstein, E., et al. (1990). Relation between beta-adrenergic blocker use, various correlates of left ventricular function and the chance of developing congestive heart failure. *Journal of the American College of Cardiology, 16,* 1327-1332.

Lindley, C.M., et al. (1992, July). Inappropriate medication is a major cause of adverse drug reactions in elderly patients. *Age and Ageing, 21,* 294-300.

Luchi, R.J., Taffet, G.E., & Teasdale, T.A. (1991). Congestive heart failure in the elderly. *Journal of the American Geriatrics Society, 39,* 810-825.

Mach, J.R., et al. (1995). Serum anticholinergic activity in hospitalized older persons with delirium: A preliminary study. *Journal of the American Geriatrics Society, 43,* 491-495.

Maltby, N., et al. (1994). Efficacy of tacrine and lecithin in mild to moderate Alzheimer's disease: Double blind trial. *British Medical Journal, 308,* 879-883.

Manolio, T.A., et al. (1993). Associations of postmenopausal estrogen use with cardiovascular disease and stroke risk factors in older women. *Circulation, 88,* 2163, 2171.

Man-Sons-Hing, M., & Wells, G. (1995). Meta-analysis of efficacy of quinine for treatment of nocturnal leg cramps in elderly people. *British Medical Journal, 310,* 13-17.

Newbern, V.B. (1991). Cautionary tales on using beta blockers. *Geriatric Nursing,* 119-122.

Oldroyd, K.G., et al. (1991). Effects of early captopril administration on infarct expansion, left ventricular remodeling and exercise capacity after acute myocardial infarction. *American Journal of Cardiology, 68,* 713-718.

O'Riordan, T.G., Tobin, A., & O'Morain, C. (1991). Helicobacter pylori infection in elderly dyspeptic patients. *Age and Ageing, 20,* 189-192.

Ouslander, J.G., et al. (1995). Does oxybutynin add to the effectiveness of prompted voiding for urinary incontinence among nursing home residents? A placebo-controlled trial. *Journal of the American Geriatrics Society, 43,* 610-617.

Park, K.C., Forman, D.E., & Wei, J.Y. (1995). Utility of beta-blockade treatment for older postinfarction patients. *Journal of the American Geriatrics Society, 43,* 751-755.

Parmelee, P.A., Katz, I.R., & Lawton, M.P. (1991). The relation of pain to depression among institutionalized aged. *Journal of Gerontology: Psychological Sciences, 46,* P15-P21.

Patt, R.B. (1992). PCA: Prescribing analgesia for home management of severe pain. *Geriatrics, 47,* 69-84.

Penn, N.D., et al. (1991). The effects of dietary supplementation with vitamins A, C, and E on cell-mediated immune functions in elderly, long-stay patients. *Age and Ageing, 20,* 169-174.

Peura, D.A. (1995). Helicobacter pylori: A diagnostic dilemma and a dilemma of diagnosis. *Gastroenterology, 109,* 313-315.

Physicians Desk Reference. (1995). Montvale, NJ: Medical Economics Data Production.

Pinkowish, M.D. (1995, October). Practical briefings—Clinical news you can put into practice now. *Patient Care,* 16-21.

Prince, R.L. (1991). Prevention of post-menopausal osteoporosis—A comparative study of exercise, calcium supplementation, and hormone-replacement therapy. *New England Journal of Medicine, 325,* 1189-1195.

Psaty, B.M., et al. (1994). The risk of myocardial infarction associated with the combined use of estrogens and progestins in postmenopausal women. *Archives of Internal Medicine, 154,* 1333-1339.

Ray, W.A., et al. (1991). Cyclic antidepressants and the risk of hip fracture. *Archives of Internal Medicine, 151,* 754-756.

Rhymes, J.A. (1991). Clinical management of the terminally ill. *Geriatrics, 46,* 57-67.

Riemersma, R.A., et al. (1991). Risk of angina pectoris and plasma concentrations of vitamins A, C, and E and carotene. *Lancet, 337,* 1-5.

Robinson, D., et al. (1994). Estrogen replacement therapy and memory in older women. *Journal of the American Geriatrics Society, 42,* 919-922.

Rovner, B.W., et al. (1990). Research and reviews—The prevalence and management of dementia and other psychiatric disorders in nursing homes. *International Psychogeriatrics, 2*(13), 22.

Rummans, R.A., et al. (1993). Learning and memory impairment in older, detoxified, benzodiazepine-dependent patients. *Mayo Clinic Proceedings, 68,* 731-737.

Saltz, B.L. (1992). Tardive dyskinesia in the elderly patient. *Hospital Practice, 27,* 167-184.

Saltz, B.L., et al. (1991). Prospective study of tardive dyskinesia incidence in the elderly. *Journal of the American Medical Association, 266,* 2402-2406.

Sanderson, P. (1990). Antibiotics and the elderly. *Practitioner, 234,* 1064-1066.

Scherr, P.A., et al. (1992). Light to moderate alcohol consumption and mortality in the elderly. *Journal of the American Geriatrics Society, 40,* 651-657.

Schuler, G., et al. (1992). Regular physical exercise and low-fat diet: Effects on progression of coronary artery disease. *Circulation, 86,* 1-11.

Shankel, S.W., et al. (1992). Acute renal failure and glomerulopathy caused by non-steroidal anti-inflammatory drugs. *Archives of Internal Medicine, 152,* 986-990.

Sheikh, J. (1995, October). The pharmacological treatment of depression in older patients. *1995 Annual Meeting—Symposia Highlights—American Geriatrics Society,* 6.

Slataper, R., et al. (1993). Comparative effects of different antihypertensive treatments on progression of diabetic renal disease. *Archives of Internal Medicine, 153,* 973-980.

Smith, G.D., et al. (1993). Cholesterol lowering and mortality: The importance of considering initial level of risk. *British Medical Journal, 306,* 1367-1373.

Stampfer, M.J., et al. (1991). Postmenopausal estrogen therapy and cardiovascular disease: Ten year follow-up from the Nurse's Health Study. *New England Journal of Medicine, 325,* 756-762.

Stroke Prevention in Atrial Fibrillation Investigators. (1994). Warfarin versus aspirin for prevention of thromboembolism in atrial fibrillation: Stroke prevention in atrial fibrillation II study. *Lancet, 343,* 687-691.

Swedish Aspirin Low-Dose Trial Collaborative Group. (1991). Swedish aspirin low-dose trial (SALT) of 75 mg aspirin as secondary prophylaxis after cerebrovascular ischemic events. *Lancet, 338,* 1345-1349.

Systolic Hypertension in the Elderly Program Cooperative Research Group. (1991). Prevention of stroke by antihypertensive drug treatment in older persons with isolated systolic hypertension: Final results of the systolic hypertension in the elderly program (SHEP). *Journal of the American Medical Association, 265,* 3255-3264.

Tariot, P.N., et al. (1994). Carbamazepine treatment of agitation in nursing home patients with dementia: A preliminary study. *Journal of the American Geriatrics Society, 42,* 1160-1166.

Tariot, P.N., et al. (1995). Lack of carbamazepine toxicity in frail nursing home patients: A controlled study. *Journal of the American Geriatrics Society, 43,* 1026-1029.

Thiessen, B.Q., et al. (1990). Increased prescribing of antidepressants subsequent to beta-blocker therapy. *Archives of Internal Medicine, 150,* 2286-2290.

Thompson, M.P., & Morris, L.K. (1991). Unexplained weight loss in the ambulatory elderly. *Journal of the American Geriatrics Society, 39,* 497-500.

Thun, M.J., et al. (1991). Aspirin use and reduced risk of fatal colon cancer. *New England Journal of Medicine, 325,* 1593-1596.

Vega, G.L., & Grundy, S.M. (1994). Lipoprotein responses to treatment with lovastatin, gemfibrozil, and nicotinic acid in normolipidemic patients with hypoalphalipoproteinemia. *Archives of Internal Medicine, 154,* 73-82.

Verdery, R.B., & Goldberg, A.P. (1991). Hypocholesterolemia as a predictor of death: A prospective study of 224 nursing home residents. *Journal of Gerontology: Medical Sciences, 46,* M84-M90.

Voight, L.F., et al. (1991). Progesterone supplementation of exogenous estrogens and risk of endometrial cancer. *Lancet, 338,* 274-277.

Wallentin, L.C., et al. (1991). Aspirin (75 mg/day) after an episode of unstable coronary artery disease: Long-term effects on the risk for myocardial infarction, occurrence of severe angina and the need for revascularization. *Journal of the American College of Cardiology, 18,* 1587-1593.

Warram, J.H., et al. (1991). Excess mortality associated with diuretic therapy in diabetes mellitus. *Archives of Internal Medicine, 151,* 1350-1356.

Weinberger, M.H. (1992). Hypertension in the elderly. *Hospital Practice, 27,* 103-120.

Whelan, A.M., et al. (1992). The effect of aspirin on niacin-induced cutaneous reactions. *Journal of Family Practice, 34,* 165-168.

Willcox, S.M., et al. (1994). Inappropriate drug prescribing for the community-dwelling elderly. *Journal of the American Medical Association, 272*(4), 292-295.

Winter, M. (1988). *Basic clinical pharmaco-kinetics* (2nd ed., pp. 13-21). Vancouver, WA: Applied Therapeutics.

Yao, Y., et al. (1992). Prevalence of vitamin B_{12} deficiency among geriatric outpatients. *Journal of Family Practice, 35,* 524-528.

Yassa, R., & Nair, N.P. (1992). A 10 year follow-up study of tardive dyskinesia. *Acta Psychiatrica Scandinavica, 86,* 262-2.

Age is opportunity no less
Than youth itself, though in another dress.
And as the evening twilight fades away
The sky is filled with stars, invisible by day.

HENRY WADSWORTH LONGFELLOW

Sexuality

■ Learning Objectives

On completion of this chapter, the reader will be able to do the following:

1. Describe sexuality as an integral component of the older adult's personality.
2. Identify age-related changes and health deviations that affect sexual function in older adults.
3. Describe demographic, physiologic, and social factors that affect the sexual function of older adults.
4. Discuss older adults' needs for closeness, touch, warmth, and sharing.
5. Conduct a sexual health assessment and formulate nursing diagnoses related to sexual function and sexual integrity of older adults.
6. Identify intervention strategies implemented by nurses to foster older patients' sexual function and sexual integrity.

Sexuality is a complex human characteristic that pervades the whole of an individual's life from birth to death. Every person has sexual feelings, attitudes, and beliefs; yet each person's experience of sexuality is unique because it is realized through a personal perspective.

■ Normal Function

Adult sexual feelings, behavior, and attitudes are influenced by learning and experiences of early childhood. What people learn about physical closeness and touching, and how they come to feel about themselves and others are major deter-minants of adult sexuality. Thus expression as a sexual being is manifested in many ways and is the result of ongoing life experiences. Although it is reasonable to expect considerable continuity over the adult life span in the expression of sexuality, new meanings may emerge as one's life situation changes.

Sexuality encompasses the biologic, psychologic, social, cultural, and spiritual aspects of sexual feelings and expression. It designates one's identity as a sexual being: the experience of maleness or femaleness; the way a person dresses, moves, speaks, and relates to others. It includes the needs for love, warmth, sharing, closeness, intimacy, sensuality, touching, and being touched.

Healthy expression of sexuality, described as sexual integrity, is promoted by the person's acceptance and comfortable recognition of himself or herself as a sexual being (McFarlane & Rubenfeld, 1983). Sexual integrity implies an integration of the physical, intrapersonal, social, cultural, and spiritual self in ways that are enriching and that enhance personality, communication, and love. Sexual integrity is individually defined as an optimal concept of self with the ability to carry out the usual sex role activities.

Sexual expression may include both genital and nongenital activities, with verbal and nonverbal expression of sexuality (Shippee-Rice, 1990). The genital (intercourse) sexual response usually consists of four stages: excitation, plateau, orgasm, and resolution. Sexual expression is essential to the human experience; for some people, age may alter certain aspects of sexual expression, but age does not affect the personal enrichment that comes from the affirmation of a sense of self as a sexual and vital person.

■ Age-Related Changes Affecting Sexuality

PHYSICAL CHANGES

Most of the published work in the area of sexuality and aging suggests that there are no known age limits to sexual activity and that there is nothing in the biology of aging that automatically shuts down sexual function (Masters et al., 1988). Furthermore, healthy older adults who want to have sexual activity are likely to be sexually active into late adulthood.

The climacteric, a transitional period in the lives of men and women, is a period when reproductive function undergoes significant change. The median age for menopause in women is 50 to 51 years, and menopause begins and ends for most women between the ages of 45 and 55 (Levy, 1994; Odom et al., 1990). Current thinking holds that the loss of hormones does not directly affect libido (Levy, 1994). The male climacteric is less well marked or understood, but it is believed that most men do experience a transitional period. Physiologic changes in both men and women that have an effect on the stages of the sexual response are listed in Table 6-1.

CHANGES IN WOMEN

Because of increased longevity the majority of women today will experience the postmenopausal state and will spend a third or more of their life after menopause. The literature contains mixed views of menopause, ranging from the view that menopause is a medical disease to the view that menopause is a welcome and anticipated freedom from childbearing. This freedom can result in increased sexual enjoyment. For most women menopause begins with a change in the pattern of menses. Even though most women experience minor symptoms, some find the symptoms temporarily distressing.

A woman is considered postmenopausal when menses has ceased for a year. Cessation of ovarian secretion of estrogen and progesterone is the major physiologic event of menopause. Decreases in estrogen production lead to reduced elasticity in the walls of the vagina and reduced vaginal lubrication. The vaginal mucosa becomes thin and the vagina shortens in length and width. During menopause women may experience vaginal itching, burning, and discomfort. As the rate and quantity of vaginal mucus secretion during sexual arousal is reduced, the result can be painful intercourse and vulvovaginitis. Vaginal dryness is easily alleviated by the use of a water-soluble lubricant. Also, women can visit their gynecologic provider and obtain a topical estrogen cream, but estrogen cream is not to be used as a lubricant (Levy, 1994). Regular vaginal exercises can be helpful to women having problems with vaginismus (involuntary constriction of the outer third of the vagina). Sexually active older women have less shrinkage of the vagina and higher levels of androgens than sexually inactive women; therefore sexually active women tend to experience less vaginal irritation (Leiblum et al.,

TABLE 6-1 Physiologic changes associated with aging

Phase	Male	Female
Excitement	More direct stimulation and longer time period required to attain full penile erection	Decreased vaginal lubrication
	Penile erection less firm	Time required for vaginal lubrication lengthened
	Sex flush less frequent	Vasocongestion of labia minora decreased
		Vaginal ballooning delayed
		Vasocongestion of breasts diminished
Plateau	Testicular elevation diminished	Elevation of labia majora decreased
	Scrotal wall vasocongestion reduced	No sex flush present
		Levels of muscle tension decreased
		No elongation or widening of vaginal barrel
Orgasm	Ejaculatory strength decreased	Vasocongestion of orgasmic platform decreased
	Number of penile contractions decreased	Number of vaginal contractions decreased
	Sensation of ejaculatory inevitability diminished	Intense or even painful uterine contractions possible
	Psychosexual pleasure of orgasm with ejaculation diminished	
Resolution	Rapid penile detumescence	Delayed areola detumescence
	Prolonged refractory period	Rapid shrinking of vaginal balloon
		Possible urinary urgency immediately after coitus
		Increased complaints of dysuria

From Shippee-Rice, R. (1990). Sexuality and aging. In C. Fogel & D. Lauver (Eds.), *Sexual health promotion.* Philadelphia: W.B. Saunders.

1983). One important symptom that should never be neglected is postmenopausal bleeding. Any woman with postmenopausal bleeding should be referred for medical evaluation to rule out a possible malignancy.

Of postmenopausal women, 30% to 80% experience vasomotor instability (hot flashes) and up to 80% will experience hot flashes for more than 1 year. Although some women experience hot flashes for significantly longer periods, hot flashes are rare after a 5-year period. Many women will experience minor sleep disturbances related to the occurrence of hot flashes (Odom et al., 1990). Another significant age-related change in all postmenopausal women

involves bone loss, which increases significantly after menopause.

Estrogen replacement therapy (ERT) is at times an alternative for treatment of symptoms that women experience during menopause. Any woman who contemplates beginning ERT should evaluate her individual risks and benefits in regard to this type of therapy with her gynecologic professional.

CHANGES IN MEN

As men age, erectile ability undergoes significant changes. Specifically, it takes longer to achieve an erection; erections tend to be less firm; the amount of semen is reduced; the intensity of ejaculation is lessened; there is less physical need to ejaculate; and the refractory period is longer (Masters et al., 1988). There is no definite end to male fertility, although after 50 years of age there is a slow increase in the percentage of men estimated to experience impotence—from 5% to 10% at 60 years of age to 20% at 70 years of age, to 30% to 40% at 80 years of age, to as much as 50% by 90 years of age (Korenman, 1994). It is not clear whether the increase in impotence is age dependent or related to the increase in chronic illness in the older population.

■ Sexual Dysfunction

At any age, sexual integrity is interwoven with total health and dependent on adaptation between physical and emotional capacities, societal mores, and individual desires. Disruptions in sexual integrity, such as sexual dysfunctions, are common throughout adult life, probably occurring at some time in the lives of at least 50% of all couples (Masters et al., 1988). Changes in sexual function are inevitable events in the lives of older adults resulting from a combination of factors: the aging process, loss of partners, the onset of chronic illnesses, and the concomitant treatments. Sexual problems in later life also include those that can occur at any age.

Sexual dysfunction is characterized by disturbances in the sexual desire and in the psychologic changes that characterize the sexual response cycle, and these disturbances cause marked distress and interpersonal difficulty. These disorders are characterized by the state of hypoactivity and/or aversion; by problems in arousal and orgasm phases; and by the presence of conditions that are causal such as general medical conditions and substance abuse–induced disorders (American Psychiatric Association, 1994).

Sexual dysfunction is the state in which an individual experiences a change in sexual function that causes that function to be viewed as unsatisfying, unrewarding, or inadequate (Thompson et al., 1989). One criterion for assessment and iden-

tification of a dysfunction is the satisfaction level of the older patient and/or the partner. In most cases of sexual dysfunction there is more than one factor contributing to the problem. A myriad of factors can lead to the development of sexual dysfunction, organic (physical or medical factors such as illness, injury, or drug effects) and/or psychosocial (including psychologic, interpersonal, environmental, situational, and cultural) (Masters et al., 1988). The precise cause of a specific dysfunction cannot always be identified. It is generally estimated that 10% to 20% of sexual dysfunctions are related to organic factors (Masters et al., 1988). As a general rule, a primary sexual dysfunction that has always been present is more likely to be psychogenic than is a secondary disorder that occurs after a period of satisfactory functioning. Organic causes should be suspected in an individual whose sexual functioning has been satisfactory for a significant period, especially when there is a change in ejaculatory or orgasmic process (Thompson et al., 1989). Research has shown that between 30% and 70% of erectile failures result from organic causes (Melman et al., 1984).

One of the most common causes of lowered potency in older men is the side effects of medically prescribed drugs. Medications may adversely affect sexual function through interference with the central nervous system and through hormonal release systems. See Box 6-1 for a list of drugs that may affect sexual function. Use of alcohol may lead to sexual dysfunction, despite the fact that older adults may use alcohol to relax and may feel that they are not drinking to excess. The tolerance for alcohol decreases with age, and alcohol can act like other drugs in that it may produce negative effects on sexual function (Butler et al., 1994).

■ Chronic Illness and Sexuality

There is increasing recognition of a reciprocal relationship between most illness and sexual functioning of affected individuals. Transient disinterest or lack of desire in sexual activity

BOX 6-1 MEDICATIONS AND SUBSTANCES AFFECTING SEXUAL FUNCTION

Anticholinergics
Antidepressants
  Tricyclics
    Amitriptyline
    Desipramine
    Doxepin
    Imipramine
    Nortriptyline
    Trazodone
  Monoamine oxidase inhibitors
    Parygline
    Phenelzine
Antihistamines and H$_2$ blockers
  Cimetidine
  Diphenhydramine
  Hydroxyzine
  Ranitidine
Antihypertensives
  Beta-blockers
  Clonidine
  Enalapril*
  Guanethidine
  Hydralazine
  Methyldopa
  Prazosin
  Reserpine
  Spironolactone
  Verapamil
Antiepileptics
  Carbamazepine
  Phenytoin
Phenothiazines
  Chlorpromazine

Haloperidol
Thioridazine
Thiothixene
Trifluoperazine
Sedatives and hypnotics
  Alprazolam
  Barbiturates
  Diazepam
Other medications
  Amphetamines
  Cancer chemotherapeutic agents
  Digoxin
  L-dopa
  Lithium
  Metoclopramide
  Morphine
  Naproxen
Commonly abused substances
  Alcohol
  Caffeine
  Cocaine
  Heroin
  Marijuana
  Nicotine
Cardiovascular agents
  Guanethidine
  Reserpine
  Timolol
  Clonidine
  Hydralazine
  Digoxin
  Thiazide
  Beta-blockers

Modified from Kligman. (1991). Office evaluation of sexual function and complaints. *Clinics in Geriatric Medicine*, 7(1). Miller, C. (1995). Medications and sexual functioning in older adults. *Geriatric Nursing*, **16**, 84, 94, 105.
*Less frequently.

occurs in most people when they are preoccupied with the symptoms of illness. Sexual problems often disappear when the illness improves. The primary reason given for cessation of sexual intercourse in older adults is the physical illness of one or both partners. Chronic illnesses tend to develop slowly over a period of years; resultant changes in sexual functioning may develop slowly and may be mistakenly attributed to the aging process rather than to the chronic disease. Of all the emotional problems that can affect an older person's interest in sexual expression, depression is most commonly reported. Depression may be a cause of lessened sexual interest, as well as a consequence.

Illness can affect sexual function in direct and indirect ways:

1. Illness can disrupt the human sexual response cycle.
2. The treatment for an illness (such as medication) can create a sexual problem.
3. The general effects of the illness (such as weakness, fatigue, immobility, pain, and depression) can affect sexual function.
4. If the condition is life threatening (such as stroke or cardiovascular disease), anxiety and fear about death may affect sexual function.
5. Illness may cause changes in the sense of self. Disease and illness that disfigure the body can alter the affected person's body image and affect sexual function.

The potential effects on sexual function of the chronic illnesses most commonly experienced by those over 75 years of age are summarized in Table 6-2.

ARTHRITIS

The symptoms of arthritis (pain, joint stiffness, weakness, and fatigue) can directly affect mobility and thereby affect sexual function in older adults. In addition, people who take steroids to help control the rheumatoid arthritic process may find that the drug decreases their interest in sexual activity. Arthritis does not appear to directly affect the individual's physiologic sexual response. The assault on body image by the progressive disfiguring elements of the disease may lead to feelings of unattractiveness.

CEREBROVASCULAR ACCIDENT (STROKE)

Causes for sexual dysfunction in poststroke patients are multiple and complex. The profound negative effect of stroke on patients' sexuality is well documented (Burgener & Logan, 1989). Erectile difficulties are extremely common in men; sequentially there is a decrease in frequency of intercourse and in sexual relating (mutual verbal and nonverbal responsiveness, caressing, and touching). Changes in role function for both the patient and partner are considered significant contributors to impaired sexual function. The partner may avoid sexual interaction, believing that sexual activity may cause another stroke. Antihypertensive drugs prescribed after the stroke may contribute to erectile dysfunction.

CARDIOVASCULAR DISEASE

Twenty percent of patients admitted to coronary care units with myocardial infarctions, or MIs, are over the age of 70. The incidence in men and in women is about equal (Kane et al., 1989). Treatment of the older patient with MI is similar to that of the younger patient, with particular attention to early mobilization. A major concern for older post-MI patients who have been sexually active before the event is their ability to resume sexual activity. The most common barriers to sexual integrity for these patients are fear and avoidance. Many cardiac patients fear experiencing another MI or death if they attempt intercourse. These fears are often experienced by the partner as well. The strain of intercourse and orgasm is roughly equivalent to the exertion of climbing two flights of steps. Typically it is safe to recommend that sexual relations be gradually resumed after a successful recovery period of 3 months. Furthermore, a side position should be encouraged; men who have had MI should avoid

TABLE 6-2 Potential effects of chronic illnesses on sexual function

Disorder	Potential effect on sexual functioning	Presumed pathogenic mechanism
Arthritis	No direct effect on sexual function; arthritic symptoms can inhibit sexual function.	—
	Steroid treatment to control arthritis may decrease sexual interest or desire (Katzin, 1990).	Opposition to stimulating action of androgen on brain and/or sex organs (caused by steroid treatment)
	Progressive disfigurement may cause body image changes.	—
Cerebrovascular accident (stroke)	No direct impairment of sexual function, but erectile disorders are common; decreased frequency of intercourse and sexual relating (Korenman, 1994).	Changes in role function of patient and/or partner; fear of relapse or sudden death
Cardiovascular disease	Impaired sexual functioning limits the quality of life in 34% to 75% of post–myocardial infarction (MI) patients (Rosal et al., 1994). No direct physical effect on sexual function in men, but only 25% of post-MI patients return to pre-MI level of sexual activity; 25% never resume sexual activity (Papadopolous, 1987). Women are less likely to experience sexual problems (Masters et al., 1988).	Depression; anxiety; fear of relapse or sudden death on part of patient or partner
Prostatectomy	Effect dependent on type of surgical procedure. 458 men with prostate cancer underwent radical prostatectomy; 51 were potent after surgery and 32% of those had bilateral nerve-sparing prostatectomy (Geary et al., 1995). After TUR, 15% to 40% of men have erectile disorder; the majority experience retrograde ejaculation (Bolt et al., 1987).	More psychologically than physiologically mediated; surgical resection of bladder neck; surgical severing of nerves
Gynecologic disorders	Vaginal or urethral infection, bleeding, or itching.	Decreased estrogen production

TABLE 6-2 Potential effects of chronic illnesses on sexual function—cont'd

Disorder	Potential effect on sexual functioning	Presumed pathogenic mechanism
Chronic obstructive pulmonary disease (COPD)	No direct impairment, but sexual activity is affected by exertional dyspnea or coughing spells (Katzin, 1990). Erectile difficulties.	Activity intolerance; anxiety or fear related to dyspnea; coughing
Diabetes	Sexual interest or desire is unaffected in men. 60% of men have erectile disorder (Korenman, 1994). Some men regain erectile ability, seemingly related to how well each individual accepts diagnosis (Jensen, 1985). In women, reduced sexual desire and/or decreased vaginal lubrication (Masters et al., 1988). Decreased orgasmic capacity or less frequent sexual activity in women (Schreiner-Engel et al., 1987). Also in women, there is a lower rate of sexual dysfunction associated with disease acceptance (Jensen, 1985).	Neuropathy and/or vascular damage
Malignancies, breast	No direct effect, but psychologic effects can be profound: depression, loss of sexual desire, and sexual dysfunction (Masters et al., 1988).	Body image change; depression; reaction of partner
All other cancers (Schover, 1988a, 1988b)	Both men and women may lose sexual desire temporarily.	Anxiety; depression; pain; nausea
	In women, vaginal dryness.	Chemotherapy
	In women, dyspareunia.	Radiation; pelvic surgery; antiestrogen therapy
	In men, decrease in sexual desire.	Removal of testicles; hormone therapy
	In men, erectile disorders.	Radiation; pelvic surgery; removal of testicles; hormone therapy
	In men, dry ejaculation or retrograde ejaculation.	Nerve damage after pelvic surgery

a position above their partner (Levy, 1994). Fatigue associated with exertion may also affect sexual integrity. The patient should be educated about the warning signals of heart strain: increased heart rate, palpitations, or shortness of breath that persists longer than 15 minutes after intercourse; chest pain, tightness, or sleeplessness following intercourse; or extreme fatigue on the day after intercourse (Moore et al., 1984).

Hypertension does not directly affect sexual function. However, the drug treatment for hypertension may have negative effects on libido, arousal, and erectile function. These effects are reversible when the drug therapy is changed, but are a significant causative factor in noncompliance in hypertensive patients. See Box 6-1 for a list of drugs that affect sexual function.

PROSTATECTOMY

Approximately one half of older men develop benign prostatic hypertrophy; half of these will be treated surgically. Recent studies on transurethral prostatectomy suggest that postsurgical effects on sexual function are very individualized and are affected by psychosocial factors. From 5% to 14% of men experience erectile dysfunction 12 months after surgery despite reporting no sexual dysfunction preoperatively (Barry, 1989; Bolt et al., 1987). Most experts consider postprostatectomy erectile dysfunction more likely to be psychologic than physiologically mediated. Hogan (1980) discusses three reasons for the difficulty: the surgery may provide an excuse for some men to terminate intercourse in the face of previously decreasing desire and performance; erectile dysfunction may be in response to the physician's attitude that suggests it is a frequent sequela; or the man may be concerned that intercourse will in some way endanger his health.

Retrograde ejaculation, the passage of sperm into the bladder rather than out through the penis, occurs in most men after surgical removal of the prostate for benign prostatic disease. Although the sensation of orgasm is unchanged, the experience of retrograde ejaculation can be quite upsetting if unexpected. The likelihood of retrograde ejaculation needs to be explained preoperatively so that the patient understands that this change in ejaculation is not harmful and does not necessarily diminish the pleasure of intercourse. The patient should be instructed that the first passage of urine after intercourse will appear cloudy.

A total prostatectomy for removal of prostatic cancer, which involves cutting the nerves controlling penile erection, may lead to permanent erectile dysfunction. However, recent reports indicate that nerve-sparing modifications of the surgical technique are being used for patients with focal, well-differentiated tumors. Sexual potency is reported to be preserved for many of these patients (Geary et al., 1995).

GYNECOLOGIC CONDITIONS AFFECTING WOMEN

Disorders affecting older women are those associated with decreased estrogen production. Thinning of the vaginal wall may predispose the older woman to infection, bleeding, and itching. Urinary tract infections are more likely to occur in women who resume sexual activity following periods of abstinence. Attention to adequate fluid intake and voiding before and immediately following intercourse may help to alleviate this problem.

CHRONIC OBSTRUCTIVE PULMONARY DISEASE

The most common problems affecting sexual expression of patients with chronic obstructive pulmonary disease, or COPD, include activity intolerance related to exertional dyspnea and anxiety related to frequent coughing spells (Katzin, 1990). Anxiety and fear related to exertional dyspnea can lead to fear of suffocation and make sexual activity stressful instead of enjoyable.

DIABETES

Sixty percent of men with diabetes have erectile dysfunction. Retrograde ejaculation occurs in

10% of diabetic men, but the desire for sex is usually unaffected (Korenman, 1994). Diabetic women may experience orgasmic dysfunction and reduced sexual desire and/or decreased vaginal lubrication. Neuropathy is the primary cause of these changes in the sexual response. Unfortunately, the sexual problems tend to be permanent and untreatable. Some men do regain erectile ability; this is seemingly related to how well they accept their diagnosis and how they view the quality of their intimate relationship or relationships. Both men and women with good disease acceptance seem to be at lower risk for sexual dysfunction.

MALIGNANCIES

The diagnosis and treatment of cancer may have adverse effects on body image, sexual response, and sex roles. Alteration or removal of body parts, changes in their function, and psychologic responses to these changes such as anxiety, depression, or guilt may result in sexual dysfunction. Many sexual problems experienced after cancer treatment are temporary, but some are permanent. When cancer is far advanced, a person's needs for affection, sharing of feelings, and touch may be heightened.

PENILE IMPLANTS

When illness causes complete inability to have erections, sexual function can be partially restored by use of a mechanical device surgically implanted in the penis. These devices can provide erections that last long enough for intercourse to take place, but they cannot restore sensation to the penis or cause ejaculation (Masters et al., 1988). For some men, penile implants can restore a sense of masculinity and may provide some restoration of sexual function. Mechanical difficulties and infection are common problems occurring in 40% of patients who have penile implants. These problems require removal of the device or additional surgery to correct the problem (Masters et al., 1988).

■ Social Changes That Affect Sexual Function: Demographics and Gender

Demographics have a limiting impact on sexual fulfillment of older adults. It seems to be the biologic fate of many women to outlive men; consequently, older women outnumber older men. The ratio of women to men varies dramatically with age. In the under-20 age group, men outnumber women; at 30 to 34 years the age group is evenly balanced; for the 65 plus age group, women exceed men three to two. This disparity becomes more marked in the upper age ranges because women have a 7-year longer life expectancy than men (U.S. Department of Health and Human Services, 1993). There are 74 men between the ages of 70 and 74 for every 100 women, and among those 85 and over, there are only 40 men for every 100 women (Table 6-3).

The implications of these facts for older adults is that the surviving man has the opportunity to expand his sexual choices, whereas the older woman is restricted by the male-female imbalance.

Older adults' marital status and living arrangements vary tremendously by sex. Most men spend their older years married and in family settings, whereas most older women spend their later years as widows outside of family settings. Men who lose a spouse through divorce or death

TABLE 6-3 Number of men per 100 women by older age group: 1986

Age	Men per 100 women
65-69	83
70-74	74
75-79	64
80-84	53
85+	40

From U.S. Bureau of the Census. (1987). *Estimates of the population of the United States by age, sex, and race: 1980-1986* (Current Population Reports, Series P-25, No. 1000). Washington, DC: U.S. Government Printing Office.

are more likely to remarry than are women in the same situation. More often than not, older men marry or remarry women younger than themselves. Men remarry sooner (in about 3 years), whereas those widows who remarry do so in about 7 years (Corby & Solnick, 1980). Older widowed men have remarriage rates over 8 times higher than those of women (U.S. Bureau of the Census, 1987).

■ Sexual Function and Aging

Over the past 25 years the impact of aging on sexual response and function has received increased attention from investigators. Research has tended, though, to focus rather narrowly on the frequency of older adults' genital sexual activities and has underemphasized the relational and emotional content of sexuality.

Throughout adulthood women and men develop distinctively different sexual styles. Men are more sexually active than women throughout life, with the exception of the very old age groups (85 years and older), in which there is no difference. Women report lower orgasmic frequency than men throughout the life span. Although orgasmic frequency in women reaches a peak in middle age and remains constant into the 60s, it falls steadily among men in this age group. Women may be more likely than men to report increased sexual interest and activity with increasing age. In general, for both sexes, the greater the interest in sexual activity when young, the greater the interest and activity when old.

Society has differing views concerning appropriate sexual behavior for older men and women. The sexual activity of an older man is more likely to be sanctioned than that of an older woman. Older men continue to be perceived as sexually attractive, whereas older women are not. Older men usually marry younger women; society perceives this as acceptable. In contrast, sexual interest by an older woman in a younger man is less likely to be condoned. For older women, single, divorced, or widowed, the only socially sanctioned partner is an older man. Thus the population imbalance of the sexes and societal expectations combine to make the unavailability of a partner a significant factor in the sexual fulfillment of older women. For both women and men a marked change in sexual activity in old age is most frequently attributed to a new partner (an affair or remarriage) or the end of a sexual relationship through death or divorce (Turner & Adams, 1983).

Research refutes the pervasive cultural myth that the old are not interested in sex. According to Janus and Janus (1993), approximately 93% of older men and 50% of older women often or always have orgasms when they have sex. Fifty-three percent of older men and 41% of older women report sexual frequency of a few times a week (Janus & Janus, 1993).

The best predictor of sexual activity for men in old age is sexual activity and interest at a younger age, whereas for older women marital status is the best predictor. Unavailability of a partner is the primary reason in both sexes for discontinuation of sexual expression. Starr and Weiner (1981) studied 800 persons between 60 and 91 years of age and found that 36% said that sex was better for them at the time of the study than when they were younger. Of this group, about 80% were sexually active, and most had experienced an increase in spontaneity of sexual expression as they grew older. Being able to spend a long time in sexual encounters whenever they wanted was seen as a major advantage of age. Bretschneider and McCoy (1988) studied 202 healthy retirement home residents, age 80 to 102. Eighty-eight percent of the men and 72% of the women fantasized or daydreamed about being sexually intimate. The most frequently reported sexual activity was touching and caressing without intercourse. Sixty-two percent of the men and 38% of the women experienced intercourse; 72% of the men and 40% of the women experienced sexual pleasure through self-stimulation. Masturbation, or sexual self-stimulation, among older people has tended to be a highly personal topic and is surrounded by taboos. Recent research reports that only 23% of older men and 35% of older women *never* masturbate (Janus & Janus, 1993). Nurses need to accept the normalcy of this behavior in both sexes and assume the responsibility of educating other health care workers about privacy needs.

Some women who were thought to be single have in fact been in discreet lifelong relationships with other women that for reasons of public opinion had to be kept secret. Some women, after years as wives and mothers, turn to a lesbian relationship (Doress & Siegal, 1987). It is estimated that gays and lesbians make up about 10% of the U.S. population; approximately the same proportion of the older adult population can be assumed to be homosexual (Butler & Lewis, 1991). The increasing information available in recent years about sexuality and aging has served to dispel many of the myths about this stage of life. However, many people, young and old, including nurses, physicians, clergy, and family members, are astonished at the idea of people in their 70s, 80s, and 90s having sexual feelings, needs, and experiences with their own sex.

Although young and middle-aged adults have become more sexually permissive in regard to their own generations, they may have difficulty accepting an older person who has continuing sexual interest. This negative opinion may stem from a feeling that sex for most older people is unimportant, negative, distasteful, or taboo (Butler & Lewis, 1991). See Box 6-2 for myths regarding sexuality and aging.

NEED FOR TOUCH

People use their sense of touch to communicate with others. To say that one is touched by a warm thought or touched by a beautiful painting or the sound of a familiar melody is an example of the use of the word *touch* to connote positive emotions. How powerful then is the actual physical experience of touch, the act of reaching out to touch the body and spirit of another in the human expression of love and caring. Intimacy needs persist to the end of life no matter what a

> ### BOX 6-2 MYTHS OF AGING AND SEXUALITY
>
> 1. Intercourse is debilitating and will tend to hasten old age and death.
> 2. Masturbation by an older person is a sign of serious emotional disturbance.
> 3. Coital satisfaction decreases after menopause.
> 4. Older men lose their ability and desire to have sex.
> 5. Older women who still enjoy sex were probably nymphomaniacs when they were young.
> 6. Older men are subject to sexual deviations such as child molesting.
>
> Adapted from Gibson, H.B. (1992). *The emotional and sexual lives of older people: A manual for professionals.* London: Chapman and Hall.

Older adults sharing a special togetherness. *Courtesy Loy Ledbetter, St. Louis.*

person's physical or cognitive abilities are. Especially important are the needs for closeness, touch, and being valued as a man or a woman. In old age, people begin to touch less and are touched less. Many older people who are frail may experience sensory deprivation because they are so seldom touched and have decreasing opportunities to touch. Touch has the potential to be a therapeutic tool to maintain contact and reduce anxiety for many older adults.

Expression of sexual feelings by older adults may add pleasure to their lives and provide relief from anxiety. Nurses have the opportunity to provide many older people with positive affirmation of their sense of self as a viable sexual person. A positive comment about a good-looking tie or a well-done hairstyle and the reaching out to touch a hand—these small acts may affirm an older man's or an older woman's sexuality.

INSTITUTIONALIZATION AND SEXUALITY

Sexuality is important to the lives of older adults who reside in institutions. Frail older adults in institutions such as hospitals or nursing homes have a capacity for sexual pleasure, which includes the need to touch and be touched and to feel warmth and caring. The gerontology literature supports the regrettable reality that nursing home staff pay little attention to the sexual needs of residents (McCartney et al., 1987). Yet certain sexual behaviors manifested by older patients in acute care units or in nursing home settings are considered by staff to be a disturbing management problem. This may be an indication of the taboo against sexual expression by older adults and a measure of staff members' lack of knowledge about sexuality. Sexual behaviors may be perceived by staff as harmful and disruptive when in fact the behavior is normal and harmless and is an expression of the older person's need for intimacy or closeness. In the absence of opportunity for direct sexual gratification, the need for sexual expression may take on many forms. Older adults may resort to clinging to possessions that can be handled or that evoke memories of lost contact with loved ones as spouse and

Touching or hugging has a therapeutic effect on both the young and the old alike.

friends die and children move away (Ebersole & Hess, 1994). Or they may use sexual jokes as a way of drawing attention to themselves as sexual beings. The sexual behaviors most frequently labeled as "problems" by staff are sexual talk—describing past or present sexual experiences; requesting staff to enter into some form of sexual activity; sexual acts—exposing genitalia, touching, or grabbing staff inappropriately; and implied sexual behavior—removing clothes, masturbating publicly, or making suggestive comments. Sexual behaviors that staff consider acceptable are limited physical contact between staff and residents such as hugging, hand holding, and kissing on the cheek or forehead, and perhaps masturbation in private.

Nursing home staff should have opportunities to participate in classes that discuss the sexual needs of older residents. It is helpful for staff to understand that sexual interest in old age is a reflection of prior levels of activity and interest. If this expression has been a significant method of coping in the past, it is likely to remain so.

■ Nursing Process

ASSESSMENT

Sexual function and integrity of older adults should be a concern for nurses and can be first approached by conducting a sexual assessment.

Aging Alert

1. Age is no barrier to satisfying expression of sexuality and fulfillment of sexual needs.
2. Regular sexual activity may provide some protection against physiologic changes of aging for women.
3. The best predictor of sexual activity and interest in old age is sexual activity and interest at a younger age.
4. Chronic illnesses tend to develop slowly over a period of time; resultant changes in sexual functioning may develop insidiously and may be mistakenly attributed to the aging process rather than to the chronic disease process.

The purpose of an assessment is to determine the individual's degree of satisfaction or dissatisfaction in fulfilling sexual needs. Early discussion of patient concerns assures the patient that sexual health is an important and an acceptable topic to discuss. Some older people are willing to talk about sexuality with a nurse if the nurse projects ease and openness. Other patients will be reluctant to initiate discussion about a sexual concern with a nurse or any health professional. Instead, they may express generalized somatic complaints such as back pain, fatigue, headache, or pelvic and abdominal pain (Sheahan, 1989). When individuals feel ill or are in pain, they usually are not interested in discussing sexual matters. However, sexual difficulties can be concerns that lead to physical depletion and emotional pain. The professional nurse must be willing to become knowledgeable about and to take responsibility for dealing with the sexual aspects of the patient's illness experience. The nurse must be aware of the unique and specific sexual problems caused by various chronic illnesses.

The scope of sexual assessment will be dictated by the nurse's preparation and experience, as well as by the patient's health problems. Sexual health assessment requires special skill. Whether or not the initial assessment elicits sharing of sexual problems is not always an indicator of the true situation. Perhaps no sexual problem exists, or perhaps it will take time for the patient to develop sufficient comfort and trust to share a problem. The patient may confide in a nurse when a problem does arise. Assessment should include a description of the older person's past patterns of sexual expression, recent changes in the pattern of sexual activity, knowledge of age-related changes in sexual functions, knowledge of illness-related changes in sexual functions, and beliefs about sexual expression. An individual's concern about sexuality may or may not be associated with a change in sexual function. Guidelines that can be used to facilitate an assessment of sexual concerns include the following:

- Provide privacy while conducting the assessment; assure the patient of the assessment's confidentiality.
- Prepare the patient for the assessment with an introductory statement that briefly explains the purpose of the interview. For example: "To help plan care for your health needs, I am going to ask you for some information. You may find these questions personal, but these are issues about which older individuals often have concerns."
- Help patients identify clearly and specifically any sexual concern or concerns they are experiencing. Assessment can begin with the question "Has your illness caused a change in sexual functioning?" If the patient answers yes, the next question can be "Is that a concern for you?" Those who reply yes may be invited to describe the concern.
- Allow the patient to refuse to answer. You might say, "You seem reluctant about answering that question. Would you prefer I bring it up later?"

- Give the older person a chance to ask questions: "What questions about sexual health would you like answered?"

Some suggested questions are included in Box 6-3.

If sexual activity has not been a concern for the older adult in earlier life, and is not at present, the nurse should not impose problems or needs on the individual. As important as sexual fulfillment is for some people, it is not a major concern for all. The nurse should be alert for covert signs of unmet sexual needs such as repeated references to sex, repeated inappropriate attempts to touch staff members, or reports of sexually inappropriate behavior from friends or family members.

The single most important factor in helping people with sexual concerns and questions is the ease and comfort with which the clinician handles sensitive and value-laden sexual topics. To be effective, nurses must first achieve a healthy attitude toward their own sexuality. Sexuality is an area to which many people attach strong emotions, religious ideas, and rigid opinions. Sexual attitudes, values, and behaviors that are acceptable to one person may be uncomfortable for another. Nurses must be able to clarify and acknowledge their own feelings, attitudes, and opinions about sexual issues. This self-understanding helps nurses to develop an atmosphere of acceptance and respect for the sexual beliefs and practices of others.

NURSING DIAGNOSES

Once the data collection has been completed, an analysis of the data, problem identification, and formulation of nursing diagnoses can take place. Nursing diagnoses represent actual or potential areas of alterations in patterns of human functioning that nurses are licensed to treat.

The diagnoses of sexual dysfunction and *altered sexuality patterns* encompass all situations in which an individual expresses concern regarding sexuality because of actual or perceived difficulties, limitations, or changes in sexual behavior (Korb & Kupperberg, 1993). These nursing diagnoses cover a wide range of defining characteristics and contributing risk factors. Defining characteristics are the cluster of subjective and objective signs that validate the presence of a diagnostic category. Contributing risk factors are those clinical and personal situations that can change or influence health status or problem development.

Defining characteristics are the patient's verbalization of sexual difficulties, limitations, or changes; impaired expression of one's sexuality; or expression of fear of potential limitations of sexual performance. The contributing risk factors can be grouped into two categories—those related to physical or medical conditions and those related to psychosocial factors. Any disease process or illness experience can cause or contribute to an altered sexuality pattern. Psychosocial factors include psychologic, interpersonal, environmental, situational, and cultural factors such as the following:

- Past experiences with sexuality (restrictive upbringing, traumatic sexual experiences)
- Death of or separation from partner or spouse
- Disability of patient or partner
- Poor communication with partner
- Lack of privacy
- Lack of opportunity for touching or being touched
- Stressors (financial worries, conflicting values)

Three frequent diagnoses that may coexist in older patients who are experiencing an alteration in sexuality pattern are the following:

Knowledge deficit
Self-esteem disturbance
Body image disturbance

It is highly unlikely that an older person would only have a diagnosis concerning sexual functioning; rather, multiple conditions and diagnoses are the norm. Because of this complexity many health professionals either ignore or overlook the

BOX 6-3 SUGGESTED QUESTIONS TO ASSESS SEXUAL CONCERNS

SEXUAL SATISFACTION

- Have you experienced any changes in your sexual relationships lately?
- To what do you attribute this change?
- What types of sexual activities have you usually enjoyed the most, including things such as hugging, kissing, sleeping together, intercourse, masturbation, and so on?
- Do you or your partner take any prescription medications? What are they? How often do you take them? Have you experienced any changes in your level of energy since you started them? What about overall feelings of well-being? Any changes in sexual desire or activity?

For men

- Have you noticed any changes in the intensity of your ejaculations, orgasms, or ability to attain or maintain an erection?
- Have you ever had orgasms without ejaculations?
- Has your level of enjoyment from sexual relations altered as a result of these changes?
- Have you had any problems with urethral discharge or urination?

For women

- Have you experienced any vaginal soreness or irritation after sexual intercourse? How long does it last? Any problems with urgency or with burning on urination after intercourse? Have you experienced abdominal contractions or back pain after intercourse?
- Have you had any problems with vaginal discharge or itching?
- Have any of these problems interfered with your sexual pleasure?
- Have you or your partner experienced any changes in your health status recently? How have these changes affected your sexual relationship?

ALTERATIONS IN SELF-PERCEPTION

- How has growing older changed your lifestyle or things you enjoy doing?
- How has the change in your health or your partner's health altered your lifestyle or your goals?
- How do you rate your general health?
- On a scale of 1 to 10, how would you describe your satisfaction with your life?
- On a scale of 1 to 10, how would you describe your satisfaction with your sexual relationships?

RELATIONSHIPS WITH OTHERS

- Have you ever discussed sexual topics with your spouse, friends, family, or health care professional?
- Whom do you talk to when you have problems of any kind or just want someone to talk to?

ENVIRONMENT

- With whom do you live?
- Do you have a chance for privacy? To be alone? To talk with others privately if you want to?

problems in sexuality that threaten the well-being of the older person. Many times the nurse who is knowledgeable and sensitive will be the first health professional to uncover older adults' concerns regarding their sexuality.

PLANNING AND GOAL IDENTIFICATION

The following are examples of diagnoses and goals that might be formulated for sexuality problems in older adults.

Alteration in sexual patterns related to loss of husband

A long-term goal would be expression of satisfaction in sexual fulfillment.

Short-term goals would be the following:

1. Verbalization of loss of sexual pleasure (feelings of warmth, love, and intimacy)
2. Resumption of social contacts with age peers
3. Involvement with adult children and grandchildren
4. Decision making regarding living arrangements

Knowledge deficit related to physical changes of the aging process or medical treatment

A long-term goal would be acceptance of age-related physical changes.

Short-term goals would be the following:

1. Understanding of impact of medications and surgical treatment on sexual functioning
2. Verbalization to health professionals of concerns with sexual functioning
3. Participation in decision making regarding sexual health

IMPLEMENTATION

One intervention model is the P-LI-SS-IT model developed by Annon (1976). The model includes four levels of intervention: P—permission giving; LI—limited information; SS—specific suggestions; and IT—intensive therapy. The nurse can use this approach for varying levels of patient need. The model assumes that many sexual problems can be managed by using educational methods that do not require intensive therapy. Comfort (1980) states that sexual counseling and therapy depend almost entirely on permission giving and correction of false attitudes toward sexuality and aging. Some patients may need information and permission to reverse sexual problems; others benefit from direct suggestions to alleviate problem areas; and others benefit from validation that their sexual behavior is normal. For some patients, more intensive therapy is necessary to resolve problems, and the nurse may act as a referral source for these patients. It is important for nurses to be cognizant of their own comfort and skill level in order to determine how to intervene and when to refer.

In the acute care setting

The myriad of acute and chronic illnesses that bring older people to hospitals often threaten sexual health. Both medical and surgical treatments for these illnesses can present hazards to sexual functioning. The patient and spouse need to have accurate information regarding the particular illness process, the treatment interventions, and the side effects of medications. The nurse educates the patient and spouse, corrects misconceptions about normal aspects of aging, and validates normalcy of sexual feelings and behavior.

Previously held attitudes, beliefs, and religious mores regarding sexual behavior need to be explored before specific suggestions regarding sexual activities can be addressed. Not all nurses are adequately prepared to intervene at this level, and referral may be the best course of action. Specific suggestions—if appropriate for the patient and within the nurse's knowledge base—can be offered, such as the following: gradually resuming sexual activities after illness; planning sexual activity to take advantage of drug effects; promoting relaxation and pain relief by taking a warm bath or shower before sexual activity; and considering options for sexual expression other than intercourse. The nurse should always be alert to factors that may jeopardize the sexual health of older hospitalized patients.

Specific intervention strategies include the following:

- Assess patient's level of knowledge and understanding regarding sexuality
- Include partner in discussions of sexual issues; facilitate communication between partner and patient
- Encourage discussion of factors that may interfere with partner relationship or expression of sexual feelings
- Act as referral source when necessary

In the nursing home

Respect for the dignity and sexual identity of nursing home residents is the primary task of the professional nurse who responds to the enormous need for high-level nursing care in our nation's nursing homes. It is crucial to the wellbeing of the nursing home resident that staff members realize that sexuality is a lifelong need and it does not cease to exist because a person becomes a resident of a nursing home. Most older people stop having sex for the same reasons they stop activities such as riding a bicycle: a decline in physical abilities, fear that people will think them foolish, and for most, the lack of a bicycle (Comfort & Dial, 1991).

The staff should be educated regarding behaviors that signal possible sexual frustration, including the following: undue need for touching; vague, generalized somatic complaints; inappropriate sexual demands; and sexual jokes. Staff need to articulate their concerns and feelings regarding certain nursing home residents' desire to masturbate both in public areas and within the private confines of the resident's room. Public masturbation creates a disturbance in nursing homes because most older residents and some staff members have been taught that masturbation is a vice, sinful, and physically harmful. Staff

---

BOX 6-4 MAINTAINING SEXUAL INTEGRITY IN NURSING HOME RESIDENTS

1. The need for intimacy and touching may be especially critical for nursing home residents who are experiencing diminished meaningful relationships.
2. Concern related to sexual difficulties can drain patients of energy that might be used for more constructive activities.
3. The nurse should assume that the nursing home resident has unmet sexual needs.
4. Integrated living units should be arranged so that an opportunity is provided for more normal relationships, thus encouraging socially acceptable communication, warmth, and touch.
5. Nursing home staff should have opportunities to participate in classes that discuss the sexual needs of older residents.

From Hillman, J. & Stricker, G. (1994). A linkage of knowledge and attitudes toward elderly sexuality: Not necessarily a uniform relationship. *Gerontologist, 34*(2), 256-260.

---

members may scold and demean a resident who engages in any form of masturbation. Nurses need to be sensitive to the complexity of this issue. There must be a regard for the older resident's sexual expression, but also respect for the other residents' values and the accepted social expression of sexuality. (See Box 6-4.)

No one should demean an older nursing home resident for any form of masturbation, but if public masturbation offends other residents, the staff can assist the resident to a private space, preferably the resident's room, where no one will pass judgment on the resident's sexual behavior. The older person may then choose to return to social activity after masturbatory activity ceases. The nurse thereby models both the acceptance of the sexual need of the individual resident and acceptance of the societal norm that calls for fulfilling the need for a private setting (Shippee-Rice, 1990).

In the private or family home

Medicare financing of home health care has increased yearly by an average of 23% from 1990 to 1993. Although projected growth is lower, the demand for home care demonstrates the high level of need for home health services (Burr & Waldo, 1995). Sexual problems will rarely be the primary reason for a home visit, but sexuality should always be part of a comprehensive assessment. A major issue to consider when assessing sexual health is the availability of privacy, as well as the availability of a partner (Mulligan & Modigh, 1991).

Many older adults reside independently in their own homes, although 13% of people over age 65 live in the homes of their children or other family members. Many people over 80 live alone, and many of these older people have an informal system of social support: family that visits on a regular basis, neighbors, community services such as Meals on Wheels, or paid helpers. The nurse should always assess the adequacy of the individualized system of care.

Older adults living with adult sons and daughters may have initiated the change in living arrangements, which may be temporary or permanent, for a myriad of reasons, such as physical changes that resulted in a permanent or temporary inability to take care of themselves. With the increasing numbers of shorter hospital stays, more and more older people will need temporary assistance to allow themselves sufficient time to return to their pre-illness level of function. Other reasons that older adults live with their adult children may include financial considerations, loss of a spouse, fear of living alone, loneliness, and loss of cognitive abilities necessary to maintain independent living. In these living arrangements, older people may experience an unantici-

pated loss of independence and privacy that threatens their sense of self as an adult and as a healthy, attractive, sexual person.

The nurse needs to use interpersonal skills to (1) show sensitivity to the older person's need for sexual expression, (2) find opportunities to affirm the older person's attractiveness, (3) encourage the person's expression of femininity or masculinity, and (4) promote social interactions with age peers.

A critical area for nursing intervention is within the family system that is providing care and sharing their home with the older parent. The adult child, although well meaning, may have difficulty in recognizing an older parent's sexual needs. The emphasis on normalcy of sexual health throughout the life span will assist most people in overcoming their initial reluctance to accept the legitimate sexual needs of their aging parent. The nurse is able to model behaviors that affirm the sexual health of the older person and encourage discussion of factors that may interfere with the expression of sexual feelings. Most importantly, the nurse should treat all sexual concerns of the older person with the utmost respect for the person's dignity.

EVALUATION

Evaluations of nursing interventions are related to criteria identified in the planning phase and articulated in the patient's short- and long-term goals. The nurse must continually evaluate the many relationships that are established with the patient and the patient's caregivers. These relationships are critical to the nurse's ability to be an effective clinician and to assist the older adult in enjoying sexual health.

Because there are sexually active people in every decade of life, including the eighth and ninth decades, nurses who work with older adults must assume active roles in promoting sexual integrity. Three areas of special importance are the education of patients, families, and staff regarding the impact of normal aging and chronic illness on sexual function; advocacy for sensitivity to older adults' needs for closeness, touch, warmth, and meaningful relationships; and competence and comfort in conducting a sexual health assessment. Nurses who assume active roles in this area will be rewarded with new understandings of behavior.

REFERENCES

American Psychiatric Association. (1994). *Diagnostic and statistical manual of mental disorders* (4th ed.). Washington, DC: Author.

Annon, J. (1976). The P-LI-SS-IT Model. *Journal of Sex Education and Therapy, 2,* 1-15.

Barry, M.J. (1989). Pre-operative guidance for men facing prostatectomy. *Medical Aspects of Human Sexuality, 23,* 25-30.

Bolt, J.W., Evans, C., & Marshall, V.R. (1987). Sexual dysfunction after prostatectomy. *British Journal of Urology, 59,* 319-322.

Bretschneider, J.G., & McCoy, N.L. (1988). Sexual interest and behavior in healthy 80-to-102 year olds. *Archives of Sexual Behavior, 17,* 109.

Burgener, S., & Logan, G. (1989). Sexuality concerns of the post-stroke patient. *Rehabilitation Nursing, 14,* 178-181, 195.

Burr, S., & Waldo, D. (1995). Data view: National health expenditure projections 1994-2005. *Health Care Financing Review, 16*(4), 221-242.

Butler, R.N., & Lewis, M.I. (1991). *Aging and mental health* (4th ed.). St. Louis: Mosby.

Butler, R.N., Lewis, M., Hoffman, & Whitehead. (1994). Love and sex after 60: How physical changes affect intimate expression. *Geriatrics, 49*(9), 20-27.

Comfort, A. (1980). Sexuality in later life. In J.E. Birren & R.B. Sloane (Eds.), *Handbook of mental health and aging* (pp. 885-892). Englewood Cliffs, NJ: Prentice Hall.

Comfort, A., & Dial, L. (1991). Sexuality and aging. *Clinics in Geriatric Medicine, 7*(1), 1-5.

Corby, N., & Solnick, R.L. (1980). Psychosocial and physiological influences on sexuality in older adults. In J.E. Birren & R.B. Sloane (Eds.), *Handbook of mental health and aging* (p. 893). Englewood Cliffs, NJ: Prentice Hall.

Doress, P.B., & Siegal, D.L. (1987). *Ourselves growing older: Women aging with knowledge and power.* New York: Simon and Schuster.

Ebersole, P., & Hess, P. (1994). *Toward healthy aging: Human needs and nursing response* (4th ed.). St. Louis: Mosby.

Geary, E., Dendinger, T., Freiha, F., & Stamey, T. (1995). Nerve sparing radical prostatectomy: A different view. *Journal of Urology, 154*(1), 145-149.

Gibson H.B. (1992). *The emotional and sexual lives of older people. A manual for professionals.* London: Chapman and Hall.

Hillman J. & Stricker G. (1994). A linkage of knowledge and attitudes toward elderly sexuality: Not necessarily a uniform relationship. *Gerontologist 34*(2), 256-260.

Hogan, R. (1980). *Human sexuality: A nursing perspective.* New York: Appleton-Century-Crofts.

Janus, S., & Janus, C. (1993). *The Janus report on sexual behavior.* New York: John Wiley and Sons.

Jensen, S.B. (1985). Sexual relationships in couples with a diabetic partner. *Journal of Sex and Marital Therapy, 11,* 259-270.

Kane, R.L., Ouslander, J.G., & Abrass, I.B. (1989). *Essentials of clinical geriatrics* (2nd ed.). New York: McGraw-Hill.

Katzin, L. (1990). Sexuality. *American Journal of Nursing, 90*(1), 55-59.

Korb, C., & Kupperberg, C. (1993). Sexual dysfunction: Altered sexuality patterns. In G. McFarland & E. McFarlane (Eds.), *Diagnosis and interventions: Planning for patient care* (2nd ed.). St. Louis: Mosby.

Korenman, S. (1994). Erectile dysfunction: Impotence. In W.M. Hazzard, E. Bierman, J. Blass, W. Ettinger, & J. Halter (Eds.), *Principles of geriatric medicine and gerontology.* New York: McGraw-Hill.

Leiblum, S., Bachman, G., Kemman, E., Colburn, D., & Swartzman, L. (1983). Vaginal atrophy in the postmenopausal woman: The importance of sexual activity and hormones. *Journal of the American Medical Association, 249,* 2195-2198.

Levy, J. (1994). Sexuality and aging. In W.M. Hazzard, E. Bierman, J. Blass, W. Ettinger, & J. Halter (Eds.), *Principles of geriatric medicine and gerontology.* New York: McGraw-Hill.

Masters, W.H., Johnson, V.E., & Kolodny, R.C. (1988). *Human sexuality* (3rd ed.). Glenview, IL: Scott, Foresman, and Company.

McCartney, J.R., Izeman, H., Rogers, D., & Cohen, N. (1987). Sexuality and the institutionalized elderly. *Journal of the American Geriatrics Society, 35,* 331-333.

McFarlane, E.A., & Rubenfeld, M.G. (1983). The need for sexual integrity. In H. Yura & M.B. Walsh (Eds.), *Human needs 3 and the nursing process* (pp. 185-233). Norwalk, CT: Appleton-Century-Crofts.

Melman, A., Kaplan, D., & Redfield, J. (1984). Evaluation of the first 70 patients in the Center for Male Dysfunction of Beth Israel Medical Center. *Journal of Urology, 131,* 53-55.

Moore, K., Folk-Lighty, M., & Nolen, M.J. (1984). Counseling the cardiac patient. *Nursing 84, 14,* 105.

Mulligan, T., & Modigh, A. (1991). Sexuality in dependent living situations. *Clinics in Geriatric Medicine, 7*(1), 153-160.

Odom, M.J., Carr, B.C., & MacDonald, P.C. (1990). The menopause and estrogen replacement therapy. In W. Hazzard, R. Andres, E. Bierman, & T. Blass (Eds.), *Principles of geriatric medicine and gerontology* (pp. 777-782). New York: McGraw-Hill.

Papadopoulos, C. (1987). Sexual problems of the CAD patient. *Medical Aspects of Human Sexuality, 21,* 53.

Rosal, M., Downing, J., Littman, A., & Ahern, D. (1994). Sexual functioning post-myocardial infarction: Effects of beta-blockers, psychological status and safety information. *Journal of Psychosomatic Research, 38*(7), 555-567.

Schover, L.R. (1988a). *Sexuality and cancer: For the man who has cancer and his partner.* New York: American Cancer Society.

Schover, L.R. (1988b). *Sexuality and cancer: For the woman who has cancer and her partner.* New York: American Cancer Society.

Schreiner-Engel, P., Schiavii, R.C., Vietorisz, D., & Smith, H. (1987). The differential impact of diabetes type on female sexuality. *Journal of Psychosomatic Research, 31,* 23-33.

Sheahan, S.L. (1989). Identifying female sexual dysfunctions. *Nurse Practitioner, 14,* 25-34.

Shippee-Rice, R. (1990). Sexuality and aging. In C. Fogel & D. Lauver (Eds.), *Sexual health promotion.* Philadelphia: W.B. Saunders.

Starr, B.D., & Weiner, M.B. (1981). *Sex and sexuality in the mature years.* New York: Stein and Day.

Thompson, J.M., McFarland, G.K., Hirsch, J.E., Tucker, S.M., & Bowers, A.C. (1989). *Mosby's manual of clinical nursing* (2nd ed.). St. Louis: Mosby.

Turner, B.F., & Adams, C. (1983). The sexuality of older women. In E.W. Markson (Ed.), *Older women: Issues and prospects* (pp. 55-72). Lexington, MA: Lexington Books.

U.S. Bureau of the Census. (1987). Estimates of the population of the United States by age, sex, and race: 1980-1986, *Current Population Reports* (Series P-25, No. 100). Washington DC: U.S. Government Printing Office.

U.S. Department of Health and Human Services. (1993). *Vital and health statistics* (Series 3, No. 27).

BIBLIOGRAPHY

Bishop, G. (1989). Sex and UTI in older women. *Medical Aspects of Human Sexuality, 23,* 65-69.

Catalona, W.J., & Bigg, S.W. (1990). Nerve-sparing radical prostatectomy. *Journal of Urology, 143*(3), 538-543.

Frank, D., et al. (1978). Mastectomy and sexual behavior: A pilot study. *Sexuality and Disability, 1,* 16-26.

CHAPTER 7

In fact, there's nothing that keeps its youth,
So far as I know, but a tree and truth.
There are traces of age in the one-hoss shay,
A general flavor of mild decay . . .

OLIVER WENDELL HOLMES, JR.

Sensation

■ Learning Objectives

On completion of this chapter, the reader will be able to do the following:

1. Identify age-related changes in vision, hearing, smell, and taste.
2. Assess the senses of sight, hearing, smell, taste, and touch of the older adult.
3. Recognize psychologic and sociocultural factors that interact with sensory functioning.
4. Understand the causes of sensory impairment in older people.
5. Develop a plan of nursing care for an older person with sensory impairment.
6. Provide appropriate nursing interventions for older adults with sensory impairment.

The richness of the human experience is perceived through the senses, especially through vision and hearing. Often, as people age, their ability to perceive the information received from their senses is impaired or distorted. Aging dulls the senses, and older adults must find ways to compensate for that change. A decline in sensory functioning is a silent, unnoticed process, which may occur undetected by both older adults and their families. This chapter encourages the reader to be aware of the physical, psychologic, and sociocultural indicators of sensory impairment. The senses discussed herein are sight, hearing, smell, taste, and touch.

■ Sight: Vision

Normal aging brings changes to the eye and to the sense of sight (Box 7-1). These changes affect the functional level of sight referred to as "vision." Aging brings an increase in the susceptibility to pathologic conditions that affect vision. It has been estimated that 1.3 million older adults have some loss of vision. A National Health Interview Survey of older people reported that close to 95% wore glasses, and for those over 85 years of age, only 45% reported that glasses corrected all of their vision problems (National Center for Health Statistics, 1986). For those over 85 years of age who report vision problems, 12% are legally blind.

BOX 7-1 AGE-RELATED CHANGES
IN THE EYE AND IN VISION

- Cornea flattens
- Sclera becomes yellow and less elastic
- Intraocular pressure increases
- Accommodation of lens decreases
- Retina receives less light
- Capability for tearing diminishes
- Ability to gaze upward decreases
- Ability to maintain convergence diminishes
- Vitreous floaters may appear
- Arcus senilis may appear
- Visual acuity decreases
- Night vision decreases

Older adults report greater dissatisfaction with their level of visual function than do members of other age groups. The visual complaints reported by older adults are problems with seeing under low lights, difficulty processing rapidly changing displays, difficulty focusing on near-vision tasks, difficulty searching in the environment, and problems with glare and decreased night vision (Schleber, 1992).

There is a need for early intervention and rehabilitation, because many of the visually impaired older adults have conditions that are amenable to treatment. The role of the nurse is in prevention of treatable vision loss through education and screening, and rehabilitation of older adults who are subject to visual impairment.

NORMAL STRUCTURE AND FUNCTION

Vision is the result of the sense of sight being stimulated by patterns of light that are external to the person. Human sight is limited by a field of vision that excludes approximately 40% of the surrounding environment: people cannot see what is behind them at the same time that they can see what is in front of them. Light enters the eye and travels first through the cornea, the major refractive surface of the eye responsible

for most of the focusing power. The light then travels through the anterior chamber, to the pupil. The pupil regulates the amount of light entering the eye through the process of constriction and dilatation. The light rays from the visual stimulus next encounter the crystalline lens. Through the process of accommodation, the lens is able to change its shape and thereby alters its focusing power and increases the imaging power of the eye, thereby enabling individuals to view near objects. Light next passes and is imaged on the retina, where the cones and rods transduce light energy into nervous system activity (Schleber, 1992). The optic nerve then transmits impulses from the retina through the visual pathway to the occipital cortex. There, in the higher centers of the brain, the impulses from the external light rays are transformed into data that can be processed and recognized as the unique human sensation of vision for a particular moment in time and space (Figure 7-1). Vision is an amazing process that happens so quickly and so easily that it is taken for granted until it is threatened by the slow but predictable process of aging.

AGE-RELATED CHANGES

The normal eye undergoes significant age-related changes (see Box 7-1). The eye's external changes give evidence of advancing age. These changes result from multiple normal changes, such as loss of orbital fat, loss of elastic tissue, and decreases in muscle tone. The skin around the eye darkens, and wrinkles referred to as "crow's feet" appear. Some older adults lose the lateral aspect of their eyebrows; this is not a classic sign of disease, as it would be in younger adults (hypothyroidism), but rather a normal occurrence of aging. Xanthomas, cutaneous deposits of lipid material, are sometimes found at the inner portion of the lid; these may indicate elevated bloodlipid levels.

These age-related changes may give rise to two conditions: senile entropion (a condition in which the lid margin turns inward) and senile ectropion (a condition in which the eyelid mar-

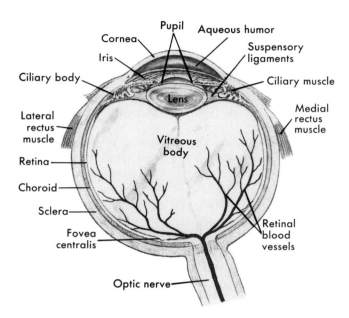

FIGURE 7-1 Cross-section of the eye. (From Thompson, J.M., et al. [1993]. *Mosby's manual of clinical nursing* [3rd ed.]. St. Louis: Mosby.)

A   B

FIGURE 7-2 A, Entropion, with lashes invading the cornea; B, ectropion, in which the lower lid falls away from the globe so that the punctum can no longer function as the exit portal for tears. (From Stein, H.A., Slatt, B.J., & Stein, R.M. [1994]. *The ophthalmic assistant: Fundamentals and clinical practice* [6th ed.]. St. Louis: Mosby.)

gin turns outward) (Figure 7-2). Although not threatening to vision, these conditions may cause the older person discomfort and may become severe enough to cause psychosocial problems because of cosmetic effects. In senile entropion the turning inward of the eyelid may cause the lashes to rest against the conjunctiva, often resulting in ocular irritation. This can be corrected by a surgical procedure if the severity warrants. In contrast, senile ectropion exposes the conjunctiva and may lead to inflammation of the affected eye.

The eye itself undergoes major changes because of the aging process. The cornea, as a result of the aging process, tends to flatten, which reduces its refractory power. Also, the sensitivity of the cornea decreases, limiting its protective function. The sclera, although it remains white throughout the life span, becomes more transparent and may take on a yellow coloration because of dehydration (Michaels, 1994). The anterior chamber becomes progressively shallower. The pupil becomes smaller, and the response to different levels of illumination is lessened because of the loss of range of pupil dilation and constriction. The retina of an older individual becomes thinner because of fewer neural cells and receives only one third the amount of light that the retina of a younger person receives. This age-related change necessitates a higher level of illumination for reading. Adaptation to dark occurs more slowly and to a lesser total extent. Older people also have difficulty with color perception, especially the blue-green distinctions.

The lens of the aging eye loses its elasticity and increases in density. Surprisingly, both eyes change at the same time and the same variance (Michaels, 1994). The ability of the lens to accommodate leads to a decrease in the ability to focus near objects. By the time they are in their fifth decade, most people require glasses to be able to read fine print. This frequent condition,

resulting from the age-related changes in the human eye, is called *presbyopia.* Corrective lenses are extremely helpful in assisting the older person in maintaining visual function. Because of the change in the lens, glare becomes a more severe adaptive problem for older adults, which increases their need for sunglasses. Depth perception is also affected by the increased susceptibility to glare and the decreased contrast sensitivity (Heath, 1993). *Floaters,* opacities occurring in the vitreous humor, may appear in the older person's field of vision and may be a cause of alarm. Although floaters can be considered a normal process of the aging eye, in some instances they may be a harbinger of a serious problem, such as retinal detachment. Therefore if floaters are observed, the patient should see an ophthalmologist.

The most common, although not universal, clinical change in the cornea is *arcus senilis,* in which a grayish-yellow ring forms around the iris (Figure 7-3). This usually begins on the upper portion of the eye. It then continues to develop until the entire iris is encircled. It is caused by a

FIGURE 7-3 Arcus senilis in a patient with a peripheral iridectomy. (From Stein, H.S., Slatt, B.J., & Stein, R.M. [1994]. *The ophthalmic assistant: Fundamentals and clinical practice* [6th ed.]. St. Louis: Mosby.)

fatty invasion of the corneal margin, which blurs demarcation between the cornea and the sclera (Kasper, 1989). Arcus senilis is common in people over age 65, has no pathologic implications, does not cause any visual problems, and is not a cosmetic problem.

An accompanying age-related change that affects many minor eye problems is diminished tear secretion. Tearing, a natural protective device of the human body, slows in its ability to defend the eye against the pollution of the environment. This predisposes the eye to more infections of the conjunctiva. Many older adults use over-the-counter preparations of hydroxyethyl cellulose in solution (brand names include Hypotears, Tears Natural, and Artificial Tears) to assist in replacement of naturally occurring tears. These solutions should be used only for mild, self-limiting conditions (e.g., dry eyes) and never for infections or inflammations.

As people grow older, normal age-related changes in vision necessitate changes in behavior. These changes are minor, and most people readily adapt by taking the measures listed in Box 7-2.

COMMON HEALTH DEVIATIONS

The major pathologic causes of visual impairment in older adults are (1) cataracts, (2) glaucoma, (3) senile macular degeneration, (4) diabetic retinopathy, and (5) temporal arteritis.

Cataracts

Cataracts are the most frequent ocular disease to occur with aging, with about 50% of adults over the age of 40 years showing some signs of clouding of the lens (Heath, 1993). Any opacification of the lens is considered to be a cataract and may be the result of multiple causes (i.e., congenital, toxic, metabolic, traumatic, or senescent). This condition is a common complication of aging; although it is bilateral in nature, one eye may be involved months before the other (Michaels, 1994).

Although 95% of those over 65 years of age have some degree of cataract formation, in very

---

BOX 7-2 MEANS OF ADAPTING TO NORMAL AGE-RELATED VISUAL CHANGES

1. Wear eyeglasses
2. Increase the amount of light when reading
3. Allow extra time for eyes to accommodate to darkness
4. Avoid nighttime driving of vehicles
5. Wear dark glasses to reduce the impact of the sun's glare

---

few of that large number is the process advanced enough to cause visual disability. The process of lens opacification develops over time, with the beginning of cataract formation occurring at the periphery of the eye. This beginning phase of cataract formation usually has no significant impact on vision. However, the mature cataract is widespread, involves the pupillary area, and leads to a slow decrease in vision. The entire lens may become opaque.

The functional implications of cataracts are twofold: (1) The ability to see detail is diminished, because of the reduction in the amount of light available to the retina; this depends on the severity of the cataract. (2) The difficulty in adjusting to glare increases, so the older person with cataracts will experience significant problems with adjusting between light and dark environments. This can create major safety problems in poorly lighted environments. Interestingly, the initial development of a cataract may cause an improvement in near vision for some older adults, but this also fades as the cataract becomes more clouded (Heath, 1993).

When cataracts interfere significantly with vision, thereby diminishing the quality of life for the individual, surgery may be appropriate. Many aspects need to be considered before surgery is performed: the degree of correctable visual acuity in each eye, the physical and psychologic ability of the patient to withstand the stress of the surgery, the type of work or leisure activities in which the patient is involved, and whether the patient has a social support system available to provide immediate monitoring and care, if necessary.

After cataract removal, there are three methods of restoring vision: eyeglasses, contact lens, and intraocular implant. Special eyeglasses, rarely used after surgery, are thick and heavy, and although they allow excellent central vision, they increase object size by about 25% and seriously impair peripheral vision. Individuals must learn to turn their heads to accommodate for peripheral vision loss, and most people have difficulty adjusting to the 25% increase in image size. In fact, if one eye is normal, eyeglasses cannot be used to restore vision lost from the afflicted eye because of the resulting disparity in image size.

The second of the three methods for post-surgical restoration of vision is the use of a contact lens. The contact lens corrects the focus of the eye, permits both central and peripheral vision, and only increases object image size by 6%, which is usually a more manageable difference. Although vision is restored, the older person must be able to add the new task of handling and caring for contact lenses to the presurgical activities of daily living. Not every older person is able or willing to insert contact lenses, and only 50% to 60% of older adults are said to be capable of wearing contact lenses (Kasper, 1989).

The most frequent cataract surgery is intraocular implantation of an artificial lens. The benefits in terms of vision restoration far outweigh the minimal risk associated with having a foreign body in the eye. Careful attention to intraocular pressure and repair of adhesions with laser procedures have resulted in dramatic improvements in vision (Heath, 1993). Most of the surgeries are done in outpatient surgical units using local anesthesia, with the older patient returning home the same day. The postoperative care usually entails periodic use of eyedrops, some restrictions in activities (such as bending and lifting), and return visits to the surgeon. Most older people need another person to assist them with their postoperative care, and many may not have a readily available family member or friendly neighbor. Therefore they may not seek or may defer treatment because they lack this important human support system.

Glaucoma

Glaucoma, the leading cause of blindness throughout the world, is an eye disorder that is characterized by a significant increase in intraocular pressure, damage to the optic nerve, and a loss in the visual field. There are two major types of glaucoma: primary open-angle glaucoma and primary closed-angle glaucoma. Primary open-angle glaucoma occurs more frequently in the older population than does primary closed-angle glaucoma. Older adults with primary open-angle glaucoma may have no symptoms, and the condition is usually discovered in a routine examination checking intraocular pressures (Michaels, 1994).

Primary open-angle glaucoma develops slowly over time, so subtly that the patient is not aware of any changes. Signs and symptoms that indicate glaucoma are an increase in intraocular pressure, family history of glaucoma, blurred vision not corrected with lenses, and a halo effect around lights. The functional impairment in vision caused by glaucoma is a loss of peripheral vision. This can cause problems for the affected person, especially in driving a car.

Medical treatment consists of eyedrops that decrease the intraocular pressure or drugs such as acetazolamide (Diamox) that decrease aqueous formation. Surgical treatment is usually reserved for difficult-to-control situations.

Primary closed-angle glaucoma is characterized by an acute, rapid-onset, painful attack of increased intraocular pressure, with a marked decrease in vision. Affected patients should be referred immediately to an ophthalmologist. Medical treatment consists of first normalizing intraocular pressure by the application of eyedrops. After

BOX 7-3 STEPS FOR SELF-ADMINISTRATION OF EYEDROPS

1. Wash your hands.
2. Use adequate light.
3. Sit, stand, or lie down in front of a mirror.
4. Tilt your head back.
5. Extend your lower lid outward to make a "pocket" into which the drops can fall, and look up.
6. Insert the drops into the pocket.
7. Release your eyelid, and close your eye.

pressure is normalized, surgical treatment is required. A peripheral iridectomy is performed on the affected eye to ensure free flow of aqueous humor.

Eyedrops as a medical treatment create problems for older adults living at home, especially those who live alone. The ability to instill drops into one's own eye calls for a high level of fine-motor skill and hand-to-eye coordination, which, because of other conditions (such as arthritis or parkinsonism), may be beyond the capacity of some older adults. Nurses must skillfully assist older adults in practicing application of the drugs so as to ensure safe and appropriate care (Feinburg, 1988) (Box 7-3).

Although drugs instilled in the eye are applied topically as eyedrops, they still may be systemically absorbed and may cause side effects. It is easy to forget that these topical drugs are absorbed into the system, so the nurse must take care to note that eyedrops can be a source of adverse side effects. Table 7-1 lists major drugs used in eyedrops and their potential side effects.

Macular degeneration

Macular degeneration, an age-related disease, involves the loss of central vision and occurs over time. There is a prevalence rate of 30% in those over 75 years of age, but with only 10% experiencing any vision loss. Onset is usually earlier, at about 65 years, with the initial involvement of only one eye; within a 4-year period the second eye is involved (Heath, 1993; Michaels, 1994). The pathogenesis is little understood, and at present there is little hope for a definitive cure. However, a theory of leakage of retinal membranes has given rise to the use of laser photocoagulation with mixed results (Michaels, 1994).

The affected older adult usually will report a loss of visual acuity or distorted vision. Distortion and subsequent loss of the center of the visual field is the usual severe symptom. The patient should be referred immediately for medical care. Peripheral vision remains intact, so the patient does not lose total vision. Vision rehabilitation consists of attempts to magnify the central vision defect area. The larger the field, the less information is lost to the individual. This can be accomplished through inexpensive ocular lenses or with video enlargement (Wasson et al., 1990). It is important to refer older adults with macular degeneration to formal vision rehabilitation services (Heath, 1993).

Diabetic retinopathy

As people with diabetes mellitus live longer, the incidence of diabetic retinopathy rises, causing a significant increase in the number of people with this form of visual loss. It occurs at a rate of 7% in people who have had diabetes for less than 10 years, 26% in those who have had diabetes for 10 to 14 years, and 63% in those who have had diabetes for more than 15 years (Stefansson, 1990). Currently, in the United States, diabetic eye changes are the leading cause of blindness in the adult population (Heath, 1993). The patient with diabetic retinopathy may experience transient blurring, loss of central vision, and significant shifts in vision. On funduscopic examination, the retina of an individual with diabetic retinopathy will exhibit irregular small hemorrhages and yellow-white exudates.

At present, bilateral involvement generally occurs 10 to 15 years after the onset of diabetes.

TABLE 7-1 Ophthalmic drugs and possible side effects

Drug	Class	Side effect
Pilocarpine	Cholinergic	Bronchospasm
Timolol	Beta-blocker	Bradycardia, hypotension, confusion
Epinephrine and phenylephrine	Adrenergic	Palpitation, hypertension

Adapted from Kane, Ouslander, & Abrass. (1988). *Essentials of clinical geriatrics* (2nd ed.). New York: McGraw-Hill.

The control of the individual's diabetes does not preclude the development of diabetic retinopathy. Laser photocoagulation as a treatment has helped to alleviate some aspects of diabetic retinopathy, but definitive treatment has not yet been devised.

Temporal arteritis

Temporal arteritis, a vascular disease of older age, is an inflammatory disease of the temporal arteries and is characterized by headache, preauricular tenderness, an enlarged temporal artery, and a complaint of general malaise. The symptoms of temporal arteritis may be overlooked by the patient and family members, who may think that the symptoms are characteristics of aging rather than of disease. One half of older patients with this disease will suffer visual loss that could have been prevented. This condition is treated via steroids.

The nurse's role in the detection of temporal arteritis is to follow up on the patient's complaints, to do an accurate assessment, and to collaborate with the physician to ensure proper medical and nursing care.

■ Nursing Process

Integration of the scientific knowledge concerning age-related changes and pathologic conditions that affect the aging eye enables the nurse to use this knowledge to provide wholistic nursing care to older adults.

ASSESSMENT

Nursing assessment of vision requires an accurate history, a functional assessment of visual acuity, and a physical examination of the eye and surrounding tissue. Psychosocial and environmental assessments are critical components of a wholistic approach to the nursing care of an older adult patient with a visual impairment.

History

Impairment of vision is usually a slow, insidious process that may go unnoticed by the older patient. The nurse must also consider that the older patient may think that nothing can be done to improve vision or that it is best not to complain about what the patient considers his or her minor problem. Taking an accurate history requires both interpersonal skill and scientific knowledge about normal aging and about particular conditions that affect vision.

Some older patients are excellent historians, but others require more time and more direct questioning to elicit needed information. Suggested questions include two types: open ended and direct. An open-ended question may have any number of correct answers and is open to the interpretation and concerns of the patient. An example of an open-ended approach is "Tell me what is different now about your vision." This is an appropriate way to begin the history taking. When completing the vision history, it is wise to conclude with an open-ended question such as "Is there anything else you can tell me about your vision?" If the patient is residing in the community, it is important to ascertain whether other health providers have been consulted and, if so, the approximate dates of the patient's most recent visits.

Direct questions, on the other hand, ask the patient to provide specific answers. Examples of direct questions concerning the patient's visual acuity would be the following:

1. When did you last see a physician about your vision?
2. When was the last time the prescription for your glasses was changed?
3. When did you last purchase glasses?
4. Are you experiencing any difficulty seeing?
5. Are you experiencing any difficulty seeing at night?
6. Do you see rings around lights?
7. Is your vision blurred?
8. Have you changed any of your activities because of your vision?
9. Have you experienced loss of vision in one eye?
10. Have you experienced a lack of tears or any minor irritations of your eyes?

When gathering information concerning the patient's visual difficulties, it is important to determine time of onset, duration (how long has it lasted?), quality of the experience (such as a yellow halo around lights), what makes it better or worse (is it worse at night?), and associated factors (a particular posture or a time of day). Has the patient experienced any eye pain, and if so, what type of pain? This information is important in understanding the specific experience of the older patient in regard to vision. The nurse who has established rapport with the patient and has made the time available to listen will be able to gather significant pertinent data.

Visual acuity

The most common test for far vision is the Snellen chart. This chart contains rows of letters of various sizes and standardized numbers at the end of each line, which indicate a degree of visual acuity. The patient stands or sits 20 feet from the chart and is tested first without glasses and then with glasses (if the patient wears eyeglasses other than just reading glasses). One eye is covered, and the other is tested by having the patient read the letters, beginning with the small-est print first. Each line of the chart is marked with a fraction (i.e., 20/20, 20/30, 20/40, etc., up to 20/200). Visual acuity is recorded as a fraction, with the numerator of 20 indicating the distance of the patient from the chart. The distance at which a person with normal vision would see the line is the number assigned to the second position in the fraction, or the denominator. This is the significant number, which indicates the degree of vision lost. The higher the denominator, the more impaired the vision.

In many settings, this chart may not be available to the nurse for testing visual acuity. A readily available alternative test of gross vision involves using one's fingers. Patients are asked to count the number of fingers that the examiner holds up within their field of vision. The examiner can test each eye separately. After checking the patient's literacy level, have the patient read from printed material such as a newspaper. This will allow you to assess ability to read different sizes of type, such as headlines, headings, and regular newspaper print. In addition, ask the patient to describe your appearance (what color is my shirt?). This type of assessment provides a rough estimate of visual acuity and is readily achievable in all settings.

Physical examination of the eye

For the physical examination of the eye, necessary equipment includes an ophthalmoscope, a Snellen chart, and a printed card with reading material. The first step in any physical examination is observation. When observing the eyes of an older person, be sure to pay close attention to the following:

1. The skin and tissue surrounding the eyes
2. The condition of the eyelids as observed when they are closed
3. The conjunctiva, particularly any signs of irritation
4. The pupils, to see whether they are usually small and show a slowed reflex response

Aging Alert

Correction of vision problems

1. Adaptation to visual changes is a socially acceptable aspect of aging.
2. Correction mechanisms (e.g., eyeglasses) are effective and socially acceptable, with no attached stigma of disability.
3. Medicare does not reimburse older people for their purchase of prescribed glasses.

When examining the eye, be sure to test with the ophthalmoscope for the red reflex. This will be impossible to visualize if the patient has a mature cataract.

Always obtain permission from the patient to perform any part of a physical examination. When examining the eye, be sure to tell the patient what you are doing. This will alleviate fears and increase the patient's cooperation during the exam. This screening examination assists the nurse in gathering data for use in clinical judgments concerning the patient's visual ability.

Psychosocial assessment

A psychosocial nursing assessment focuses on the strengths of the older person. Unfortunately, without such a focus, the vitality and resilience of the older person is often unrecognized. To maintain this focus, nurses should acknowledge individual patients and their unique abilities to cope with different levels of sensory impairment.

Psychosocial assessments of sensory functioning, for both vision and hearing, include questions that ask patients how they perceive themselves coping with their impairments and what strengths they utilize to adjust to their levels of sensory impairment. When a patient's family members are available, ask the patient whether these family members should be consulted before you obtain the opinions of relatives who might not even be knowledgeable about the

patient (Box 7-4). Nonetheless, it is important to establish which individuals provide significant care of the older patient and to utilize them to corroborate information gained from the patient.

The assessment creates a picture of the patient's lifestyle by use of specific questions. The following questions facilitate gathering of lifestyle information: What is a normal day like for you? Tell me what you did yesterday. Have you changed anything about your life in the past week? And so on. When asking these kinds of questions, it is important to be aware of the patient's mood while responding to each question and to allow time for the patient to reflect and remember. Accept the patient's lifestyle with a willingness to see in it the strengths that have fostered a long life.

Family assessment

Assessment of family members is important because their attitudes will have a significant impact on the older person's ability to maintain an independent lifestyle. Items to assess include the following:

1. What are the perceptions of the family concerning the patient's visual abilities?
2. Does the family need information concerning the patient's functional level?
3. If medical treatment is necessary, such as eyedrops every 4 hours, does the family have the resources, knowledge, and motivation to assist the older patient in accomplishing the task?
4. Does the family identify a primary caregiver?
5. What is done by the caregiver to assist in the patient's visual functioning?
6. Is the caregiver open to professional assistance?

The nurse should be aware of the difficulties that arise for caregivers. Providing care for older parents or an older spouse can be extremely stressful and demanding. The caregiver is an important part of the patient's milieu and should always be included in the process of assessment.

BOX 7-4 PSYCHOSOCIAL ASSESSMENT OF VISION

QUESTIONS FOR PATIENT AND/OR FAMILY MEMBERS

1. In what respect has your (the patient's) vision changed?
2. Has the change in your vision affected your ability to walk around your home? Walk outside your house? Go grocery shopping?
3. Has the change in your vision affected the manner in which you are able to take care of yourself, such as getting dressed? Bathing and grooming? Using the bathroom?
4. Have you noticed any changes in the way your family treats you?
5. Have you had family members or friends who have had visual impairment? What was it like for them?
6. Have you changed your social engagements because of your visual problems?
7. Do you worry that somehow your visual problems are related to something you did or didn't do?
8. Are you worried about your safety as a result of your visual problems? Is there anything else that frightens you about your change in vision?
9. Have you felt sad or depressed because of your visual loss?
10. Can you tell me how you are handling this difficult situation?
11. Is there anything else you would like to tell, or something I've forgotten to ask?

Often, the caregiver of an older person may be an informal patient of the nurse, especially if the nursing care is delivered in the home.

Environmental assessment

The environmental assessment consists of two distinct portions: (1) the assessment of the living arrangement and (2) the resource assessment.

Living arrangement assessment Box 7-5 highlights several environmental features to assess when considering the needs of an older person with a visual impairment. Assessment of the environment depends on the living arrangement of the patient. Older adults in need of nursing care may be found in any one of three environments: the private or family home, the hospital, or the nursing home. The most difficult of these to assess properly is the private home. Many older people live alone in the community. They may reside in single-family homes or they may live alone in apartment buildings that are primarily occupied by older residents.

Assessment of an apartment residence should include both the apartment and the area of the apartment building that the older patient uses. One aspect that calls for daily use may be an elevator. This may present a hazard for some older adults with visual impairment. They may have difficulty determining when the elevator arrives, especially if the doors and the interior are gray. Getting off the elevator at the correct destination may be difficult for the visually impaired unless there are markings designating the number of the floor placed at eye level, in bright colors, and visible from the elevator.

The opening and closing of elevator doors presents a possible hazard for older adults. To see when the door opens, to decide if there is room in the elevator, and then to walk into the elevator before the door closes is a difficult task for an older person with a visual impairment. Daily use of elevators and their hazards are also part of the living arrangements for most nursing home residents.

The assessment of the environment has added significance when the patient has a visual impairment. It is helpful to understand how the things most of us take for granted, such as using

BOX 7-5 ENVIRONMENTAL ASSESSMENT FOR VISUAL IMPAIRMENT

1. Adequate lighting is available.
2. Light switches are conveniently located.
3. Stairways are well lighted.
4. Night-lights are used, especially in bathrooms and bedroom.
5. Handrails are available where there could be a sudden change of light, such as on outside steps.
6. Glare from windows is controlled by use of drapes and/or shades.
7. No furniture is placed in entryways.
8. Bright nonskid tape is on top and bottom steps to indicate beginning and end of stairs.
9. Shiny surfaces, such as shiny waxed floors, are avoided.
10. Contrasting colors are used in decorating (very dark colors or very light pastels are avoided).

an elevator, call for extra energy and fortitude for the older person with a visual impairment. Old age is not for the weak of spirit. Express your respect for the abilities of older adults as they go about their daily tasks of maintaining themselves as independent citizens in a difficult environment.

A home visit is necessary to adequately assess living arrangements, although information concerning common household hazards for the visually impaired can be given to patients who are attending a clinic and do not want their home to be assessed. The hospital and the nursing home need to be assessed by nurses, to be sure that the environment is supportive of the visually impaired older patient. All significant parameters of the environment should be assessed. The nurse has a responsibility to ensure a safe environment in hospitals or in nursing homes. The needs of the patients are the professional con-

cern of the nurse, and at times these needs may conflict with the demands of the institution. The nurse must be able to state the high-priority needs of the patients, such as increased lighting at night, and then to serve as an advocate to promote and protect the safety of the patients.

Resource assessment The resource assessment is the second portion of the environmental assessment. This assessment is critical for older adults already living outside of an institutional environment, and for those older patients who are about to be discharged from either the hospital or the nursing home. Suggestions for lighting for the aging eye may include the following (Rosenberg, 1994):

1. Only one light source should be in a work area, and it should be out of the visual field of the worker.
2. The strongest light should be directly on the task; areas farther from the task should be well lighted, but at a lower density.
3. Luminous ceiling light should be avoided.
4. Watching television in the dark should be avoided.

Often this process of resource assessment may be an interdisciplinary function, but the nurse must be actively involved. The patient and the patient's family and/or caregiver need information regarding what resources are available within their community and how to obtain the services both initially and over time. Within the assessment of resources, look for the following:

1. Special resources of the community and the nation to assist visually impaired older adults, such as The Lighthouse National Center for Vision and Aging
2. Availability of aids for limited vision
3. Patient's financial ability to obtain and maintain needed services

NURSING DIAGNOSES

A diagnosis is always made by analysis of the data gained through the assessment process. This process includes accessing the patient's total health care record, an in-depth nursing assessment, and conferences with family members and other health care providers. A nursing diagnosis is always made by the clustering of data that define and support the diagnosis.

Nursing diagnoses to be considered when caring for a patient with a visual impairment include the following North American Nursing Diagnosis Association (NANDA) diagnoses:

1. Alteration in sensory/visual perception
2. Impaired social interaction and/or social isolation
3. Risk for injury

The diagnosis of alteration in visual perception may be related to pathologic or other conditions, as evidenced by the following:

1. Low scores on visual screening test
2. Self-reports of limited vision
3. Inability to see near or far objects
4. Inability to recognize familiar people at a distance
5. Loss of a particular part of the visual field
6. Medical diagnosis

The diagnosis of impaired social interaction and/or social isolation may be related to visual impairment, as evidenced by the following:

1. Failure to attend usual social meetings, such as meetings of Gray Panthers, church groups, and bridge clubs
2. Failure to attend usual forms of entertainment, such as movies or concerts
3. Failure to attend usual family gatherings, such as grandchildren's birthday parties
4. Failure to visit friends

The diagnosis of risk for injury may be related to impaired vision, as evidenced by the following:

1. Hazardous living arrangement
2. Lack of cautious behavior
3. Denial of visual loss
4. Refusal to adhere to medical regimen
5. Lack of use of aids for limited vision
6. Additional functional deficits, such as limited mobility

PLANNING AND GOAL IDENTIFICATION

The planning phase of the nursing process consists of establishing realistic short- and long-term goals, based on data obtained in the assessment phase. Whenever possible, goals should be developed with the patient included as an equal member of the health care team.

Alteration in visual perception

A long-term goal is that the patient will adapt to visual loss. Short-term goals include the following:

1. Patient will be able to compensate for loss of peripheral vision by recognizing appropriate times to turn head to increase range of visual field.
2. Patient or caregiver will demonstrate ability to insert eyedrops.
3. Patient will wear clean and properly placed eyeglasses during periods of ambulation.

Impaired social interaction due to visual impairment

A long-term goal is that the patient will resume a normal range of activities. Short-term goals include the following:

1. Patient will attend Gray Panther meeting, being driven to meeting by Mr. Jones, a friend.
2. Patient will attend church services with daughter.
3. Patient will attend bridge social on Thursday evening.

These two examples illustrate the planning associated with specific diagnoses, to facilitate the reader's understanding of the specific and individualized patient-centered nature of planning.

IMPLEMENTATION

Nursing interventions that assist the older patient with visual impairment need to be specific to the defined goals, etiologies, and the defining characteristics that have been identified in the assessment phase. They also address the defining characteristics and causes that are amenable to change through interventions.

Three settings are considered to be the typical environments in which older adults receive nursing care. Two settings are institutions: (1) an acute care setting, usually a large teaching hospital or a community hospital, and (2) a nursing home. The third setting and the least restricted environment is the older person's private home. Most older people experience nursing care in at least two of these settings, and some of those who experience nursing care over a long period do so in all three settings.

In the acute care setting

Nursing care of the older adult patient with visual impairment is guided first by the condition of the patient and then by the setting in which the care is given. If the nursing care is rendered in an acute care setting, such as a hospital, the patient is probably in the setting primarily for surgical treatment, such as cataract surgery. Because most cataract surgery is performed on an outpatient basis, the nurse's role in the preoperative care and the postoperative care and teaching is important to the well-being of the patient. Both the patient and the caregiver need instruction. A caregiver will usually accompany the older patient to the surgical center and will be available after the surgery for the first 24 hours of home care. The postoperative care usually entails periodic application of eyedrops and some minor limitations on the patient's activity. The nurse needs to allow sufficient time for teaching and for answering any questions of the caregiver, who may also be an older adult.

Often when an older patient is admitted for an emergency situation that is unrelated to vision, the patient's visual deficit will go unnoticed. Glasses may have been left at home or by the bedside in the nursing home. Nurses in the hospital should be alert when they see an older patient without glasses because of the high incidence of visual impairment in the older population. The loss of corrected vision may add to the stress of a hospital stay and may deprive the older hospitalized person of the ability to see

clearly and to make sense of a strange and somewhat hostile environment.

The nurse is familiar with the sights in the hospital—the food on the dinner tray, the screen on the monitor, the person delivering pills or fixing an intravenous (IV) bag that hangs near the bed, and the faces and white coats of the medical team making rounds. For the older visually impaired patient, each new person who comes into the hospital room may pose a threat. The alert nurse can make a significant difference in the older patient's ability to maintain a sense of control and a sense of reality by making sure that eyeglasses are readily available, clean, and used by the patient.

In the nursing home

In the nursing home the nurse must be vigilant to changes that occur in the older resident's vision, must be aware of the resident's need for annual visits to an ophthalmologist, and must have an understanding of the significance of medications and their potential side effects. The care of the resident's eyeglasses should be supervised by the nurse, to ensure that they are cleaned and properly worn. It may be wise to label the glasses with the resident's name, to ensure that if they are lost, they will be returned. Residents who are confused may become more confused if their eyeglasses are lost and not replaced. The importance of maximizing the resident's visual ability should be emphasized to the staff, to the physicians, and to the resident's family.

In the private or family home

Generally, the nurse will assist the patient who lives in a private or family home in creating a barrier-free environment that allows the patient to continue to function independently. Safety is a high priority in the nurse's interventions with such patients. Besides assisting with the environment, the nurse must create a caring milieu that will facilitate the patient's acceptance of the visual impairment and will strengthen coping abilities that allow adaptation to the demands of the visual deficit.

In the private or family home, as in the nursing home, the nurse is the primary provider and must take responsibility for ensuring that all the strengths of the older person are maximized. Vision, even though it may not be the reason for the formal nursing visit, should always be assessed. The opportunity to teach older adults or couples how to improve their living environment should not be overlooked. Nurses have a responsibility to their patients to provide services that not only treat their physical conditions but also provide them with information and a caring milieu that allows continued growth, an encouraged spirit of hope, and a safe environment.

EVALUATION

In the evaluation phase the nurse examines the nursing interventions in terms of patient outcomes. Have the specific patient-centered, short-term goals been accompiished? Were these accomplished through the intervention of the nurse, or was some other unforeseen event responsible for the meeting of the goals? To what does the patient attribute the change? What about the long-term goal—has enough time passed that progress should have been made toward meeting that goal? What does the patient think? Do any of the etiologies or defining characteristics of the diagnosis still exist, and if so, how are they affecting the patient? Does the plan of care need to be revised, or has the problem been resolved?

Has the plan of care made a difference? Does the nursing documentation clearly delineate the assessment, the diagnosis, the plan of intervention, and the method of evaluation of the nursing care received by this older person? The evaluation phase of the nursing process should never be left unfinished or undocumented. Documentation is a critical factor in development of a scientific foundation for nursing practice, particularly in the compiling of data on sensory deficits such as vision or hearing impairments.

■ Hearing

The prevalence of hearing loss in the older population in the United States is significant. In the longitudinal Framingham Heart Study of adults age 63 to 95, the prevalence of hearing loss for the most important frequencies was 42% (Gates et al., 1990). Hearing loss is the third most frequently reported chronic problem in the over-65 population, and for people age 65 to 74, 24% have hearing loss, whereas in those over the age of 75, 38% experience hearing loss. In all older age groups, men have more hearing impairment than women (Jerger et al., 1995). The number of hearing-impaired adults is estimated at about 7 million people, and the number is expected to increase to at least 11 million by the year 2000 (Rees et al., 1994). In nursing home residents the prevalence of significant impairment in hearing is as high as 70% (Jerger et al., 1995). It is safe to say that hearing loss is a major factor that influences the quality of life for significant numbers of older nursing home residents.

NORMAL STRUCTURE AND FUNCTION

Hearing is a process of the transmission of sounds from the external environment through the mechanism of the ear and the auditory neural pathways to the brain's cortex (Figure 7-4). The human ear consists of three interrelated parts. The outer ear is made up of the pinna, the tragus, and the external ear canal; the middle ear contains the tympanic membrane and the three ossicles (malleus, incus, and stapes); and the inner ear is made up of the cochlea, the vestibule, and the semicircular canals. Hair cells, the auditory receptors, are located within the cochlea.

The normal auditory process includes sound entering through the external ear, proceeding through the canal, and striking the tympanic membrane. The sound then vibrates and is transmitted as neural impulses through the inner ear by the three ossicles. The purpose of the middle ear is to transform energy from the sound waves in the ear into the mechanical force needed to activate the fluid in the cochlea. The cochlea, the sensory organ of hearing, is snail shaped, filled with fluid, and located in the temporal bone. The sensory hair cells in the cochlea play a significant role in the transmission of the neural impulses to the brain along the auditory (eighth cranial nerve) neural pathway. The cochlear por-

FIGURE 7-4 Components of the ear. (From Thompson, J.M., et al. [1993]. *Mosby's manual of clinical nursing* [3rd ed.]. St. Louis: Mosby.)

tion of the auditory nerve consists of about 30,000 nerve fibers, which carry information to the brain. The central auditory system is where the processing of speech occurs in the auditory cortex in the temporal lobe (Jerger et al., 1995).

The auditory process allows specific external sounds to be interpreted as meaningful communication. Hearing is fundamental to human interaction. Without the ability to hear, the older person is deprived of the total experience of life. There may be a loss of intimacy, friendship, and significant roles, such as musician or teacher. Hearing also allows the individual to discern the sounds of the external environment and to judge whether the sounds convey any danger, such as the ringing of a smoke alarm.

AGE-RELATED CHANGES

Although hearing loss is not a universal age-related occurrence, many older people experience hearing loss. Age-related changes and mani-festations of diseases that lead to hearing loss are not well understood at this time. In spite of our lack of complete scientific understanding of this common condition, the nurse needs to know the different types of hearing loss and the terms that define hearing loss.

Common complaints of older adults concerning itching in the external ear and increase in cerumen impaction are related to changes in the number of sweat glands. Cerumen glands are modified sweat glands. Their reduction, along with a decrease in other types of sweat glands, results in dry skin and dry and hard earwax. The itching can be controlled by regular and small amounts of baby oil if there is no infection. Cerumen ear impaction can be averted by careful monitoring to avoid buildup.

Although there is a degenerative process involving the ossicular chain, middle ear changes are minimal and not clinically significant (Rees et al., 1994). Inner ear changes affecting the auditory processing system seem to increase with age and lead to an auditory processing disorder and a peripheral hearing sensitivity loss. An age-related loss of cochlear hair cells is thought by many to be a significant source of hearing loss (Rees et al., 1994). Cells of the auditory pathway have a highly specialized function and have limited regenerative ability. The length of their cell life is determined by a myriad of variables: heredity, environmental insults (noise), nutrition, cholesterol, and the body's adaptation to stress (Rees et al., 1994).

COMMON TERMS

Presbycusis is a global term used to describe hearing loss associated with normal aging. Hearing loss includes decreased hearing sensitivity caused by peripheral cochlear defects. A secondary feature of hearing loss is a defect in central auditory processing. This loss leads to (1) impairment of hearing for high-frequency tones, (2) impairment of frequency discrimination, (3) impairment of sound localization, and (4) impairment of speech discrimination (Jerger et al., 1995).

Presbycusis has been further delineated and classified based on the clinical manifestations and the current but limited understanding of the degenerative process of hearing loss.

Sensory presbycusis usually begins in middle age and is slowly progressive, and it is characterized by a loss of ability to hear high-frequency sounds (Mulrow & Lichtenstein, 1991).

Neural presbycusis is hearing loss characterized by loss of speech discrimination in excess of what would be expected in terms of loss of frequencies; it is a disorder of central processing of auditory information.

This comprehensive problem with central processing of auditory information is characterized by difficulty in understanding speech in spite of the ability to hear sounds. This type of hearing loss is related to aging changes in the auditory centers of the brain. Although not universal, it is a problem for a significant number of older adults (Jerger et al., 1995).

To be *deaf* means either to have been born without the ability to hear or to have suffered hearing loss before the advent of speech.

Tinnitus is a continuous or intermittent sound that is perceived but that is not caused by external sources; the sound is perceived in various ways, such as whistling or blowing. Frequently, people who experience hearing loss complain of tinnitus.

Approximately 20% of the population experiences tinnitus at some time in their life. The etiology of tinnitus is not clear, but factors that have been known to cause or worsen tinnitus are noise exposure, wax buildup, medications (aspirin), ear or sinus infections, allergies, and head or neck trauma. Treatments that may provide some relief are use of a hearing aid, masking of noise, biofeedback, and cognitive-behavioral therapy. Overexposure to noise, alcohol, nicotine, caffeine, and stress are all factors that have the potential to worsen tinnitus (American Tinnitus Association [ATA], 1993). The American Tinnitus Association, Post Office Box 5, Portland, OR 97207-0005.

HEARING LOSS

Hearing loss can occur at any age, as a result of many causes (e.g., otitis media, intense noise exposure, head trauma, and some drugs, such as streptomycin and gentamicin, which may have ototoxic effects) (see Box 7-6 for a list of ototoxic drugs). However, age itself also seems to be a cause of hearing loss. A loss of hearing acuity begins for most people in about the third decade of life (Heath, 1993). The functional ability of hearing is one of the fundamental skills that enables people to communicate with one another and therefore to live within a community. Without the ability to hear and to differentiate the meaning of sounds, hearing-impaired older adults are at risk for a loss of communicative skills and for resulting social isolation. Often hearing loss is undetected because the early, insidious signs and symptoms go unrecognized and untreated. For many older people with hearing loss, consonants such as *sh, f, v, t, p,* and *b* are

BOX 7-6 OTOTOXIC DRUGS (THAT CAN PRODUCE HEARING LOSS)

1. Aspirin
2. Chloroquine
3. Cisplatin
4. Erythromycin
5. Furosemide (Lasix)
6. Gentamicin
7. Indomethacin
8. Kanamycin
9. Neomycin
10. Quinidine
11. Quinine
12. Streptomycin
13. Tobramycin
14. Vancomycin

Adapted from Weinstein, B. (1989). *Geriatrics, 44*(4), 42-49.

frequently misheard, leading many times to misunderstanding (Jerger et al., 1995).

Behaviors such as withdrawal from usual social activities, increased fatigue at social gatherings, suspiciousness, and loneliness are many times considered to be normal age-related changes rather than symptoms of hearing loss that may be amenable to treatment (Bess, 1989). These significant behavioral clues to the insidious onset of hearing loss may go unnoticed by older patients and their families. This is because of the gradual, noncrisis characteristic of these behaviors and the prevailing belief that aging brings negative changes in lifestyle.

Older adults who are hard of hearing lose the ability to understand information from media sources (e.g., radio and television). They miss the intimacy of a quick and friendly comment. Establishing new friendships is increasingly difficult when communication is hindered by hearing loss, and affected people worry that they will embar-

rass themselves by responding inappropriately. It is not surprising that studies show that hard-of-hearing people are more dissatisfied with life and more depressed than are people with no hearing problems. A study conducted with a sample of older people living in their own homes found a significant relationship between hearing loss and depression (Mulrow & Lichtenstein, 1991).

The symptoms of hearing loss include gradual loss of auditory sensitivity, with perception of high-frequency sounds diminishing first. Also, there is difficulty in localizing signals and a problem in understanding speech in unfavorable situations. This loss leads to a distortion of words, and sounds become jumbled. The resultant effect is poor speech discrimination. This is characterized by the often heard remark of the hearing-impaired person, "I can hear you but I can't understand what you are saying."

Hearing loss is not uniform; some sounds are heard, whereas others are not. For example, hearing loss is worse for high frequencies than for low frequencies and is greater for consonants than for vowels. This pattern of loss makes word discrimination extremely difficult. The sentence "The thinner cat is red" may be heard as "The dinner hat is red," leading to an inappropriate response, ensuing embarrassment, and perhaps social withdrawal for the hard-of-hearing older person.

Hearing loss can have a profound effect on intimate relationships. Chmiel and Jerger (1993) found that older people with hearing loss judge their auditory handicap less severely than do their spouses. This finding supports the notion that hearing-impaired older people may not recognize the problems their hearing loss causes for those with whom they share their lives.

One form of hearing loss is referred to as "loudness recruitment." In this hearing impairment, the sounds of normal speech cannot be understood and must be made more intense to be heard; however, if the sounds exceed the individual's hearing threshold, they are heard with disturbing loudness. Thus there occurs the classic situation in which the older patient asks

Aging Alert

1. Adaptation to changes in hearing is difficult.
2. Hearing loss may be unrecognized.
3. Corrective devices (e.g., hearing aids) are not always effective.
4. Many older people consider hearing aids to be a negative sign of aging and disability.

the nurse to speak up but then bitterly complains after the request is granted, saying that it is not necessary to yell to be heard. The solution is to find the individual patient's threshold and to try to speak at that level. Another nursing intervention is to teach patients about their hearing impairment and to assist them in taking an active part in structuring communications with others.

AURAL REHABILITATION

Older people who enter an aural rehabilitation process have typically experienced hearing loss for an average of at least 10 years (Weinstein, 1989). Everyone with a hearing disorder should have an ear, nose, and throat medical evaluation to rule out a treatable condition. One common, recurring, often overlooked, compounding factor that increases hearing loss for older patients is impacted cerumen. After this and all other treatable conditions have been ruled out as causing or contributing to the hearing loss, an evaluation by an audiologist is essential for assessment of the appropriate steps for aural rehabilitation (Jerger et al., 1995). Assisted listening devices (hearing aids), instruction in speech reading (lipreading), and motivational counseling are important components of a rehabilitation program.

Only 20% of hearing-impaired people own hearing aids; older users are much less satisfied than younger people, and use of hearing aids decreases with age (Schum, 1992). The presence of auditory processing disorder causes increased dissatisfaction with hearing aid use (Stach & Jerger, 1991). Other factors implicated in the rejection of hearing aids by older adults are denial of the condition, high cost of hearing aids (not covered by Medicare or most insurance policies), difficulty in managing the controls, and the perception that hearing aids are a stigma (Weinstein, 1989).

Despite limitations, hearing aids do improve the quality of life for many hard-of-hearing older adults. Advances in technology include mechanisms to reduce background noise and digital switching devices to accommodate different listening situations (Chmiel & Jerger, 1995). Often, older people do not know when a hearing aid will help or how to begin the process of obtaining a hearing aid. Recent literature is available from the American Association of Retired Persons (AARP) in the form of two booklets: *Have You Heard? Hearing Loss and Aging* and *Product Report: Hearing Aids*. A 1992 article entitled "How to Buy a Hearing Aid" appeared in *Consumer Reports*. Many older adults will find this article helpful, and this periodical can be obtained in most public libraries.

■ Nursing Process

ASSESSMENT

Physical examination

Examination of the external ear canal is performed by use of the otoscope. It is important to use the largest-sized speculum that the ear will accommodate to facilitate optimal visualization of the canal. The external ear canal is a narrow, winding canal, not a straight line. Before inserting the speculum, pull the auricle slightly upward and backward; this will facilitate entrance into the canal. It is best to have patients tilt their heads to the opposite shoulder; this allows a better view of the canal. The canal is sensitive, so the examiner should exercise skillful control of the otoscope and should stabilize the patient's head with the free hand to minimize unnecessary movement.

Cerumen in the canal may be seen as a brownish-yellow material, with varying degrees of consistency. The most common compounding cause of conduction hearing loss is an accumulation of cerumen. If there is no obstruction in the canal, the examiner will be able to observe the pearly gray tympanic membrane. The outline of the malleus may be seen, and a light reflex known as the "cone of light" may also be seen during the otoscopic examination of a normal ear.

Hearing assessment

Screening for hearing acuity consists of three tests: the spoken word test, the Rinne test, and the Weber test. To perform both the Weber and Rinne hearing tests, the nurse will need a 500-Hz tuning fork. The nurse should be sure that the fork is vibrating before applying it to the patient. Avoid touching the vibrating surfaces.

The spoken word test The spoken word test consists of simply standing a few feet from the patient, placing a hand in front of the mouth to conceal its movements, and whispering a short sentence. This should be done on both sides of the patient to test hearing in both ears. The patient should be asked to repeat the sentence. It is important to change the sentence when testing the second ear.

The Weber test Strike the tuning fork, check the vibration, and place the handle of the fork on the center of the patient's forehead firmly in touch with the skull bone. Ask the patient where the sound of the vibration is heard. People with sensorineural hearing loss will hear the sound in the better ear, those with conductive loss will hear the sound in the impaired ear, and those with normal hearing will hear the sound equally in both ears.

The Rinne test Strike the tuning fork, check the vibration, and place the handle of the fork firmly on the mastoid process. Ask the

Healthy People 2000 Objectives

17.17 Increase to at least 60% the proportion of providers of primary care for older adults who routinely evaluate people aged 65 and older for impairments of vision and hearing.

From U.S. Department of Health and Human Services. (1990). *Healthy People 2000: National health promotion and disease prevention objectives* (DHHS Pub. No. [PHS] 91-50212). Washington, DC: U.S. Government Printing Office.

patient to say when the sound of the vibration is no longer heard. At that point, place the still-vibrating tuning fork next to the anterior surface of the external ear. Again, ask the patient to signal when the sound is no longer heard. The principle that guides this test is that air conduction is greater than bone conduction.

Normal-hearing patients will report hearing the sound longer when the tuning fork is held in the air next to the ear. Normal-hearing patients also will report no difference in the loudness of the sound. In conductive hearing loss, the sound of the vibrating tuning fork is heard more loudly and longer at the mastoid process.

Psychosocial assessment

The psychosocial assessment for patients experiencing hearing loss is similar to that for visual loss (Box 7-7). Denial or lack of understanding may be more pronounced in a patient with hearing loss than in a patient with visual loss. The increased denial of hearing loss may be attributed to negative stereotypic images of older people not hearing well, consequently losing social status, and not being able to compensate for this loss. This image persists in spite of the many successful hard-of-hearing older adults.

BOX 7-7 PSYCHOSOCIAL ASSESSMENT OF HEARING

1. Is there any specific problem you are experiencing that is related to your hearing loss?
2. Have you changed in any way your communications with family or friends?
3. Are you having difficulties listening on the telephone or listening to the radio, television, or movies?
4. At times, does your hearing problem cause you to avoid groups of people?
5. Do you feel a loss of self-confidence because of your hearing problem?
6. At times, does your hearing problem cause you to feel depressed?
7. Is there any information you need to help you live with your hearing problem?
8. Is there anything that I have not covered that you would like to tell me about your hearing?

Nurses need to focus on the ability of hard-of-hearing older people to manage their deficit and to continue meaningful lives.

Another factor that contributes to the negative view of hearing loss is the fact that hearing aids have not been as successful in correcting hearing loss as glasses have been in correcting visual loss. Furthermore, many older patients have had experiences with relatives or friends who were unable to use a hearing aid effectively. These factors, plus the insidious nature of hearing loss, contribute to the denial of loss and increase the reticence of many older people in seeking treatment.

The nurse conducting a psychosocial assessment needs to consider the patient's attitude. Even though an attitude may be prevalent in society, one cannot assume that every individual patient subscribes to that attitude. It is also good

to recall the high level of association between depression and hearing loss and to be alert for any symptoms of depression.

With the patient's permission, include family members in the psychosocial assessment. The attitudes and behaviors of family members regarding the patient's hearing loss should always be assessed. If possible, it is also wise to ask family members the same questions asked of the patient regarding the patient's response to the hearing loss. The older patient with hearing loss has experienced a significant sensory ability loss that often goes unrecognized by both the patient and the patient's family. The nurse has an opportunity to make a contribution to the quality of life for many older adults by providing screening and early detection of hearing loss.

Environmental assessment

Because hearing loss can create communication difficulties, any environmental factor that impedes or facilitates human communication should be assessed. The major areas to assess are the placement and use of radios, televisions, and telephones. Assessment data should be obtained concerning the normal noise level and the changes in the noise level influenced by environmental factors.

The hospital and the nursing home can be difficult places for older patients who have hearing losses. Staff should be aware of the significance of hearing loss in its effects on the communication abilities of the patient. The volume of the radio or television, especially in the nursing home, needs to be adjusted to the level that is comfortable for the patient. Also, all staff should be instructed in and reminded of the procedures necessary to facilitate communication with a hearing-impaired person. Nurses must always model the correct techniques in communicating with the older patient who has a hearing loss.

Resource assessment

The use of a hearing aid is addressed in this portion of the assessment. Ask open-ended ques-

BOX 7-8 HEARING AID ASSESSMENT

1. How have you managed with your hearing aid?
2. On a normal day, how long do you wear your hearing aid?
3. Are you having any difficulties using your hearing aid?
4. Can you show me how you put in your hearing aid and how you adjust the controls?
5. Do you need assistance in using the aid? If so, is a person living with you able to help?
6. How often do you change the batteries in your hearing aid?
7. Do you have spare batteries available?
8. Where do you keep the aid when it is not in use?
9. At night, do you disengage the battery?

BOX 7-9 HINTS FOR FIRST-TIME HEARING AID USERS

1. Begin by using the aid for short periods of time, and add 30 minutes each day.
2. Start by using the aid when listening only to one person. Avoid using it when in large groups until accustomed to the aid.
3. Before placing the aid into the ear, be sure that the switch is off.
4. Practice inserting the aid and using the controls before purchasing the aid.
5. Higher volume is not always better.
6. Whistling sounds or squeals indicate too high a volume or a loose-fitting earmold.
7. Have patience, and allow for enough time to get accustomed to using the aid.

tions, such as "How have you been doing with using your hearing aid?" This type of question allows the skillful nurse to obtain pertinent data without threatening the patient (Box 7-8). Attentive listening to answers to the open-ended questions, coupled with responses to a few direct questions, will help the nurse to assess how well the older patient is adjusting to living with a hearing aid.

During this interview the nurse needs to be empathetic concerning any difficulties the patient may experience in using the hearing aid. Encouragement and positive reinforcement of behaviors that demonstrate acceptance and utilization of the hearing aid are important nursing interventions that may increase the older person's ability to overcome a hearing deficit (Box 7-9).

The economic status of the older patient will have a significant impact on the patient's ability to purchase a hearing aid, because the current Medicare provisions do not cover either eyeglasses or hearing aids. Purchase and maintenance of hearing aids can be quite expensive.

Prices and options vary, with a low of $500 to $700 for a behind-the-ear aid, and with the most sophisticated aid being digitally programmed and costing $2500 ("How to Buy," 1992). The constant replacement of batteries is both an added cost and an added chore, which may be difficult for many older adults to manage.

In addition, a hearing aid for hearing loss is not equivalent to eyeglasses for vision loss. Eyeglasses are made specifically for individual vision loss, whereas most hearing aids do not have that type of specificity. Adjustment to a hearing aid takes time and patience.

Some older adults, because of physical, cognitive, or social conditions, will be unable to use a hearing aid successfully. For example, the person may be unable to manipulate the controls of a hearing aid successfully because of arthritis, may be unable to understand instructions because of dementia, may be unable to afford the high cost of the hearing aid, or may even be unwilling to accept the necessity of wearing a hearing aid. These are reasons frequently given for not purchasing and using hearing aids. Another reason may be that the hearing aid is not effective in particular situations, such as listening to television or listening in noisy environments.

Assistive listening devices (ALDs) can be used in addition to hearing aids or even as an alternative to them. These devices enhance the older person's ability to understand speech in difficult situations. An inexpensive and easy-to-use ALD is a hard-wired system, which includes (1) a microphone that is held close to the sound source, (2) an amplifier, (3) a transducer, and (4) a headphone (Figure 7-5). The ALD (hard-wired) system can be used to facilitate interviews and history taking for hearing-impaired older adults who may have chosen not to use a conventional

FIGURE 7-5 Assistive listening device (hard-wired) system from Radio Shack.

hearing aid. The low cost and the commercial availability of these devices make them an attractive alternative for some older people. The ALD (the hard-wired system) is available from Radio Shack and from the telephone company (Weinstein, 1989).

NURSING DIAGNOSES

NANDA diagnoses that should be considered when caring for a patient with a hearing loss include the following:

1. Alteration in auditory perception
2. Impaired verbal communication
3. Self-esteem disturbance
4. Impaired social interaction and/or social isolation

The diagnosis of alteration in auditory perception may be related to physical changes, as evidenced by the following:

1. Results of audiology testing
2. Self-reports of hearing loss
3. Reports of others concerning the patient's hearing loss

The diagnosis of impaired verbal communication may be related to hearing loss, as evidenced by the following:

1. Test results
2. Self-reports and reports by others
3. Avoidance of people individually and in groups
4. Denial of hearing difficulties
5. Reluctance to use a hearing aid
6. Blaming others for hearing difficulties
7. Increased arguments
8. Withdrawal from family

The diagnosis of self-esteem disturbance may be related to hearing loss, as evidenced by the following:

1. Expression of feelings of diminished self-worth
2. Avoidance of people
3. Suspiciousness of others

The diagnosis of impaired social interaction may be related to hearing loss, as evidenced by the following:

1. Diminished activity level
2. Avoidance of people

PLANNING AND GOAL IDENTIFICATION

The planning phase consists of compiling all the data gathered during the assessment phase and deciding on priorities of care. After the priorities have been designated, the planning team will plan appropriate nursing interventions that will ameliorate or alleviate the condition. The nursing intervention may be a referral or a consultation with a representative of another health discipline. Each planned nursing intervention is goal specific, not random.

Alteration in auditory perception

A long-term goal is that the patient will adapt to hearing loss. Short-term goals include the following:

1. Patient will accept use of hearing aid.
2. Caregiver and support system will encourage and assist patient in the beginning stages of hearing-aid use.
3. Patient will be able to care for and correctly use hearing aid.

Impaired verbal communication

A long-term goal is that the patient's verbal communication with others will be appropriate and untroubled. Short-term goals include the following:

1. Patient will not avoid communication with family and friends.
2. Arguments within the family will diminish.
3. Patient will be able to verbalize the personal reality and consequences of having a hearing loss.

Impaired social interaction

A long-term goal is that the patient will regain and maintain a pre–hearing-loss level of social interaction with family, friends, and community organizations. Short-term goals include the following:

1. Patient will attend family functions.
2. Patient will engage in personally chosen social activities.

IMPLEMENTATION
In the acute care setting

Hospitalization of older people occurs for many reasons, but usually not for treatment concerning their hearing loss; instead, the hearing loss may go undetected or disregarded. Not all older people are hard of hearing, but the functional status of hearing should be part of every nursing assessment. Also, if there is a hearing loss, the nurse must assess both how well the patient understands and accepts the loss, and how well the patient communicates, in order to be able to formulate a plan of care.

When an older patient is undergoing diagnostic testing, particularly in a hospital, the patient may be engaged in multiple interactions with a wide array of people, from the transport personnel to the technicians conducting the tests. These interactions take place in a dynamic, complex, and even frenzied environment, including crammed corridors and crowded elevators. For the older patient in a wheelchair—or worse, on a stretcher or a gurney—the environment may be frightening. In addition, for the hard-of-hearing patient, it may be difficult to understand instructions. In these situations the nurse can intervene by taking the time to explain to the patient in detail the reason for the test, the procedures involved in the test, and any other helpful information about the experience. The nurse may also intervene to alert other hospital staff to the patient's level of hearing loss; this nursing intervention often improves the diagnostic testing experience for all concerned.

When developing interventions for communicating with hard-of-hearing older patients, it is critical to allow time for the patient to process information. Without sufficient time for the inter-

> ## BOX 7-10 STEPS TO EFFECTIVE COMMUNICATION WITH HEARING-IMPAIRED OLDER ADULTS
>
> 1. Be sure you have the person's attention before beginning to speak.
> 2. Face the person to whom you are speaking, and stand reasonably close to the listener.
> 3. Avoid standing in the glare of bright sunlight or other lights.
> 4. Lower the pitch of your voice.
> 5. Speak clearly and slowly.
> 6. Use short sentences.
> 7. Avoid background noise.
> 8. Encourage the use of nonverbal communication, such as touch.
> 9. Use written communication if you are unable to communicate verbally.

action and without knowledge and compassion on the part of the nurse, effective nursing care will not occur. Several measures can be taken to communicate effectively with hearing-impaired older adults, as seen in Box 7-10.

In the nursing home

With the large numbers of hearing-impaired people who are living in nursing homes, it is crucial that all nursing home personnel be aware of appropriate ways to communicate with hard-of-hearing residents. In addition, hearing loss may exacerbate the confusional states of many nursing home residents. Residents with dementia may also be hard of hearing. Therefore nurses must continually assess both the hearing function and the communication ability of the residents. Nurses must also use a high level of skill to communicate effectively with older residents who are afflicted with both dementia and hearing loss.

Nurses need to emphasize to the staff members the importance of (1) allowing time for the resident to respond, (2) recognizing each resident's unique abilities, and (3) acquiring and constantly using communication skills that facilitate dialogue with people who suffer from hearing loss. All levels of nursing staff should be instructed in the different ways in which hearing loss is manifested. Such awareness may help to minimize complaints that residents are just stubborn or only hear what they want to hear. The staff must understand the symptoms associated with the loss of the ability to discriminate sounds and speech, as well as those accompanying a simple loss of hearing of gross sounds. If necessary, repeatedly explain the differences to the nursing staff responsible for the daily personal care of nursing home residents. The professional nurse plans, guides, and supervises the care of the resident, and the nonprofessional staff members are educated and supervised by the professional nursing staff.

One physical aspect of hearing loss that needs constant assessment and treatment is the accumulation of cerumen (earwax). Mahoney (1993) observed impacted cerumen in 26 out of 104 nursing home residents, and 78 other residents had a large accumulation of cerumen without impaction. Although small, this study does suggest a high incidence of impacted cerumen in nursing home residents. Nurses can improve the quality of life for these older people. After checking with each patient's physician to be sure that there are no contraindications (e.g., punctured tympanic membrane), the nurse may cleanse the patient's ears. Irrigation as a method of cleansing cerumen from the external canal is usually considered a nursing function. An effective method of cerumen removal is to use either a dental waterpik or a bulb syringe for irrigation. The water should be tepid; hot or cold extremes will distress the resident. If the cerumen is difficult to dislodge, it may be necessary to use drops, such as mineral oil or a mixture of hydrogen peroxide and mineral oil, to soften the accumulation. The irrigation should be done with the resident's shoulder draped with a towel, the head tipped toward the shoulder, and an emesis basin positioned to catch the draining water. The ear canal will need to be viewed with an otoscope both before and after the irrigation. The goal of the irrigation is a clear canal. Some improvement in hearing may result from this procedure. It is best to assess for accumulated cerumen on a monthly basis.

In the private or family home

Many of the interventions cited for the acute care and nursing home settings have relevance to the private or family home setting. The teaching of specific communication skills should focus on the family caregivers. Some caregivers may find it extremely difficult to accept any type of instruction in communication. Family members usually have a long history of communication patterns that might not be amenable to change. As is the case with hospitalized older patients, the primary reason for a home visit seldom relates to the patient's hearing loss. Nonetheless, the nurse can use expert knowledge in assessing, diagnosing, and intervening to make a significant contribution to the quality of life for the hearing-impaired older person.

Family members need an understanding of the type of hearing loss the older patient is experiencing and how it affects daily living. Also, techniques for improving communication with the older patient may be taught by the nurse both to interested family members and to the hard-of-hearing patient. Often, the authentic concern of the nurse creates a therapeutic milieu that allows and encourages older adults and their families to continue to maintain an independent living arrangement.

EVALUATION

Evaluation of nursing interventions is an essential component of the nursing process that often goes unnoticed and unrecorded. It is crucial for nurses always to include an evaluative statement in the documentation of care. For one thing, evaluation may help to determine the accuracy of assessment data, as well as to substantiate the nursing diagnoses. Often, reassessment is the appropriate outcome of the evaluative process. The plan of care may need to be updated if the patient's hearing impairment changes—whether the change represents improvement or deterioration.

The long-term and short-term goals are the guideposts for the evaluative phase: Have these goals been met? Is the patient satisfied with the outcome of the care received? Is the family satisfied? Are the health care providers sure that everything has been done, to the best of their ability, to resolve the patient's particular problems? Wholistic, patient-oriented evaluation of nursing care is an obligatory component of the nursing process.

■ Smell and Taste

Imagining the smell of a wood fire in a campground evokes other sensory memories—images of companions and the taste of burnt marshmallows. The smell of coffee in the morning prompts a conscious anticipation of the taste of the hot coffee. That sense of awareness and anticipation of taste are denied to older adults who experience a diminished sense of smell. Aging generally reduces, though it does not extinguish, the sense of smell (Chauhan et al., 1989).

The research literature dealing with age-related changes in the sense of taste is not as clear as that pertaining to the sense of smell. There are many methodologic problems because of the complexity of the sense of taste. Psychologic, cultural, and social factors influence a person's perception of taste. In spite of the methodologic problems, current research does suggest that older people have a higher threshold for sensing sour, bitter, and salt tastes (Chauhan, 1989) and that the taste for sweet does not seem to undergo any age-related change (Bartoshuk et al., 1986). A *higher threshold* means that it takes more sensory stimulation to trigger the sensory experience of taste. Thus in the case of salt intake, older adults would use more salt than they did when they were younger to experience the same level of salt taste.

ASSESSMENT OF SMELL

Assessment of the sense of smell is performed during the testing of the cranial nerves. The olfactory (first cranial) nerve is tested by having patients close their eyes, compress one of their nostrils, and sniff through the other nostril to identify odors such as those of coffee or cloves.

ASSESSMENT OF TASTE

Taste buds are located in the tongue. The sense of taste is tested during the assessment of the facial (seventh cranial) nerve and the glossopharyngeal (ninth cranial) nerve. The tongue is tested for discernment of salty, sweet, sour, and bitter tastes.

NURSING DIAGNOSES

The diagnosis of sensory-perceptual alterations, specifying either gustatory or olfactory, may be related to the aging process, as evidenced by the following:

1. Changes noted on physical examination
2. Self-reports of change in sense of smell and/or taste
3. The lack of any known pathologic cause for change in sense of smell and/or taste

PLANNING, IMPLEMENTATION, AND EVALUATION

The decline in the senses of taste and smell has nursing implications in the area of nutrition, which the chapter on nutrition addresses extensively. Further, the diminished sensory experience of the older person influences the person's daily life. The nurse must be constantly on the alert for ways to fortify and to encourage use of the individual's remaining sensory capacity. Also, the knowledge of age-related changes in the senses of smell and taste may help health professionals to understand why so many older patients complain about the quality of the food they receive in health care institutions. Efforts should focus on ways to improve the attractiveness of meals and to work with dietary staff to plan tasteful but appropriate diets for older adults.

■ Touch

The importance of touching and being touched is established in humans during infancy. Without some form of touch, a newborn infant cannot survive; so it is in all stages of life. Touching allows physical connections among people. Mulaik et al. (1991), in a study of 98 hospitalized patients, reported that 95% of their sample believed that touch conveyed affection and caring. Similarly, in a study of nursing home residents, Moore and Gilbert (1995) found that comforting touch used by nurses communicated affection and immediacy. However, the significance that older adults ascribe to touch cannot always be assumed to be positive, and touch does have the potential to convey impending harm rather than comfort. The perception and the interpretation of touch are influenced not only by physical properties but also by a complex web of psychologic and sociocultural factors. The nurse must respect the older adult's need for touch but must also be mindful of the verbal and nonverbal cues concerning the level of touch appropriate for each older person.

ASSESSMENT

Testing for the physical properties of the sense of touch is part of the neurologic examination. When testing the fifth cranial (trigeminal) nerve, the perception of light touch is assessed by touching the patient with a wisp of cotton at three facial locations: ophthalmic, maxillary, and mandibular. A brief screening of the sensory system will include assessment of perception of light touch at the extremities by comparing the distal with the proximal regions. The psychologic and sociocultural aspects of touch are the major foci of the nursing assessment. These areas are difficult to assess, because the variability between patients in their expression of touch

and in their expression of the need to be touched is immense. Clinical experience will heighten the nurse's ability to assess the variables that influence the patient's sense of touch. Psychologic and sociocultural variables that influence touch are physical condition, level of trust, cultural significance of touch, and level of self-esteem.

NURSING DIAGNOSIS

Self-esteem disturbance related to tactile deprivation may be evidenced by (1) expressed feelings of diminished self-worth and (2) documented or stated lack of touching or being touched.

PLANNING AND GOAL IDENTIFICATION

The planning is specific to the diagnosis of self-esteem disturbance. A long-term goal is that the patient will express feelings of self-worth. A short-term goal is that the patient will experience daily evidence of caring through the sense of touch. The planning will also include development of specific nursing interventions that will contribute to meeting the short- and long-term goals developed earlier in the planning phase. An intervention directed at meeting the short-term goal of having the patient experience caring through the sense of touch might be that all nursing staff, when approaching the patient, will extend their hand to touch the patient's hand, to express positive regard. This intervention is also aimed at the long-term goal of raising self-esteem. Planning is essential to well-thought-out, systematic nursing care that meets the needs of the patient. Reflection and thought are indispensable in the development of a nursing plan.

IMPLEMENTATION

The bond of human interaction calls for a physical connection between people. The nurse who reaches out to touch an older patient's hand reaches across the interpersonal barriers of language and across the experience of illness and high-technology health care, across to the fear of being sick, old, and alone. The nurse has an obligation to bring a discernable presence of caring. This type of caring may be communicated by appropriate touch. Nurses are allowed, through the social mandate of caring for others, the privilege of touching others. Few professions are granted this unusual status, and nurses must acknowledge the responsibility that touching entails, especially with the vulnerable. Many times older adults are vulnerable and need acceptance and affirmation of their personhood from the people who share their lives.

There are variations in the way that people experience touch, and the nurse must skillfully assess the older person's need for the expression of touch. To develop a skill level that facilitates touching and caring for the frail older person, nurses must also know a great deal about themselves. Self-knowledge is fundamental to the ability to engage in professional nursing. Questions to consider when caring for older adults include the following:

1. What do I think and feel about touching others?
2. Do I react with appropriate touch when contacting physically unattractive frail older adults?
3. Am I frightened by older adults?
4. Do older people threaten me in some special personal way?
5. What negative and positive experiences have I had with older adults?

With touch, as with all other forms of communication, the receiver's interpretation of the message is an important link in the communication process. How the older patient responds to the nurse's communication of caring through the physical act of touching will be influenced by many of the psychologic and sociocultural factors that have been discussed in the assessment portion of this chapter.

These complex variables influence the communication of caring through the medium of touch but should not deter the nurse from initiating a message of caring by touching the older patient. If the patient seems unreceptive to such spontaneous forms of touching, consider offering to massage the patient's feet or back. This type of directed and physical touching may be more acceptable to some older patients.

EVALUATION

The evaluation of nursing care is always focused on the short- and long-term, patient-centered goals developed during the planning phase. The need to follow through on the plan of care is a paramount concern for those involved in the care of older adults. Often, the plan of care is developed by the professional nurse but carried out by nonprofessional assistants. Nonetheless, the care remains the responsibility of the professional, licensed nurse and not that of the nursing assistants. This responsibility requires managerial and supervisory skills, which nurses must develop in order to ensure implementation of the plan of care and to evaluate it.

REFERENCES

American Tinnitus Association. (1993). *Tinnitus family information pamphlet.*

Bartoshuk, L.M., et al. (1986). Taste and aging. *Journal of Gerontology,* 41-51.

Bess, F. (1989). Hearing impairment as a determinant of function in the elderly. *Journal of the American Geriatrics Society, 37*(2), 123-128.

Chauhan, J. (1989). Relationships between sour and salt taste perception and selected subject attributes. *Journal of the American Dietetic Association, 89*(5), 652-656.

Chauhan, J., et al. (1989). Age-related olfactory and taste changes and interrelationships between taste and nutrition. *Journal of the American Dietetic Association, 87*(11), 1543-1550.

Chmiel, R., & Jerger, J. (1993). Some factors affecting assessment of hearing handicap in the elderly. *Journal of the American Academy of Audiology, 4,* 249-257.

Chmiel, R., & Jerger, J. (1995). Quantifying improvement with amplification. *Ear Hearing, 16,* 166-175.

Feinburg, M. (1988). *Eye medications: May be more than meets the eye.* Baltimore: University of Maryland School of Pharmacy, Elder Health Program. Morris Plain, NJ: Parke-Davis.

Gates, G., et al. (1990). Hearing in the elderly: The Framingham cohort 1983-1985. *Ear Hearing, 11,* 247.

Heath, J.H. (1993). Vision. In R. Hamm (Ed)., *Primary care geriatrics*. St. Louis: Mosby.

How to buy a hearing aid. (1992). *Consumer Reports, 57,* 716-721.

Jerger, J., et al. (1995). Hearing impairment in older adults: New concepts. *Journal of the American Geriatrics Society, 43,* 928-935.

Kasper, R. (1989). Eye problems. In W. Reichel (Ed.), *Clinical aspects of aging* (3rd ed.). Baltimore: Williams & Wilkins.

Kovar, M.G. (1986). *Aging in the '80s: Preliminary data from the supplement on aging to the National Health Interview Survey, United States, Jan-June, 1984* (Advance data from Vital and Health Statistics of the National Center for Health Statistics, No. 115, DHHS Pub. No. [PHS] 86-1250). Hyattsville, MD: Public Health Service.

Mahoney, D. (1993). Cerumen impaction: Prevalence and detection in nursing homes. *Journal of Gerontological Nursing, 19*(4), 23-30.

Michaels, M. (1994). The Eye. In W.M. Hazzard, E. Bierman, J. Blass, W. Ettinger, & J. Halter (Eds.), *Principles of geriatric medicine and gerontology* (3rd ed.). New York: McGraw-Hill.

Moore, J., & Gilbert, D.A. (1995). Elderly residents' perceptions of nurses' comforting touch. *Journal of Gerontological Nursing, 21*(1), 6-13.

Mulaik, J.S., et al. (1991). Patient's perceptions of nurses' use of touch. *Western Journal of Nursing Research, 13*(3), 306-323.

Mulrow, C.D., & Lichtenstein, M.J. (1991). Screening for hearing impairment in the elderly: Rationale and strategy. *Journal of General Internal Medicine, 6,* 249-258.

Rees, T., Duckert, L., & Milczuk, H. (1994). Auditory and vestibular dysfunction. In W.M. Hazzard, E. Bierman, J. Blass, W. Ettinger, & J. Halter (Eds.), *Principles of geriatric medicine and gerontology* (3rd ed.). New York: McGraw-Hill.

Rosenberg, R. (1994). Lighting and the aging eye. *Aging and Vision News, 6*(1), 3-4. (Available from The Lighthouse, 800 Second Avenue, New York, NY 10017)

Schleber, F. (1992). Aging and the senses. In J. Birren, R.B. Sloane, & G. Cohen (Eds.), *Handbook of mental health and aging*. San Diego: Academic Press.

Schum, D. (1992). Responses of elderly hearing aid users on the hearing aid performance inventory. *Journal of the American Academy of Audiology, 3,* 308-314.

Stach, B., & Jerger, J. (1991). Special hearing aid considerations in elderly patients with auditory processing disorders. *Ear Hear, 12*(suppl.), 131S-138S.

Stefansson, E. (1990). The eye. In Hazzard, W., Andres, R., Bierman, E., & Blass, J. (Eds.), *Principles of geriatric medicine and gerontology*. New York: McGraw-Hill.

Wasson, J.H., et al. (1990). The prescription of assistive devices for the elderly. *Journal of General Internal Medicine, 5,* 46-54.

Weinstein, B. (1989). Geriatric hearing loss: Myths, realities, resources for physicians. *Geriatrics, 44*(4), 42-49.

C H A P T E R 8

The faces of the old are like old houses;
every line's a highway from the past.

R. McKuen, *Valentines*

Integument

■ Learning Objectives

On completion of this chapter, the reader will be able to do the following:

1. Identify age-related changes in the integument and in the oral mucous membranes.
2. Assess the older adult's integument and oral mucous membranes.
3. Recognize risk factors that lead to impaired skin integrity and alterations in oral mucous membranes.
4. Describe the causes of integumentary impairment, and oral mucous membrane impairment in older adults.
5. Develop a plan of nursing care for an older adult with integumentary impairment or with alterations in oral mucous membranes.
6. Implement appropriate nursing interventions for older adults with integumentary impairment and with alterations in oral mucous membranes.
7. Evaluate the effectiveness of nursing interventions carried out to resolve integumentary and oral mucous membrane problems.

Although the skin provides a protective barrier between the body and the environment, diseases of the skin and subcutaneous tissue do occur. Furthermore, some age-related changes in the skin and oral mucous membranes can lead to delayed healing of wounds, decreased sweating, altered temperature regulation, wrinkles, loss of dentition, and increased susceptibility to disease. These skin conditions and diseases account for high morbidity and high treatment costs. Despite advances in dental hygiene, the average person has lost ten teeth by the age of 70; more than 65% of older adults have an edentulous jaw (Kresevic & Lincoln, 1995). This chapter presents information regarding age-related skin and oral mucous membrane changes, the major causes of skin and oral mucous membrane impairment, and the nursing requirements to manage these integumentary problems when they occur among older adults.

■ Skin

NORMAL STRUCTURE AND FUNCTION

The skin is the largest organ of the body and comprises three layers: the epidermis, the dermis, and the subcutaneous. The *epidermis* is the outermost layer and consists of stratified squamous epithelium cells (keratinocytes and melanocytes). The main functions of the epidermis are to protect the body against invasion by environmental substances, to restrict water loss, and to synthesize keratin cells. Two divisions make up the epidermis: the superficial papillary dermis (connecting with the epidermal layer) and the reticular dermis (connecting with the subcutaneous fat layer). Appendages of the epidermis are the eccrine and apocrine sweat glands, sebaceous glands, hair, and nails. The *dermis* comprises the papillary layer and the reticular layer. Blood vessels and nerve elements are in the *papillary layer,* which extends into the epidermis. Elastin fibers, collagen fibers, and reticulin fibers form the *reticular layer.* The *subcutaneous layer* is composed of loose connective tissue and fat cells. Its main functions are to provide heat, insulation, and caloric reserves and to act as a shock absorber. A cross section of the skin is shown in Figure 8-1.

The major functions of the skin include protection, minimization of body fluid loss, excretion of some waste materials and toxins, temperature regulation, blood pressure regulation, tissue repair, synthesis of vitamin D, sensory perception, and expression of feelings. Increasingly, intact skin is being recognized as a key element in the prevention of disease; disruption in skin integrity provides a site for pathogens to enter (Beare & Myers, 1994). Each of these functions is described in Table 8-1.

AGE-RELATED CHANGES

As humans age, two types of predictable changes occur in the skin: (1) intrinsic aging and (2) photoaging. In intrinsic aging, there is a systemic

TABLE 8-1 Functions of the skin

Skin function	Mechanism
Protection	Intact skin covering creates a physical barrier against bacteria, minor physical trauma, and foreign substances
Synthesis of keratin	Keratinocytes are produced in the basal layer, develop, and then move to the surface of the skin
Excretion of wastes	Sweat, sodium chloride, urea, and lactic acid are excreted through the skin
Blood pressure regulation	Skin blood vessels can constrict, which promotes venous return and increases the cardiac output and blood pressure
Fluid regulation	Skin keeps fluids contained in the body
Temperature regulation	Skin blood vessels can (1) dilate to promote heat loss or to prevent tissue freezing (radiation); (2) constrict to conserve heat; or (3) regulate temperature by conduction, convection, and evaporation
Tissue repair	Skin replaces damaged skin cells and forms scar tissue
Production of vitamin D	In the presence of ultraviolet light, a precursor of vitamin D is converted to vitamin D in the skin
Sensory perception	Special sensors in the skin respond to touch, pain, heat, cold, pressure, vibration, tickling, itching, wetness, oiliness, and stickiness
Expression of emotional feelings	Surface of the skin can respond to emotions through sweating, pallor, or flushing.

decrease in circulation, a loss of cells, and a loss of elastic collagen fibers and muscle mass. The number of pressure and light-touch sensors decreases with age, which predisposes older adults to mechanical and thermal injuries. Subcutaneous fat atrophies on the face, hands, shins, and soles, whereas it hypertrophies on the abdomen (in men) and thighs (in women). Locally, the skin decreases production of sweat, sebum, and vitamin D. There is delayed or diminished cell replacement, response to injury, barrier function, chemical clearance, and sensory perception. Immune, vascular, and thermoregulatory responses of the skin decrease with age (Klein, 1988).

As aging progresses, there is loss of hair color and a thinning of pubic, axillary, and scalp hair. The nails thicken, develop longitudinal lines, and decrease in growth rate. These changes may result in dryness, wrinkling, laxity, uneven pigmentation, and the occurrence of skin lesions (both benign and malignant), age spots, and skin tags (acrochordons).

In photoaging the effects of environmental damage become more evident and there is more profound aging in skin areas exposed to sunlight. Many of the changes related to photoaging are preventable or, in some cases, reversible. All of these changes may affect individuals in unique ways and may occur at varying rates within and among individuals (Bruno & Craven, 1982). There are clinical changes in photoaging such as "fine and coarse wrinkling, yellow, lax, leathery texture, blotchiness and pigmentary changes, telangiectasia, actinic keratoses, and elastotic skin with giant comedones" (Kurban & Kurban, 1993, p. 35).

It is estimated that 60% of older adults have a skin disorder (Kurban & Kurban, 1993). The incidence of pressure ulcers in older adults ranges from 4% in home health care patients to 66% in older adult patients admitted for femoral fracture (Bergstrom et al., 1992). The most common skin disorders seen in older adults are acrochordons, seborrheic keratoses and skin cancers, fungal infections, dermatitis, pigmentary disturbances, psoriasis, and urticaria. Senile warts, senile purpura, lentigines, nevi, astheoses, cherry angiomas, and comedones are also frequently encountered (Beare & Myers, 1994).

COMMON HEALTH DEVIATIONS
Acrochordons

Acrochordons (skin tags) are the most common benign skin lesion seen in older adults (Figure 8-2). They are usually found in the armpit or groin and beneath the breasts in women. They do not pose a great risk and can be easily removed by curettage or with liquid nitrogen in the primary care provider's office.

Xerosis

Xerosis is the most common skin problem in the older adult. Decreased moisture content and altered functioning of the eccrine and sebaceous glands, accompanied by dry air and heat in the winter, contribute to the problem. If the dryness is severe, itching may occur, leading to inflammation. Emollients containing urea or lactic acid can be used to promote hydration and the removal of excess keratin. After application of an emollient, the skin should be blotted but not wiped completely dry. If cracking has occurred, a cortisone cream can be applied, followed by application of an emollient. Some cosmetic moisturizers actually increase dryness and should be avoided. Increased humidity may provide some relief. The use of bath oils is controversial because of the danger of slipping in the tub.

Keratoses

Seborrheic keratotic lesions are frequently seen on aging skin (Figure 8-3). This benign epidermal growth consists of keratinocytes and melanocytes. They are genetically transmitted as an autosomal dominant trait and occur most frequently in white-skinned people. Keratotic lesions are yellow to brown or black and occur most often on the face, scalp, trunk, and upper extremities. They begin as small papules or plaques and gradually become rough or warty in appearance. They are harmless and treatment is not mandatory, but because they are visibly disfiguring, the older adult may be embarrassed by or ashamed of their appearance. Treatment usually consists of the application of topical steroids or cryosurgical removal, which can usually be accomplished in the physician's office without anesthesia. The occurrence of new or increased numbers of seborrheic keratoses has been linked with internal malignancies and should be investigated (Habif, 1996).

Actinic keratotic lesions, the most frequent skin tumor in older adults, occurs in fair-skinned individuals who have been exposed to sun damage (Figure 8-4). The lesions appear as small, scaly patches, are light pink to reddish, and range from a few millimeters to centimeters in size. The lesion may grow into a hyperketotic mass with dark pigmentation. Approximately 1% of actinic keratoses develop into squamous cell carcinoma. The typical lesion does not change over long periods but must be watched carefully. Treatment consists of cryosurgery, liquid nitrogen therapy, or topical treatment with fluorouracil solution or cream over a 2- to 4-week period. Thereafter, the patient needs to avoid sun exposure or to use a sunscreen, if one can be tolerated (Weiss, 1989).

Skin cancers

The aging skin is particularly prone to development of skin cancers. Basal cell carcinoma accounts for 80% of all skin cancers. Squamous cell carcinomas and malignant melanomas make up the remaining 20% (Fenske et al., 1989). Older adults should be alerted to the fact that cancerous skin lesions develop more slowly than in the young and that changes in a mole or a skin lesion may be gradual.

Basal cell carcinoma A basal cell carcinoma forms in the germinative layer of the epidermis, is usually slow growing, and is frequently detected and treated in the early stages; metastasis is rare (Figure 8-5). This form of cancer is strongly associated with chronic sun exposure (solar ultraviolet radiation), although scars, exposure to x-ray irradiation, and chemical carcinogens are often implicated as causative agents. The lesions usually begin as papules, and the tumor border is raised and waxy in appearance. Frequently the lesions appear on the nose, eyelid, or cheek, although tumors are also seen on the trunk. Treatment is based on the location, the tumor's characteristics, and the patient's age. The goal is to eliminate the tumor while preserving the surrounding tissue. This is accomplished through surgical excision, curettage-desiccation, radiation therapy, cryotherapy, microsurgery, or laser treatment.

Micrographic surgery, as a technique for the removal of basal cell carcinomas, offers many advantages for older adults. It provides the highest cure rate, conserves normal tissue (which enhances cosmetic results), requires only local anesthesia, and can be less expensive than hospital operating room surgery (Habif, 1996). This surgery is indicated for recurrent skin cancers and large, poorly differentiated cancers (Figure 8-6). Sun avoidance is necessary to reduce the incidence of new basal cell cancers (Tierney et al., 1995).

Squamous cell carcinoma Squamous cell cancer is usually slow growing and is first observed as a scaly, slightly elevated lesion consisting of squamous epithelial cells (Figure 8-7). The lesion may bleed or may have an irregular shape. This carcinoma has a good prognosis if detected and treated early; however, if not treated early, squamous cell carcinoma can metastasize. The treatment for basal cell carcinoma is also used for squamous cell carcinoma. A preexisting area of actinic keratoses may be the site of the lesion, or the lesion can arise from areas of chronic trauma or irritation, such as the lower lip.

Malignant melanoma A malignant melanoma develops from melanocytes, some of which occur in nevi or other pigmented lesions (Figure 8-8). Any change in a mole or development of bleeding areas should be investigated. In older adults the back and lower extremities are often targets. About 70% of melanomas are classified as superficial spreading melanomas, 10% as lentigo melanoma (on skin areas exposed to sun), 8% as acral lentiginous melanoma, and 15% as nodular melanoma (Kurban & Kurban, 1993). Following confirmation of the melanoma by biopsy, the patient is examined for evidence of metastasis. Treatment involves deep surgical removal of the lesion, chemotherapy, and possibly radiation therapy. Follow-up examinations are essential because recurrence of malignant melanomas is common.

Radiation therapy for treatment of cancer causes damage to the normal skin and to mucous membranes. These can be classified as local or systemic effects. Locally, the effects are related to the area of skin irradiated and may include alopecia (loss of hair) and localized skin reactions. Three stages of skin reactions are (1) erythema, (2) dry desquamation with flaking, and (3) moist desquamation with shedding of surface epithelium (Beare & Myers, 1994). Treatment of radiation effects on the skin includes (1) avoiding further trauma, (2) reducing friction and exposure to the sun, (3) using nonadhesive dressings, (4) keeping the skin warm and dry, and (5) avoiding harsh chemicals and soaps. Use of over-the-counter (OTC) skin products should be discouraged, because they may contain harmful ingredients.

Pressure ulcers

A *pressure ulcer* is an area of cellular necrosis, which is an endemic problem in the debilitated patient population. In skilled care nursing home facilities, the prevalence is approximately 23% (Panel for the Prediction and Prevention of Pressure Ulcers in Adults, 1992). Pressure ulcers develop when the external pressure on the skin covering bony prominences exceeds capillary hydrostatic pressure. Generally there is agreement that local tissue perfusion and oxygenation are compromised in the pressure ulcer patient. Patients who are immobile, dependent, malnourished, and subject to friction and shearing force

are most likely to develop pressure ulcers (Kashyup, 1989). A pressure ulcer can be described in terms of stages for purposes of treatment. (See Figure 8-9 for a description of the four stages of pressure ulcers.) Sites for pressure ulcers are the sacrum, greater trochanter (hip), ischial tuberosity (buttocks), lateral malleolus (ankle), ears, and tuberosity of the calcaneus (heel) (Tierney et al., 1995). These sites account for more than 95% of all pressure ulcers; in immobile older adults the most frequent site for a pressure ulcer is the sacrum.

Assessment Numerous pressure ulcer risk assessment tools are available to identify the high-risk older adult. Two validated pressure ulcer risk assessment tools are the Braden scale (Box 8-1) and the Norton scale (Box 8-2) (Panel for the Prediction and Prevention, 1992).

Generally the assessment should focus on clustering clinical cues to provide a guide for interventions. In Sparks's study (1990), 11 assessment parameters and 20 clinical cues were identified as being characteristic of the patient who develops a pressure ulcer. See Table 8-2 for a description of the assessment parameters and clinical cues.

Pressure ulcer risk assessment using established instruments such as the Braden scale or Norton scale should be performed initially and repeated at frequent intervals to detect changes requiring implementation of pressure ulcer prevention protocols.

Family assessment Discuss the impact of skin problems with family members or significant others. Determine the adequacy of their knowledge base and the need for patient or family education to carry out prescribed skin regimens.

Environmental assessment Determine the nature of the patient's living environment and daily activity patterns. If frequent sun exposure occurs, advise the use of sunscreen and protective clothing. Find out about environmental hazards, such as wrinkled bed linen, improperly fitting shoes or clothes, uncovered heat vents, and exposure to radiation. If the patient is immobile,

BOX 8-1 BRADEN SCALE FOR PREDICTING PRESSURE ULCER RISK

Patient's Name _____ Evaluator's Name _____ Date of Assessment _____

Category	1	2	3	4
SENSORY PERCEPTION Ability to respond meaningfully to pressure-related discomfort	**1. Completely limited:** Unresponsive (does not moan, flinch, or grasp) to painful stimuli, due to diminished level of consciousness or sedation. OR limited ability to feel pain over most of body surface.	**2. Very Limited:** Responds only to painful stimuli. Cannot communicate discomfort except by moaning or restlessness, OR has a sensory impairment which limits the ability to feel pain or discomfort over ½ of body.	**3. Slightly Limited:** Responds to verbal commands but cannot always communicate discomfort or need to be turned, OR has some sensory impairment which limits ability to feel pain or discomfort in 1 or 2 extremities.	**4. No Impairment:** Responds to verbal commands. Has no sensory deficit which would limit ability to feel or voice pain or discomfort.
MOISTURE Degree to which skin is exposed to moisture	**1. Constantly Moist:** Skin is kept moist almost constantly by perspiration, urine, etc. Dampness is detected every time patient is moved or turned.	**2. Moist:** Skin is often but not always moist. Linen must be changed at least once a shift.	**3. Occasionally Moist:** Skin is occasionally moist, requiring an extra linen change approximately once a day.	**4. Rarely Moist:** Skin is usually dry; linen requires changing only at routine intervals.
ACTIVITY Degree of physical activity	**1. Bedfast:** Confined to bed.	**2. Chairfast:** Ability to walk severely limited or nonexistent. Cannot bear own weight and/or must be assisted into chair or wheelchair.	**3. Walks Occasionally:** Walks occasionally during day but for very short distances, with or without assistance. Spends majority of each shift in bed or chair.	**4. Walks Frequently:** Walks outside the room at least twice a day and inside room at least once every 2 hours during waking hours.
MOBILITY Ability to change and control body position	**1. Completely Immobile:** Does not make even slight changes in body or extremity position without assistance.	**2. Very Limited:** Makes occasional slight changes in body or extremity position but unable to make frequent or significant changes independently.	**3. Slightly Limited:** Makes frequent though slight changes in body or extremity position independently.	**4. No Limitations:** Makes major and frequent changes in position without assistance.
NUTRITION Usual food intake pattern	**1. Very Poor:** Never eats a complete meal. Rarely eats more than ⅓ of any food offered. Eats 2 servings or less of protein (meat or dairy products) per day. Takes fluids poorly. Does not take a liquid dietary supplement, OR is NPO and/or maintained on clear liquids or IVs for more than 5 days.	**2. Probably Inadequate:** Rarely eats a complete meal and generally eats only about ½ of any food offered. Protein intake includes only 3 servings of meat or dairy products per day. Occasionally will take a dietary supplement, OR receives less than optimum amount of liquid diet or tube feeding.	**3. Adequate:** Eats over half of most meals. Eats a total of 4 servings of protein (meat, dairy products) each day. Occasionally will refuse a meal, but will usually take a supplement if offered, OR is on a tube feeding or TPN regimen, which probably meets most of nutritional needs.	**4. Excellent:** Eats most of every meal. Never refuses a meal. Usually eats a total of 4 or more servings of meat and dairy products. Occasionally eats between meals. Does not require supplementation.
FRICTION AND SHEAR	**1. Problem:** Requires moderate to maximum assistance in moving. Complete lifting without sliding against sheets is impossible. Frequently slides down in bed or chair, requiring frequent repositioning with maximum assistance. Spasticity, contractures, or agitation leads to almost constant friction.	**2. Potential Problem:** Moves feebly or requires minimum assistance. During a move skin probably slides to some extent against sheets, chair, restraints, or other devices. Maintains relatively good position in chair or bed most of the time but occasionally slides down.	**3. No Apparent Problem:** Moves in bed and in chair independently and has sufficient muscle strength to lift up completely during move. Maintains good position in bed or chair at all times.	
				Total Score

© Copyright Barbara Braden and Nancy Bergstrom, 1988.

BOX 8-2 NORTON SCALE

NORTON RISK ASSESSMENT SCALE

		Physical Condition		Mental Condition		Activity		Mobility		Incontinent		
		Good	4	Alert	4	Ambulant	4	Full	4	Not	4	TOTAL
		Fair	3	Apathetic	3	Walk/help	3	Sl. limited	3	Occasional	3	SCORE
		Poor	2	Confused	2	Chairbound	2	V. limited	2	Usually/Urine	2	
		Very Bad	1	Stupor	1	Bed	1	Immobile	1	Doubly	1	
Name	Date											

Reprinted with permission, Norton D., McLaren R., and Exton-Smith A.N.: *An investigation of geriatric nursing problems in hospital*, 1962, reissue 1975, Churchill Livingstone, Edinburgh.

TABLE 8-2 Pressure ulcer assessment parameters and clinical cues

Assessment parameters	Clinical cues
Activity status	Confinement to bed; confinement to chair; paralysis
Circulation	Decreased
Incontinence	Bladder; bowel
Infection	Localized infection in pressure-supporting areas
Mechanical factors	Friction; external pressure; shearing forces
Mental status	Comatose
Mobility status	Dependent
Musculoskeletal status	Skeletal prominence; loss of tissue; loss of muscle
Nutritional status	Cachexia or debilitation; dehydration; low serum albumin
Self-care ability	Dependent
Skin condition	Maceration

suggest the use of materials to prevent skin breakdown, such as cushions, mattresses, lotions, and positioning devices.

Once the nurse identifies a patient as requiring intervention for pressure ulcers (either to prevent or to treat such ulcers), the nurse must plan, implement, and monitor the appropriate interventions. The management and treatment of pressure ulcers can be divided into two categories: (1) preventive therapy and (2) treatment of existing pressure ulcers.

Preventive therapy Preventive pressure ulcer therapy requires adequate nutrition (increased protein and vitamins) and hydration, keeping the skin clean and dry, and reducing friction, shearing forces, and the amount of pressure exerted on any

Aging Alert
Warning signs
of malignant melanoma
in a pigmented lesion
- Asymmetry
- Border irregularity
- Color variation or dark border color
- Diameter greater than 6 mm

From Kurban, R. S., & Kurban, A. K. (1993). Common skin disorders of aging: Diagnosis and treatment. *Geriatrics, 48* (4), 30-42.

body part. Reduction of pressure may be accomplished by moving and turning the patient at least every 2 hours and by using pillows, flotation devices, special mattresses, and positioning devices.

To prevent tissue trauma from shearing force or friction, the patient must be lifted, not pulled, when repositioned in bed or in a wheelchair. Small shifts of body weight are also effective in reducing pressure. Using a "pull sheet" or reusable underpad may aid in moving the patient without causing additional tissue trauma. Shearing force can be reduced by limiting the amount of time the patient spends at an angle of 30 degrees or higher. The use of pressure-reducing devices such as foam mattresses, water mattresses, and gel-filled cushions should follow local institutional guidelines. The key to prevention is relief of pressure.

Treatment Treatment of existing pressure ulcers depends on their location and severity and the patient's condition. Pressure ulcers must be constantly monitored to detect changes in healing and the onset of infection. Pressure ulcers can be grouped into stages, according to their characteristics, and treatment may be provided according to general guidelines for each stage. It is essential to recognize that pressure relief is the key element in any treatment plan. (See Table 8-3 for an overview of treatment strategies related to the stage of pressure ulcer development.)

Two publications dealing with the prediction, prevention, and treatment of pressure ul-

TABLE 8-3 Pressure ulcer treatments

Stage	Goal	Treatment
0	Prevention of skin breakdown	Relief of pressure
		Eliminate shear and friction
		Maintain adequate nutrition/fluid
		Use pressure-relieving devices
		Turning frequently
1	Erythema resolves	All of the above
	No epidermal breakdown	+ Transparent adhesive dressings
		+ Padding bony prominences
2	Epidermis heals	All of the above
	No necrotic tissue	+ Hydrocolloidal dressings
		Polyurethane foam dressings
3	Ulcer heals	Same as for stage 0
	Free of eschar	+ Treat infection
	No infection	Debridement—surgical or enzymatic
4	Ulcer heals	Surgical closure (skin graft or skin flap)
	No osteomyelitis	

Aging Alert
Prevention of pressure ulcers

- Increase mobility; move or turn frequently
- Examine skin daily for areas of redness or tenderness
- Maintain nutritional status and hydration
- Reduce pressure on bony prominences
- Avoid friction and shearing forces
- Keep skin dry; pat skin, do not rub

cers are available to clinicians and patients. The first, *Pressure Ulcers in Adults: Prediction and Prevention* (Panel for the Prediction and Prevention, 1992), provides guidelines for identifying patients at risk for pressure ulcers and recommends early interventions for the prevention of pressure ulcers. *Treatment of Pressure Ulcers* (Bergstrom et al., 1992) makes recommendations in six areas: assessment, managing tissue loads, ulcer care, managing bacterial colonization and infection, operative repair, and education and quality improvement. Both publications are available as a quick reference guide for clinicians and as a patient's guide, which is available in English and Spanish. To order copies of the guidelines, call the Agency for Health Care Policy and Research (AHCPR) Publications Clearinghouse at 1-800-358-9295 or write to AHCPR Publications Clearinghouse, Post Office Box 8547, Silver Spring, MD 20907.

Venous ulcers

Venous ulcers occur when venous blood pools in the lower extremities, causing skin lesions and infections (Figure 8-10). In older adults this is most frequently caused by venous insufficiency. The incidence of venous ulcers is estimated to be 0.2% to 0.4% among the general population; the incidence is probably higher in the older adult segment of the population. These ulcers are commonly located on the medial aspect of the leg, whereas ulcers caused by arterial insufficiency are found on the lateral aspect of the leg or the malleoli (ankles). Research has shown that diffusion and exchange of nutrients are impaired following the occurrence of unrelieved venous pressure.

Preventive treatment includes education about meticulous foot care and use of aseptic technique. Strategies to improve circulation and maintain cellular nutrition, such as elevation of the feet and use of compression stockings to reduce edema, are also recommended. "Compression should achieve a pressure of 30 mm Hg below the knee and 40 mm Hg at the ankle. The stockings should not be used in patients with arterial insufficiency ... Pneumatic sequential compression devices may be of great benefit" (Tierney et al., 1995). When ulcers occur, treatment is aimed at correction of factors that impair wound healing. This includes nutritional therapy, with particular emphasis on vitamin C and zinc, if the patient is malnourished. Control of systemic diseases such as anemia, congestive heart failure, and diabetes mellitus is essential.

The ulcer is cleansed, treated with a steroid ointment, and covered with an occlusive dressing or a polyurethane foam dressing, and an Unna zinc paste boot is applied (changed weekly). The ulcer should heal in 2 to 3 months; if healing does not occur, pinch grafts may be necessary. Newer techniques, using cultured epidermal cell grafts, are being used in some cases not successfully treated with other therapy (Tierney et al., 1995).

Antibiotic therapy is usually avoided unless there are signs of cellulitis. If there *are* signs of cellulitis, hospitalization or specialized home care may be required for the administration of intravenous antibiotics. Because many patients have allergies, the nurse must exercise caution in selecting and using both topical preparations and those with systemic effect. Contact dermatitis might occur, causing pruritus and erythema, which further delay healing.

Synthetic occlusive dressings for venous ulcers are helpful in reducing pain and in stimulating granulation tissue. This type of treatment also allows the patient to be monitored in an outpatient setting. Occlusive dressings may become filled with exudate, and an unpleasant odor is often present; nonetheless, in most cases the patient is instructed *not* to remove the dressing. The dressing usually remains in place for 2 to 3 weeks, after which time it is removed and replaced with a standard dressing. If the surrounding skin is very fragile or there is extensive dermatitis, occlusive dressings cannot be used. For patients who are unable to do their own dressing changes, Unna boots may be used to dress ulcers; they are changed only once a week and are a form of occlusive therapy.

Arterial ulcers

Arterial ulcers are usually caused by atherosclerosis. They occur on the legs, ankles, and feet and are characterized by pallor, patchy bluish-purple mottling of the skin, and cold, clammy skin. Absence of arterial pulses and distortion of the toenails (onychogryposis) are also clinical signs of arterial ulcers. The ulcers are smaller than venous ulcers and are sharply defined, and muscle or tendon is often exposed. Cues for distinguishing arterial and venous ulcers are presented in Table 8-4.

Treatment is aimed at reducing peripheral vascular disease risk factors. Smoking should be strongly discouraged because the nicotinic acid in tobacco causes arteries to constrict. Hypertension, diabetes mellitus, hyperlipemia, and obesity should be controlled. Meticulous foot care is essential. The patient should be referred to a podiatrist for management of corns, calluses, and nail dystrophies. Protective foot pads may be needed to prevent injury.

Fungal infections

Fungal infections occur frequently in the compromised older adult. *Candida albicans,* a yeastlike fungus, is normally found in the body; moist skin, use of antibiotics or corticosteroids, and poor general health can lead to candidiasis (Figure 8-11). It is manifested by pruritus, burning, and red, eroded patches of skin. Treatment consists of topical and systemically acting antifungal agents such as nystatin (Mycostatin). Cool Burrow's compresses may be recommended to relieve inflam-

TABLE 8-4 Cues for distinguishing arterial and venous ulcers

Cue	Arterial ulcer	Venous ulcer
Previous history	Arteriosclerosis	Thrombophlebitis
Pain	Severe	Moderate
Characteristics		
Margins	Well defined	Ragged
Location	Tips of toes, heels, phalangeal heads, above lateral aspect of malleolus	Malleolus, pretibial area
Depth	Deep	Shallow
Tissue	Necrotic	Granulated
Skin	Shiny, dry	Edematous
Nails	Thick	Unchanged
Skin temperature	Variable	Cool or hot
Dependent position	Rubor	Unchanged
Edema	None	Common

mation. The patient should be taught to keep the skin clean and dry and to change into clean clothing frequently, to avoid reinfection. Use of cotton underwear and stockings may also be helpful.

Toenails may be infected with *Trichophyton rubrum*. Affected nails are thickened, discolored, and dystrophic; debris may be found under the nail. Creams or lotions such as miconazole, clotrimazole, or ciclopirox may be used as topical agents. In some cases the infection cannot be cured but can be kept under control. If the nail plate is involved, systemically acting antifungal agents may be used for a 2- to 4-week course of therapy (Tierney et al., 1995).

Herpes zoster

Herpes zoster is an acute, painful infection of a sensory nerve and its nerve path. It is caused by the varicella-zoster virus, which resides in most people. The incidence is closely related to age (e.g., 80% in 80-year-olds).

The initial lesions appear as vesicles along a dermatome; pain frequently precedes the lesions by 3 to 4 days (Figure 8-12). Most commonly, the thoracic region is affected, although the cervical, trigeminal, lumbar, and sacral regions may be the site. The acute stage lasts approximately 3 weeks and may require analgesics. Acyclovir (Zovirax) may hasten healing and reduce pain. It is given orally, and the patient should be encouraged to drink fluids (Weaver, 1995). The pain accompanying herpes zoster is often severe, and systemically acting steroids may be used. Patients may apply calamine lotion or vinegar solution (¼ cup white vinegar to 2 qt water) to reduce discomfort. Herpes zoster may recur, and in immunosuppressed patients it can lead to other complications and even death.

Postherpetic neuralgia, a dermatomal pain syndrome, occurs in about 10% of people (especially older adults) after herpes zoster infection. It is treated with analgesics; if these are ineffective, the patient may be given amitriptyline and phenothiazine. A topical cream containing capsaicin is thought to block painful stimuli from the periphery to the spinal cord. Systemically acting corticosteroids may reduce the incidence of postherpetic neuralgia but are contraindicated in immunosuppressed patients (Thiers, 1989).

Dermatitis

Dermatitis, or inflammation of the skin, can manifest itself as eczema, allergic contact dermatitis, or seborrheic dermatitis. These inflammations cause erythema, edema, exudate, erosion, itching, and scabs or scales.

Eczema (eczematous dermatitis) can be acute, subacute, or chronic. In the acute stage the skin is erythematous and there are exudates, weeping vesicles, and crusts. Itching of the affected area is a major complaint of older adults with dermatitis. Treatment includes use of systemically acting medications to reduce itching, corticosteroids to control the inflammatory response, and anti-infective agents to treat secondary infections. Local treatment includes the application of topical corticosteroids, antibacterials, and antifungal agents. Frequently, soaks and dressings are applied to the affected areas to provide relief of pain and itching. The patient should be instructed in good hygiene measures to prevent infections and in the application of ointments and dressings.

In the subacute and chronic phases the patient should be instructed in the use of stronger corticosteroids and the use of compresses, occlusive dressings, and tar preparations. Because eczema is difficult to treat and often causes concerns with body image changes, patients should be encouraged to ventilate their thoughts and feelings about these skin changes and to discuss how such changes affect their lifestyles.

Allergic contact dermatitis is not related to age, but when it does occur in older adults, it may be more severe and generalized than in the younger population. Allergies to medications, rubber, cosmetics, and *Rhus* plants (poison ivy, poison oak, etc.) are the most common causes. Patients being treated with neomycin for stasis dermatitis or ulceration often develop contact dermatitis. Medications free of ethylenediamine and neomycin should be used in the treatment of allergic contact dermatitis in the older adult; for example, nystatin (Mycolog II cream), Myocream, and Tri-Statin.

The emergence of transdermally delivered drugs (e.g., nitroglycerin, scopolamine, and clonidine) has led to an increase in allergic contact dermatitis. Other agents, such as hair dyes, fragrances, preservatives, and sunscreens containing paraaminobenzoic acid (PABA) or glycerol PABA are frequent causes of allergic contact dermatitis.

Seborrheic dermatitis is seen around the scalp, eyebrows, eyelids, and back (Figure 8-13). It is a chronic, recurrent, erythematous scaling eruption of cells. It is usually treated with a daily dandruff shampoo using a product containing 1% selenium sulfide or 2% pyrithione zinc. A topical corticosteroid solution may be added, if needed. If the dermatitis is resistant to this treatment, a selenium sulfide 2.5% suspension may be used once a week—shampoo scalp using fingertip massage, rinse, shampoo again, leave solution on for 5 to 10 minutes, then rinse (Tierney et al., 1995).

With facial seborrheic dermatitis, low-dose topical corticosteroid may be used twice daily until the condition is controlled, then continued daily or every other day. Sometimes, antimicrobial creams such as sulfacetamide lotion or iodochlorhydroxyquin may be selected to avoid the use of steroids. When the eyelids are involved (seborrheic blepharitis), they can be treated with daily applications of baby shampoo on a cotton swab.

Pigmentary disturbances

Pigmentary disturbances include nevi and vitiligo. *Nevi* contain melanin and are usually benign (Figure 8-14). They usually require no treatment unless they occur in areas of the body where they are subject to trauma or unless changes occur in their appearance. Surgical removal may be accomplished by cryosurgery or by punch biopsy and usually does not require hospitalization.

Vitiligo manifests itself as a localized area of depigmentation (Figure 8-15). Initially, vitiligo appears in areas exposed to the sun, but it may also involve the hands, axillae, perineum, and periorbital areas. It may be associated with diabetes mellitus, thyroid dysfunction, Addison's disease, and pernicious anemia (Thompson, et al., 1993). There is usually no treatment, although the affected areas should be protected from the sun by use of sunscreen, wearing protective clothing, or avoidance of exposure. Some mixed success has been achieved in repigmentation with photosensitizers, skin dyes, and depigmenting agents.

Pruritus

Pruritus, generalized itching, is frequently encountered in the older adult population. It is sometimes caused by drug reactions and skin sensitivity to dyes in clothing. In some cases, systemic disease or psychogenic factors may have a role. Frequently, dry skin is associated with pruritus because of decreased sweat gland activity; frequent bathing and low humidity in the environment increase the problem. Treatment is symptomatic and includes removal of the offending agent, decreasing the frequency of baths, and substituting mild soap products for stronger ones, as well as the use of lotions and emollients to reduce the itching. In severe cases, medications such as antihistamines may be needed. The patient may also get comfort from sitz baths (for itching of the perineum or buttocks) and from cool compresses.

Psoriasis

Psoriasis, a chronic disease of keratin synthesis, is seen in 3% to 5% of the general population (Figure 8-16). In older adults it often appears as a plaque-type psoriasis vulgaris. The other forms, exfoliative psoriasis and generalized pustular psoriasis, may also occur in older adults. Outbreaks are sometimes precipitated by stress, drugs (e.g., beta-blockers or lithium), and infection. Psoriasis manifests itself with dry, well-circumscribed, silvery, scaling papules and plaques. It usually involves the back, buttocks, and extensor surfaces of the extremities (knees and elbows). There is rapid mitotic activity, faulty keratinization of the horny skin layer, and dilation of the upper dermal vessels. Treatment is directed toward the minimization of stress and the use of medications—such as topical corticosteroids—to reduce inflammation, control lesions, and reduce discomfort. Emollients are used after bathing; petroleum gel is inexpensive and works well. Ultraviolet B phototherapy is used and may be combined with coal tar applications. For patients with resistant psoriasis, use of psoralens plus long-wave ultraviolet A (PUVA) is advised. This treatment requires a fluorescent bed unit and cannot be used in patients with a history of skin cancer or cataracts because of the photosensitization risk. Specialized facilities may provide daily treatment with methoxsalen. Patients with extensive psoriasis may require systemic treatment.

Synthetic retinoids such as etretinate may be used before and concurrent with phototherapy. The patient needs to be monitored closely and evaluated for skeletal hyperostosis. The toxic effects of etretinate (such as dry mucous membranes, thirst, fatigue, muscle and bone pain, and diffuse alopecia) should be discussed before treatment. Methotrexate, azathioprine, and hydroxyurea are other agents used in psoriasis treatment; all are potent medications and require close monitoring (Lowe, 1989).

Senile purpura

Senile purpura is an area of bruising, usually on the forearms, that occurs either spontaneously or with little or no trauma. It is caused by loss of subcutaneous tissue and subsequent loss of support for capillaries close to the skin surface. There is no medical treatment, but care should be taken to avoid injury to delicate tissues.

Wrinkles

Wrinkles occur as the skin becomes less elastic and the epidermis loses collagen and elastic fibers. Smoking has been associated with facial wrinkling caused by decreased capillary and arteriolar blood flow; patients should be advised to quit smoking (Grady & Ernster, 1992). Because so much of a person's self-concept is related to appearance, millions of dollars are spent each year to retain a youthful (i.e., wrinkle-free) look. Advances in pharmaceuticals and cosmetics have encouraged many older adults to believe that normal aging changes can be reversed or minimized.

Topical tretinoin (Retin-A) may reverse wrinkles and other skin damage caused by the sun. Treatment of photodamaged skin with tretinoin has produced an 80% increase in collagen I formation (Griffiths et al., 1993). Tretinoin cream (0.05%) is applied very sparingly to clean, dry, photodamaged areas of the skin. A gel product (0.01%) is available for people with oily skin. No medication should be placed on open wounds, in deep skin folds, or on the eyes or eyelids because of the possibility of severe burning. The patient should be advised to avoid the use of toners, astringents, exfoliants, and abrasive scrubs. The patient should be instructed to use a sunscreen with a sun protection factor (SPF) of a minimum of 15 on a daily basis.

New treatments such as injection of botulism toxin A are being used to reduce facial wrinkles and provide cosmetic improvement (Keen et al., 1994). A permanent implant using a synthetic polymer (Gore-Tex expanded polytetrafluoroethylene soft-tissue patch) is being used to correct deep wrinkles and folds. Because these treatments and products are new, long-term results of their use are not known, and the patient should be educated to remain cautious about extravagant claims and to use products prudently.

NURSING PROCESS

Synthesized knowledge of skin changes in older adults forms the basis for providing comprehensive nursing care. The prevention of skin breakdown and the treatment of existing skin disorders are integral nursing care components.

ASSESSMENT
History

Obtain a history from the patient covering skin problems, trauma, chronic disease, or debilitating illness. Assess the patient's knowledge level, and determine the patient's ability to carry out a skin care regimen. Inquire about the patient's past exposure to the sun or other radiation. Ask questions about the impact of any skin changes on the patient's self-concept and body image. Try to determine the level of support from family or other social support systems.

Physical examination

Inspect the entire body surface; describe characteristics of rashes, cuts, wounds, scratches, scales, lice, bruises, and nails. Describe any lesions present; include the size, color, texture (raised or flat), crustiness, dryness, or weeping of the area of skin being described. Use a millimeter or centimeter ruler to increase accuracy in reporting lesions. Check health records for serum albumin, hemoglobin, and hematocrit results to assess nutritional status. Observe the quantity and distribution of hair to determine areas of decreased circulation such as in the lower extremities. Check pulses in all extremities; a diminished pulse or absence of a pulse may indicate venous or arterial insufficiency.

Arterial insufficiency is characterized by coolness, sensitivity to cold, pallor on elevation of the extremities, redness on lowering of extremities, cyanosis or mottling, loss of hair on limbs, and tight, shiny skin. Other characteristics include thickened, brittle nails, delayed capillary filling, decreased or absent peripheral pulses, and ulceration on the extremities.

Venous insufficiency is characterized by swollen, ropelike, or ruptured superficial leg veins, edema of the lower extremities, atrophy of skin and soft tissue, gangrenous changes, and nocturnal cramping.

NURSING DIAGNOSES

Data gathered during the assessment phase are analyzed, and appropriate nursing diagnoses are made. Each diagnosis must be supported by subjective and/or objective clinical data obtained from the patient, family, health records, and health team members. The following nursing diagnoses approved by the North American Nursing Diagnosis Association (NANDA) may apply to the older adult with skin integrity problems:

High risk for impaired skin integrity: pressure ulcer
Impaired skin integrity
Impaired tissue integrity
Knowledge deficit: skin care

Risk for impaired skin integrity: Pressure ulcer

The condition may be evidenced by the presence of risk factors, which may be either external and/or environmental or internal and/or somatic.

External and/or environmental risks
Pressure
Shearing forces
Friction
Moisture
Physical immobility

Internal and/or somatic risks
Poor nutritional status (cachexia or debilitation, dehydration, decreased serum albumin)
Decreased circulation
Comatose state, altered level of consciousness, or confusion
Musculoskeletal alterations (skeletal prominences, loss of subcutaneous tissue, loss of muscle, paralysis)
Poor skin condition (maceration)
Incontinence (bowel and bladder)

Impaired skin integrity

The condition may be evidenced by the following defining characteristics:

Disruption of skin surface
Destruction of skin layers
Invasion of body structures

Impaired tissue integrity: Venous ulcer

The condition may be evidenced by the following defining characteristics:

> Ulceration of the lower extremity
> Normal pulses
> Edema

Knowledge deficit: Skin care

The condition may be evidenced by the following defining characteristics:

> Verbalization of need for information about skin condition
> Inaccurate follow-through on instructions for management of skin problem
> Incomplete resolution of the skin problem
> Readmission for the same skin problem

PLANNING AND GOAL IDENTIFICATION

The outcome identification phase of the nursing process consists of setting realistic long- and short-term goals based on nursing diagnoses. The patient is an integral member of the health care team and, if able, should be closely involved in the development of these goals.

Risk for impaired skin integrity: Pressure ulcer

A long-term goal is that the patient will have no skin breakdown. Short-term goals include the following:

1. Patient or family will verbalize an understanding of preventive skin care measures.
2. Patient or family will demonstrate preventive skin care measures.
3. Patient or family will be able to describe the relationship between risk factors and skin breakdown.

Impaired skin integrity

A long-term goal is that the patient will have healed lesions or wounds. The following may be appropriate short-term goals:

1. Patient will explain skin care regimen.
2. Patient will carry out skin care regimen correctly.

3. Patient will understand the relationship between various risk factors and skin breakdown.
4. Patient will discuss impact of skin changes on body image and self-concept.

Impaired tissue integrity

A long-term goal is that the patient will follow the skin care regimen after discharge from the hospital. Short-term goals include the following:

1. Patient will verbalize an understanding of the relationship between various risk factors and skin changes.
2. Patient will maintain peripheral circulation at baseline level (specify parameters for individual patient).
3. Patient will carry out skin care regimen, including exercise, foot care, avoidance of dependent positions, and use of anti-embolism stockings.

Knowledge deficit: Skin care

A long-term goal is that the patient will verbalize an understanding of skin condition and its relationship to risk factors. Short-term goals include the following:

1. Patient will follow instructions for skin care correctly.
2. Patient will demonstrate correct skin care regimen.
3. Patient will state intention to use skin care consultants.

IMPLEMENTATION

Nursing interventions are planned to achieve the goals established for the skin care plan. They should focus on the etiology of the problem and should be specific. Interventions are carried out wherever the patient may be found—in the acute care setting, the nursing home, or the patient's private home environment. Because of the frequency of skin problems in older adults, it is likely that most or all of the measures discussed will be needed in at least one setting.

Health Promotion
Skin protection

- Examine skin daily for any changes, and report any changes in moles or lesions. Report any lesion that fails to heal.
- Avoid scratching of dry skin.
- Avoid daily hot baths or showers. Bathing 2 to 3 times per week is sufficient. Daily sponge bathing is permissible.
- Use superfatted, nondeodorant soaps.
- Use bath or mineral oils with extreme caution. These can cause slipping in the shower or tub.
- Apply emollients or lotions after bathing.
- Drink several glasses of water every day.
- Do not use rubbing alcohol on skin. This causes drying.
- Consider the use of a humidifier in winter, if dry skin is a problem.

Health Promotion
Sun exposure

- Protect skin from overexposure to the sun. Avoid being in the sun between the hours of 10 a.m. and 3 p.m.
- Wear protective clothing, such as light-colored, long-sleeved shirts, long pants, and wide-brimmed hats, when out in the sun.
- Apply sunscreen with an SPF of at least 15 before exposure to the sun. Wear sunscreen even on cloudy days (clouds do not block ultraviolet rays).
- Avoid sunburn. There is no such thing as a healthy tan!

The focus of each intervention is on achieving a specific goal. For purposes of discussion, each section describes physical care measures, psychosocial care measures, and educational measures carried out by the nurse, patient, and/or family to resolve skin problems.

In the acute care setting

The primary way to prevent skin breakdown is to decrease pressure. This can be accomplished through frequent changes in position, the use of pressure-relieving devices, and regular inspection of the skin for signs of early damage. Position changes should be made at least every 2 hours, and small shifts of body weight should be encouraged. *Bony prominences should not be massaged.* Avoid drying agents such as alcohol or alcohol-based rubs. Use moisturizing agents to

prevent skin dryness. To avoid shearing force when moving patients, lift—do not pull. A complete bath can be given every 3 to 4 days, and a sponge bath can be given daily, to prevent drying of the skin. The skin should be patted dry, not rubbed, to avoid tissue trauma. Good nutrition and adequate hydration are integral components of a skin care program to maintain skin integrity. All skin surfaces should be inspected daily so that corrective action, if needed, can be initiated immediately.

Compresses or wet dressings using Burrow's solution (Domeboro powder) are sometimes used to treat skin problems. The packet is mixed with 1 qt of water, and the solution is applied using sterile gauze dressings for 30 minutes 3 times a day. The wet dressing should be wrapped with a nonporous covering to protect the rest of the patient's skin.

Pressure-relieving devices usually consist of mattresses, cushions, and body part supports (see further discussion of pressure-relieving devices in Table 8-5). For the patient at minimal

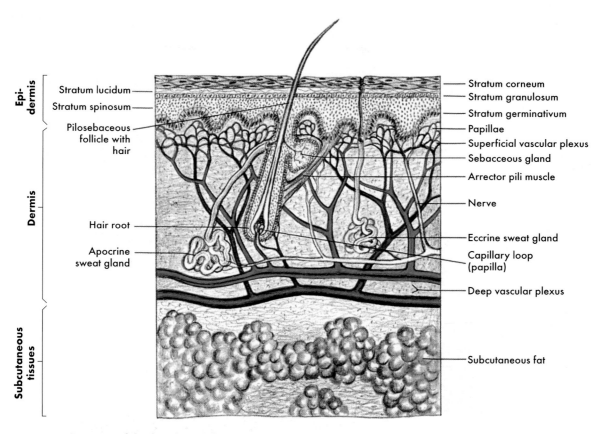

Epi-dermis

Stratum lucidum
Stratum spinosum

Pilosebaceous follicle with hair

Dermis

Hair root

Apocrine sweat gland

Subcutaneous tissues

Stratum corneum
Stratum granulosum
Stratum germinativum
Papillae
Superficial vascular plexus
Sebacceous gland
Arrector pili muscle
Nerve
Eccrine sweat gland
Capillary loop (papilla)
Deep vascular plexus

Subcutaneous fat

FIGURE 8-1 Structures of the skin. (From Thompson, J.M., et al, [1993]. *Mosby's manual of clinical nursing,* St. Louis: Mosby.)

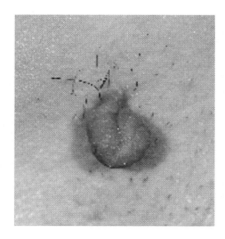

FIGURE 8-2 Acrochordon (skin tag). (From Habif, T.P. [1996]. *Clinical dermatology,* [3rd ed.]. St. Louis: Mosby.)

FIGURE 8-3 Seborrheic keratosis. (From Habif, T.P. [1996]. *Clinical dermatology,* [3rd ed.]. St. Louis: Mosby.)

FIGURE 8-4 Actinic keratosis. (From Habif, T.P. [1996]. *Clinical dermatology,* [3rd ed.]. St. Louis: Mosby.)

FIGURE 8-5 Basal cell carcinoma. (From Habif, T.P. [1996]. *Clinical dermatology,* [3rd ed.]. St. Louis: Mosby.)

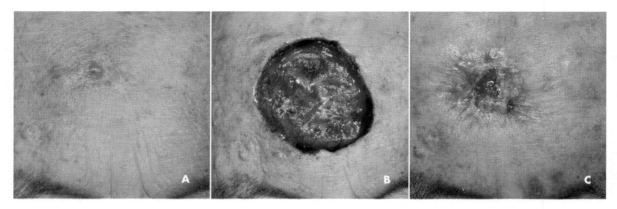

FIGURE 8-6 Basal cell carcinoma before, immediately after surgery, and 6 weeks after surgery using Mohs' micrographic surgical technique. (From Habif, T.P. [1996]. *Clinical dermatology,* [3rd ed.]. St. Louis: Mosby.)

FIGURE 8-7 Squamous cell carcinoma. (From Habif, T.P. [1996]. *Clinical dermatology,* [3rd ed.]. St. Louis: Mosby.)

FIGURE 8-8 Lentigo malignant melanoma. (From Habif, T.P. [1996]. *Clinical dermatology,* [3rd ed.]. St. Louis: Mosby.)

Pressure Ulcer Staging

Stage 1

Nonblanchable erythema of intact skin; the heralding lesion of skin ulceration. Discoloration of skin, warmth, or hardness may also be indicators.

Stage 3

Full-thickness skin loss involving damage or necrosis of subcutaneous tissue that may extend down to, but not through, underlying fascia. The ulcer presents clinically as a deep crater with or without undermining of adjacent tissue.

Stage 2

Partial-thickness skin loss involving epidermis and/or dermis. The ulcer is superficial and presents clinically as an abrasion, blister, or shallow crater.

Stage 4

Full-thickness skin loss with extensive destruction, tissue necrosis, or damage to muscle, bone, or supporting structures (eg, tendon, joint capsule).

FIGURE 8-9 Stages of a pressure ulcer. (From the National Pressure Ulcer Advisory Panel and the Agency for Health Care Policy and Research.)

FIGURE 8-11 Candida intertrigo. (From Habif, T.P. [1996]. *Clinical dermatology,* [3rded.]. St. Louis: Mosby.)

FIGURE 8-10 Venous stasis ulcer. (From Habif, T.P. [1996]. *Clinical dermatology,* [3rded.]. St. Louis: Mosby.)

FIGURE 8-12 Herpes zoster. *A,* A common presentation with involvement of a single thoracic dermatome. *B,* A group of vesicles that vary in size. Vesicles of herpes simplex are a uniform size. (From Habif, T.P. [1996]. *Clinical dermatology,* [3rded.]. St. Louis: Mosby.)

FIGURE 8-13 Seborrheic dermatitis. (From Habif, T.P. [1996]. *Clinical dermatology,* [3rded.]. St. Louis: Mosby.)

FIGURE 8-14 Dermal nevus. Surface speckling. Examination of the surface of this pigmented lesion with a hand lens reveals uniform speckling over the surface, a characteristic of a benign pigmented nevus. (From Habif, T.P. [1996]. *Clinical dermatology,* [3rded.]. St. Louis: Mosby.)

FIGURE 8-15 Vitiligo. (From Habif, T.P. [1996]. *Clinical dermatology,* [3rded.]. St. Louis: Mosby.)

FIGURE 8-16 Psoriasis. (From Habif, T.P. [1996]. *Clinical dermatology,* [3rded.]. St. Louis: Mosby.)

FIGURE 8-17 *A*, External pressure on the parotid gland of this client with acute bacterial sialadenitis produces pus at the parotid duct orifice. *B*, Fordyce spots–normal sebaceous glands just under the buccal mucosa. *C*, Sublingual varicosities. (From Cawson, R.A., Binnie, W.H. & Eveson, J.W. [1994] *Color atlas of oral disease: Clinical and pathologic correlations,* [2ⁿᵈ ed.]. London: Wolfe Publishing.)

A

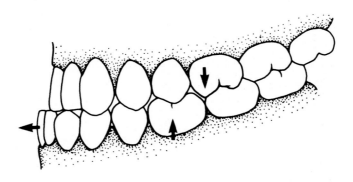

B

C

FIGURE 8-18 Occlusion. *A*, Class I–neutroclusion. *B*, Class II–distoclusion. *C*, Class III–mesioclusion. (From Brand, R. & Isselhard, D. [1990]. *Anatomy of orofacial structures,* [4ᵗʰed.]. St. Louis: Mosby.)

FIGURE 8-19 Phenytoin-induced gingival hyperplasia. (From Cawson, R.A., Binnie, W.H., & Eveson, J.W. [1994]. *Color atlas of oral disease: Clinical and pathologic correlations,* [2nd ed.]. London: Wolfe Publishing.)

FIGURE 8-20 Squamous cell carcinoma. Several ulcerated lesions are present on the lower lip of this patient who has spent years working outdoors. (From Habif, T.P. [1996]. *Clinical dermatology,* [3rd ed.]. St. Louis: Mosby.)

FIGURE 8-21 Oral candidiasis. (From Habif, T.P. [1996]. *Clinical dermatology,* [3rd ed.]. St. Louis: Mosby.)

TABLE 8-5 Types of pressure-relieving devices

Interventions	Inventory	Limitations and considerations
Pressure-relieving devices		
Static (nonmoving)	Footboard Footcradle Sheepskin Adhesive foam Pads Bed overlays Wheelchair cushions	1. Adhesive foam may be applied in a circle (bull's-eye fashion) around the wound after applying a skin barrier. 2. Linen should always be tucked loosely over pads and mattresses. 3. Incontinence pads should not be placed between the patient and the device unless they permit airflow. 4. Foam overlays should be strictly avoided for patients who smoke in bed because of the overlays' flammability when wet or soiled. Approximately 4 inches of foam is required for pressure relief.
Dynamic (moving)	Mattresses Low–air loss beds (LALBs) or air-fluidized beds (AFBs) Air Fluidized Support System (Skytron) Biogard (Bio Clinic) KinAir (Kinetic Concepts) Akros (Lumex)	1. LALBs are used for intermediate-to high-risk patients, and as a step-down bed for patients no longer requiring AFBs. 2. AFBs are designed to treat and prevent tissue trauma in high-risk patients.

Reprinted from Thomason. (1988, Summer). Pressure ulcers: Considerations of intervention strategies. *Ostomy/Wound Management*, pp. 49-50.

risk for skin breakdown, the sheets should be kept clean, dry, and free of wrinkles.

Psychosocial measures include discussion about changes in body image that may have been caused by the skin condition. Patients should be encouraged to ventilate related feelings and to seek ways to improve their self-esteem. The patient may be referred to a psychiatric or mental health specialist if needed.

In the nursing home

In the nursing home the patient is more apt to be confined to a bed or a wheelchair. The proper selection and use of therapeutic beds, mattresses, and cushions are of the utmost importance. Vigilance in the identification and early treatment of potential problems is essential to preventing extensive skin damage. Paraprofessionals should be skilled in recognizing and reporting significant skin changes in the patients they care for, but the professional nurse remains accountable for the condition of the residents' skin.

In the private or family home

Confinement to bed often leads to impaired skin integrity. Conservative estimates of the cost of pressure ulcer care in the home setting put the cost at $60 million (Bergstrom et al., 1992). Meticulous attention to maintaining skin integrity will prevent some skin problems. The family needs to ensure that the older adult is bathing once or twice a week, to inspect skin areas that are hard to see, and to obtain professional advice if there are questions about skin conditions. The patient and family should use over-the-counter skin preparations judiciously, always watching for skin reactions.

The nurse should instruct the patient and family in the skin care regimen and provide ample time for them to demonstrate, under supervision, their ability to employ the newly learned techniques. For patients with chronic skin problems, include their usual home regimen in the plan of care, to avoid confusion and to reinforce the importance of patient and family participation in the plan of care.

Special Medicare requirements apply to the use of skin care products in the home. For example, reimbursement is currently limited to postdebridement ulcer care (Medical Technology and Practice Patterns Institute [MTPPI], 1989). The home health care team is responsible for teaching the patient and primary caregiver the skin regimen to be followed. Other important aspects of home management include evaluation of nutritional status and the identification and selection of home care equipment.

EVALUATION

Evaluation of nursing care consists of two parts. The first part involves determining whether the patient outcomes have been achieved (e.g., is the skin intact?). The second part involves evaluating whether the care that is planned and executed meets established standards of care. The nurse evaluates each diagnosis and each goal and makes a judgment about the extent to which the goal has been achieved and the problem has been resolved. To make available all information needed for evaluation, both nursing interventions and goal achievement must be documented. The patient and the family should be involved in this process. Ask them whether the planned interventions have been carried out. Is there a need to revise the plan of care or the goals? The evaluation of care provides feedback

necessary to revise the plan of care, document resolution of the problem, or identify new problems.

■ Oral Mucous Membrane

NORMAL STRUCTURE AND FUNCTION

Healthy, intact oral mucous membranes allow the individual to speak, chew, taste, and maintain a normal physical appearance. In general the oral mucous membrane should be moist, smooth, and pinkish. Adults normally have 32 teeth, although the third molars (wisdom teeth) are often removed (leaving 28 teeth). The crown of the tooth is visible and should be shiny, white (although yellow to gray coloration is common), smooth edged, and free of caries, plaque, and chipped enamel. The lips should be free of cracks, fissures, dry crusts, scales, and edema. Examination of the buccal cavity reveals the status of the Stensen ducts (openings of the parotid glands) and Fordyce spots (sebaceous glands), and tissue changes (Figure 8-17). Normal gums are pink to orange, are moist, and fit tightly to the teeth. The mouth should be free of foul odor. Mucous membranes covering the tongue have salivary glands and the lingual papillae, which contain the taste buds. The tongue's dorsal surface is slightly rough and moist, whereas the ventral surface is smooth with prominent veins.

AGE-RELATED CHANGES

Changes in the oral mucous membrane during aging may include loss of dentition, decreased salivary secretion, atrophy of oral tissues, gum diseases, and degenerative changes in the masticatory apparatus. The protective tooth enamel thins, and the dentin becomes translucent. These changes may cause malocclusion, erosion, and abrasion, as well as halitosis. It is estimated that three fourths of the taste buds may be lost by age 70; the tongue becomes smooth, and there is loss of the filiform papillae. Decreased salivary production leads to dry mouth and diffi-

Healthy People 2000 Objectives
Oral health

Reduce to no more than 20% the proportion of people age 65 and older who have lost all of their natural teeth.

Extend to all long-term institutional facilities the requirement that oral examinations and services be provided no later than 90 days after entry into these facilities.

Increase to at least 60% the proportion of people age 65 and older using the oral health care system.

From U.S. Department of Health and Human Services. (1990). *Healthy People 2000: National health promotion and disease prevention objectives* (DHHS Pub. No.[PHS] 91-50212). Washington, DC: U.S. Government Printing Office.

culty swallowing and chewing. The atrophy of oral tissues leads to a reduction in host resistance, rendering older adults more susceptible to infections and oral cancer.

Perhaps the greatest oral mucous membrane impairment in the older adult is gum disease, which leads to gingivitis, gingival hyperplasia, halitosis, and periodontal disease. The loss of dentition leads to malocclusion, which results in excessive bone resorption, muscular imbalances, and temporomandibular arthritis.

It is estimated that one out of two retired people are edentulous. More than 30 million Americans are suffering from gum-related diseases. Improved dental techniques allow permanent implantation of false teeth and replacement teeth, and correction of malocclusion. Despite these advances, oral mucous membrane disturbances will cause pain and suffering for many older adults.

COMMON HEALTH DEVIATIONS
Oral trauma

The mouth can be traumatized by loss of dentition. The loss of teeth contributes to malocclusion of the jaw and causes stress on the remaining teeth. These changes are shown in Figure 8-18. These stresses can lead to increased bone resorption and muscle imbalances. Temporomandibular joint pain is common, characterized by headaches and pain in the pharynx and tongue. Chronic temporomandibular joint disease can lead to arthritic changes and osteoarthritis. Preventive treatment includes annual visits to the dentist, daily brushing and flossing, and prompt attention to symptoms of headache or pain in the mouth. Dental appliances can be made to correct malocclusion deficits, and temporary or permanent tooth replacement can stop the bone resorption. Treatment for arthritic changes consists of symptomatic relief of pain and swelling, usually with antiinflammatory agents such as ibuprofen.

Gingivitis

Gingivitis, inflammation of the gums, is a common problem in older adults (Figure 8-19). It can manifest itself as chronic desquamatous gingivitis, in which there is sloughing of the oral mucosa. Inflammatory gingival hyperplasia is related to improperly fitting dentures. Plaque contributes to gingivitis, and the gums become darker in color, edematous, and soft and bleed easily. Poor dental hygiene practices must be corrected and a vigorous oral hygiene program implemented. In severe cases the dentist must remove plaque and treat the local oral infection with antibiotics sensitive to the specific organism. If gingivitis is not successfully treated, the client may develop periodontitis and eventually lose teeth.

Oral cancer

Oral cancers can take the form of squamous cell carcinoma (90%), sarcomas, and striated and smooth muscle tumors; lymphomas and melanotic and amelanotic tumors are also seen in older adults (Figure 8-20). Some of these cancers are caused by the trauma of constant irritation (e.g., cheek biting or a tooth hitting on the gum). Others are related to the use of tobacco (smoking or chewing) and alcohol, which causes traumatic changes in the mucosal membrane. As with most cancers, early detection and treatment are the keys to a positive outcome. Surgical excision and removal of the tumor can be performed, along with radiation therapy and chemotherapy. These treatments often cause more oral mucous membrane irritation, and the mouth becomes painful, with open sores and lesions. Extreme caution should be used in providing mouth care, and irritating substances such as alcohol-based mouthwash should be avoided.

Malnutrition

Malnutrition can cause significant oral mucous membrane problems. B-complex avitaminosis can lead to bald tongue, to erythematous, multiple ulcerations inside the cheeks, and to cracked, crusted, and tender lips. All of these can lead to *glossodynia* (burning sensation of the tongue) and/or *dysphagia* (difficulty swallowing). Treatment involves correction of the underlying nutritional deficiency and symptomatic relief of sores and lesions. Local measures include mouth rinses, lip emollients, and frequent oral hygiene with a soft-bristled toothbrush. A waterpick with a mild antiseptic solution may provide gum stimulation and may increase oral comfort. Systemically, vitamins are administered, and dysphagic patients are evaluated for the need for special feeding measures.

Contact dermatitis

Contact dermatitis of the oral mucosa can be caused by sensitivity to acrylic dentures. Patients who wear dentures should always be examined for signs of inflammation or irritation. Sometimes a liner can be inserted between the buccal cavity and the denture to reduce this problem.

Schmutz pyorrhea

Schmutz pyorrhea is an accumulation of debris around the neck of each tooth. There is characteristically a foul mouth odor, and the gums separate from the tooth. Treatment usually consists of meticulous oral hygiene after the plaque has been removed by the dentist.

Oral moniliasis (candidiasis)

Candidiasis, a yeast infection, is frequently seen in the oral mucosa of older adults as saliva production decreases and there is atrophy of the oral mucosa. This causes the oral flora to change and white plaques to form on the gums, tongue, and buccal cavity (Figure 8-21). Oral candidiasis is treated with anti-infective agents such as nystatin (Mycostatin), both systemically and locally. Candidiasis causes stomatitis (ulceration of the mouth), which is painful and may require the use of locally acting anesthetic agents and frequent mouthwashes for comfort.

NURSING PROCESS

With knowledge of the normal anatomy and physiology of the oral mucous membrane and the major health-related problems encountered by the older adult, the nurse is able to apply the nursing process to an individual patient. The essential elements for providing care to the older adult with oral mucous membrane problems are presented in this section.

ASSESSMENT

Examination of the oral cavity and gathering of information about oral hygiene practices form the basis of the assessment for oral mucous membrane problems. In addition, information is obtained about the psychosocial adjustment of the patient, the effect of environmental variables, and the patient's resources in terms of family, community, and financial support.

History

Ask the patient what type of toothbrush is used and whether dental floss is used. Does the patient wear dentures regularly? If not, why not? Are they painful or ill fitting? Obtain a tobacco history (cigars, cigarettes, or chewing tobacco). What is the intake of alcohol? Is there any pain, burning, numbness, paresthesia, or temperature change in the oral cavity? Is there impaired taste sensation? Are there any swallowing difficulties or voice changes? Does the patient have annual dental examinations?

Physical examination

Open the patient's mouth and observe for presence of teeth, then inspect the patient's bite, observe for decayed teeth (caries), and inspect the gum line. Use a penlight to aid in seeing into the oral cavity. Be especially careful to look for plaque, which leads to calculus formation and causes the gums to recede, subsequently leading to bone regression and loss of teeth. Observe for signs of trauma related to toothbrushing, such as bleeding gums. Palpate for lip indurations. Look inside the cheek for Stensen's ducts. Observe for changes in the tongue, such as swelling, ulceration, coating, or changes in size, texture, or color, movement of the tongue, breath odor (halitosis), saliva production, Wharton's duct, and swelling or varicosities on the ventral surface of the tongue. Examine the hard and soft palate, pharynx, and regional lymph nodes.

Psychosocial assessment

If there is evidence of oral mucous membrane impairment, determine what effect it has had on the patient and family. Interview family members to ascertain changes in the patient's behavior. Has the patient withdrawn from social events or refused to attend group activities? How is the patient coping with body image changes and making adjustments to the illness?

Environmental assessment

Determine whether there are any environmental hazards such as tobacco in the home. What financial resources does the patient have to obtain dental services and dental hygiene supplies? Does the patient participate in any support groups?

NURSING DIAGNOSES

A nursing diagnosis is made by analyzing data obtained during the assessment process. Clusters of data define and support the selected diagnoses. The following are examples of NANDA-approved nursing diagnoses that might be developed by the nurse caring for an older adult with alterations in oral mucous membranes.

Oral mucous membrane alteration related to dehydration

The condition may be evidenced by these defining characteristics: decreased moisture (xerostomia, viscous saliva, or fissure), inflammation, edema, or halitosis.

Oral mucous membrane alteration related to mechanical trauma

Trauma may be evidenced by any of these defining characteristics:

> Sensory changes (pain, burning taste, paresthesia, numbness, temperature sensitivity)
> Lesions or ulcers (leukoplakia)
> Ill-fitting dentures
> Inflammation or edema (mucositis, stomatitis)

Oral mucous membrane alteration related to pathologic conditions

A pathologic condition may be evidenced by any of the following defining characteristics:

> Sensory changes (pain, burning taste, paresthesia, numbness, temperature sensitivity)
> Decreased moisture (xerostomia, viscous saliva, or fissure)
> Color changes (erythema, pallor, pigmentation, coated tongue, exudate)
> Lesions or ulcers
> Bleeding, hyperemia, or hemorrhage
> Induration

Inflammation or edema (mucositis, stomatitis, gingivitis, glossitis, desquamation)
Halitosis

PLANNING AND GOAL IDENTIFICATION

Outcome identification consists of setting realistic short- and long-term goals based on the nursing diagnoses and related factors identified during the assessment process. The patient should be an equal partner in establishing these goals whenever possible. The interventions to be carried out are discussed in the next section.

A long-term goal is that the patient will demonstrate correct oral hygiene practices. Short-term goals include the following:

1. Patient will be free of oral exudate and halitosis.
2. Patient will have pink and moist oral mucous membranes.
3. Patient will have no sores, lesions, or blisters in the mouth.

IMPLEMENTATION

Nursing interventions to manage oral mucous membrane problems revolve around the maintenance and preservation of intact oral tissue (Kresevic & Lincoln, 1995; Sparks & Taylor, 1995). This is accomplished through meticulous oral hygiene, using a soft-bristled toothbrush, using a fluoride dentifrice, and routine dental flossing. A waterpick may be used to remove food particles and provide gum stimulation. In addition, normal saline mouthwashes may soothe the oral mucosa. Alcohol-based mouthwashes should be avoided, because they are drying and may irritate the sensitive mucosa. Self-applied fluoride gels, available by prescription, contain about 0.5% fluoride. These gels may be used by patients with "high caries activity, orthodontic appliances, salivary flow problems caused by drugs or radiation therapy . . . and recurrent decay around the margins of existing restorations" (Miller & Truhe, 1994, p. 34). These fluoride gels are most effective when used at bedtime because salivary flow is decreased during sleep. The patient should be instructed not to eat or drink for 20 minutes following a fluoride gel application.

Providing appropriate oral care remains a nursing priority in all settings. Specific measures on which to focus in the acute care setting, the nursing home, and the private or family home are discussed in the following sections.

In the acute care setting

For patients with thick mucus or dried secretions, mechanical debridement of the mouth with a mixture of hydrogen peroxide and normal saline may be helpful (Lehman, 1995). Oral care may need to be given every 2 hours for some patients.

If saliva production is greatly diminished, medications may need to be changed to increase salivary secretion. Sugar-free lemon drops may increase saliva production. In some cases, artificial saliva products are ordered to simulate normal salivary action. To prevent further oral mucous membrane damage, the patient should use fluoride dentifrices and fluoride mouthwashes (Miller & Truhe, 1994). Careful attention should be given to maintaining an adequate fluid intake.

The patient experiencing pain may require local and/or systemic analgesia. Locally, topical anesthetic agents such as 1% lidocaine oral gel may reduce discomfort. For moderate to severe pain, nonsteroidal anti-inflammatory agents or narcotic analgesics may be prescribed. Some pain relief may also be obtained by avoiding hot, acidic, and spicy foods. In some instances, nasogastric or gastrostomy feedings may be needed to provide adequate nutrition.

The confused or comatose patient may require oral care with a special toothbrush that has attached suction. The patient should be positioned to minimize the risk of aspiration. An alternative intervention is for the nurse to put on gloves, wrap a 4- by 4-inch gauze pad around the hand, wet it with saline, and mechanically cleanse the oral cavity. Lemon and glycerin swabs should not be used because they are drying to the oral mucosa. A water-soluble lubricant can be applied to the lips to prevent blisters, cracking, and sores. Dentures should be cleaned at least daily using a commercial denture cleaner. If stored overnight, they must be placed in a well-identified denture container. Dentures should never be put in tissues or laid on the patient's tray. If the patient has lost or gained more than 20 pounds, the dentures should be checked for fit and altered if necessary.

In the nursing home

In addition to regular oral hygiene, the nursing home resident should be scheduled for periodic oral examinations. An oral evaluation should be performed every 6 months by the nurse practitioner or physician, and visits to the dentist should be planned on an annual basis. If the patient has significant oral changes, the diet may need to be revised from a soft diet to a pureed diet. Also, the nurse must regularly observe the older adult's oral hygiene habits and provide assistance if self-care practices are ineffective.

In the private or family home

There are no real differences in providing oral care at home. Follow the general guidelines for oral hygiene. Advise caregivers that it may be necessary to use a bulb syringe to remove fluid if the patient is unable to swallow. The family should be instructed to place the patient on his or her side to minimize the risk of aspiration. Frequent removal of oral secretions using a tissue may be necessary.

EVALUATION

To evaluate the effectiveness of oral hygiene measures, the nurse determines whether the patient's health care goals have been achieved. Is the mouth free of odor? Is the oral cavity free of plaque or gum irritation? Is the buccal tissue pink and free of lesions? Has there been a reduction in oral discomfort? Is the patient or family able to demonstrate correct oral hygiene practices? If the answer to these questions is yes, the interventions have been successful and the oral mucous membrane impairment is being controlled.

REFERENCES

Beare, P. C., & Myers, J. L. (1994). *Principles and practices of adult health nursing* (2nd ed.). St. Louis: Mosby.

Bergstrom, N., Bennett, M. A., Carlson, C. E., et al. (1992). *Treatment of pressure ulcers* (Clinical Practice Guidelines, No. 15; AHCPR Pub. No. 95-0652). Rockville, MD: U.S. Department of Health and Human Services, Public Health Service, Agency for Health Care Policy and Research.

Bruno, P., & Craven, R. F. (1982). Age challenges to wound healing. *Journal of Gerontological Nursing, 8*(12), 687-691.

Fenske, N. A., Grayson, L. D., & Newcomer, V. D. (1989, April 15). Common problems of aging skin. *Patient Care, 23,* 225-238.

Grady, D., & Ernster, V. (1992). Does cigarette smoking make you ugly and old? *American Journal of Epidemiology, 137,* 839-842.

Griffiths, C. E., Russman, A. N., Majmudar, G., Singer, R. S., et al. (1993). Restoration of collagen formation in photodamaged human skin by tretinoin (retinoic acid). *New England Journal of Medicine, 329,* 530-535.

Habif, T. P. (1996). *Clinical dermatology* (3rd ed.). St. Louis: Mosby.

Kashyup, P. K. (1989). Pressure ulcers. In V. D. Newcomer & E. M. Young (Eds.), *Geriatric dermatology: Clinical diagnosis and practical therapy.* New York: Igaku-Shoin.

Keen, M., Blitzer, A., Aviv, J., Binder, W., et al. (1994). Botulism toxin A for hyperkinetic facial lines: Results of a double-blind, placebo-controlled study. *Plastic and Reconstructive Surgery, 94*(1), 94-99.

Klein, L. (1988). Maintenance of healthy skin. *Journal of Enterostomal Therapy, 15*(6), 227-231.

Kresevic, D. M., & Lincoln, R. A. (1995). Nursing practice with elders. In W. J. Phipps, V. Cassmeyer, J. Sands, & M. K. Lehman (Eds.), *Medical-surgical nursing: Concepts and clinical practice* (5th ed.). St. Louis: Mosby.

Kurban, R. S., & Kurban, A. K. (1993). Common skin disorders of aging: Diagnosis and treatment. *Geriatrics, 48*(4), 30-42.

Lehman, M. K. (1995). Fluids and electrolyte imbalance. In W. J. Phipps, V. Cassmeyer, J. Sands, & M. K. Lehman (Eds.), *Medical-surgical nursing: Concepts and clinical practice* (5th ed.). St. Louis: Mosby.

Lowe, N. J. (1989). Psoriasis. In V. D. Newcomer & E. M. Young (Eds.), *Geriatric dermatology: Clinical diagnosis and practical therapy.* New York: Igaku-Shoin.

Medical Technology and Practice Patterns Institute. (1989). *Public policy implications related to use of the air-flotation bed treatment in the home care setting.* Washington, DC: Author.

Miller, M., & Truhe, T. (1994). Fluoride: An update for the year 2000. *Dentistry Today, 13*(10), 34-41.

Panel for the Prediction and Prevention of Pressure Ulcers in Adults. (1992). *Pressure ulcers in adults: Prediction and Prevention* (Clinical Practice Guidelines, No. 3; AHCPR Pub. No. 92-0047). Rockville, MD: Agency for Health Care Policy and Research, Public Health Service, U.S. Department of Health and Human Services.

Sparks, S. M. (1990). Nurse validation of pressure ulcer risk factors. *Dissertation Abstracts International.*

Sparks, S. M., & Taylor, C. M. (1995). *Nursing diagnosis reference manual* (3rd ed.). Springhouse, PA: Springhouse.

Thiers, B. H. (1989). Herpes zoster and postherpetic neuralgia. In V. D. Newcomer & E. M. Young (Eds.), *Geriatric dermatology: Clinical diagnosis and practical therapy.* New York: Igaku-Shoin.

Thompson, J. M., McFarland, G. K., Hirsch, J. E., Tucker, S. M., & Bowers, A. C. (1993). *Mosby's manual of clinical nursing* (3rd ed.). St. Louis: Mosby.

Tierney, L. M., McPhee, S. J., & Papadakis, M. A. (1995). *Current medical diagnosis and treatment.* Norwalk, CT: Appleton and Lange.

Weaver, V. (1995). Management of persons with problems of the skin. In W. J. Phipps, V. Cassmeyer, J. Sands, & M. K. Lehman (Eds.), *Medical-surgical nursing: Concepts and clinical practice* (5th ed.). St. Louis: Mosby.

Weiss, S. R. (1989). Actinic keratoses. In V. D. Newcomer & E. M. Young (Eds.), *Geriatric dermatology: Clinical diagnosis and practical therapy.* New York: Igaku-Shoin.

CHAPTER 9

If I'd known I was going to live so long,
I'd have taken better care of myself.

LEON ELDRED

Regulation: Endocrine, Temperature, and Infection

■ Learning Objectives

On completion of this chapter, the reader will be able to do the following:

1. Discuss age-related changes in the endocrine system.
2. Recognize the prevalence of diabetes in the older adult population.
3. Describe the nursing care of the older diabetic patient.
4. Discuss the vulnerability of an older adult to disorders of temperature regulation.
5. Recognize signs and symptoms of hypothermia and hyperthermia in an older adult.
6. Identify age-related changes and environmental factors that increase susceptibility to infection in the older adult.
7. Describe the nursing care of the older person with an infection.

To regulate is to strive for equilibrium. This chapter addresses the human physiologic mechanisms that allow the older person to compensate for age-related changes and still maintain biophysical equilibrium. This chapter focuses on three aspects of regulation. First, it describes age-related changes in the endocrine system, the effects of those changes on older adults, and the nursing care of older diabetic patients. Next, it addresses the age-related changes that affect thermoregulation and the response to external ex-

tremes of temperature. Finally, the chapter discusses the older person's susceptibility to and response to infection.

■ Endocrine System

NORMAL STRUCTURE AND FUNCTION

Nurses and other health care professionals view endocrinology in a very broad sense, as both the study of the relationship of the endocrine system and its hormones to other aspects of human physiology, and the study of the impact of the endocrine system on human health and human behavior. In conjunction with the neurologic system, the endocrine system maintains the body's ability to regulate its response to the internal and external environment. The endocrine system (1) regulates the body's response to stress and injury; (2) maintains growth, development, and reproduction; (3) adjusts ionic homeostasis; and (4) modulates and maintains energy metabolism. The endocrine system is composed of glands that secrete specific hormones, and each hormone has a specialized function and relationship to receptor sites throughout the body (Table 9-1). Most hormones are produced

and dispersed in a regular diurnal or circadian rhythm, except that the reproductive female hormonal rhythm is on a monthly rather than a daily release cycle. Though the exact relationship between human hormones and human behavior remains largely unknown, and the wide variations in individual behaviors make it difficult to ascertain that relationship, scientists continue to be intrigued by the study of endocrinology and human behavior. Regarding the relationship between the hormones produced by the body organs and the behavior of the individual, the keen student can be certain to find much in the literature to pique an interest in the dilemmas that have plagued researchers for many years.

AGE-RELATED CHANGES

As it does in all body systems, the aging process causes changes in the endocrine system—some essentially benign and silent, others more bothersome and clinically significant, and perhaps others not now known or understood. A decreased secretion of the growth hormone during sleep, a decrease in dopamine, an increased release of somatostatin, a lessening of the feedback inhibition of adrenocorticotropic hormone (ACTH) by glucocorticoids, a decrease in estrogen production, a diminished availability of testosterone, a decrease in sperm production, and an increase in follicle-stimulating hormone (FSH) and luteinizing hormone (LH) are examples of silent, age-related changes that occur in the aging endocrine system (Terry & Halter, 1994).

Some age-related endocrine changes produce noticeable change in many older adults. Both female and male gonadal functions are affected by the aging process. In the older woman, the capacity for reproduction ceases with the occurrence of menopause, caused by the deficiency in estrogen production. Male gonadal age-related change may vary from individual to individual, more so than in the older female population, but usually sperm production decreases and the blood level of follicle-stimulating hormone increases.

TABLE 9-1 Endocrine system

Gland	Hormone
Pituitary	Growth hormone
	Thyrotropin
	Adrenocorticotropin
	Follicle-stimulating hormone (FSH)
	Luteinizing hormone (FH)
	Prolactin
	Antidiuretic (vasopressin)
	Oxytocin
Pineal	Melatonin
Thyroid	Thyroxine (T4)
	Triiodothyronine (T3)
	Calcitonin (thyrocalcitonin)
Parathyroid	Parathormone
Pancreas	Insulin
	Glucagon
	Somatostatin
Adrenal	Mineralocorticoids
	Glucocorticoids
	Androgens
	Epinephrine
	Norepinephrine
Ovaries	Estrogen
	Progesterone
Testes	Testosterone

Aging Alert

Older adults who complain of fatigue and decreased energy should be screened for thyroid malfunction; these symptoms should not be minimized and carelessly attributed to increasing age.

Two abnormal conditions of the thyroid gland can occur in the older person and can be difficult to recognize. Hyperthyroidism, long thought of as a disease of younger people, has been shown to be a significant factor in the care of older people; prevalence rates in people 60 years and older are significantly higher than the rates in younger people. At times, hyperthyroidism and hypothyroidism are misdiagnosed or overlooked in older people. Symptoms—such as feeling unwell, weight loss, slowed mental functioning, loss of energy, and slowed physical movement—are thought of by many, including older adults themselves, their families, and inexperienced health professionals, as being "just signs of growing older" (Gregerman & Katz, 1994). Thus correctly assessing and diagnosing thyroid conditions is an important aspect of the care of older adults.

The aging process also brings a decline in glucose tolerance. Fasting blood glucose increases after the age of 40 years and continues to rise with increasing age. Insulin can still be secreted from the pancreas, but aging brings an insulin insensitivity that is not well understood (Mersey, 1989). The care of the older patient with diabetes mellitus (DM) is discussed in the following section of this chapter.

COMMON HEALTH DEVIATION: DIABETES MELLITUS

As early as the first century A.D. *diabetes mellitus* was described by Aretaeus, a physician; his vivid word-picture portrayed clearly an illness that we know today by the same name, but for which the prognosis has markedly improved. Today diabetes can be controlled and managed successfully. Aretaeus spoke of the disease as "being a melting down of the flesh and limbs into urine . . . the patients never stop making water; the flow is incessant, as if from the opening of aqueducts. The nature of the disease is chronic . . . the death is speedy" (Galloway, 1973). Changes in the level of knowledge about diabetes have been numerous since the first century, yet much remains to be learned about this complex and puzzling illness.

Diabetes mellitus is a chronic health problem that is not limited to any age group. The pathology that involves a defect in the production and/or use of insulin, is not unique to the very young, to the middle aged, or to the very old. For many years, scientists and researchers have been trying to solve the mystery of diabetes, and there is every indication that the search will continue for some time to come. A recent report noted that Sherlock Holmes was a mystery solver, too, but that unlike Holmes, who locked himself away from people to try to find answers to his mysteries, diabetes researchers meet with many other scientists to share information and to try to define clues that will lead them all to the solution of the diabetes mystery. Actually, diabetes is more accurately described as several mysteries overlapping each other.

Complicating the mystery of some defect in the production or the use of insulin is the fact that the gland that produces insulin is the pancreas, an endocrine gland (Radak et al., 1990), and the functioning of endocrine glands confounds scientists. At present, the science of endocrinology is viewed very broadly, as encompassing the total body metabolism. Rather than studying a single gland to the exclusion of the others, scientists now tend to look at the interrelationship among glands, hormones, and the various effectors in the body system. Although much information can be found in the scientific literature, it is also true that of all the health problems experienced by humans, diabetes is still the most frequently encountered of the endocrinology problems (Solomon, 1980).

Definition

Diabetes mellitus (DM) is a "syndrome characterized by generalized metabolic dysfunction and a variety of clinical disorders" (Goldberg et al., 1990, p. 69). It develops when the body's ability to produce or to use insulin breaks down, and it is viewed as a genetically heterogenous group of disorders characterized by glucose intolerance. It is a "condition of relative or absolute lack of insulin, affecting carbohydrate, protein and fat metabolism" (Thompson et al., 1993, p. 816).

Physiology of the pancreas

The pancreas, a body organ located in the abdomen, has both exocrine and endocrine functions. One part of the pancreas, about 20% of the gland, contains the islets of Langerhans, on which are located beta cells that secrete insulin, a powerful hormone. The remainder of the gland functions as an exocrine gland and secretes enzymes for food digestion.

Insulin plays a major role in the metabolic processes of the body by controlling the storage and metabolism of ingested metabolic fuels. Three functions of insulin can be identified:

1. Insulin facilitates the uptake, use, and storage of glucose, amino acids, and fats.
2. More specifically, in relation to glucose, insulin promotes
   a. The storage of glycogen in the liver
   b. The use of glucose in muscles
   c. The storage of fat in adipose tissues by enhancing the transport of glucose across cell membranes
3. Insulin regulates the level of blood glucose that is formed from ingested carbohydrates or from conversion of amino acids and fatty acids into glucose by the liver (gluconeogenesis).

Normally, insulin is released from the pancreas according to the level of glucose in the blood. Beta cells in the pancreas stimulate or withhold insulin secretion minute by minute, according to the changing blood glucose levels.

Pathophysiology

In people with DM, insulin is not secreted according to the blood sugar levels, possibly because of one or more of the following:

- A deficiency in the production of insulin by the beta cells
- Insensitivity of the insulin secretory mechanism of beta cells
- Delayed or insufficient release of insulin produced by the beta cells
- Excessive inactivation of the insulin by chemical inhibitors or "binders" in the circulation

In some diabetic patients there is excess insulin present, but it is not being used because of an inadequate number of insulin receptors on the body's cells. This has been observed in obese, non–insulin-dependent diabetic patients. With weight loss, the number of insulin receptors on the cells appears to increase, thereby allowing the glucose to enter the cell.

Elevated blood glucose levels reflect a decreased glucose uptake by the tissues (increased gluconeogenesis). If blood glucose concentration is high enough, the kidneys may not reabsorb all the filtered glucose, and the glucose appears in the urine. In the presence of increased gluconeogenesis, protein and fats are no longer stored or deposited in the cells. With a deficiency of insulin, the muscles cannot use glucose. Free fatty acids are then mobilized from adipose tissue cells and are broken down by the liver into ketone bodies to produce energy.

Diabetic ketoacidosis is characterized by excessive amounts of ketone bodies in the blood. Patients with diabetic ketoacidosis show hyperventilation and a loss of sodium, potassium, chloride, and water. The net result of acute, uncontrolled diabetes mellitus is a loss of fat stores, liver glycogen, cellular protein, electrolytes, and water. The complications of long-term diabetes involve both large and small blood vessels, particularly the large vessels of the brain, the heart, the kidneys, and the extremities, as well as the small vessels of the eyes, the kidneys, and the nerves. The exact mechanism underlying the pathology of diabetes is not known, although a number of hypotheses exist as to why diabetes occurs and how insulin utilization malfunctions (Goldberg et al., 1990).

Types of diabetes

Diabetes is classified as type I or type II. *Type I diabetes* is known as insulin-dependent diabetes mellitus (IDDM). It usually develops abruptly, and symptoms include polyuria, polydipsia, polyphagia, and weight loss. It is thought that IDDM may be caused by an autoimmune destructive process in the beta cells of the islets of Langerhans in the pancreas. A very small percentage of older diabetic patients, and 5% to 10% of all diabetic patients, have IDDM (Goldberg et al., 1990); these are usually people who are genetically susceptible to the development of diabetes. However, environmental factors can also play a role in the development of this condition. In fact, the cause of IDDM is not completely understood. Hypotheses include the probability of genetic influence, or viral etiology, as well as the aforementioned possibility of an autoimmune response of the person. Any of these can be studied alone, or a combination of these causes can be examined.

Type II diabetes is known as non–insulin-dependent diabetes mellitus (NIDDM). Approximately 90% to 95% of all diabetic patients have a diagnosis of NIDDM. Among this group, about 20% are nonobese and 80% are obese.

NIDDM is the more prevalent form of diabetes in older people. In Western societies it affects about one out of every ten white people over the age of 65; among people over 85 years of age,

Aging Alert

Complaints of polyuria, polydipsia, polyphagia, and unexplained weight loss from an older person may signal an abrupt onset of IDDM.

NIDDM affects about one out of every four people.

Age-, gender-, and race-adjusted guidelines are not available at present. Clinicians are faced with the challenge of considering only one set of criteria for diagnosis and treatment of the NIDDM patient, whether that person is male or female; whether young, middle aged, or old; and no matter what the race or country of origin. Until guidelines are available, diagnosticians and therapists will be forced to cope with a number of questions. For example: Should the hypoglycemia of a 20-year-old be treated the same as that of an 80-year-old? Can one expect the same outcomes of treatment in the different age groups? Is one age group more at risk for development of complications than is the other? How can treatment be determined for people of varying ages?

Reasons for the increased number of diagnosed cases of diabetes are the improved methods of screening presently available and the improved and more widely available information about diabetes being provided to the public. As screening reveals people who have diabetes, the outlook becomes more promising for controlling and managing the condition and for preventing the complications of uncontrolled diabetes. As more and better information becomes available to the public, the life span of the older diabetic patient can be lengthened, and an enhanced quality of life can be realized.

Aging Alert

People especially prone to developing diabetes mellitus are those who are over 65 years of age, who are overweight, and whose family members may be diabetic.

Risk factors and incidence

Diabetes can occur in people of any age, race, or gender, although some older adults may be more at risk than others. The chance of becoming diabetic doubles with every decade of life (Blainey, 1986). Although scientists have not defined precisely the cause or cure for DM, significant strides have been made in the scientific community in identifying risk factors in the development of this troublesome problem (Box 9-1).

Awareness of these factors can encourage the alert and observant person to undergo regular checkups for diabetes mellitus. When DM is identified early, the patient can usually respond more positively to treatment and can have greater hope for avoiding or at least delaying the onset of the complications that often accompany blood sugar alterations. Programs to educate the public about signs and symptoms of diabetes are becoming more prevalent (Abbey, 1990), and health-conscious people are responding more promptly to the presence of signs that suggest that they may be experiencing alterations in blood sugar metabolism. The signs and symptoms of type I and type II DM are presented in Table 9-2.

Although both types of DM present an alteration in blood sugar utilization, there are important differences in the symptoms that can be observed in each type. All of the symptoms are significant. The public needs to know the symptoms of diabetes, and health care personnel need to be especially alert to the presence of any of the symptoms when caring for the older adult.

Symptoms

Early signs and symptoms of DM are usually related to metabolic defects; late signs are frequently linked with complications that result from vascular defects. Patients with IDDM usually have a history of glucosuria, weight loss, and anorexia. As a rule, these people are thin, and they usually have ketoacidosis (Goldberg et al., 1990). Symptoms of type II diabetes are not readily apparent, and often the condition is not detected or diagnosed until some other pathology occurs and the elevated blood glucose is discovered. By the time it is detected, especially in the older person, complications are often present. The linkage between genetic mechanisms and diabetes is not as obvious with NIDDM as it is with IDDM; this is true despite the fact that more than 90% of patients with NIDDM have a family history of diabetes (Goldberg et al., 1990). There is an age-related increase in the prevalence of DM and in impaired glucose tolerance; this may be associated with a genetic factor. However, independent processes also influence the decline in glucose tolerance that is present in aging people. Factors that contribute to compromised glucose tolerance include overeating, adherence to a low-carbohydrate, high-fat diet, and physical inactivity. Factors that assist in improving the glucose tolerance are modifications of the diet, reduction of body weight, and increased physical activity.

It is critical to recognize and to differentiate two clinical manifestations: diabetic ketoacidosis (DKA) and hyperglycemic hyperosmolar nonketosis (HHNK). *Diabetic ketoacidosis* is an acute insulin deficiency that causes metabolic acidosis as a result of fat breakdown (Thompson et al., 1993). DKA is usually caused by the experience of a stressful event, either physiologic or emotional; by a failure to take regularly scheduled insulin; by a failure to take an adequate amount of insulin; or by some type of infection. It is not unusual for the patient to experience DKA during the initial stages of DM, when efforts are underway to diagnose the illness.

BOX 9-1 DIABETIC RISK FACTORS

- Age—People over 65 years of age are more at risk; 26% of people 85 and older have diabetes
- Race—Nonwhites are about 20% more likely to develop diabetes than are whites
- Sex—Women are 50% more likely than men to develop diabetes
- Genetic predisposition, such as having a diabetic blood relative
- Infections, especially viral infections
- Stress or anxiety that results in lowered blood sugar
- Prolonged bed rest
- Obesity

TABLE 9-2 Signs and symptoms of diabetes mellitus

Type I	Type II
Abrupt onset	Gradual development; can exist for some time before detection
Polyuria	—
Polydipsia	—
Polyphagia	Tendency to overeat, especially high-fat, low-carbohydrate diet
Weight loss	Obesity
History of glycosuria	—
Susceptibility to ketoacidosis	Susceptibility to nonketotic hyperosmolar dehydration

DKA can develop rapidly when there is an inadequate amount of insulin, with the end result being hyperglycemia (Thompson et al., 1993). As a result of the inadequacy, there is a reduced amount of glucose entering the cells, and the body metabolizes fat instead of carbohydrates. Free fatty acids are mobilized from adipose tissue, and liver oxidases act upon the fatty acids to produce ketone bodies. When the ketone bodies escape into the bloodstream, metabolic acidosis results. The overall picture becomes life threat-ening, with manifestations of hyperglycemia, water and electrolyte loss, acidemia, and eventually coma. Prompt and vigorous treatment with insulin and fluids is necessary.

DKA occurs more commonly in people with IDDM and is considered a serious complication of the illness. Early manifestations of DKA include *polyuria* (excessive urination), *polyphagia* (excessive appetite), and *polydipsia* (excessive thirst). Dehydration and electrolyte depletion occur as a result of osmotic diuresis. Oliguria develops gradually, as do symptoms of malaise, vision changes, headache, muscle aches, abdominal pain, nausea, and vomiting. A distinguishing symptom is the development of a sweetish odor to the breath, as the result of acidemia.

Hyperglycemic hyperosmolar nonketosis is severe hyperglycemia and hypertonic dehydration without significant ketoacidosis. Most victims of HHNK are elderly and infirm; they are frequently institutionalized or mentally impaired. This syndrome does not include ketosis, as a rule, but there are possible alterations of the sensorium (sense of awareness). People who are most prone to develop HHNK are older and have no history of diabetes. The onset of HHNK can be either abrupt or gradual. Obvious symptoms of HHNK include hyperglycemia, profound dehydration, and possibly a sleepy confusion that can result in eventual coma. The patient usually exhibits hypotension, dry mucous membranes, poor skin turgor, fever, tachycardia, and neurologic signs. This is a very serious condition that requires attention as soon as it is detected.

The complexity of correctly diagnosing HHNK is compounded by the fact that both hyperglycemia and hyperosmolarity are also present in the person with DKA, and the precipitating factors are usually the same.

Diagnostic tests

A number of tests can be performed to establish the diagnosis of diabetes. Often, detection of sugar in the urine is the first indication of a potential problem with glucose metabolism. This clinical sign is a signal for further diagnostic studies to be carried out, including the glucose tolerance test, strip tests, urine tests for glucose, urine tests for ketones, and the glycohemoglobin assay.

Glucose tolerance test Preceding the glucose tolerance test, the patient ingests a high-carbohydrate diet for 3 days. After the patient fasts overnight, a blood sample is obtained; then the patient consumes a 75-gm carbohydrate drink. Blood samples are then obtained at ½-, 1-, and 2-hour intervals. Results of the test are compared with normal values.

The nurse should bear in mind the following when reviewing a patient's glucose tolerance test results:

- Older patients, especially those over 50 years of age, usually demonstrate a higher glucose tolerance curve than do younger patients.
- Variations in the glucose tolerance curve can be altered by diet, activities, and medications, despite careful attempts to control these variables.

Strip tests The use of strip tests permits initial diagnosis and continued monitoring of blood glucose levels. A number of convenient reagent kits are available for diabetic screening and testing purposes. Some can be read visually;

others can be read with more precision through the use of a meter that provides a digital display of the glucose level, as evidenced by the reagent strip.

Following the diagnosis of diabetes, patients may use the reagent strips to determine the level of blood glucose on a regular basis. The diabetic patient's development of a pattern for testing the blood glucose level is critical to learning the foods, exercise, and medications that enhance the patient's control of blood sugar, as well as to discover those factors that interfere with control.

Urine testing for glucose Urine tests for glucose are no longer relied on as diagnostic tests for diabetes. Aging tends to raise the renal threshold, so the absence of sugar in the urine cannot rule out the possibility of diabetes. After NIDDM has been diagnosed in a patient, urine testing may be adequate for subsequent monitoring of that patient because his or her diabetes is fairly stable; however, it is not accurate enough for IDDM patients.

Urine testing for ketones Because ketosis is a dangerous complication of diabetes, urine testing for ketones is important. Ketones in the urine signal a deterioration of control; the body is breaking down stored fat to obtain energy. If elevated blood glucose levels persist, or if the patient just does not feel well, the patient should be tested for ketone bodies in the urine. One of two tests can be done to check for acetone in the urine:

1. "Acetest"—the use of a reagent that reacts with urine to yield a color; the depth of the color correlates with the ketone body concentration
2. "Ketostix"—the use of a reagent strip that is dipped into the urine; the resulting color is compared with a color chart

Glycohemoglobin assay The glycohemoglobin assay provides the primary care provider with important information about the patient's average blood sugar level for the 2- to 3-month period before the test. The test is not altered by a recent ingestion of food, recent exercise, or recently administered medication. Rather, the assay provides information about the time-averaged blood glucose values.

Glycohemoglobin (glycosylated hemoglobin) is a type of minor hemoglobin that exists in everyone's bloodstream and was discovered in the red blood cells of diabetic patients in 1969; it is defined as the blood glucose that is bound to hemoglobin. Initially the glycohemoglobin assay was quite complicated and was performed only in the research laboratory. Since 1977 a simpler method of measuring glycohemoglobin has been available and is of benefit in a qualitative patient assessment for diabetes. The amount of glycohemoglobin formed and stored in a red blood cell depends on the amount of glucose available to the cell over a 120-day life span. It is of significant value to determine this information when the examiner wishes to know a diabetic patient's average blood glucose level.

Complications in older adults

As diabetic patients learn more about diabetes management, and as they respond to the prescribed exercises, diet, and medication to control blood glucose levels, they experience longer life spans. However, because they are living longer, they are also more likely to experience some of the long-term complications of diabetes. The parts of the body most frequently involved in these complications are the eyes, the nervous system, the vascular system (heart and blood vessels), and the urinary system (kidneys). To compound the challenge of coping with complications individually, it is not unusual for diabetic patients to experience one or more complications simultaneously (Box 9-2). The incidence of complications is directly related to the length of time that a patient has had DM and directly related to prolonged hyperglycemia. These complications may be delayed or prevented by the following:

- Diagnosing diabetes mellitus early—before the complications can develop
- Maintaining blood glucose levels within a normal range
- Adhering conscientiously to prescriptions for exercise, diet, and medication

The eyes Diabetes is one of the four leading causes of blindness in the United States. Of the patients with diabetes, 25% have some form of retinopathy, and the prevalence increases with the duration of the disease.

People with diabetes also experience an increased risk of cataracts. Early intervention is important here, too; safe extraction of the cataract and surgical implant of lenses has proven very effective in preventing blindness in diabetic patients.

The sense of sight is important for everyone, but it is especially important for the older diabetic patient. Many of the tasks associated with managing diabetes require vision. For example, the diabetic patient needs to be able to see the syringe to measure insulin, to read glucose levels when testing blood and/or urine, to read prescriptions, to read the labels on various foods, and to read literature about diabetes.

The nervous system Because the autonomic (involuntary) nervous system may become involved in diabetic neuropathy, there may be incomplete emptying of the urinary bladder, leading to urinary infections. Sometimes the gastrointestinal system is affected, resulting in early satiety, bloating, vomiting, constipation, or diarrhea; a long-term problem may be fecal incontinence.

The heart and blood vessels There is an increased incidence of heart disease and hypertension in diabetic patients, although the reason for this has not been well defined. Although some older adults may be firmly committed to lifelong habits, such as smoking and the use of alcohol, these should be strongly discouraged.

As a result of the potential for complications, the diabetic person can expect to experience long-term detrimental effects of hyperglycemia

---

BOX 9-2 COMPLICATIONS OF DIABETES MELLITUS

EYES

- Diabetic retinopathy is caused by changes in the small blood vessels, especially the vessel walls of the retina.
- Loss of visual acuity depends on the location of the retinal lesion.
- Frequent eye examinations should be done (at least once each year) for early detection of retinopathy.

NERVOUS SYSTEM

- Motor, sensory, and autonomic peripheral nerves are susceptible to diabetic neuropathies.
- Diabetic neuropathies include pupillary changes, orthostatic hypotension, sexual dysfunction, lower extremity discomfort (including pain, which may be dull, aching, cramping, burning, or crushing), and paresthesia (tingling, burning, coldness, numbness).

VASCULAR SYSTEM

- In the presence of DM, changes occur in the blood vessels that lead to long-term complications. In the larger vessels, these involve the heart and peripheral circulation, especially the legs. In the smaller vessels, these involve the eyes, kidneys, and nervous system.
- Numbness and reduced pain perception in the lower extremities can lead to complex foot injuries; an initial, minor injury can develop into major and even overwhelming trauma.
- Cellulitis can lead to decreased circulation.
- Ischemia can cause gangrene.
- Absence of sweating can lead to cracked skin, which enables entry of bacteria.

URINARY SYSTEM

- Persistent elevation of blood glucose results in a thickening of the glomeruli, so filtering functions are less efficient.
- The thicker glomeruli become more permeable, and blood proteins are improperly eliminated in the urine.
- Patients with diabetic nephropathy have increased morbidity and mortality.

---

and hyperinsulinemia on the blood vessels. Data from the Framingham study suggest that the hypertensive diabetic patient is at heightened risk for vascular complications, including myocardial infarction and stroke, especially as diabetic people age and experience increased duration of diabetes (McKee et al., 1971). In NIDDM patients the risk for coronary disease is more pronounced in women than in men, probably related to the distribution of upper body fat in older women.

Circulation problems are often demonstrated in the diabetic patient in the form of foot problems. Meticulous care of the feet should be included in every diabetic patient's instruction sessions. Guidelines for foot care in the diabetic patient include the following (Blainey, 1986):

- Careful daily inspection of the feet, to detect any abnormality (blisters, breaks in the skin, bruises, calluses)

- Regular cleansing of the feet with mild soap and water
- Protecting the feet from injury by wearing properly fitting shoes and hose (stockings)
- Avoiding the use of garters or tight shoes
- Cutting toenails carefully; they should be cut straight across to avoid ingrown toenails (regular visits to the podiatrist are advised)

The kidneys Kidney complications usually occur in diabetic patients who have had the disease for a long time. Late symptoms of kidney involvement include anemia, lethargy, nausea, and high blood pressure. The goal of diabetic control is to prevent renal complications, or resolve them before end-stage kidney disease develops. Strategies for care include maintenance of blood sugar level as close to normal as possible, blood pressure control, and restriction of protein in the diet (Fisch, 1990).

Scientists have not been able to determine with precision the extent to which early detection of diabetes can reduce morbidity and prolong survival of the diabetic person. Despite this uncertainty, there is concerted effort on the part of health care personnel to control and to effectively maintain the normal balance of blood glucose in the patient with a diagnosis of diabetes.

■ Nursing Process

Two types of challenges confront the nurse who is responsible for guiding the care of older diabetic patients: (1) caring for the patient with a recent diagnosis of diabetes and (2) caring for the older patient who has been known to be diabetic for some time. The adaptation problems will differ between these two groups of patients, and the goals of self-management will be different. The collective needs of each of the two groups of people will differ because of the differences in the length of time they have experienced diabetes; also, the needs of the individuals within each group will differ because each person is unique. The major nursing responsibility for both groups will entail careful and continual assessment, collaborative planning, and implementation of measures that foster the patients' use of self-care abilities to keep their own blood glucose levels under control. The nurse is urged to make diligent use of creative teaching techniques to motivate older diabetic patients to care for themselves.

ASSESSMENT

While considering how recently the patient has received a diagnosis of diabetes, the nurse includes the following questions in the assessment of the older diabetic patient.

What does the patient know about diabetes?

Discussion with the patient should reveal to the nurse whether the patient knows something about the role of the pancreas and the role of insulin in causing the condition of diabetes. Although the layperson is not expected to achieve a knowledge base equivalent to that of a clinician, the diabetic patient should understand that diabetes involves either an inadequate amount of insulin or an improper use of insulin in the body.

What does the patient understand about food, diabetic diets, and weight control through dietary management?

Diet is an area of instruction that will receive a great deal of attention in the care of the diabetic patient. To provide appropriate instruction for the patient, the nurse assesses the patient's existing knowledge about food and its management. Some level of knowledge about food will have been acquired whether or not the patient has been diabetic for a long time. It is important for the nurse to identify what is known by the patient, as well as to identify the gaps in knowledge and the areas of need for information.

In how much activity is the patient involved?

As some people get older, their levels of physical activity tend to decrease, and with valid reason.

Some changes in mobility and some unsteadiness in walking may have occurred; some painful joints may make it difficult to change body positions; some family and/or environmental factors may reduce or interfere with motivation to be active. The nurse can assess these and a number of other possibilities to gain insight into each patient's situation. All of these factors must be considered to identify where the older diabetic patient needs assistance, advice, and support.

Is there a stigma associated with the condition in the mind of the patient? How do the family and/or peers feel about diabetes? Are they upbeat about the management and control of this health problem, or do they feel depressed and negative about diabetic care?

In the presence of comorbidity, the older diabetic patient may need help in coping with diabetes as one more thing to think about in an array of health problems. The nurse must identify how the patient feels about the diagnosis of diabetes mellitus. Conversations with the patient and significant others may help the nurse to identify the relationship that exists among them. Also, observation of the patient's home environment, when possible, may provide important clues for the nurse who is gathering data about the patient's status.

What other medications have been prescribed for the patient, and how reliable is the patient in taking medications?

If it is necessary for the older diabetic patient to take insulin or one of the oral hypoglycemic agents, the nurse identifies what other medications the patient is taking and the conditions for which medications have been prescribed. How reliable has the patient been in taking the medications? What is the patient's pattern of reliability? Can the nurse predict the patient's reliability in self-administration of insulin if it is necessary, or in the regular self-administration of a prescribed hypoglycemic agent? Answers to these questions will guide the development of a plan for the patient's care and will suggest the way that strategies for care can be defined.

NURSING DIAGNOSES

After completion of the assessment activities, the data about the patient will have been gathered, organized, and clustered according to the patient's needs and priorities. These activities will have provided an excellent opportunity for nurse-patient trust to have become well established. Further assessment will be an ongoing activity, in which meetings between the nurse and the patient will become regular events. Emphasis will be on continued assessment of progress and on changes needed to manage and control blood glucose levels.

The diabetic patient, whether the diagnosis of diabetes is recent or not, can experience a wide variety of nursing diagnoses. One possible nursing diagnosis for a diabetic patient is "altered nutrition: more than body requirements"—that is, a situation in which the patient eats more food (nutrients) than is needed. This situation may be evidenced as the patient experiences difficulty in adjusting to the dietary regimen prescribed as a result of diabetes. The patient may experience stress in adjusting to the new regimen; as a result, a resorting to the previous eating patterns may occur.

The following additional diagnoses may be made:

- Activity intolerance
- Impaired physical mobility
- Impaired home maintenance management (diet and medication)
- Knowledge deficit about the administration of diabetes medication
- Body image disturbance
- Self-esteem disturbance
- Impaired adjustment to exercise, diet, and medication

PLANNING, GOAL IDENTIFICATION, AND IMPLEMENTATION

Having identified the areas in which the patient has need for knowledge, the nurse and the

Aging Alert

Three critical components of care for the older diabetic patient are exercise, diet, and medication.

patient collaboratively plan a program of care, which strongly emphasizes the self-care responsibilities of the patient, though the nurse accepts responsibility for teaching and supporting the patient in the management of diabetes. The goals of care include the following:

- Adherence to diet, exercise, and medication regimens
- Continued acquisition of knowledge about diabetes
- Maintenance of blood glucose levels within a normal range
- Prevention of DM complications

Exercise

Exercise enhances the ability of the body to use glucose, although scientists have not been able to define the mechanism by which this happens. Regular exercise improves the level of blood glucose, and it improves circulation, helps digestion, and encourages a feeling of well-being. Because of the positive effect of exercise, this aspect of treatment is strongly recommended. However, each exercise program must be individualized according to the abilities and limitations of the person. As people age, the presence of comorbidity influences treatment and care for all illnesses. From a positive standpoint, the exercise that is recommended for diabetes may also benefit the person who suffers from arthritis or from osteoporosis. In any case, however, the selection of exercises is critical. Low-impact exercises, such as walking and swimming, are usually recommended for older people and are quite

effective for them. As the older people gradually become more impaired, a home program of stretching and range-of-motion activities can be designed and taught to the patient. As with all forms of treatment, before any particular exercise program is started, the patients should be examined for any potential hazards relating to the fitness activity; they should also be advised to start slowly and to increase their level of activity very gradually.

Diet

Diet is another important factor in the care of older diabetic patients. Usually the older person has established lifelong routines and preferences for eating particular foods, in particular amounts, and at particular time intervals. Often the dietary requirements for diabetic management and control differ from those long-established eating and dietary patterns of the older diabetic patient. This aspect of diabetic care presents an immediate and major challenge to the nurse. The patient has to be convinced that adjustments in foods and dietary habits are necessary. Teaching the patient about foods and dietary habits is one challenge; an even greater challenge is to get the patient to accept and to comply with the prescribed diet and food preparation requirements. The nurse encourages the patient to believe the following: a reasonable goal is to achieve a well-balanced, consistent diet.

The food plan recommended by the American Dietetic Association (ADA) for the diabetic diet consists of wholesome food and a well-balanced selection of foods from the six food groups.

In all likelihood, patients with diabetes can eat the same food as that prepared for others in the family. However, the diabetic patient must eat the proper foods at the proper time and in the amounts recommended. The American Dietetic Association and the American Diabetes Association have prepared extensive literature about food exchanges for diabetic patients. The *food exchange* is a selection system in which the patient can choose the foods to eat at each meal from a variety of foods in each of six food groups. The following lists the food groups and the number of servings from each group to be selected for a 1500-calorie daily diet:

Food group 1: Starch and bread list   8 servings/day
Food group 2: Meat list   5 servings/day
Food group 3: Vegetable list   4 servings/day
Food group 4: Fruit list   3 servings/day
Food group 5: Milk list   2 servings/day
Food group 6: Fat list   3 servings/day

Consultation with a qualified dietitian to review food selection and to discuss food preparation can be invaluable to the diabetic patient. In fact, a positive experience related to the dietary aspect of diabetic care can sometimes make the difference in ensuring compliance that is consistent with the patient's needs and preferences, as well as specific food likes and dislikes. The variety of food choices (exchanges) available in the food exchange system can provide an arrangement of meals and snacks that will be satisfying for the patient, as well as compatible with the diabetes. See Box 9-3 for examples of food selections on each list.

If there are obstacles to the purchase or the preparation of a nutritious diet, the diabetic patient may seek the services provided by Meals on Wheels or congregate feeding programs. These programs are available to those in need of warm, nutritious meals and will assist the diabetic patient in achieving a prescribed diet regimen.

In addition to the selection and preparation of prescribed foods, the regularity of eating scheduled meals and snacks is very important for the diabetic patient. This is one means of maintaining a balanced blood glucose level.

Medication

The third essential component of self-care for the diabetic patient is medication, though diet is the cornerstone of therapy, and control of the blood glucose level by adjustment of diet is often the treatment of choice. In some instances diabetic patients can comply with a prescribed diet and can keep blood glucose levels within normal limits through food adjustment alone.

Type I (IDDM) diabetic patients Though diet, exercise, and medication are crucial to both types of diabetic patients, some differences between the two should be addressed. Type I (IDDM) diabetic patients require careful instruction and regular support to learn about insulin administration. Monitoring and support must be provided for the IDDM patient for as long as necessary if the patient is to become able to function independently in giving the subcutaneous injections of insulin on a daily basis. Clear instructions and patient demonstrations of the technique of insulin administration will enable the patient to achieve self-care and will reassure the patient and the caregiver that self-care is a reasonable, positive goal in health care.

When the type and dosage of insulin have been prescribed, the nurse assumes responsibility for teaching the patient the technique of administering the medication and making the needed regular observations. The diabetic patient must know how to detect or monitor two conditions, and how to respond if they are detected: hyperglycemia and hypoglycemia.

Hyperglycemia is a state of high blood sugar that occurs when the patient has too much food or too little insulin. Symptoms include extreme thirst, increased urination, itching, drowsiness, headache, and sometimes nausea. The onset of this complication is rather gradual. Blood glucose tests reveal a high blood glucose level. The physician should be called in the case of this reaction.

Hypoglycemia is a state of low blood sugar that occurs when the patient has too little food, too much insulin (or oral hypoglycemic medication), or too much exercise. Symptoms include shaking, tachycardia (fast heartbeat), sweating, dizziness, and hunger. The onset of this complication is sudden, and tests will reveal a very low blood glucose level. As soon as symptoms of hypoglycemia appear, the patient should drink a

BOX 9-3 SELECTED FOODS ON THE EXCHANGE LIST

Starch and bread list (One-half cup of cereal, grain, or pasta is one exchange; a 1-oz bread product is one exchange.)

Cereals, grains, and pasta
Bran flakes	½ cup
Cooked cereals	½ cup
Grits (cooked)	½ cup
Pasta (cooked)	½ cup
Rice (cooked)	⅓ cup

Dried beans, peas, and lentils
Beans and peas (cooked)	⅓ cup
Lentils (cooked)	⅓ cup
Baked beans	¼ cup
Chick peas	⅓ cup

Starchy vegetables
Corn	½ cup
Corn on cob—6 inches long	1
Lima beans	½ cup
Potato—baked	1 small (3 oz)
Potato—mashed	½ cup
Squash—winter	1 cup

Bread
Bagel	½ (1 oz)
English muffin	½
Pita—6 inches across	½
Pumpernickel, rye	1 slice (1 oz)
White	1 slice (1 oz)

Meat list (The list is divided into three parts, depending on the amount of fat and calories: lean, medium fat, and high fat. The following exchanges are taken from the lean meat list.)

Beef	1 oz
Ground round, flank steak, tenderloin, chipped beef	
Pork	1 oz
Fresh ham, lean pork	
Veal	1 oz
Cutlets, chops, roasts	
Poultry	1 oz
Chicken, turkey	
Fish	
All fresh or frozen fish	1 oz
Oysters	6 medium
Tuna—canned in water	¼ cup
Cheese	¼ cup
Any cottage cheese	
Other	1½ oz
95% fat-free luncheon meat	

Continued

BOX 9-3 SELECTED FOODS ON THE EXCHANGE LIST—cont'd

Vegetable list (Serving size for one vegetable exchange is ½ cup of cooked vegetables, 1 cup of raw vegetables.)

Asparagus	Beets
Beans—green, wax	Cabbage
Carrots	Sauerkraut
Eggplant	Spinach (cooked)
Leeks	Tomato— 1 large
Onion	Turnips
Peppers—green	Zucchini (cooked)

Fruit list

Apple—raw, 2 inches across	1
Applesauce—unsweetened	½ cup
Banana— 9 inches long	½
Cantaloupe— 5 inches across	⅓
Grapefruit	½ medium
Grapes	15 small
Orange— 2½ inches across	1
Pear	1 small
Strawberries—raw, whole	1¼ cup

Juice

Cranberry juice cocktail	⅓ cup
Orange juice	½ cup
Pineapple juice	½ cup
Prune juice	⅓ cup

Milk list

Skim milk	1 cup
½% milk	1 cup
1% milk	1 cup
Lowfat buttermilk	1 cup
Plain nonfat yogurt	8 oz
Whole milk	1 cup

Fat list

Unsaturated fats

Margarine	1 tsp
Mayonnaise	1 tsp

Nuts and seeds

Almonds	6 whole
Pecans	2 whole
Peanuts	20 small
Walnuts	2 whole
Olives	10 small

Saturated fats

Butter	1 tsp
Bacon	1 slice
Coconut—shredded	2 tbsp
Cream—light, coffee	2 tbsp
Cream—sour	2 tbsp

Adapted from American Diabetic Association and American Dietetic Association. (1989). *Exchange lists—For meal planning*. Virginia and Illinois: Author.

glass of orange juice (8 oz) or should eat several (about five or six) Lifesavers, one or two pieces of medium-sized hard candy, or 2 tsp of sugar or honey. With this prescribed treatment, the blood sugar levels usually return to normal within 20 to 30 minutes. When the symptoms have disappeared, the patient may appreciate having a glass of milk and a peanut butter sandwich if mealtime is not near.

IDDM patients are urged to wear an identification bracelet or to carry an identification card to notify appropriate people of the diabetic condition and insulin dependency. It is also important for IDDM patients to carry extra carbohydrate supplies with them at all times so that they can respond if symptoms of hypoglycemia appear.

Type II (NIDDM) diabetic patients   Type II (NIDDM) diabetic patients are also challenged to maintain blood glucose levels within a normal range, and they, too, need to comply with adjustments in food intake. Often, NIDDM patients are coping with an obesity problem, too, so guidance in weight reduction, as well as blood glucose control, is provided. Usually, NIDDM patients are treated with one of the sulfonylureas; these are chemical compounds that have been available to diabetic patients as oral medications since 1956. Their purpose is to stimulate insulin secretion, and if the response to these drugs is positive, patients can maintain adequate control of their diabetes with just the oral medication. The majority of diabetes patients enjoy a good response to these drugs, and this method of maintaining a normal blood glucose level has been welcomed by many diabetic patients. Regular monitoring of blood glucose levels, regular examinations to detect potential complications of diabetes, and strict adherence to prescribed diets are essential to successful control of this complex illness.

Family support

Older patients face a unique challenge in exercising control over this health problem. Some people experience diminished vision as they age, so the selection of food in the grocery store and the preparation of food at home present potential problems. Diabetic patients must carefully read food labels to determine the ingredients so that they do not buy foods that have unwanted sugar. Most diabetic patients who have recently received their diagnosis find it difficult to change from their accustomed food patterns, having to adjust or even delete some favorite recipes from their diets. Caregivers of older adults can support the older diabetic patient during the days when these adaptations are being made. Patients, families, and caregivers should be encouraged to give the assistance needed during the early days of adjusting to the illness, which will aid the compliant, interested, and motivated patient in assuming self-care.

EVALUATION

The liaison between the diabetic patient and the nurse is never ending. Positive management and control of DM depends on conscientious attention to diet, exercise, and medications. The nurse remains available to the patient, as needed, and also schedules regular meetings with the patient, to reassess patient needs and to reinforce information about diabetes and about specific self-care activities. The nurse thoroughly evaluates the extent to which specific patient problems have been and are being resolved according to the nursing diagnoses that were established at the outset of care.

The nurse assumes a heavy responsibility for teaching the DM patient how to provide the self-care that is required for DM management and why it is essential. The nurse must diligently assess the patient's need for information, as well as the patient's ability and intention to adhere to the prescriptive plan that is offered. "Nursing is a primary force for helping older [diabetic] persons comply with programs designed to enhance their health status" (Dellasega, 1990).

With adequate instruction, reasonable support, and sincere help, the older diabetic patient can usually manage the exercise, diet, and medication self-care of the diabetic regimen. The nurse provides information about these aspects of diabetes treatment so that the patient will know about the health problem and will know what to do, how to do it, and when to do it. Determining the secret to compliance for each individual patient will be a continuing challenge for those who are caregivers for older adults with diabetes.

DM poses one of the most challenging health care problems with which many older patients are coping. Whether the condition is that of IDDM or NIDDM, it usually requires major adjustments in the patient's lifestyle. The patient who has recently received the diagnosis of DM must learn to maintain an ideal body weight, must learn to regulate blood glucose levels through dietary adjustment and/or medication administration, must learn the technical skill of self-administration of insulin, and must learn to engage in activities and exercises on a regularly scheduled basis, all of which require deliberate attention and planning. Many activities of daily living (ADLs) that were performed automatically and without deliberate planning in the past now require careful consideration to ensure that all aspects of diabetic self-care are included in the activities of each day. In their effort to prevent the complications that are known to accompany increased blood glucose levels, diabetic patients are usually motivated to learn all that they need to know about diabetes and about self-care requirements. With assistance and support from nurses who know about diabetic care, most patients can successfully cope with the diagnosis of DM. Those patients who have difficulty adhering to the prescribed care regimen present a major but not impossible challenge to the nurse.

■ Temperature

COMMON HEALTH DEVIATION: DIFFICULTY IN TEMPERATURE REGULATION

Temperature is controlled through the processes of sweating, shivering, vasoconstriction, vasodilation, and hypothalamic and nervous system functions. Difficulties in temperature regulation in older adults are probably related to an increasing inability to respond adequately to change in temperature and a narrowing of homeostatic mechanisms (Abrass, 1994). Shivering decreases in older adults (Collins et al., 1981), as does the function of their sweat glands (Balin, 1990). Decreased sensitivity, sedentary lifestyle, and disorders of the cardiovascular, endocrine, and nervous systems all contribute to the vulnerability of the older person to experiencing *hypothermia* (low body temperature) or *hyperthermia* (high body temperature) (Natsume et al., cited in Abrass, 1994).

Hypothermia

Many older adults may unknowingly be quite susceptible to developing a mild hypothermia, which, unrecognized, may progress to a more severe condition. During the winter season, hypothermia, which is underreported and underdiagnosed, contributes to morbidity and, to a lesser extent, to mortality in the older adult population (MacLean & Emslie-Smith, 1977; Rango, 1984). There is evidence that in the older adult population, hypothermia (core body temperature less than 34° C) occurs during the winter season in northern climates such as in Great Britain, Canada, and the northern United States. Two large-scale surveys were conducted in Great Britain among older adults who lived in private or family homes (outside of acute care or nursing home settings), and the results demonstrated that 10% of the subjects had experienced some degree of hypothermia (Fox et al., 1973).

Because body fat contributes to the body's ability to insulate itself against the cold, thin older men are at high risk for developing hypothermia (Thorne & Wahren, 1990). Furthermore, malnutrition caused by mental confusion, homelessness, or chronic alcohol abuse increases the risk of hypothermia. These alterations, along with drugs that interfere with normal thermoregulation, account for older adults' poor adjustment to extremes in environmental temperature.

A particularly hazardous behavior in cold weather is the ingestion of alcohol. The use of alcohol blocks the vasoconstrictive response to cold and actually makes a person physically colder, contrary to the perceived sense of warmth. Factors that predispose an older adult to hypothermia are extremes of temperature (although hypothermia can occur in moderate temperatures), poor or no housing, malnutrition, increased age, multiple diseases, alcohol use, and impaired mental functioning (Robbins, 1989).

■ Nursing Process

ASSESSMENT

During a period of cold weather, when an older patient with a history of exposure to the cold or with a history of poor socioeconomic living conditions seeks treatment, the nurse caring for the patient considers the possibility of hypothermia. The older person in the early stages of hypothermia may appear fatigued, complain of weakness, have cool skin, and exhibit signs of confusion.

Early symptoms of severe hypothermia may be increased confusion and increased sensation of being cold. Consciousness is usually lost when the body temperature descends to between 30° and 28° C. The most important clinical sign is the recording of low body temperature.

NURSING DIAGNOSIS

Hypothermia related to exposure to a cold environment is evidenced by body temperature of less than 34° C and altered mental state.

PLANNING AND GOAL IDENTIFICATION

A long-term goal is that the patient will be knowledgeable concerning risk factors of hypothermia and will engage in health-promoting activities. A short-term goal is that the patient will be monitored closely until body temperature returns to the normal range.

IMPLEMENTATION

The first aspect of treatment is to remove the patient from the cold environment. If clothing is wet, it should be removed immediately and the patient should be covered top and bottom with

Aging Alert

- Older adults need protection from extremes of temperature.
- Exposure to a cold environment is especially hazardous for older people if they are malnourished, dehydrated, or wearing inadequate clothing.
- Exposure to a very warm environment can result in heat stroke for the older person.
- Ingestion of alcohol and/or medications can contribute to hypothermia or hyperthermia in the older person.

blankets. Care needs to be taken when moving these patients, because rough handling may cause arrhythmias. In mild hypothermia (32° to 34° C), treatment consists of passive warming and monitoring. More severe hypothermia is a medical emergency and requires hospitalization of the patient. Mortality for severe hypothermia is 50% or higher in older adult populations. Underlying infections are a frequent condition in older patients admitted to the hospital with hypothermia (Darowski et al., 1991).

Prevention of hypothermia is the best treatment. In the winter, any older adult who is at risk for hypothermia requires indoor temperatures that are higher than 70° F. Good nutrition, increased fluid intake, decreased alcohol intake, and adequate clothing will help protect the older person from hypothermia (McGough, 1983). Many older adults in the homeless population of large cities in the United States are at risk for hypothermia during severe winter weather.

EVALUATION

The determination of successful treatment of hypothermia is based on the clinical sign of body temperature readings that range above 34° C, and on the older patient's exhibiting diminished symptoms of confusion and sensations of cold. The need to decrease the threat of recurring hypothermia may call for a change in the living arrangements of the older person, and social services may be the appropriate referral. The care of the older person is a team effort, and all members of the health care team are utilized to bring about optimal care and to ensure the return to health of the older person.

Hyperthermia

Over 3000 deaths occur on a yearly basis in people over 60 years of age as a direct result of heat stroke. The degrees of heat illness can range from a mild state (heat exhaustion), in which symptoms include muscle cramps and volume depletion, to the more severe state of heat stroke (Robbins, 1989). Heat exhaustion often occurs when a person has engaged in exercise during days of extreme temperature and high humidity.

Hyperthermia or "heat stroke," is defined as an acute condition in which body temperature rises above 40.6° C (105° F) (Abrass, 1994). Heat stroke in the older adult is usually nonexertional and occurs in a warm climate. Death from heat stroke is not an element of the past. Studies done in the 1980s reported that in the 1984 New York City heat wave, deaths increased by almost 50% in people 75 years old and over. Women were more prone to succumbing to heat stroke than men by a three-to-two margin in heat waves in New York, St. Louis, and Georgia (Centers for Disease Control, 1984; Hope et al., 1984). A more recent experience was the heat wave of 1995 in Chicago, in which large numbers of deaths of older adults stunned the city and the nation.

The major causes of heat stroke are (1) impairment of heat loss caused by diminished sweating or the absence of sweating and (2) environmental factors. Physiologic age-related changes, disease processes, and extremes in climate all contribute to the increased risk of heat stroke in the older person. Often, cardiovascular disease in the older person is aggravated during a time of intense humidity and heat. The older person may not be physically able to respond to the stress caused by the heat wave, and death may result.

Risk factors for heat stroke are being older, being female, living alone, being mentally confused, having poor sensitivity to temperature changes, being alcoholic, having heart disease or diabetes, having reduced fluid intake, and taking tranquilizers and anticholinergic drugs (Abrass, 1994).

■ Nursing Process

ASSESSMENT

The older patient who has an elevated temperature may not be recognized as suffering from heat illness. The elevated temperature may be attributed to another factor, such as an infection. Factors that contribute to occurrence of heat illness are a prolonged heat wave, a history of exposure (such as a broken air conditioner during a heat wave), and a sensation of being warm. The patient may complain of general nonspecific types of symptoms, which can include headache, dizziness, and weakness.

Heat stroke is a serious, life-threatening condition and is manifested by classic signs and symptoms; loss of consciousness, headache, weakness, nausea, and hot skin with an elevated body temperature are the signs that will lead the clinician to consider heat stroke. The complications of heat stroke are severe and often lead to death if not corrected quickly.

NURSING DIAGNOSIS

Hyperthermia related to exposure to extreme temperature and depletion of fluid volume is evidenced by a temperature of 40.6° C.

PLANNING AND GOAL IDENTIFICATION

Long-term goals include the following: (1) the patient will be knowledgeable concerning the importance of hydration and the risks of exposure to extremes of temperature, and (2) the patient will also engage in health-promoting behaviors that reduce the risk of hyperthermia. A short-term goal is that the patient will be monitored and treated appropriately until temperature returns to the normal range.

IMPLEMENTATION

Hyperthermia is considered a medical emergency and requires immediate hospitalization and treatment that will lower body temperature. Treatment consists of lowering the body temperature—through cold water sponging of the body surface or through baths. The core body temperature should be brought to 39° C (102° F) within the first treatment hour (Abrass, 1994). There is a significant risk of shock, and many older adults do not survive an episode of severe hyperthermia. Constant monitoring is an essential nursing action during this emergency situation.

EVALUATION

Evaluation is a continuous, patient-centered, goal-oriented process. Determination of the successful achievement of the short-range goal of restoring the older person to a normal temperature range is the first step in the evaluative process. The long-term goal of educating the patient, the family, and the community is a joint goal of all health professionals.

Evaluation of achievement of the long-term goal will focus on the nurse's particular patient population: the individual patient, if the nurse has been the provider for a particular patient with hyperthermia; the nursing home residents, if the nurse is the director of nursing in a nursing home; the community, if the nurse is a public health nurse in a particular community; and the nation, if the nurse is a consultant to the federal government. Evaluation of nursing care provides a systematic, empirically based method for appraisal of interventions and for the development of standards of care that are recognized by the profession and by society as effective and appropriate for special populations.

HEALTH PROMOTION

The best treatment for both hypothermia and hyperthermia is prevention. The nurse must increase the awareness of older adults regarding their physical vulnerability to extremes of environmental temperature. The nurse's educational focus for the prevention of heat illnesses is on teaching older adults and their caregivers to engage in appropriate behaviors during warm weather, such as decreasing exercise, increasing intake of fluids, avoiding alcohol, and wearing loose-fitting clothing.

■ Infections

The risk of acquiring a serious infection increases as people age. Older adults have poorer outcomes from the treatment of infections and subsequently have higher rates of morbidity and mortality than do younger people. This section of the chapter discusses age-related changes in the body's defense system; other physical, social, and environmental factors that contribute to the increased risk of infection; and the nursing care of the older person who is at risk for infection.

THE BODY'S DEFENSE SYSTEM
First lines of defense

The mechanical barriers of the skin and the mucous membranes are the first lines of human defense against noxious agents. Once these barriers are broken and penetrated, the human body can activate two other intrinsic mechanisms to protect the person: the inflammatory process and the immune response. These are part of the body's reaction whenever cells or tissues are injured or a foreign material is introduced into body tissue.

Inflammatory process

The inflammatory process is an acute, immediate, generalized response to cell injury, which results in vasodilation and delivery of fluid and cellular material to the damaged area. The cardinal manifestations of inflammation, although muted in older adults, are redness, heat, pain, swelling, and altered function. The role of the inflammatory process is to localize, destroy, and remove injurious agents to allow for the healing process to occur.

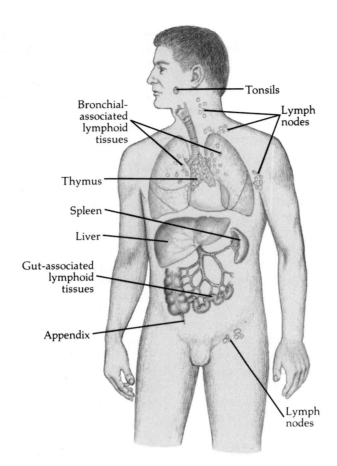

FIGURE 9-1 Organization of the immune system. (From Thompson, J.M. et al. [1993]. *Mosby's clinical nursing* [3rd ed.]. St. Louis: Mosby.)

Immune response

The immune system is a complex organization of groups of cells and tissues that function to protect the body against invasion by microorganisms, to maintain internal homeostasis, and to guard against the development of tumor cells (Thompson et al., 1993) (Figure 9-1). The immune response can be one of two types: humoral immune response or cell-mediated immune reaction. Both types of immune response are activated by the introduction of antigens into the body. *Antigens* are usually protein structures that exist as part of the complex orga-

nization of bacteria, viruses, or foreign living tissues. Immunoglobulin antibodies are formed as part of the humoral immune response to attack those antigens. Cellular immunity, a function of the cell-mediated response, occurs through the development of specifically sensitized lymphocytes. T cells (T lymphocytes) are crucial for cellular immunity, and B lymphocytes are active participants in humoral immunity. The combined immune response functions to eliminate the offending antigen. A more extensive explanation of the body's defense system is beyond the scope of this text, but the reader is advised to consult an appropriate text, if necessary, to understand the complex workings of this intricate system.

AGE-RELATED CHANGES IN THE BODY'S DEFENSE SYSTEM

There is debate in the field concerning age-related changes that are universally experienced by the human immune system. Although the older adult population shows an increase in both the number of infections and the incidence of certain diseases such as cancer, there is still not complete understanding of how age affects the immune system. There is agreement among scientists that with age there is a loss of functional cells, a decrease in the proliferation ability of T cells, a change in the ability to respond to an event, and basic changes in the pattern of response to an activation event (Adler & Nagel, 1994). There is, however, a high degree of variability of immune function among the older adult population, with some older adults having an immune function comparable to that of a younger person.

On the other hand, there is a remarkable stability in the total white count and in the number of lymphocytes of most older individuals (Adler & Nagel, 1994). One important clinical result of age-related changes in the body's defense system is a slowed response to antibiotic therapy (Yoshikawa et al., 1989). Furthermore, the element of time, the slowed response of the older immune system to events, may be the most significant factor in the increased rate of mortality and morbidity in older people. The fact remains that an older adult is more vulnerable to infection and its complications than is a younger person.

CONTRIBUTING FACTORS TO INFECTION
Physical changes

Age-related physical changes in the older person that increase susceptibility to infection are atrophic skin, decreased gastric acid, decreased pulmonary function and cough reflex, decreased mucociliary activity, and decreased elasticity of the bronchiolar musculature.

Nutrition

The nutritional status of older patients is particularly pertinent to their ability to withstand and recover from an infectious process. Depletion of protein reserves interferes with the function of the immune system. There is a consensus that serum albumin shows a steady decline throughout adult life. The normal range of serum albumin for adults is 3.8-5.0 g/dl, and the range for older adults is hypothesized to be 3.3-4.9 g/dl (Hodkinson, 1990). This age-related change might not be significant, but it is well understood that the diet of the older person is a critical factor in the prevention of and recovery from infectious illness.

Chronic disease and medications

The coexistence of chronic diseases with the need for medications that may suppress the immune response is another significant factor that affects the vulnerability of the older person to infection. Certain corticosteroid, antibiotic, non-steroidal anti-inflammatory, and cytotoxic drugs have the potential to cause immunosuppression. Also, radiation therapy, a frequent treatment modality for cancer, destroys lymphocytes. These drugs and treatments, combined with age-related changes, decrease the ability of the older person to respond effectively to an infectious illness.

Psychosocial factors

Other factors that influence the older person's susceptibility to infection are a long history of smoking, living in an air-polluted community, having been engaged in a hazardous occupation, alcoholism, poor access to health care, and poor social support systems. In addition, mental confusion is a significant risk factor because the confused older person may not recognize signs and symptoms of a progressing infection, which may delay early detection and treatment.

The same problem of delay in seeking treatment occurs with an older adult who has an inadequate support system. Delay increases the potential for a serious infection and may be the direct result of a lack of available transportation. Gaining access to health care is difficult if there is no transportation. Usually the older person is expected to go to the health care provider, as opposed to a more reasonable treatment arrangement, which would bring the provider to the patient.

Fever

An age-related change that affects the clinical manifestation of an infection in an older adult is the increased significance of a fever. Often the older person will not have a high fever, but will have a low-grade fever that may be overlooked by the inexperienced nurse or physician. Any level of fever in an older patient is to be considered a sign of a bacterial infection until proven otherwise.

Often the older person with a serious infection may have no sign of a fever, but will show atypical signs of weakness, anorexia, and, most significantly, a change in functional status. Knowing the importance of taking an in-depth history and knowing about age-related changes that affect the well-being of the older patient are two major components of the knowledge base that guides the practice of the gerontologic nurse.

TYPES OF INFECTIONS

Infections are a leading cause of morbidity and death in those 65 years of age and older, with pneumonia and influenza being the fifth leading cause of death in this age group (U.S. Bureau of the Census, 1992). In the United States fewer than 1000 people a year die of vaccine-preventable diseases of childhood. In contrast, between 50,000 and 70,000 adults die of influenza virus infections and pneumococcal bacterial infections (National Vaccine Program, 1994). The most commonly acquired bacterial pneumonias among community-dwelling older adults are caused by *Streptococcus pneumoniae, Hemophilus influenza,* and *Mycoplasma pneumoniae.* Nosocomial pneumonias contracted in institu-

tional settings are commonly caused by *Staphylococcus aureus* and by gram-negative coli such as *Escherichia coli, Klebsiella pneumoniae,* and *Pseudomonas aeruginosa.* Older adults are also particularly susceptible to pneumonia from *Legionella* and *B. catarrhalis.* Older adults also represent a disproportionally large share of reported active tuberculosis cases, primarily cases of reactivation of previous infections (Fraser, 1993).

More than 70% of the tetanus cases reported annually are in people 50 years of age or older, and nearly all of the 1 to 5 cases of diphtheria reported annually occur in unimmunized adults (*National Vaccine Program,* 1994).

Older adults are also more susceptible to urinary tract, intraabdominal, and skin and soft-tissue infections. Asymptomatic bacteriuria occurs in 20% of women over the age of 65 and in about 10% of the men (Baldasarre & Kaye, 1991). Acute diverticulitis, gastroenteritis, and appendicitis are frequent sources of intra-abdominal infections in the older adult. Alterations in skin integrity can be caused by age-related thinning of the dermis and increased susceptibility of the dermis to shear forces. Skin integrity can also be disrupted by pressure injuries, ischemia, and maceration. Immobility and fecal and urinary incontinence are major factors leading to disruption of skin integrity.

Age-related alterations in skin and mucosal barriers, decreased ciliary activity and diminished cough reflex, and decreased bone marrow reserve and diminished cellular and humoral immunity contribute to older adults' increased susceptibility to infection and increase infection-related morbidity. Diminished homeostatic reserve mechanisms, such as age-related decreased catecholamine response and decreased concentrating ability of the kidneys, also contribute to the infection-related morbidity (Fraser, 1993). The risks are even greater when malnutrition, smoking, alcohol or drug abuse, immobility, chronic disease, altered skin integrity, poor hygiene of the older adult or caregivers, and impaired cognitive function are present.

In hospitals and long-term care facilities, nosocomial infections are a significant threat to the older person's safety. Visitors and staff, equipment, and the older person's own flora (integumentary, nasopharyngeal, perineal) are reservoirs for infectious agents. The respiratory, gastrointestinal, urinary, and integumentary systems are most frequently involved (Stolley & Buckwalter, 1991).

When setting goals or outcomes for individual patients, it is important to keep in mind key risk reduction objectives set forth in *Healthy People 2000* that target older adults (U.S. Department of Health and Human Services, Public Health Service, 1991) (see *Healthy People 2000 Objectives* box).

Health teaching, guidance, and counseling interventions to meet the year 2000 goals should include providing information on vaccine-preventable diseases; the effectiveness and safety of adult vaccines; proper food handling, storage, and preparation, and risks associated with improper handling, storage, or preparation; and modification of behavior that will lead to healthy lifestyles.

■ Nursing Process

ASSESSMENT

The patient's general appearance is the first consideration in assessing the risk of infection. The possibility of infection in an older patient is always to be considered, no matter what the reason for seeking treatment may be. It is far safer to be overcautious, always thinking, Does this patient have an infection? Could an infection be responsible for the fatigue, for the loss of function, or for the loss of appetite?

The minimal assessment measures needed to identify data indicating the threat of infection are a careful history and general physical examination. Information on existing medical conditions and their past and current treatment is needed, especially in relation to infections, respiratory disease, genitourinary problems, cardiovascular disease or sequelae, immune system disorders,

Healthy People 2000 Objectives

20.11 Increase pneumococcal and influenza vaccination levels among institutionalized chronically ill or older people: at least 80%; pneumococcal pneumonia and influenza immunization among noninstitutionalized, high-risk populations, as defined by the Immunization Practices Advisory Committee: at least 60%. (Baseline: 10% estimated for pneumococcal vaccine and 20% for influenza vaccine in 1985.)

21.2f Increase to at least 40% the proportion of adults aged 65 and older who have received, as a minimum within the appropriate interval, all of the screening and immunization services and at least one of the counseling services appropriate for their age and gender as recommended by the U.S. Preventive Services Task Force.

From U.S. Department of Health and Human Services. (1990). *Healthy People 2000: National health promotion and disease prevention objectives.* (DHHS Pub. No. [PHS] 91-50212). Washington, DC: U.S. Government Printing Office.

endocrinopathies, and/or chronic integumentary system problems. Radiation therapy and chemotherapy can compromise the immune system, as well as depressing normal protective mechanisms. Immunization history should be obtained, with particular attention to influenza, pneumococcal, and tetanus/diphtheria vaccines, as well as information on tuberculin skin testing and allergies. Over-the-counter, prescription, or illicit drug use should be noted. Drugs such as decongestant, neuroleptic, antidepressant, and cholinergic agents can cause xerostomia with subsequent dental caries and alteration of the normal buccal flora (Terpenning & Bradley, 1991). To-bacco and alcohol use must be determined, be-cause both can dry the mucous membranes and interfere with mucociliary protective mecha-nisms. Information related to usual dietary intake with special attention to caloric and protein adequacy is also important, because protein ad-equacy affects various aspects of the specific and nonspecific immune systems.

On the other hand, many older adults seek treatment because they know about their health—for example, the infection site is observ-able, such as with a skin infection, or the infec-tion is recurring, such as a urinary tract infection—in which case the patient is aware of early symptoms and able to seek treatment.

Health history

A complete history, a physical examination, and laboratory test results are required when there is a suspicion of infection. The patient's health history is an important component of the assess-ment. It is well known by health care profession-als that a comprehensive history will provide 95% of the data needed to determine the success-ful treatment for most conditions. The ability to listen to, direct, reassure, and question older patients concerning their health is a remarkable skill. The nurse is the health care provider most able to elicit a comprehensive history from an older person because of the educational process and the knowledge base of professional nursing.

Physical examination and laboratory tests

The physical examination data should provide information on the older person's overall appear-ance, energy level, and cognitive functioning. Diminished cognitive function may not only in-crease the person's risk of infection, but may also herald impending infection. Any alterations in skin integrity should be noted. The ability to cough, deep breathe, and effectively clear the airway, and an adequate gag reflex are also needed to protect against the invasion of bacteria and should be assessed during the physical ex-amination. Urine retention and poor fluid intake may contribute to an increased risk of bladder in-fections, making assessment of hydration status and the genitourinary system essential. The pres-ence of urinary catheters, nasogastric tubes, or in-travenous lines must also be noted, because they not only provide a reservoir for infectious agents but also bypass usual body defense systems.

Laboratory data for initial assessment include a complete blood count (CBC) and a culture of the suspected site of infection, if this is feasible. The collection of sputum for culture in an older pa-tient is difficult because of the decreased ability to cough. An elevated white count is expected if the patient has an infection; lymphocytes are usually elevated with a viral infection, and neutrophils are elevated with a bacterial infection.

Immunization history

Immunization history should be obtained. Particu-lar attention should be directed toward the immu-nizations received for the respiratory tract infec-tions of influenza and pneumococcal pneumonia. Recent studies have shown the pneumococcal vaccine to be both efficacious and cost-effective (Shapiro et al., 1991). The pneumococcal vaccine should be given every 5 to 6 years, whereas the influenza vaccine is given every year. Also, the status of tetanus immunization should be re-viewed; 10-year intervals are the recommended schedule for the tetanus vaccine.

Cognitive status examination

The cognitive status of the older patient may be a critical factor in the development of an infection. If a mental status examination reveals poor func-tional ability, it is prudent to ask family members or other caregivers about the patient's performance of personal hygiene activities and activities of daily living. The older person may not have family, or may be living in a nursing home, in which case the nursing home staff may be more knowledgeable about the patient than are family members. It is important to obtain accurate information concern-ing the patient's ability to perform self-care.

Environmental assessment

The environment plays a significant role in the older person's acquisition of an infection. Hospital-acquired (nosocomial) infections occur in older adults at a much higher rate than in younger age groups (Saviteer et al., 1988). Urinary tract infections associated with catheters are the most common type of nosocomial infections, with wound infections second in number and severity. The increased physical vulnerability of older patients contributes to their susceptibility to nosocomial infections. Nearly 75% of nursing home residents develop at least one nosocomial infection. Poor hand washing, use of equipment such as humidifiers and catheters (intravenous or urinary), and food handling and preparation are all factors that can contribute to the risk of infection in both home and institutional settings (Ferri, 1994).

The nurse can be instrumental, however, in the development of infection control policies and procedures and in the prevention of nosocomial infections both in the hospital and in the nursing home.

NURSING DIAGNOSES

After data have been collected, clustered, and analyzed, the nurse uses clinical decision-making skills, based on knowledge obtained through observation and on scientific knowledge, to arrive at a nursing diagnosis. Such a diagnosis is necessary to guide the nurse in planning appropriate nursing interventions that provide patients with the best solution to their health problems. Interventions are also designed to promote the patient's health and to enhance the patient's quality of life.

Three diagnoses are suggested to allow the reader to plan care for older adults who are at risk for an infection and to take into account the influence of the different settings in which patients are located.

1. Risk for infection related to advanced age and elective surgical procedure

2. Risk for infection related to advanced age, urinary incontinence, poor cognitive ability, and residence in a nursing home
3. Risk for infection related to advanced age, living alone, and surgical wound

PLANNING, GOAL IDENTIFICATION, AND IMPLEMENTATION
Planning in the acute care setting

The nursing diagnosis is risk for infection related to advanced age and elective surgical procedure. Goals for hospitalized older patients who are having elective surgical procedures include the following:

1. Patient will not incur an infection during hospitalization or immediately after discharge from the hospital.
2. Wounds will heal in an appropriate time frame.
3. Unnecessary catheterization, especially with indwelling catheters, will be avoided.
4. Patient will receive adequate pain control medication postoperatively.
5. Patient will cooperate in postoperative therapy to decrease the risk of respiratory infection.

Intervention in the acute care setting

Preoperative risk factors such as smoking, poor nutrition, or decreased cognitive ability are recognized and corrected, if possible. Preoperative teaching includes providing information and training in deep breathing, coughing, and turning exercises. Nutritional consultations with the dietitian and with the physician are an important consideration in preventing problems in wound healing, particularly because nutritional requirements vary with the condition of the patient and the type and extent of the surgical procedure.

If the patient is admitted before surgery, the nurse may have an opportunity to allay fears and anxieties about the hospital experience. Now that Medicare cost-containing measures are in effect, older patients having elective surgery often receive preoperative teaching in a physician's office or in a special hospital unit that admits only same-day surgical patients.

In hospitals, nosocomial infections are a significant threat to the older person's safety. Visitors and staff, equipment, and the older person's own flora (integumentary, nasopharyngeal, perineal) are reservoirs for infectious agents. The respiratory, gastrointestinal, urinary, and integumentary systems are most frequently involved (Stolley & Buckwalter, 1991).

To decrease the incidence of wound infections, the patient should have three consecutive showers or baths within a 24-hour period before surgery (Palmer, 1990). Postoperatively, the staff nurse is more likely to be effective if the preoperative teaching can be reinforced and the patient is free of pain. To decrease the risk of a postoperative respiratory tract infection, the nurse uses sterile catheters and gloves when suctioning secretions. The vulnerability of the older patient to incurring a nosocomial infection necessitates strict adherence to all infection control procedures.

The anxiety of the patient and family is alleviated if the nurse (1) takes time to explain the importance of monitors and other technical equipment, (2) assists with procedures such as coughing and deep breathing, and (3) provides the patient with timely medications to relieve pain.

Planning in the nursing home

The nursing diagnosis is risk for infection related to advanced age, urinary incontinence, poor cognitive ability, and residence in a nursing home. This diagnosis is suggested by the patient's frequent, uncontrolled urination, history of urinary tract infection, and the fact that the professional staff are considering placement of a Foley catheter.

The goals are specific to the nursing diagnosis and to treatable etiologic factors. Nursing care cannot change advanced age, but the care can ameliorate some of the effects of advanced age. Goal setting includes the resident, or a family member if the resident is unable to participate. The long-term goal is that the resident will not experience any urinary tract infection during a 3-month period. Short-term goals include statements that address the problem of incontinence and the resident's ability to perform toileting activities with a degree of safety. For example, a short-term goal might be "Resident will void in the appropriate place and will wash hands after voiding."

Intervention in the nursing home

Interventions in the nursing home include vigilance by the professional nurse to see that hand washing is a part of the routine activities of all members of the nursing staff. Infection control measures and basic antiseptic procedure need to be constantly attended to, taught, and reinforced.

Some cognitively impaired older adults are at increased risk for infection as a result of their behaviors. The inability to recognize and respond appropriately to an urge to void increases the likelihood of incontinence and of infection. Also, the inability to perform daily personal hygiene tasks, such as timely hand washing, adds to the risk of infection. Often these very behaviors or similar health-threatening behaviors are the reason that the cognitively impaired older adult became a nursing home resident. The nurse is the major provider of care and is responsible for individualized interventions that (1) monitor and augment the toileting activities of the resident, (2) enable personal hygiene tasks to be performed, (3) improve nutritional and fluid status, (4) provide for dry skin, (5) include family members in planning for patient care, and (6) maintain the dignity of the resident.

Planning in the private or family home

The nursing diagnosis is risk for infection related to advanced age, living alone, and surgical wound. This diagnosis is suggested by poor nutritional status, poor personal hygiene, and the incisional site. The older person living in a private or family home is certainly less at risk for acquiring an infection than those who are in health care institutions, but such risk is still substantial. Many home care visits by the nurse are for dressing changes, and these dressings are often for a surgical wound.

The long-term goal might be that the wound will heal within 6 weeks, and the short-term goal might be to have Meals on Wheels deliver meals for 1 month. Adequate nutrition is critical for wound healing, and many older adults living alone and recuperating from hospitalizations are unable to prepare adequate meals. The need for community services is apparent, and the nurse works with the social worker to provide needed services to the older patient.

Other outcomes that may pertain to both the older adults and their caregivers include the following:

- Will be able to describe the risk of infection and potential outcomes
- Will use appropriate hand washing techniques and personal hygiene measures
- Will use only the antibiotics prescribed and in the manner prescribed
- Will have age-appropriate vaccinations
- Will wash fruits and vegetables thoroughly and use proper refrigerated storage
- Will demonstrate proper food handling and preparation techniques
- Will specify ways to minimize contact with infected individuals
- Will promptly report potential signs and symptoms of infection to the health care provider
- Will practice appropriate cleaning and maintenance procedures for humidifiers, catheters, respiratory equipment, or other devices used in daily personal care or treatment
- Will have a plan for alternative care if the caregiver develops an infection

Intervention in the private or family home

The role of the nurse as a teacher and promoter of health and well-being is a major consideration in home care nursing. The nurse assesses how the patient manages personal hygiene, and teaches the patient the importance of hand washing. Personal hygiene is an important aspect of the prevention of infection in the older person. Daily cleansing of skin, thorough drying with a clean towel, and daily use of clean, cotton undergarments decrease the likelihood of infections. The visiting home care nurse provides reassurance and support, along with the technical expertise necessary to monitor the progress of wound healing, and the ability to access community-based services.

EVALUATION

Evaluation of all nursing care is ongoing and relates to specific goals in terms of patient outcomes. For example: Was an infection prevented? Did the wound heal in the appropriate time frame? Were new methods of teaching the nursing home resident to control voiding successful? Did the patient cough and deep breathe effectively during the first 24 hours postoperatively? The answers to these kinds of questions must be legally documented in medical records. Systematic, observable evaluation must be recorded and documented appropriately.

REFERENCES

Abbey. (1990). *Diabetes care guide.* Unpublished project, Catholic University of America, School of Nursing, Adult Nurse Practitioner Program, Washington, DC.

Abrass, I.B. (1994). Disorders of temperature regulation. In W. Hazzard, et al., (Eds.), *Principles of geriatric medicine and gerontology* (2nd ed., pp. 383-412). New York: McGraw-Hill.

Adler, W., & Nagel, J. (1994). Clinical immunology. In W. Hazzard, et al., (Eds.), *Principles of geriatric medicine and gerontology* (2nd ed., pp. 60-71). New York: McGraw-Hill.

Baldasarre, J.S., & Kaye, D. (1991). Special problems of urinary tract infections in the elderly. *Medical Clinics of North America, 75*(2), 375-389.

Balin, A. (1990). Aging of the human skin. In W. Hazzard, et al., (Eds.), *Principles of geriatric medicine and gerontology* (pp. 383-412). New York: McGraw-Hill.

Blainey, C. (1986). Diabetes mellitus. In D.L. Carnevali & M. Patrick (Eds.), *Nursing management for the elderly* (2nd ed., pp. 403-422). Philadelphia: J.B. Lippincott.

Centers for Disease Control. (1984). Heat associated mortality—New York City. *Morbidity and Mortality Weekly Report, 33*, 430.

Collins, K.J., et al. (1981). Shivering thermogenesis and vasomotor responses with convective cooling in the elderly. *Journal of Physiology, 320*, 76.

Darowski, A., et al. (1991). Hypothermia and infection in elderly patients admitted to hospital. *Age Ageing, 20*, 100.

Dellasega, C. (1990, January). Self-care for the elderly diabetic. *Journal of Gerontological Nursing, 16*(1), 16-19.

Ferri, R.S. (1994). Health perception-health management pattern. In R.S. Ferri (Ed.), *Care planning for the older adult: Nursing diagnosis in long term care.* Philadelphia: W.B. Saunders.

Fisch, M.D., Jr. (1990, June). Complications of diabetes, other than those of vision, in older patients. *Aging and Vision News, 3*(1).

Fox, R.H., et al. (1973). Body temperatures in the elderly: A national study of physiological, social, and environmental conditions. *British Medical Journal, 27*, 200-206.

Fraser, D. (1993). Patient assessment: Infection in the elderly. *Journal of Gerontological Nursing, 19*(7), 5-11.

Goldberg, A.P., Andres, R., & Bierman, E.L. (1990). Diabetes mellitus in the elderly. In W. Hazzard, et al., (Eds.), *Principles of geriatric medicine and gerontology* (pp. 60-71). New York: McGraw-Hill.

Gregerman, R., & Katz, M. (1994). Thyroid diseases. In W. Hazzard, et al. (Eds.), *Principles of geriatric medicine and gerontology* (2nd ed., pp. 719-737). New York: McGraw-Hill.

Hodkinson, H.M. (1990). Alterations of laboratory findings. In W. Hazzard, et al. (Eds.), *Principles of geriatric medicine and gerontology* (pp. 241-244). New York: McGraw-Hill.

Hope, W., et al. (1984). Illness and death due to environmental heat: Georgia and St. Louis. 1983. Leads from the MMWR. *Journal of the American Medical Association, 252*, 209.

MacLean, D., & Emslie-Smith, D. (1977). *Accidental hypothermia.* London: Blackwell Scientific.

McKee, P.A., et al. (1971). The natural history of congestive heart failure: The Framingham Study. *New England Journal of Medicine, 285*, 1441.

Mersey, J. (1989). Diabetes mellitus in the elderly patient. In W. Reichel (Ed.), *Clinical aspects of aging.* Baltimore: Williams & Wilkins.

National Vaccine Program. (1994). *Adult immunization: A report by the National Advisory Committee.* Atlanta: U.S. Department of Health and Human Services, Public Health Service, Centers for Disease Control and Prevention.

Palmer, M.A. (1990). Care of the older surgical patient. In C. Eliopoulos (Ed.), *Caring for the elderly in diverse care settings.* Philadelphia: J.B. Lippincott.

Radak, J.T., Jewler, D., & Steinburg, C. (1990, September). Finding more clues. *Diabetes Forecast, 43*(9), 31-38.

Rango, N. (1984). Exposure-related hypothermia mortality in the United States 1970-79. *American Journal of Public Health, 74*, 1159.

Robbins, A. (1989). Hypothermia and heat stroke: Protecting the elderly patient. *Geriatrics, 44*(1), 73-80.

Saviteer, S., Samsa, G., & Rutale, W. (1988). Nosocomial infections in the elderly: Increased risk per hospital day. *American Journal of Medicine, 84*, 661.

Shapiro, et al. (1991). The protective efficacy of polyvalent pneumococcal polysaccharide vaccine. *New England Journal of Medicine, 325*, 1506.

Solomon, B.I. (1980, September). Symposium on endocrine disorders: Foreword. *Nursing Clinics of North America, 15*(3), 433-434.

Stolley, J.M., & Buckwalter, K.C. (1991). Iatrogenesis in the elderly: Nosocomial infections. *Journal of Gerontological Nursing, 17*(9), 30-34.

Terpenning, M.S., & Bradley, S.F. (1991). Why aging leads to increased susceptibility to infection. *Geriatrics, 46*(2), 77-80.

Terry, L., & Halter, J. (1994). Aging of the endocrine system. In W. Hazzard, et al. (Eds.), *Principles of geriatric medicine and gerontology.* New York: McGraw-Hill.

Thompson, J.M., et al. (1993). *Mosby's clinical nursing.* St. Louis: Mosby.

Thorne, A., & Wahren, J. (1990). Diminished meal-induced thermogenesis in elderly men. *Clinical Physiology, 10*, 427.

U.S. Bureau of the Census. (1992). *Sixty-five plus in America.* (Current Population Reports, Special Studies P-23-178RV.) Washington, DC: U.S. Government Printing Office.

U.S. Department of Health and Human Services, Public Health Service. (1991). *Healthy People 2000: National health promotion and disease prevention objectives: Full report, with commentary.* Washington, DC: U.S. Government Printing Office.

Yoshikawa, T., Castle, S., & Norman, D. (1989). Update on infection. In R. Ham (Ed.), *Geriatric medicine annual 1989*. Oradell, NJ: Medical Economics Books.

BIBLIOGRAPHY

Carroll-Johnson, R.M. (Ed.). (1991). *Classification of nursing diagnoses: Proceedings of the ninth conference*. Philadelphia: J.B. Lippincott.

Commission on Accreditation of Rehabilitation Facilities. (1992). *Standards manual for organizations serving people with disabilities*. Tucson: Author.

Hofland, S.L., & Mort, J. (1994). Infections in long-term care facilities: Issues for practice. *Geriatric Nursing, 15*, 260-264.

Keene-Payne, R. (1994). Hospitalized older adults. In M.O. Hogstel (Ed.), *Nursing care of the older adult* (pp. 250-264). Albany, NY: Delmar.

Martin, K., & Scheet, N. (1992). *The Omaha system: A pocket guide for community health nursing*. Philadelphia: W.B. Saunders.

McFarlane, E.A. (1993). Nursing diagnosis: The critical link in the nursing process. In G.K. McFarland & E.A. McFarlane (Eds.), *Nursing diagnosis and intervention* (2nd ed., pp. 10-20). St. Louis: Mosby.

Portenoy, R. (1989). Cancer pain. In R. Ham (Ed.), *Geriatric medicine annual 1989*. Oradell, NJ: Medical Economics Books.

Reynolds, C.A. (1994). Emergency care. In M.O. Hogstel (Ed.), *Nursing care of the older adult* (pp. 265-287). Albany, NY: Delmar.

Ross, J.E. (1991). Iatrogenesis in the elderly: Contributors to falls. *Journal of Gerontological Nursing, 17*(9), 19-23.

Young, R., & Olson, E.A. (1991). *Health, illness and disability in later life: Practice issues and interventions*. Newbury Park, CA: Sage Publications.

Where I was born and where and how I have lived is unimportant. It is what I have done with where I have been that should be of interest.

GEORGIA O'KEEFFE

Cardiovascular Function

■ Learning Objectives

On completion of this chapter, the reader will be able to do the following:

1. Identify age-related physiologic changes of the cardiovascular and peripheral vascular system.
2. Identify and describe the common pathophysiologic changes that affect the cardiovascular system of the older adult.
3. Assess the cardiovascular functioning of older adults.
4. Recognize the psychosocial and cultural factors that influence the nursing management of older adults with cardiovascular problems.
5. Develop a plan of care for an older adult with cardiovascular impairment.
6. Provide appropriate nursing interventions for older adults with cardiovascular impairment.
7. Identify health promotion strategies to improve the quality of cardiovascular function in the older adult.

The cardiovascular system of the older adult endures significant changes associated with aging. The line between changes caused by disease and normal changes caused by aging is often blurred. Changes that were once thought to be the result of aging, such as a decrease in cardiac output, are now considered changes brought about by disease. It is important to remember that the effects of cardiovascular disease vary widely in the older population; the effects of aging and disease can produce severe cardiovascular dysfunction in one person and minimally detectable functional compromise in another.

■ Normal Structure and Function

The main function of the heart is to circulate blood to all the tissues of the body. Blood supplies oxygen and nutrients to the cells and removes the waste products of metabolism.

Irregularly conic in shape, the heart is situated in the thoracic cavity, positioned obliquely within the mediastinal space. The skeleton plays a major role in protecting the heart: the ribs, the sternum, and the vertebral column provide a breadbasket-like enclosure for this vital organ. The heart is covered by the *pericardium,* a thin, double-walled sac that contains a small amount of lymphlike fluid. The pericardium protects the surface of the heart from infection. The fluid of the pericardium also serves to reduce friction, which occurs during the normal cardiac cycle.

The heart is a hollow, muscular organ with four chambers: the right and left atria, and the right and left ventricles (Figures 10-1 and 10-2). The right atrium receives blood from the superior vena cava, the inferior vena cava, and the coronary sinus. From the right atrium, blood flows through the tricuspid valve to the right ventricle. Blood then flows to the lungs via the pulmonary artery, to be oxygenated. This oxygenated blood then flows to the left atrium, which is smaller than the right atrium but a bit thicker. Next, blood flows through the mitral valve to the left ventricle, a thick, large muscle that contributes to cardiac contractility. Blood is

then routed through the aortic valve to be circulated to the body and coronary arteries.

Although the heart is four chambered, it functions as a two-sided pump with two cycles of action: a contraction phase, termed *systole,* during which blood is ejected from the heart; and an expansion phase, termed *diastole,* during which the heart relaxes and blood flows into the chambers. The cardiac cycles of systole and diastole are initiated by a cellular conduction system. It regulates the heart's rate and rhythm, and generates, transmits, and coordinates electrical impulses throughout the cardiac muscle cells. The heart's pumping mechanism is controlled by this electrical impulse, carried by specialized cardiac muscle fibers through the heart. The heartbeat originates in the sinoatrial (SA) node, also called the pacemaker. The electrical impulse

FIGURE 10-1 Frontal schematic view of the heart. (From Phipps, W.J., et al. [1995]. *Medical-surgical nursing: Concepts and clinical practice,* [5th ed.]. St. Louis: Mosby.)

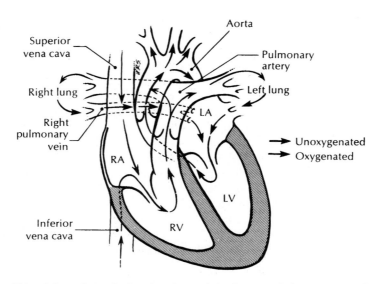

FIGURE 10-2 Route of blood flow through the chambers of the heart and the great vessels. (From Malasanos, L., et al. [1990]. *Health assessment* [4th ed.]. St. Louis: Mosby.)

travels down the specialized muscle of both atria to the atrioventricular (AV) node. From the AV node the impulse spreads across both ventricles through the tissue of the atrioventricular bundle, also known as the bundle of His, and then through the right and left bundle branches. The conduction pathway ends in a fine network of conductive tissue called the Purkinje fibers.

The electrical impulse of the heart is a result of the change in a series of charged ions crossing the cardiac cell membrane. This is called action potential. The resting cardiac cell has a charge of −90 mV. As potassium and sodium cross in opposite directions across the membrane, the electrical charge is altered. There are five phases to the cardiac cell action potential: phase 0—rapid depolarization; phase 1—change to repolarization; phase 2—stabilization period; phase 3—sudden acceleration of repolarization; and phase 4—return to the resting phase. Characteristics of the heart pacemaker cells are similar to those of cardiac muscle cells. However, the action potential of pacemaker cells in the resting state is

−40 mV and the depolarization and repolarization are more gradual (Figure 10-3).

There are many factors that influence movement of blood in the heart and body. Cardiac output (CO) is based on the amount of blood pumped from the left ventricle per minute. CO is determined by multiplying stroke volume (SV), the amount of blood ejected from the ventricles, by the heart rate (HR): CO = SV × HR. Factors that affect CO are preload and afterload. Preload is the degree of tension on the ventricle at the end of diastole, or left ventricle end-diastolic pressure (LVEDP). Afterload is the resistance against which the heart pumps. If the vascular resistance increases, the afterload increases; therefore the heart compensates to maintain SV and CO by increasing ventricular contractility. Contractility of the heart muscle is dependent on preload and afterload. Drugs and the sympathetic nerve can alter the rate (chronotropic) and force (inotropic) of contractions.

The Frank-Starling curve is described as the energy of contraction proportional to the initial

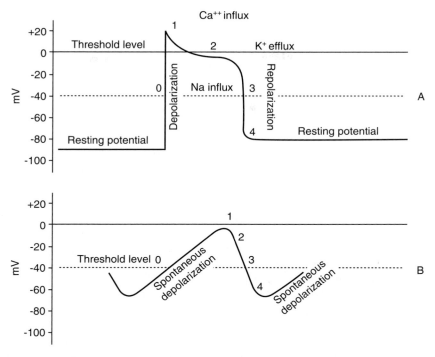

FIGURE 10-3 Cardiac action potential. (From Thompson, J.M., et al. [1993]. *Mosby's clinical nursing* [3rd ed.]. St Louis: Mosby.)

length of the cardiac muscle fiber. Preload, which is the length of the stretch of the cardiac muscle fiber, and stroke volume create the Frank-Starling curve. Blood volume, HR, SV, and peripheral resistance all contribute to the shape of the Frank-Starling curve. As one ages, the cardiac muscle begins to lose its ability to stretch and rebound as it becomes more like a worn-out elastic band, predisposing a person to congestive heart failure (CHF).

The peripheral vascular system is composed of arteries, capillaries, and veins. The oxygenated blood flows from the left ventricle of the heart into highly elastic arteries of the body, which are able to distend because of increased pressure. Constriction and dilatation of the arteries control blood flow as the body's needs change. The

arterial system holds 20% of the blood volume. Capillaries are the smallest vessels, in which the exchange of the oxygen, nutrients, and waste products occurs. The venous system collects the blood from the capillaries to return it to the heart. The venous system holds approximately 60% of the blood volume and has the ability to distend and compress as the body's needs change. One-way valves assist the veins in moving blood from the arms and legs back to the heart. Like the cardiac system described earlier, the peripheral vascular system responds to changes brought about by the autonomic nervous system and chemical agents such as drugs.

The function of the cardiovascular system is influenced by many factors. As one ages, the response to these factors is altered. The condition of an aged heart, as well as other factors such as blood volume, determines the level at which the heart will function. The following section describes the age-related changes that occur.

■ Age-Related Changes

In general, the most common change in the cardiovascular and peripheral vascular system associated with increased age is a stiffening of structures. These structural changes affect the function of both the heart and the peripheral vascular system. Lipofuscin, a yellow-brown granular material, accumulates in the myocardial cell, and amyloid deposits are seen extracellularly. As in other areas of the body, collagen and lipid deposits increase intercellularly in the heart muscle, resulting in different degrees of ventricular hypertrophy (Kenney, 1989). This decreases left ventricular (LV) stretch (compliance). The valves of the heart also become thicker and more rigid as a result of calcification. The mitral and aortic valves are most affected because of their exposure to high pressures in the vascular system. In addition, in the conduction system, the SA node is infiltrated by fat and connective tissue, resulting in a decrease in the heart's ability to regulate the rate of the sinus node, also causing a slowing of electrical impulses through the AV tissue. There is a 10% decrease in the number of pacemaker cells in the SA node by age 75 (Gawlinski & Jensen, 1991). Many of the arrhythmias seen in the older person are a result of either the decrease in pacemaker cells or the infiltration of fat in the SA node.

These physiologic and biochemical changes affect the heart's performance. Even though the resting heart rate only modestly decreases with age, there is a significant decrease in the maximum heart rate that can be achieved with exercise. Also, there is a slight increase in preload, a decline in SV, a prolonged relaxation contraction phase, and a 50% reduction in LV filling caused by stiffness (Wenger, 1992).

Data from the Baltimore longitudinal study suggests that the cardiac output during exercise remains unchanged with age. Because of the delay in diastolic filling time, there is more time for the ventricles to fill. This helps to offset, to some extent, the stroke volume decrease that occurs because of stiffening of the left ventricle. These changes associated with increased age are particularly notable when the cardiovascular system is challenged. First, the aging cardiovascular system becomes less responsive to increases in work load and has a diminished reserve capacity for managing high levels of stress. Second, resting myocardium oxygen consumption is reduced by approximately 1% per year as one ages, resulting in a decrease in exercise tolerance. The measurement of myocardium oxygen consumption is commonly used to determine functional status. Lastly, it has been shown that older people's response to beta stimulation induced by drugs or the autonomic nervous system is also decreased. A regular exercise program has been shown to improve exercise tolerance in older adults (Shephard, 1993).

The effect of normal aging on the peripheral vascular system is arterial stiffening. Vascular changes occur because of cross-linking of collagen, causing a thicker and less elastic vessel. This is related to changes in the subendothelial vascular layer, which becomes thickened with connective tissue. Fragmentation of elastin and calcification occur within the media of the vessels and contribute to increased rigidity. These changes are independent of atherosclerosis and hypertension. Generally, there is an increase in resistance in the vascular system, and the baroreceptor in the arterial tree becomes less sensitive to pressure changes (Wenger, 1992).

Overall, the age-related changes in the cardiovascular system increase the probability of disease. The rate of change with age will affect the progression of cardiovascular disease in varied and unique ways. The individual's adaptive capacity will also influence the manifestation of disease. For instance, one person with arterial

Aging Alert

1. The line between normal aging processes and disease is difficult to delineate.
2. The normal aging heart has a diminished capacity to manage high levels of stress.
3. Lifestyle influences cardiovascular function.

insufficiency may develop significant collateral circulation in the lower extremities and experience little discomfort, whereas another with the same degree of blockage in major peripheral arteries will not develop collateral circulation sufficient to prevent claudication.

The major age-related cardiovascular and peripheral vascular changes are a result of the interaction of several factors. As the vessels become thick, they are less able to respond to stressors such as illness, medications, and exercise. The following sections will review unique characteristics of common health deviations, focus on the older adult's cardiovascular and peripheral vascular concerns, and outline health promotion criteria for this population.

■ Common Health Deviations

ATHEROSCLEROSIS AND CORONARY ARTERY DISEASE

Atherosclerosis is the most commonly used term for thickening and hardening of the arteries. This condition is the leading cause of coronary obstruction, otherwise known as coronary artery disease (CAD). It is also the leading cause of death in the United States for the age group over 65 years; over 80% of all CAD is found in people over 65. Atherosclerosis is the process that leads to ischemic events. It appears to begin early in

life and progresses over the years. After menopause, women have the same rate of disease as men. Clinical manifestations of atherosclerosis of the coronary arteries include warning signs and symptoms of angina pectoris or myocardial infarction (MI), resulting in damaged heart muscle. Atherosclerosis is the common pathologic cause that leads not only to CAD but also to hypertension, stroke, renal failure, and peripheral vascular disease. These organ dysfunctions are the result of limited blood supply caused by narrowing of the arteries by atheromatous plaque. Generally, symptoms of CAD are not experienced until the vessel lumen is reduced by 50% or more. CAD is suspected in individuals who have positive cardiac risk factors such as male gender, being a postmenopausal woman, history of cigarette smoking, hypertension, hyperlipidemia, obesity, diabetes mellitus, or a family history of heart disease. Recently, physical inactivity, increased emotional stress, and type A personality have been identified as positive risk factors for CAD. Individuals who manifest signs of atherosclerotic disease elsewhere, such as those with a history of stroke or peripheral vascular disease, are likely to have CAD as well.

Many older adults, even though they may have CAD, are not symptomatic, possibly because they are sedentary or bedridden. The activity that would ordinarily produce anginal symptoms is simply not undertaken. However, symptoms may still appear if they are active or if there is a challenge, such as an infection. Angina pectoris, which is the symptomatic pain associated with the constriction of coronary arteries, is the same in the older adult population as in the younger population. However, the major complaint that drives a person to seek medical attention may be shortness of breath, syncope, sweating, or heart palpitation during exertion, rather than the traditional substernal chest tightness relieved with rest. As with angina pectoris, the older adult does not usually complain of classic symptoms for an acute myocardial infarction. The symptoms frequently reported are confusion, syncope, vertigo, weakness, progressive shortness of breath, abdominal pain, and cough. Other explanations for the lack of stated symptoms of pain are that there may be an altered pain sensation, or that the older adult may dismiss the pain as something that is normal and expected with age.

To prevent the progression of CAD, risk factor modification is the treatment of choice. Factors such as age, gender, and genetics cannot be altered, but the reversible risk factors can be reduced. There is evidence to suggest that there can be some regression of atherosclerosis with treatment (Gamble, 1994). However, the best situation is for steps to be taken early in life to prevent atherosclerosis.

Primary prevention includes a lifestyle of regular exercise, maintenance of ideal body weight, no tobacco use, limited alcohol use, a low-fat, low-cholesterol, and low-salt diet and stress reduction techniques. Secondary prevention includes screening methods, such as blood pressure (BP) measurements and cholesterol testing, to determine those at risk for CAD. Once CAD risk factors, such as elevated blood pressure, are identified, a person can control the risk factor to prevent disease progression. Other risk factor modification programs include decreasing cholesterol levels, participating in a smoking cessation program, adhering to a low-fat, low-cholesterol, and low-salt diet, and participating in a formalized exercise program (Box 10-1).

There is strong evidence that controlling one's serum cholesterol, decreasing low-density lipoprotein (LDL), and increasing high-density lipoprotein (HDL) reduce the risk of CAD. The damage from hypercholesteremia begins in middle age and continues to progress as one ages, resulting in CAD. Based on current studies, it is believed that hypercholesteremia levels of over 240 in older adults constitute a risk factor for CAD. It is recommended that all adults strive to meet the guidelines set by the National Heart, Lung, and Blood Institute's National Cholesterol Education Program (Table 10-1).

BOX 10-1 CARDIOVASCULAR RISK FACTOR PROFILE

Family history of heart disease
Sex
    Male (35 to 55 years)
    Female (over 50 years or after menopause)
Hypertension
Smoking
Excessive weight or obesity
Elevated serum level of lipids and fats
Diabetes mellitus
Physical inactivity; sedentary lifestyle
Stress
For women over 50 years: use of estrogen (i.e., birth control pills) and smoking

Obesity has been directly related to CAD, as well as to hypertension, hypercholesterolemia, and hyperglycemia. Weight reduction or maintenance of ideal body weight reduces the risk of CAD, as well as that of these other medical conditions. The American College of Sports Medicine recommends a brisk walk 4 times a week to improve cardiovascular function (U.S. Department of Health and Human Services [USDHHS], 1994). In one study, high-level physical activity (in excess of 2000 kcal per week) in people age 65 to 79 was associated with improved survival, as compared with that in peers with lower physical activity levels. In addition to preserving myocardial oxygen consumption, exercise is also beneficial in reducing LDL levels, increasing HDL levels, improving mental processing, improving glucose tolerance and insulin sensitivity, improving functional status in people with arthritis, and reducing the risk of fractures from osteoporosis (Shephard, 1993).

Diabetes mellitus is another risk factor associated with CAD. Although the genetic compo-

TABLE 10-1 Initial classification of total cholesterol, HDL cholesterol, LDL cholesterol levels*

Cholesterol level (mg/100 ml)	Classification
TOTAL	
<200	Desirable without risk factors
200-239	Borderline high
>239	High
HDL	
<35	Low (higher levels are desirable)
LDL	
<160	Desirable with two or fewer cardiac risk factors
<130-160	Desirable with two or more cardiac risk factors
<100	Desirable with cardiovascular disease

*If two or more cardiac risk factors are identified, LDL cholesterol and triglyceride levels should be analyzed.

nent of diabetes is not understood, it is believed that diabetes causes destruction of the smooth muscular cells and arterial endothelial, thus contributing to the formation of arteriosclerosis (Bierman, 1994). A significant amount of data supports the notion that control of diabetes will help prevent the vascular changes associated with the disease, reducing a person's risk of developing CAD.

Smoking is the most destructive risk factor associated with CAD, because in combination with other risk factors, it increases a person's risk of developing CAD in a multiplicative manner. Therefore a person who is hypertensive and smokes is 4 times more likely to develop CAD than a person who just has hypertension.

Although modifying risk factors is considered the initial step in slowing the progression of CAD, several available therapies have been shown to be beneficial to older adults who have symptomatic CAD. Both percutaneous transvenous coronary angioplasty (PTCA) and coronary artery bypass graph (CABG) surgery are options to alleviate symptoms and limit further damage. Opening up one or two blocked vessels using PTCA is the preferred therapy, because it is less invasive. However, because of advanced aging, many older adults may have more than three vessel stenoses and may experience overall a decrease in the symptoms if CABG is performed. Half of all the CABGs performed are on people older than 65 (Wenger, 1992). Data evaluating the difference in morbidity and mortality among those patients who have had a PTCA versus those who have had a CABG is incomplete. It is clear, however, that older adults see an improvement in their quality of life when they are symptom free. Regardless of the procedure, clinical and ethical factors need to be reviewed to address potential risks based on each older person's medical situation.

HYPERTENSION

Both primary and secondary hypertension have a high incidence in the older adult population. It is estimated that about 45% of white men and women and 60% of black men and women age 65 to 74 have hypertension (Wenger, 1992). At this time the definition of hypertension in older adults is the same as in younger age groups, as set forth by the 1993 Fifth Report of the Joint National Committee on Detection, Evaluation, and Treatment of High Blood Pressure.

A form of hypertension frequently encountered in older adults is isolated systolic hypertension, in which systolic blood pressure is greater than or equal to 160 mm Hg and diastolic blood pressure is less than 90 mm Hg ("The Fifth Report," 1993). The diastolic pressure is normal, but the systolic pressure is consistently above 160 mm Hg. About 3 million older people in the United States have isolated systolic hypertension: 1 out of every 3 older women, and 1 out of every 5 older men. (Diastolic hypertension, however, is more readily seen in the population younger than 55.) There has been a long-standing debate over what the normal range of blood pressure is for the older adult population, as well as whether or not their high blood pressure should be treated. This debate continues despite significant findings supporting the currently defined range of normal blood pressures and the benefits related to the treatment of hypertension. (For classification of arterial hypertension, see Table 10-2.) Several large studies, including the Framingham study and the European Working Party on Hypertension in the Elderly, identify significant decreases in cardiovascular and cerebrovascular events in the older adult population treated for systolic hypertension (Applegate & Rutan, 1992).

The underlying causes of essential hypertension in older adults are atherosclerosis, loss of elasticity of vessels, and a stiff aorta. These factors result in an overall increase in peripheral vascular resistance (PVR). Another possible cause of increased PVR is abnormal renal sodium excretion, which results in sodium and water retention. The mechanism is unclear but postulated to be either a decline in plasma renin levels or decreased beta-adrenergic activity in the older population. Unfortunately, the result is the same: too much intravascular volume, predisposing one to high blood pressure. A contributing factor to this is thought to be the high sodium content of the American diet.

The usual nonpharmacologic therapeutic approaches to hypertension are weight loss, salt restriction, exercise, smoking cessation, and alcohol restriction.

The various pharmacologic agents used in the treatment of older hypertensive adults are based on the premise that hypertension in older adults is caused by increased peripheral vascular resistance, low renin levels, decreased CO, and decreased sensitivity to beta-stimulation. Diuretics used to be the first step in treatment. However, beta-blockers (beta-adrenergic blocking agents), calcium channel blockers, and angiotensin-converting enzyme (ACE) inhibitors have proven effective in the treatment of hypertension in older adults. Initiation of drug therapy should be gradual and with half the recommended dose (Massie, 1994).

TABLE 10-2 Classification of arterial hypertension by arterial pressure levels*

Pressure (mm Hg)	Category
Systolic	
<130	Normal BP
130-139	Borderline isolated hypertension
140-159	Stage 1 mild hypertension
160-179	Stage 2 moderate hypertension
180-209	Stage 3 severe hypertension
>210	Stage 4 very severe hypertension
Diastolic	
<85	Normal BP
85-89	High normal BP
90-99	Stage 1 mild hypertension
100-109	Stage 2 moderate hypertension
110-119	Stage 3 severe hypertension
>120	Stage 4 very severe hypertension

The fifth report of the Joint National Committee on detection, evaluation and treatment of high blood pressure. (1993). *Archives of Internal Medicine, 153,* 154-183.
*When systolic and diastolic pressures fall into different categories, the higher category should be selected to classify the individual's BP status.

HYPOTENSION

Hypotension occurs in 20% to 30% of noninstitutionalized older adults, with a clear correlation between the incidence of hypotension and age. There is also a relationship between hypotension and an elevated basal blood pressure. The higher the resting blood pressure, the greater the fall in BP with postural change to the upright position. Several factors contribute to the increased incidence of hypotension, including a decreased baroflex response to both hypotensive and hypertensive stimuli. In addition, volume depletion, hypotensive drugs, Valsalva maneuver, and prolonged bed rest can cause significant hypotensive events. The greatest danger to older adults with orthostatic hypotension is injury from a fall. Changing from a sitting or lying position to an upright one can cause dizziness or lightheadedness and a subsequent fall.

The nurse should periodically evaluate orthostatic changes. First, the BP should be checked after the patient has been in a lying position for 5 minutes. Then the patient should be asked to stand up, and the BP should be taken after 1 minute of standing and then again after 5 minutes. A decrease in systolic BP of 20 mm Hg or more after standing is indicative of orthostatic hypotension. It is important to instruct older adults, especially sick older adults, to change positions slowly, and to go from a lying to a sitting position before standing. In addition, to enhance venous return, the patient can dorsiflex the feet before standing and can use elastic stockings. Elevation of the head of the bed at night or during naps may decrease the hypotension.

Some older adults experience a postprandial hypotension. This is a recently recognized phenomenon in which there is a decline in BP of 20 mm Hg or more 1 hour after a meal. This drop in BP does not occur in younger adults or in the absence of a meal. Another noted occurrence of sudden hypotension is seen in men after voiding. Clear instructions to void sitting down and to wait 1 to 2 minutes before standing when finished will prevent a fall.

CONGESTIVE HEART FAILURE

Congestive heart failure, or CHF, increases exponentially with age and is more common in men than in women. The prevalence of CHF increases from approximately 3% in those age 45 to 65, to 6% in those age 65 to 75, and 10% in those 75 years old and older (Luchi et al., 1991). Heart failure means that the heart cannot provide sufficient cardiac output to meet the metabolic needs of the body. CHF may result from systolic or diastolic dysfunction, or both. The dysfunction results in an elevated ventricular end-diastolic pressure, with subsequent congestion of pulmonary or systemic veins and the organs that they drain.

The major underlying causes of heart failure in older adults, as well as in younger populations, are ischemic heart disease, hypertension, and calcific degenerative valvular disease. There are several distinct physiologic responses that occur when a heart is failing. There is an increased heart rate, contractility, and venous return, and decreasing glomerular filtration. The heart begins to stretch out. Up to a point, the Frank-Starling mechanism increases stroke volume to maintain adequate heart function. When this protective mechanism can no longer maintain normal heart function, congestive heart failure will occur.

Characteristics of CHF include cardiac enlargement, increased jugular venous distention, basilar rales, S_3 heart sound (gallop), an enlarged liver, and edema. Even though fluid retention is common in CHF, neither pedal edema nor pretibial edema alone is diagnostic of CHF. In older adults, pedal edema can also be caused by venous stasis. Simply sitting for more than an hour can cause an accumulation of fluid in the feet and ankles.

Pharmacologic treatment of CHF resulting from systolic dysfunction includes digitalis, coupled with a diuretic and vasodilator. By stimulating the contractile function of the heart and decreasing preload and afterload, the Frank-Starling curve shifts to the left to maximize SV. It is not uncommon for older adults to have an acute episode of CHF and be placed on long-term digitalis therapy, although individuals who do not have an arrhythmia in conjunction with the CHF may be good candidates for having the digitalis discontinued. Discontinuation of digitalis therapy can help prevent the negative side effects related to the drug. Older adults have a decrease in lean body mass and glomerular filtration rate, which puts the older patient at high risk for developing the side effects of digitalis treatment. Nonetheless, patients with atrial fibrillation should continue to be given digitalis.

In addition to digitalis, angiotensin-converting enzyme (ACE) inhibitors, which have been of benefit in managing severe CHF, are also useful in managing mild to moderate CHF. These drugs have been shown consistently to reduce 1-year mortality of older adults with severely symptomatic heart failure (Cohn, 1992). An extra beneficial effect seen with ACE inhibitors is the reduction of potassium loss in patients who are also on loop or thiazide diuretics.

Attention to continuing patient education for people with CHF cannot be stressed enough. Management of this chronic condition requires the person to comply with medication regimens, diet restriction, and a lifestyle modification program. Continued encouragement for patients to notify their providers if symptoms such as weight gain and progressive shortness of breath occur should be reinforced by the nurse with every interaction.

VALVULAR HEART DISEASE

Valvular heart disease is another common disorder in older adults. Most valvular problems are asymptomatic or have symptoms that are difficult to assess. The valves most commonly affected are the aortic and mitral valves. Valvular problems can be classified as being related either to stenosis, a narrowing of the valve that inhibits the flow of blood, or to regurgitation, an incomplete closure of the valve that results in a back-flow of blood.

Aortic stenosis (AS) is the most frequently seen valvular lesion in older adults. As people continue to live longer, the progression of valvular degeneration and deposits of calcium increase the incidence of AS. Symptoms are difficult to assess, making the diagnosis difficult. Although a systolic murmur may be present, it is often not considered clinically significant. However, once the diagnosis of severe AS is determined by a combination of symptoms such as shortness of breath, angina, and dizziness, surgical management has been shown to be successful in decreasing the mortality, which may be as high as 50% in 2 years.

Aortic regurgitation (AR) in older adults is usually a result of hypertension, atherosclerosis, or congenital valvular deformities. Clinically, AR is suspected when a diastolic murmur is heard on physical examination. Medical treatment is frequently successful and is able to prevent the need for surgical intervention. However, in the case of acute AR as a result of trauma or infective endocarditis, emergency surgery may be indicated.

Mitral valve disease is seen less frequently in older adults as compared to other valvular disease. Mitral stenosis, many times a result of rheumatic fever, is usually diagnosed after a person experiences atrial fibrillation, pulmonary embolism, or stroke.

The clinical presentation of aortic stenosis, aortic regurgitation, mitral stenosis, and mitral regurgitation is frequently characterized by fatigue, syncope, angina pectoris, and CHF. The treatment for severe valvular disease is valve replacement. Age is not a contraindication to surgery; older adults generally have a good prognosis with valve replacement procedures. However, older adults with severe valvular disease, especially those with comorbidity, may be high-risk surgical candidates.

ARRHYTHMIAS AND CONDUCTION DISORDERS

Older adults are susceptible to cardiac arrhythmias and conduction disturbances because of a combination of age-related changes and varying degrees of commonly encountered pathophysiologic conditions.

Sick sinus syndrome (SSS), sometimes termed the "bradycardia-tachycardia syndrome," is a commonplace conduction disorder occurring episodically in a small percentage of older adults. This arrhythmia results from atrial enlargement or from fibrous and sclerotic changes occurring in or around the SA node. The components of SSS are (1) a malfunctioning SA node, (2) an unresponsive AV node, and (3) widespread conduction problems resulting from a combination of age-related changes and heart disease.

Older adults with this arrhythmia may experience syncopal episodes, when their heart rhythm changes abruptly from a bradycardia (usually less than 50 beats per minute) to a tachycardia, such as atrial fibrillation with a fast ventricular response or paroxysmal atrial tachycardia. Older adults with SSS may have one or more of the following clinical symptoms: confusion, fatigue, weakness, palpitations, syncope, presyncope, dizziness, lightheadedness, vertigo, falls, angina, CHF, or transient ischemic attacks (TIAs). Despite the serious nature of this disorder, the mortality rate associated with SSS seems to be no worse than that for people of the same age without it. Nevertheless, pacemaker insertion is recommended to control the patient's symptoms and to avoid injuries and upsets associated with falls, fainting, and dizziness.

Another significant arrhythmia that causes syncope and carries the possibility of sudden death in older people is acute Adams-Stokes syndrome. This syndrome consists of syncopal attacks caused by low cardiac output resulting from either extremely slow or extremely fast heart rates. Common precipitating heart rhythms include complete heart block, severe sinus bradycardia, SA block, ventricular tachycardia, supraventricular tachycardia, and ventricular fibrillation. These sudden blackout spells constitute a medical emergency and may require cardiopulmonary resuscitation (CPR) and electrical defibrillation, followed by the installation of a permanent cardiac pacemaker. Attacks are accompanied by dizziness, palpitations, or cerebrovascular confusion, and they may or may not be accompanied by seizures. Recovery may occur spontaneously if an escape rhythm is established in time.

With the exception of multifocal ectopic beats, atrial fibrillation is the most common arrhythmia found in older adults, occurring in approximately 5% of all people over age 60 (Laupacis et al., 1992). Atrial fibrillation occurs because of atrial enlargement, or from thickening or fatty infiltration in and around the sinus node and the internodal tracts. Although atrial fibrillation is frequently found in otherwise healthy individuals, some health disorders may predispose a person to this arrhythmia. In the United States hypertensive heart disease is the most common cause, but atrial fibrillation also commonly occurs in the context of acute disorders, such as myocardial infarction (or MI), pulmonary embolism, CHF, hypoxia, pericarditis, thyrotoxicosis, and SSS. It is associated with chronic disorders, as well as with ischemic heart disease, aortic stenosis, chronic lung disease, mitral valve disease, and cardiomyopathy.

Atrial fibrillation may be physiologically tolerable to the older patient, as long as the ventricular response rate does not exceed 60 to 90 beats per minute. With heart rates faster than this, ventricular filling is apt to be inadequate; therefore patients with untreated atrial fibrillation with a fast ventricular response may suffer from decreased cardiac output and serious cardiovascular compromise.

This arrhythmia is also associated with the formation of thrombi because of the stagnation of blood in the improperly contracting left atrium. It is this characteristic that is thought to be the cause of cerebral emboli. Evidence suggests that patients with recurrent paroxysmal atrial fibrillation have a 5-time greater risk of embolism stroke (Dalen, 1994).

In atrial fibrillation, digoxin is often used to decrease the ventricular rate to between 60 and 90 beats per minute. After digitalization, quinidine may be used to induce chemical cardioversion to normal sinus rhythm. Sotalol (Betapace), a new, promising antiarrhythmic, has been an effective pharmacologic agent in converting atrial fibrillation to normal sinus rhythm, with fewer side effects (Juul-Möller et al., 1990).

The treatment of atrial fibrillation may also involve the use of direct current (DC) cardioversion, which is effective in about 85% of euthyroid patients with normal electrolytes who do not respond to digitalis therapy (Pritchett, 1992). If the atria are enlarged, however, this arrhythmia is bound to recur. Because it is known that the incidence of stroke from atrial fibrillation is high, it is strongly recommended that all people with this arrhythmia be adequately treated with anticoagulants. People to be considered for exclusion from this therapy are those with a history of recent bleeding, alcohol abuse, poor compliance, and frequent falls (Dalen, 1994).

It is very important that older patients with recent-onset atrial fibrillation be evaluated for hyperthyroidism. Thyrotoxicosis is a reversible cause of this arrhythmia, which often manifests itself atypically with cardiac symptoms in the older patient. The treatment of asymptomatic older patients with atrial fibrillation at a reasonably normal overall ventricular rate may merely consist of treatment of the underlying cause, reassurance, and a decrease in dietary sodium.

Unlike atrial fibrillation, which often occurs in otherwise healthy older individuals, atrial flutter is unusual and is almost always a sign of disease, usually pulmonary embolism or organic heart disease. It may also result iatrogenically from the treatment of atrial fibrillation with digitalis. Atrial flutter is a less tenacious arrhythmia than is atrial fibrillation and is particularly responsive to cardioversion, which is often considered to be the treatment of choice. Other pharmacologic treatments used to reduce the heart rate in atrial flutter are verapamil, digoxin, procainamide, quinidine, propranolol, or combinations of these drugs, along with cardioversion.

Many arrhythmias are associated with the use of antiarrhythmic medications. Digitalis is a major drug that is not only used in the treatment of many tachyarrhythmias, but also is responsible for causing many arrhythmias. The myocardium of an older adult is particularly sensitive to the effects of digitalis, and even small amounts of the drug may trigger conduction disturbances. Arrhythmias commonly encountered that are caused by digitalis intoxication are ventricular premature complexes, paroxysmal or nonparoxysmal atrial tachycardias, and heart block. For this reason, digitalis should always be considered as a probable cause of any new arrhythmia occurring in a digitalized older patient. If such an arrhythmia should occur, digitalis should be discontinued or decreased, and the possibility of hypokalemia should be assessed. Medications used to treat ventricular arrhythmia may worsen the arrhythmia by triggering more ventricular beats, as documented by the CAST study (Aronow, 1995).

Rhythm disturbances are evaluated by assessing the apical and radial pulses, by interpreting 12-lead electrocardiograms (ECGs) and rhythm strips, and by use of in-hospital cardiac telemetry and 24-hour Holter monitoring. When treating the older patient with antiarrhythmic drugs, the nurse should always keep in mind that drug toxicity can very easily occur. Serum digoxin levels, for example, tend to be higher in older adults than in younger adults who receive the same dose, and the drug is also likely to remain active in the body of an older individual for a longer time. Therefore the nurse should be alert to signs of digoxin toxicity, such as gastrointestinal symptoms, bradycardia, heart block, and tachyarrhythmias. Also, the nurse needs to be wary of doses of digoxin greater than 0.125 mg or more per day.

STROKE AND TRANSIENT ISCHEMIC ATTACKS

Stroke is the third most common cause of death and a major reason for disability in the older adult population. Although the incidence of stroke has decreased over the past decade, it is clearly a disease of older adults, with the incidence increasing with age (Bruno, 1993a). The incidence of stroke is 10 times greater in people 75 to 84 years old than in people 55 to 64 years old. Approximately 75% of the 50,000 strokes that occur yearly affect those over 65 years of age.

The major risk factors for the occurrence of stroke include hypertension, diabetes mellitus, lipid abnormalities, atrial fibrillation, and congestive heart failure. Of these, hypertension is most important. Hypertension damages the lining of the vessels and increases the rate of plaque formation in the arteries. The formation of the atheromatous plaque increases the risk of thrombus formation, leading to cerebral infarction. The major causes of stroke are (1) cerebral infarction due to thrombus or embolism, (2) intracranial hemorrhage, and (3) subarachnoid hemorrhage. Approximately 80% of strokes are the result of cerebral infarction. Strokes are primarily characterized by sudden acute neurologic deficit. The most common symptoms are motor dysfunction, sensory alteration, speech or language deficit, vision disturbance, or any combination of these symptoms.

Initial medical treatment of stroke caused by cerebral infarction includes (1) control of blood pressure, (2) control of blood sugar, (3) control of stroke-related seizure activity, and (4) osmolar therapy to treat cerebral edema, in order to prevent herniation caused by increased intracranial pressure. Heparin is used for anticoagulation during the initial phase of the stroke once hemorrhagic stroke has been ruled out. Stroke prophylaxis after the initial critical period consists of both treatment of risk factors such as hypertension, smoking, and diabetes, and antiplatelet therapy or anticoagulation. Ticlopidine, an antiplatelet drug, has also been proven to reduce strokes in those patients who cannot tolerate aspirin (*1996 Physicians GenRx,* 1996). Older adults with an additional history of atrial fibrillation or valvular disease will require anticoagulation therapy such as administration of warfarin (Coumadin) for the rest of their lives. Aggressiveness of medical treatment in older adults will depend on the nature of coexisting diseases, as well as the individual's preference. Clinical trials are currently in progress to determine if a carotid endarterectomy is beneficial to patients who have had a stroke. Based on completed trials, it is believed that people with stenosis of greater than 70% will benefit from this surgical procedure (Bruno, 1993b).

Transient ischemic attacks are caused primarily by emboli that lodge in the retinal or small cerebral arteries but subsequently dissolve. The most common symptoms associated with cerebral ischemia caused by an embolus include paresis, paresthesia, and monocular or binocular visual disturbance. These symptoms usually last less than 20 minutes and resolve completely within 24 hours. Reports are varied on the relationship between TIA and stroke. Approximately 30% of people with TIA who are untreated may go on to develop a stroke (Bruno, 1993b). Treatment of older adults with TIA is similar to that described previously.

Older adults who experience the symptoms of TIA are often very fearful that they will have a stroke and become even more debilitated and dependent. They also fear injury from falling during a TIA. Often, any event that threatens further dependency becomes terrifying.

PERIPHERAL VASCULAR DISEASE

Collateral arterial circulation in the legs is often sufficient to ensure minimally adequate perfusion of the lower extremities, even in the presence of considerable narrowing of the arterial lumina of major vessels. Should arterial occlusion occur, however, it is essential that blood flow be restored within 4 to 6 hours to avoid necrosis and loss of the limb. Nurses must recognize the clinical presentation of lower extremity arterial occlusion, which includes "the six *p*'s": (1) pallor, (2) pain, (3) pulselessness, (4) paresthesia, (5) paralysis, and (6) "polar" (i.e., coldness of the limb). These symptoms represent the end point of arterial occlusion. Kelley (1989) describes two other important indicators of arterial occlusion: loss of sensation of light touch on the toes, and decreased ability to move toes, especially to dorsiflex the great toe.

A more common presentation of arterial peripheral vascular disease (PVD), however, is that of intermittent claudication. *Claudication,* a term that comes from the Latin meaning to limp, denotes ischemia with exercise. This disorder, which is commonly encountered in older patients, is especially prevalent in smokers. In this condition, there is a narrowing of the arteries that feed the lower extremities. The narrowed arteries can just compensate with a minimal blood flow under resting conditions. With exercise such as walking, however, the requirement for oxygen to the legs is increased 5 to 7 times, and this level of tissue oxygen need can no longer be met (Kelley, 1989). Lower extremity ischemia gives rise to a dull aching pain in the calf or thigh, which abates with rest. Patients often describe claudication pain as a "charley horse" or leg muscle cramp, and they can describe a particular walking distance required to bring it on (this is called the "claudication distance"). Claudication pain should subside after only a few minutes of rest. These clinical features are referred to as the walk-pain-rest cycle.

Intermittent claudication should not be confused with pseudoclaudication, a neurospinal disorder in which the walk-pain-rest cycle is not consistent from day to day. Patients affected by pseudoclaudication describe experiencing good and bad days, and relief from their leg pain is obtained by either sitting up or lying down (Thiele & Strandness, 1994).

Authentic intermittent claudication can progress to leg pain at rest, which is a much more ominous condition. In cases of pain at rest, the patient experiences severe aching of the lower extremities, usually over the foot and toes. This pain typically occurs at night while the patient is in bed, when the feet are elevated or flat. In this position, the arterial flow is more compromised than when legs and feet are dependent, as when sitting or standing. Patients with this level of arterial occlusion often describe a need to dangle their legs over the side of the bed to obtain relief from the pain. This degree of compromise of the arterial circulation to the legs can result in ulceration, gangrene, infection, tissue necrosis, and limb loss.

Conservative management of intermittent claudication is usually all that is recommended. Arteriography and possible surgery are saved for the most serious cases involving advanced symptoms. Patients are implored to stop smoking at once and are advised to maintain an optimal weight, and to walk daily up to the point of pain tolerance. Pentoxifylline, a drug used to lower blood viscosity by making the red blood cells more deformable, is the only medication proven to be beneficial for patients with claudication. Vasodilators should usually be avoided because generalized vasodilation could actually siphon blood away from the lower extremities, further compromising this critical blood supply (Giordano, 1983). Patients with intermittent claudication can usually be reassured that the risk of limb loss is relatively low (approximately 1% per year) even without treatment; among diabetic patients the incidence increases to 5% per year (Thiele & Strandness, 1994).

Older diabetic patients with arterial PVD of the lower extremities have a more serious problem because of the frequent combination of (1) arterial compromise below the knee with (2) peripheral neuropathy that often leads to infection, ulceration, gangrene, and/or osteomyelitis. Unfortunately, lower extremity vascular surgery in people with diabetes is much less likely to produce a good result than is surgery in a nondiabetic patient. Poor perfusion of the foot occurs because of the predilection of diabetes to affect the patency of the medium-sized arteries below the knee (the tibial and peroneal arteries). Therefore it is absolutely essential that diabetic patients have their feet inspected regularly, and they should be counseled about the importance of wearing comfortable, well-fitting shoes that will not create blisters or calluses. A podiatrist may be very helpful in providing foot care.

VARICOSE VEINS

Varicose veins are primarily the result of valvular incompetence occurring in the superficial system of veins, which returns about 10% of venous blood from the lower extremities to the heart. Varicosities occur because of the failure of the valves or because of distention or weakening of the venous walls, which reduces the ability of the valves to close adequately. Obesity, tight-fitting garments, and increased body fluid contribute to the development of varicose veins. This extra strain on the veins causes them to widen, lengthen, and become distended. The tortuous veins then create more distention because of the increased pressure of the fluid load within the poorly supported, superficial peripheral veins. The lower leg edema created by this increase in fluid under pressure usually subsides overnight. This disorder is very common in older women, and a positive family history is considered an important risk factor. Unless there is venous insufficiency, varicose veins tend to be asymptomatic. With true insufficiency of venous return, however, patients complain of aching in the calves of their legs, which is alleviated when the legs are elevated. Prolonged standing and sitting tend to exacerbate this condition. The use of elastic stockings, which are applied early in the day while the patient is supine, can also minimize the aching and swelling.

CHRONIC VENOUS INSUFFICIENCY

Chronic venous insufficiency, unlike simple varicose veins, is thought to result from incompetence in the deep venous system, although it is manifested in the superficial venous system. Called the "postphlebitic syndrome," the chronic aching, edema, and skin changes are usually caused by destruction of the valves because of a previous inflammatory process in the vein. Damage to the deep venous system also may follow an episode of significantly elevated intravascular venous pressure, which can lead to edema and extravasation of red blood cells

(RBCs) and plasma proteins into the superficial tissues, with discoloration and induration of the skin. The brownish discoloration tends to occur on the medial aspect of the lower leg, which may eventually lead to ulcer formation because of a deficiency in tissue oxygen. These ulcers are not only slow to heal, but also prone to infection. Patients with this disorder may benefit from application of dressings applied upward from the toes to the knee. Once healing has occurred, the patient should be fitted with support hose to prevent a recurrence of the edema and ulceration.

Many older patients, as well as younger ones, develop thrombophlebitis of the lower legs. In this disorder there is obstruction and inflammation of a leg vein, usually as a result of a thrombus, trauma, infection, or hypercoagulability; this results in the formation of a clot within the vein. Factors that predispose a person to developing thrombophlebitis are surgery (especially prostate and hip surgery), trauma to the legs, prolonged bed rest, venous stasis, and varicose veins. The patient may have the presenting symptom of a reddened leg, which is warm to the touch around the area of the inflamed vein, and which may or may not be associated with significant swelling. The patient may complain of an increasingly painful leg, which becomes even more uncomfortable when walking or standing. There may be a hard, tender, thrombosed cord along the course of the vein, and often a red streak is visible. This disorder is generally not prone to embolization and therefore will respond to conservative treatment. This treatment consists of heat, elevation of the leg, the use of elastic support stockings, and anti-inflammatory medication.

On the other hand, deep vein thrombosis (DVT) often does not manifest itself so obviously at first because the deep veins are not as available for surface examination, and the signs and symptoms may be minimal. It is not uncommon for the first indication of DVT to be in connection with a diagnosis of pulmonary embolism, when the health care provider examines the legs in a search for the cause. A pulmonary embolism results when a clot from a deep vein breaks loose and lodges in the lungs. Because DVT may manifest itself more subtly, it is very important to pursue any complaint of leg pain in an older patient. In this disorder, the affected limb may be either pale or reddened, and the leg will be normal to warm in temperature. Swelling, however, may be marked with DVT, and the superficial veins may appear to be engorged. It is important to measure the circumference of a swollen leg at the thigh, knee, and ankle, and to compare these measurements with those of the other leg over time. It is a good idea to mark on the legs where these measurements were obtained so that the data will reflect the change in circumference and not the difference in the exact area of the leg being measured.

Superficial thrombophlebitis can be treated with bed rest, compression of the vein with elastic stockings, local heat, and anti-inflammatory medication. Deep vein thrombosis

Health Promotion
Components of a health promotion education program
1. Promote healthy lifestyle
2. Promote daily exercise
3. Promote adequate nutrition
4. Promote compliance with pharmacologic therapy
5. Promote self-esteem and independence
6. Promote social and recreational participation

is more serious and, in addition to these measures, usually requires hospitalization for heparin therapy and bed rest to ward off the possibility of thromboembolization. Oral anticoagulant treatment with warfarin is continued for a time after heparin therapy has been discontinued.

Exercise is important. *Courtesy Loy Ledbetter, St. Louis.*

Other objectives target reducing use of tobacco, as outlined in the chapter on respiratory function. Counseling an older person on the benefits of physical activity, a balanced diet, maintaining an ideal body weight, and eliminating the use of tobacco and alcohol is challenging. Assessing a person's physical activity habits includes asking about organized and general activities. House and yard work, as well as walking, can be adequate forms of exercise if accumulated time is greater than 30 minutes per day, 5 days a week (USDHHS, 1994). For an organized activity such as brisk walking or swimming, the American College of Sports Medicine suggests that the goal is to maintain at least 55% of the target heart rate for 20 minutes, 4 times a week. Discussing the types of activities an older person enjoys can assist the nurse in designing an exercise program together with the patient. Table 10-3 outlines suggestions to make when counseling older patients on overcoming barriers to exercise. Many organizations have specific exercise programs to meet the needs of the older adult population. These exercise programs are designed to have more time for warm-up and cool-down periods, and they teach self-monitoring of heart rate so that the goal of 50% to 60% of maximum heart rate is achieved and maintained. Organized group programs provide a format for other education programs and risk factor screening. For those patients who may require tertiary preventive measures after they have experienced a cardiovascular event, an organized cardiac rehabilitation activity program may be suggested.

Dietary counseling is considered both a primary and secondary preventive measure. Regardless of age, a person can be educated on the components of a healthy diet. A brief questionnaire can be used to assess an older person's nutritional health (Box 10-2). If an older person is identified as having either a high-risk nutritional score or high risk for cardiovascular disease, counseling on the essential components of a healthy diet is necessary. Patients should be given the basic information as recommended by the Dietary Guidelines for Americans (Box 10-3). In addition, supportive information assisting patients in reading food labels and understanding the Food Guide Pyramid is necessary if a patient is to meet these guidelines. The nurse needs to take the time necessary to review this information with the older individual. The nurse has the ability to provide adequate assessment of the older person's understanding and to provide a forum for personal questions to address the patient's needs.

Cholesterol levels can be lowered through dietary changes or medication. To reduce the total cholesterol level (TCL), a reduction in calories is often necessary, as well as a reduction in cholesterol and saturated fat intake. The daily intake should consist of only 30% total fat, and only 10% of the fat intake should be in saturated fats. Care must be taken, however, in recommending caloric restrictions to the older adult. Caloric restrictions even in an obese older person may cause protein caloric malnutrition, putting the person at risk for immunologic compromise and possible death from an ensuing infection. Any dietary change for the older adult must be made with recognition of the fact that a change in one area can produce an adverse effect in another. In addition, the recommended dietary substitutions of fish for red meat may present a financial hardship. If dietary changes are to be effectively implemented, the individual who does the shopping or meal preparation, as well as the older individual, must be part of the planning process.

Providing time for a discussion with both the patient and the person responsible for shopping and preparing meals is necessary to formulate a meal plan that everyone will enjoy.

■ Health Promotion and Education

Adopting a specific lifestyle is a personal choice. The challenge and goals set forth by the Healthy People 2000 Objectives are designed to educate the population and promote tools to assist people in the maintenance of a healthy lifestyle.

TABLE 10-3 Overcoming barriers to exercise

Barrier	Suggested response
Exercise is hard work.	Pick an activity that you enjoy and that is easy for you.
I do not have the time.	We are only talking about three 20-minute sessions per week. Could you do without three TV shows each week?
I am usually too tired for exercise.	Tell yourself, "This activity will give me more energy." See if it doesn't happen.
I hate to fail, so I will not start.	Physical activity is not a test. You will not fail if you choose an activity you like and start off slowly.
I do not have anyone to work out with.	Maybe you have not asked. A neighbor or a co-worker may be a willing partner. Or you can choose an activity that you enjoy doing by yourself.
There is not a convenient place.	Pick an activity you can do at a convenient place. Walk around your neighborhood or do exercises with a TV show or a videotape at home.
I am afraid of being injured.	Walking is very safe and is excellent exercise. Choose a safe, well-lit area.
The weather is too bad.	There are many activities that you can do in your own home, in any weather.
Exercise is boring.	Listening to music during your activity keeps your mind occupied. Walking, biking, or running can take you past lots of interesting things.
I am too overweight.	You can benefit regardless of your weight. Pick an activity that you are comfortable with, like walking.
I am too old.	It is never too late to start. People of any age, including older people, can benefit from physical exercise.

Adapted from Project PACE, *Physician-based Assessment and Counseling for Exercise*. San Diego, CA: San Diego State University; 1991. Used with permission of the publisher; © 1991.

Primary prevention interventions educate the population in the importance of maintaining an ideal weight, eliminating tobacco use, limiting alcohol use, exercising daily, and having a healthy diet. Secondary prevention programs are to identify people who are at risk for developing CAD. Designing programs for people who have been identified as having CAD risk factors has shown to be effective in reducing mortality and morbidity from cardiovascular disease (Pearson et al, 1994). It is never too late for a person to learn new behaviors and incorporate them into his or her life. If initial time is given to educating a patient, benefits will accrue. Research supports the fact that if an older person engages in health promotion activity and becomes an active participant, the results will be positive.

Restriction of salt intake may have multiple benefits, in addition to treating hypertension. However, to maintain the older adult's interest in food, it may be more helpful to suggest limiting the amount of salt used, and not adding salt to prepared food, rather than encouraging a no-salt diet. This represents the difference between a 2- and a 4-gram sodium intake. Food can be cooked with light salt, but no additional salt should be added; and salty foods such as canned soups, ham, and bacon should be avoided. Exploring

BOX 10-2 WARNING SIGNS OF POOR NUTRITION

The Warning Signs of poor nutritional health are often overlooked. Use this checklist to find out if you or someone you know is at nutritional risk.

Read the statements below. Circle the number in the yes column for those that apply to you or someone you know. For each yes answer, score the number in the box. Total your nutritional score.

DETERMINE YOUR NUTRITIONAL HEALTH

	YES
I have an illness or condition that made me change the kind and/or amount of food I eat.	2
I eat fewer than 2 meals per day.	3
I eat few fruits or vegetables or milk products.	2
I have 3 or more drinks of beer, liquor, or wine almost every day.	2
I have tooth or mouth problems that make it hard for me to eat.	2
I don't always have enough money to buy the food I need.	4
I eat alone most of the time.	1
I take 3 or more different prescribed or over-the-counter drugs a day.	1
Without wanting to, I have lost or gained 10 pounds in the last 6 months.	2
I am not always physically able to shop, cook, and/or feed myself.	2
TOTAL	

Total Your Nutritional Score. If it's —

0-2 **Good!** Recheck your nutritional score in 6 months.

3-5 **You are at moderate nutritional risk.** See what can be done to improve your eating habits and lifestyle. Your office on aging, senior nutrition program, senior citizens center, or health department can help. Recheck your nutritional score in 3 months.

6 or more **You are at high nutritional risk.** Bring this checklist the next time you see your doctor, dietitian, or other qualified health or social service professional. Talk with them about any problems you may have. Ask for help to improve your nutritional health.

These materials developed and distributed by the Nutrition Screening Initiative, a project of:

 AMERICAN ACADEMY OF FAMILY PHYSICIANS

 THE AMERICAN DIETETIC ASSOCIATION

 NATIONAL COUNCIL ON THE AGING, INC.

Remember that warning signs suggest risk, but do not represent diagnosis of any condition. Turn the page to learn more about the Warning Signs of poor nutritional health.

Reprinted with permission by the Nutrition Screening Initiative, a project of the American Academy of Family Physicians, the American Dietetic Association, and the National Council on the Aging, Inc., and funded in part by a grant from Ross Products Division, Abbott Laboratories.

BOX 10-3 DIETARY GUIDELINES FOR AMERICANS*

1. Eat a variety of foods.
2. Maintain a healthy weight.
3. Choose a diet low in total fat (less than 30% of calories), saturated fat (less than 10% of calories), and cholesterol.
4. Choose a diet with plenty of vegetables, fruits, and grain products (five or more servings daily).
5. Use sugars only in moderation.
6. Use salt and sodium only in moderation.
7. If you drink alcoholic beverages, do so only in moderation (no more than one drink daily for women or 2 drinks daily for men). Women who are pregnant or planning to become pregnant should not drink at all.

From U.S. Department of Agriculture and U.S. Department of Health and Human Services.
*Use these dietary guidelines with the Food Guide Pyramid.

substitute seasonings can be very helpful in ensuring that food still tastes good. If the patient uses prepared foods, encourage the use of frozen foods low in salt instead of canned or packaged foods.

The zeal to control cardiovascular risk should not lead to a decrease in the overall quality of nutritional intake or to a compromise in nutritional status. The overall goal of maintaining an ideal body weight can usually be achieved if the diet and exercise guidelines described previously are observed. If an older person's weight is not within the recommended range for his or her age and height, it may be necessary to provide additional support group activities and dietary information to assist him or her in achieving this goal.

Another important part of educating older adults is providing clear and complete information regarding medications. Older people may be taking several prescribed drugs as well as several over-the-counter (OTC) medications because of multiple medical problems. Education should cover the name of the medication, dosage, interval for taking the medication, and why the medication was prescribed. Special precautions should be discussed (Box 10-4). Medications that are of timed-release form should never be broken or crushed. Ask the patient to restate medication information before leaving an office visit or hospital. This intervention provides an opportunity for questions and clarification of the specific medication regimen. Older adults may benefit from an audiotape schedule of the medication regimen, or a written schedule that can be placed on the refrigerator or medicine cabinet as a reminder. Containers should have an easy-open lid and typing on the label that is large enough to read. In addition, the older patient should have a pocket-sized list of medications to be carried daily in case of an emergency and that can be reviewed at office and home care visits.

Nurses can be very instrumental in educating patients, evaluating their progress, and offering support. Many times a creative individual program jointly designed by the nurse and the patient is necessary to ensure compliance. Building a relationship to assist older patients in incorporating new behaviors into their day-to-day activities may be a challenge, but the overall benefits are worth the effort. The use of every interaction to teach or clarify a health promotion activity will convey the nurse's interest in patients' well-being and provide an opportunity for positive feedback and encouragement on a job well done.

■ Nursing Process

Obtaining an accurate and complete picture of a problem from an older adult is challenging at times. Changes that occur in older adults are often insidious and heightened by the combina-

Healthy People 2000 Objectives

To reduce heart disease and stroke, by the year 2000 . . .

15.1 Reduce coronary heart disease deaths to no more than 100 per 100,000 people (a 26% decrease). (Age-adjusted baseline: 135 per 100,000 in 1987.)

15.2 Reduce stroke deaths to no more than 20 per 100,000 people (a 34% decrease). (Age-adjusted baseline: 30.3 per 100,000 in 1987.)

15.4 Increase control of high blood pressure to at least 50% of people with high blood pressure (a 108% increase). (Baseline: 11% controlled among people aged 18 through 74 in 1976-80; an estimated 24% for people aged 18 and older in 1982-84.)

15.6 Reduce blood cholesterol to an average of no more than 200 mg/dL (a 6% decrease). (Baseline: 213 mg/dL among people aged 20 through 74 in 1976-80, 211 mg/dL for men and 215 mg/dL for women.)

To increase physical activity and fitness, by the year 2000 . . .

1.3 Increase moderate daily physical activity to at least 30% of people (a 36% increase). (Baseline: 22% of people aged 18 and older were active for at least 30 minutes 5 or more times per week and 12% were active 7 or more times per week in 1985.)

1.5 Reduce sedentary lifestyles to no more than 15% of people (a 38% decrease). (Baseline: 24% for people aged 18 and older in 1985.)

To improve nutrition, by the year 2000 . . .

2.3 Reduce overweight to a prevalence of no more than 20% of people (a 23% decrease). (Baseline: 26% for people aged 20 through 74 in 1976-80, 24% for men and 27% for women; 15% for adolescents aged 12 through 19 in 1976-80.)

2.5 Reduce dietary fat intake to an average of 30% of the calories (a 17% decrease). (Baseline: 36% of calories from total fat and 13% from saturated fat for people aged 20 through 74 in 1976-80; 36% and 13% for women aged 19 through 50.)

From U.S. Department of Health and Human Services. (1990). *Healthy People 2000: National health promotion and disease prevention objectives.* (DHHS Pub. No. [PHS] 91-50212). Washington, DC: U.S. Government Printing Office.

tion of normal changes of aging, pathologic processes, and pharmacologic therapies. The most important concept on which to base nursing care is to remember the effect of these combined changes on the functional capacity of the older adult. As a person ages, the functional impact from cardiovascular disease can be profound.

ASSESSMENT

An appropriate assessment of cardiovascular function will include both a history and a physical examination, although the most useful data collected from the assessment will be from the history. The patient's energy available for providing historical information may be extremely limited. People with severe cardiovascular problems may suffer from both physical and mental decrements. When the patient is a poor historian, the family, friends, or other responsible parties may be of significant help. Information may also be obtained from the health record, if it is available. Some older patients may not report clear symptoms

BOX 10-4 COMMONLY USED DRUGS FOR CARDIOVASCULAR PROBLEMS

Digoxin
    Indications
        Heart failure
        Atrial fibrillation
    Actions
        Positive inotropic action
        Negative chronotropic action
        Decreases conduction through AV node
    Selected side effects
        Anorexia
        Nausea and vomiting
        Arrhythmias, both fast and slow
        Yellow or green vision disturbances
        Muscle weakness
        Central nervous system alterations; confusion and depression
    Precautions and special considerations
        Narrow therapeutic window
        Eliminated more slowly in older adults
        Hypokalemia may enhance digoxin toxicity
        Loading and maintenance dose to be started at half the recommended adult dose
        Monitor pulse rate, rhythm, edema, and changes in weight
Beta-adrenergic blockers (atenolol, metoprolol, propranolol, sotalol, timolol)
    Indications
        Hypertension
        Angina pectoris, due to coronary atherosclerosis
        Cardiac arrhythmias
        Myocardial infarction
    Actions
        Reduce myocardial work load and oxygen consumption
        Decrease heart rate, myocardial contractility, and BP
    Selected side effects
        Exacerbation of CHF, AV block
        Hypotension
        Lightheadedness
        Bronchospasm
        Masking of symptoms of hypoglycemia
    Precautions and special considerations
        Should not be used in patients with CHF, chronic obstructive pulmonary disease, asthma, heart
            block, or SSS
        Use with caution in insulin-treated diabetic patients and patients with PVD
        Should be withdrawn slowly in patients with angina
        Instruct patients to rise slowly from lying down and avoid prolonged standing

BOX 10-4 COMMONLY USED DRUGS FOR CARDIOVASCULAR PROBLEMS—cont'd

Diuretics (thiazide, hydrochlorothiazide; loop diuretics, furosemide; potassium-sparing agents, spirono-lactone)

    Indications

        Hypertension

        CHF

        Edema

    Action

        Inhibit reabsorption of sodium and water in kidneys

    Selected side effects

        Hypokalemia or hyperkalemia

        Hyperuricemia

        Glucose intolerance

        Hypercholesteremia

        Hypertriglyceridemia

        Orthostatic hypotension

    Precautions and special considerations

        Monitor serum electrolytes

        May precipitate acute gout

Angiotensin-converting enzyme inhibitors (captopril, enalapril)

    Indications

        Hypertension

        Heart failure, in addition to digitalis and diuretics

    Actions

        Inhibit the conversion of angiotensin I into angiotensin II

        Decrease action of renin, therefore sodium and fluid retention

        Prevent vasoconstriction

        Reduce preload and afterload

    Selected side effects

        Hyperkalemia

        Dry cough

        Rash

        Loss of taste sensation

        Angioneurotic edema

    Precautions and special considerations

        Can cause proteinuria and reversible acute renal failure

        Hypotension may be seen with the initial dose

Calcium antagonists (verapamil, diltiazem, nifedipine)

    Indications

        Hypertension

        Angina

        Supraventricular tachyarrhythmias

    Actions

        Inhibit entry of extracellular calcium into smooth muscle cells and myocardial cells

        Decrease AV node conduction

        Vasodilated—dilate coronary arteries and decrease PVR

        Negative inotropic action

Continued

BOX 10-4 COMMONLY USED DRUGS FOR CARDIOVASCULAR PROBLEMS—cont'd

Selected side effects
  Flushing
  Headaches
  Weakness
  Dizziness
  CHF
  Constipation
  Third-degree AV block
Precautions and special considerations
  May cause liver dysfunction
  Monitor BP and for signs of hypotension
  Assess for signs of CHF
Antiarrhythmic agents (quinidine, disopyramide, and procainamide—group I A; propranolol—II C; verapamil—IV C)
  Indication
    Arrhythmias
  Actions
    Slow conduction and prolong myocardial refractory period
    Prolong action potential period
    Slow AV conduction
    Prolong AV node refractory period
  Selected side effects
    Hypotension
    Nausea and diarrhea
    Drug-induced lupus associated with procainamide and quinidine
  Precautions and special considerations
    Caution with hepatorenal disease
    All antiarrhythmics may worsen or cause other arrhythmias
    Monitor VS and ECG
Nitrates (nitroglycerin, isosorbide)
  Indication
    Angina pectoris
  Actions
    Vasodilatation
    Decrease preload and afterload
    Decrease myocardial oxygen requirements by decreasing PVR and reducing work load
  Selected side effects
    Hypotension
    Reflex tachycardia
    Headaches
  Precautions and special considerations
    Tolerance may occur with long-term use
    Alcohol consumption may cause flushing, pallor, weakness, hypotension, and syncope
    Sublingual nitroglycerin must be stored in a cool dry place and renewed every 6 months

---

BOX 10-4 COMMONLY USED DRUGS FOR CARDIOVASCULAR PROBLEMS—cont'd

Salicylates (aspirin, such as Ecotrin)
  Indications
    Cerebral vascular accident (CVA)
    Venous emboli
    Cerebral ischemia
    Need for inhibition of platelet aggregations
  Action
    Block formation of platelet thromboxane A_2
  Selected side effects
    Gastric distress and heartburn
  Precautions and special considerations
    Patients with asthma may develop a hypersensitivity reaction
    Consider use of an enteric-coated ASA (e.g., Ecotrin), and suggest patients take ASA with food if
      they experience gastrointestinal upset
    May cause prolonged bleeding and bruising, especially in conjunction with anticoagulant therapy
Anticoagulants (warfarin)
  Indications
    Chronic atrial fibrillation
    Venous thrombosis
  Actions
    Prolong clotting time
    Prevent recurrent TIA
  Selected side effects
    Hemorrhage
    Nausea
    Dermatitis
  Precautions and special considerations
    Monitor prothrombine time or INR
    Other medications and a diet rich in vitamin K will alter blood level
    Should not be taken with aspirin or nonsteroidal antiinflammatory medication

---

because they feel that discomfort and failing health are simply an expected part of aging. The assessment of cardiovascular function must be integrated into a complete assessment, to develop a plan of care that takes into account the strengths and weaknesses of the individual. In addition, the patient or responsible party should participate in the development of the plan of care.

History

The histories of cardiovascular problems are as varied as the types of problems that can affect the cardiovascular system. The symptoms can have an abrupt onset, or a slow, almost undetectable course. Questions that are particularly important to ask include the following:

1. Do you have a history of heart or vascular problems?
2. Do you take any medication for heart or vascular problems?
3. Have you had any of the following symptoms?
   a. Shortness of breath on exertion (If so, how much exertion?)

    b. Cough

    c. Swelling of your ankles or lower legs (Or have your shoes felt tight?)

    d. Chest pain, or leg or thigh pain

    e. Disturbance of sleep because of difficulty in breathing

    f. Palpitations, irregular heartbeats, or pounding heart

    g. Leg pain with exercise (If yes, how long did it take to subside after you stopped the exercise?)

    h. Dizziness or lightheadedness on standing

4. How many pillows do you sleep on at night? If more than one, is it because of shortness of breath?

5. Do you have a history of high blood pressure, diabetes, high cholesterol, smoking, severe chest pain, heart attacks, or strokes?

6. Do you know what your normal blood pressure is?

7. Do you know what your cholesterol level was when last measured?

8. Do you exercise on a regular schedule? If so, what type of exercise do you do, and for how long?

9. When did you have your last chest x-ray examination? Your last electrocardiogram?

10. Do you eat three meals a day? Who prepares your meals?

Physical examination

The equipment necessary to assess the cardiovascular function of older patients includes a stethoscope, an ophthalmoscope (funduscope), a sphygmomanometer, a tuning fork, and a sharp object. The techniques used in examination of the cardiovascular system will primarily involve inspection, palpation, and auscultation. The following areas should be included in the physical examination:

1. The vital signs should be checked—BP, heart rate, and respiratory rate. Be sure to check the BP in both arms initially. The BP should also be taken with the individual in a supine and then a standing position to evaluate the possibility of orthostatic hypotension. The apical pulse should be counted for 60 seconds, to determine whether an arrhythmia exists.

2. Body weight should be checked daily in individuals with CHF.

3. A funduscopic examination should be performed on patients, especially those with hypertension, diabetes mellitus, hyperlipidemia, and PVD. Observe for arteriovenous nicking, small hemorrhages or tortuous vessels, and/or exudates.

4. The lungs of patients with CHF may have crackles in the bases. The level of the crackles extending upward from the bases is associated with the severity of the CHF. Instruct the person to take a deep breath through the nose and out the mouth. The lung sounds may be very difficult to hear in older patients who are bed bound, who are in persistent vegetative states, or who have significantly reduced levels of consciousness. In these cases, respirations are frequently shallow.

5. The heart sounds of S_1 and S_2, which are normally heard in the patient without cardiovascular disease, may be accompanied by an extra sound, such as the S_3 sound that is commonly heard with CHF. Extra beats or dropped beats may also be present in patients with arrhythmias or conduction disturbances. Murmurs may be present and may indicate a valvular disorder. Heart sounds are frequently difficult to hear in older adults because of an increase in the air space in the lungs, which muffles the sounds. Other sounds, such as breath sounds, vocal sounds, and gastric gurgling may interfere with accurately hearing the heart sounds. Listening for carotid bruits and inspecting for jugular venous distention are also important parts of the examination of the heart.

6. When peripheral vascular disease is a concern, palpation and auscultation of pulses in the lower extremities are important. Periph-

eral vascular examination of the lower extremities should also include assessment of the skin for color changes, decreased temperature of one limb versus the other, skin atrophy (shiny, thin skin), and a decreased distribution of hair on the lower legs and toes. The feet should also be carefully assessed for any evidence of erythema, blisters, calluses, sores, infections, or ulcerations, and the toenails should be examined for thickening or pitting. Capillary refill time elicited by pressing on the nail bed of a toe should normally be less than 15 seconds. When refill takes more than 40 seconds, severe vascular disease may be present. Pedal or lower leg edema may be present in patients with venous insufficiency or right-sided heart failure. Edema should be graded as to severity on a scale of 1 to 4, with 4 being the most severe. The level of edema should also be determined.

7. Peripheral neuropathy should be evaluated by testing deep tendon reflexes, sensory function (light touch), and motor function (pinprick, proprioception, and vibratory sense). Arterial occlusion of the lower legs should also be evaluated by assessing response to light touch on the toes, and the ability to move and dorsiflex the toes, especially the large toes.

8. A mental status examination (MSE) should be routinely performed on older patients because some changes in mental status may be important signs of disease and/or may indicate the presence of a reversible delirium.

It is important to keep in mind that in older patients, signs of cardiovascular disease may be minimal or undetectable through physical examination. This may be particularly true in the case of unsymptomatic CAD, hypertension controlled with medication, and CHF.

Psychosocial assessment

A critical component of any assessment is to ask individuals, if competent, whom they would like to have make decisions for them if they should become unable to make decisions about their care themselves. This is particularly important for individuals with cardiovascular problems because of the significant risk of their experiencing a life-threatening event, with subsequent initiation of life support treatment that may range from artificial feeding and hydration through a gastric tube to artificial ventilation. Many individuals have strong feelings about what they would and would not want to have happen to them should a massive stroke or myocardial infarction occur, and it is clearly in the patient's best interest that these wishes be explored and put in writing. Individuals in nursing homes or in private or family homes may not want to be hospitalized even if they are experiencing an acute life-threatening event. Because of the risk of cardiac arrest, an assessment of whether the patient would want to be resuscitated is very important. If possible, older adults should be encouraged to give their durable power of attorney for health to someone of their choice. If this is not possible, they should at least identify someone whom they can trust to speak for them. Careful documentation of the person's desires is extremely important.

The patient's fears concerning the possible occurrence of a stroke or heart attack, or the possibility of an amputation of a leg because of PVD, should be assessed. Many older adults fear debilitation and dependency more than death. Another common fear is that something will happen to them while they are alone and that they will remain alone and injured or ill for a long time before someone finds them.

A very broad concept of family is frequently useful when considering the family assessment of an older adult. (See Box 10-5 for considerations in assessing the patient's family.) It is not unusual for older adults to have survived their spouses, their siblings, and even their children. The closest family member may be a grandchild, a niece, or a nephew. For those living in their own

---

BOX 10-5 FAMILY ASSESSMENT

1. Are the family members whom the patient has designated to be involved in health care decisions aware of this expectation?
2. Who are the family members who provide care, and what is their role in caring for the patient's cardiovascular needs?
3. What kinds of stress does caring for the patient impose on the individual family members?
4. What is the level of knowledge among family members about the patient's condition, and who is their primary source of information?
5. How do family members feel about the patient's decisions regarding resuscitation orders and life support interventions?
6. What barriers block the participation of family members in the care of the patient?

---

homes, the home health aide may be the only "family" the older adult has. Similarly, the nursing staff of a nursing home may serve as surrogate family members for older adults needing nursing home care. Finally, a court-designated responsible party may have the decision-making prerogative that is traditionally reserved for relatives.

An individual with cardiovascular problems may need assistance in obtaining medications and in taking them correctly. If dietary modifications are part of the care plan, those who shop for and prepare food need to be included in the patient-family education and planning.

It is important to assess how cardiovascular problems have affected the patient's self-concept and ability to function. The following topics would be appropriate to discuss:

1. The patient's perceptions of the cardiovascular problem (or problems)

2. The patient's perceptions of the effects of cardiovascular problems on normal activities of daily living and on instrumental activities of daily living
3. The patient's fears about the effects of the cardiovascular problem
4. What the patient sees as his or her future
5. The cultural or spiritual meaning to the patient of the experience with the cardiovascular problem
6. The effect of the cardiovascular problem on the psychologic functioning of the patient—is there a feeling of hopelessness, anxiety, or depression?
7. What the patient does that is pleasurable each day and what the patient would like to do that he or she is not currently doing
8. The patient's knowledge of and ability to manage the medical and nursing treatments
9. How the patient's body image or feeling of attractiveness has been affected by the cardiovascular problem

Environmental assessment: Living arrangement

The environment in which the older adult with cardiovascular problems lives can either support the maximal functioning of the individual, or present barriers that may cause unnecessary dependency, especially in the patient's home. The environmental assessment for a private or family home specific to cardiovascular problems is presented in Box 10-6. Environmental assessment should also be performed for individuals in nursing homes or hospitals. The assessment in these settings specific to cardiovascular problems should include the following questions:

1. Do noise levels exist that might cause extreme stress and sleep deprivation, such as from noisy roommates or noise from patient care equipment?
2. Is the temperature level comfortable? Too warm an environment may exacerbate CHF, whereas too cold an environment may cause further circulatory compromise in someone with PVD.

BOX 10-6 ENVIRONMENTAL ASSESSMENT

1. What is the length of the hallway from the patient's apartment to the elevator or building entrance?
2. Are there stairways, and how many times a day does the patient have to climb the stairs?
3. If oxygen is needed, is there space for the equipment in the patient's bedroom? Can the oxygen be moved easily to a different room, if necessary, and can it be taken out of the home if the patient leaves?
4. Is there a suitable stool, chair, or sofa on which the patient can prop up his or her legs if pedal edema is a problem?
5. Are there sharp edges on the furniture or loose scatter rugs that could cause injury to the patient with arterial insufficiency, syncopal episodes, or orthostatic hypotension?
6. Is a telephone or other lifeline means of communication within easy reach should an emergency occur, such as severe chest pain?
7. Are the kitchen facilities designed for safety?
8. Does the bathroom have an elevated toilet seat, bars to assist in getting off the toilet, and bars in the shower or bath to assist in getting in and out of the shower, and is the bathroom free of hazards that would result in a fall?
9. Are laundry facilities accessible?
10. Is there a community environment for walking and interacting with other people?

Resource assessment

Older adults with cardiovascular problems may need the use of community resources either to stay in their homes or to return to their homes after a hospitalization. The types of community resources frequently needed are equipment, such as oxygen or a hospital bed in which the head can be easily elevated, or adaptive devices, such as a bedside commode to allow the patient to avoid strain. There may be a need for a home health aide who can do grocery shopping and meal preparation, as well as assisting with activities of daily living. There may be a need for a prosthetic device following a limb amputation due to PVD. The patient who has had an amputation also may need a physical therapist to come into the home, for further rehabilitation related to the use of a prosthesis.

The resources used will depend in large part not only on the availability of a service but also on the ability to pay for the service. Some services provided through community resources are covered through private insurance plans, Medicare, or Medicaid. To be eligible for Medicaid, an individual must meet the income requirements of the state in which the individual lives. Medicare, the federally sponsored program, pays for a number of services provided in the home. The support system of friends, family, volunteers, home health aides, and nurses and other professionals is critical for older adults, regardless of where they live, but particularly when they are living alone in their own homes or apartments.

NURSING DIAGNOSES

After completing the history and physical examination of the patient, with assistance from a family member or significant other, the clinician can formulate a diagnosis and develop a plan of care with individualized interventions to best address the needs of the older patient. The following three nursing diagnoses are frequently used to reflect cardiovascular problems in older adults:

1. Alteration in tissue perfusion due to interruptions in arterial and venous flow
2. Alteration in health maintenance due to lack of adequate resources and perceived threat to health
3. Alteration in comfort due to pain from cardiac ischemia and impaired circulation to the extremities

Alteration in tissue perfusion

The alteration may be evidenced by cardiopulmonary, cerebral, or peripheral signs and symptoms:

> Cardiopulmonary—shortness of breath, tachycardia, rales, S_3, S_4, dry cough, peripheral or sacral edema, arrhythmia, chest pain, hypotension, cold or clammy skin
> Cerebral—altered mental status, restlessness, symptoms of TIAs, syncope
> Peripheral—changes in skin color and texture, temperature, hair distribution, sensation, edema, leg pain or tenderness, intermittent claudication, diminished healing capability

Alteration in health maintenance

The condition may be evidenced by unhealthy and incompetent behavior. Defining characteristics include but are not limited to the following (McFarland & McFarlane, 1993):

- Poor diet
- Need for alcohol, drugs, or tobacco
- Lack of adequate immunizations
- Inability to take responsibility for basic health practices
- Lack of knowledge of basic health practices
- Failure to manage stress

Alteration in comfort

The alteration may be evidenced by chest pain, intermittent claudication or arterial occlusion, venous insufficiency or edema, thrombophlebitis, and/or symptomatic arrhythmias.

PLANNING AND GOAL IDENTIFICATION

The planning phase determines a plan of action to assist the patient toward the goal of optimal wellness, based on the highest level of fulfillment. Both short- and long-term goals are developed for the older patient. Expected outcomes are designed with input from the patient, the patient's family or other responsible party, and the clinician.

Alteration in tissue perfusion

The long-term goal is that the patient will alter activities of daily living to minimize the effects of alterations in cerebral, peripheral, and cardiopulmonary tissue perfusion. The outcomes can be grouped into three areas (McFarland & McFarlane, 1993):

1. There will be adequate blood flow in the affected vessels.
2. Tissue needs will be reduced.
3. Patient and family will understand the cause of the problem.

The long-term goal may be achieved by reaching the following short-term goals:

1. Patient will have adequate tissue perfusion and cellular oxygenation of the cardiovascular, cerebral, and peripheral system.
2. Patient will be able to modify lifestyle activities to prevent cardiopulmonary, cerebral, and peripheral signs and symptoms.
3. Patient or caregiver will appropriately control metabolic needs by administration of medications, understanding their actions, dosage, and common side effects, and by avoiding stress-related activities.

Alteration in health maintenance

The primary goal is for the affected patient to understand that lifestyle modification is necessary to assist in the control of the aging process response of the cardiovascular, peripheral vascular, and cerebral systems. Patients should actively participate in the planning. A long-term goal would be the following: Patient will be able to modify cardiac risk factors, incorporating new behaviors into his or her lifestyle.

Short-term goals are the following:

1. Patient will be able to verbalize fears and perception of the cardiovascular, peripheral vascular, and cerebral disease.
2. Patient will engage in health behaviors such as adherence to a low-fat and low-salt diet, compliance with the medication regimen, and follow an appropriate exercise program to improve quality of life.
3. Patient will be able to identify probable future health maintenance needs.

Alteration in comfort

The long-term goal is to control the factors that intensify the symptoms: Patient will be able to describe measures to control chest pain, claudication, and dizziness.

Short-term goals are the following:

1. Patient will take appropriate medications to control pain.
2. Patient will schedule frequent rest periods.
3. Patient will monitor activity.

IMPLEMENTATION
In the acute care setting

On admission to an acute care setting, a patient with a cardiovascular problem serious enough to warrant admission may experience anxiety. The older patient in the hospital setting is frequently not included in treatment decisions. Patients who lose control of the situation often become resentful. Other issues that can add to the anxiety are fear of death or pain, and financial complications. Calmly sitting with the patient to gain an understanding of the nature of the anxiety will assist the nurse in planning interventions to alleviate the anxiety. Individuals who have been accustomed to doing things in their lives in a particular way or to eating particular foods may resist changes. It is important to discuss with the patient any changes that are likely to affect the usual way of doing things, or any special likes and dislikes. Allowing the patient to decide what to eat and when to shower or take a walk may seem like a small thing, yet to a patient it is very important. You can also arrange for a social service representative to come by and speak to the patient regarding financial concerns.

Another commonly seen condition in a seriously ill patient admitted to an acute care setting is confusion. It is easy for the nursing staff of a hospital to assume that this person has chronic dementia and will always be confused. The multiple effects of the cardiovascular problems, medical treatment, and changes in environment frequently cause delirium. Interventions aimed at orienting patients after they have been stabilized are often successful in producing remarkable mental status improvements. Explaining the time of day at each meal and having a clock and calendar in the room can help the patient achieve orientation.

Older individuals with cardiovascular problems are more likely to die or develop adverse outcomes related to hospitalization than are members of any other age group. This is because older adults have significantly compromised reserve capacity for adapting physically or emotionally to acute illness and to the trauma of hospitalization. In the hospital setting it is important to have advance directives on record, if at all possible, particularly because cardiac arrest is a significant risk in older adults with cardiovascular disease. Family and significant others should be included in decision making about diagnostic testing and treatment.

In the nursing home

The primary interventions specific to nursing home care of the resident with cardiovascular problems are the following: (1) maintaining or improving a resident's functional abilities, (2) enhancing the resident's sense of autonomy while fostering a safe environment, (3) monitoring the conditions related to the cardiovascular problems of the resident, and (4) providing specific therapies that will improve the resident's cardiovascular functioning. The reason that the older adult is in a nursing home may not necessarily be related to a cardiovascular problem. The reason usually relates to the effect of the multiplicity of disease processes linked with the normal effects of aging to diminish the person's functional capacity to such an extent that the person can no longer live in a private or family home without assistance. Many older individuals may not have family members living or may not have family members available who can provide the often extensive care needed to maintain someone in the private or family home.

Assisting residents with cardiovascular problems in maintaining autonomy should include supporting those activities that they can do themselves. It may include ensuring that a portable oxygen tank is available so that the resident can attend activities that are enjoyable. A sense of autonomy is usually clearly linked to making decisions about oneself. This includes being involved in the resident care conference, being informed about the status of the cardiovascular problem, and participating in care-planning decisions.

Monitoring the resident is critical in early detection of acute problems related to the cardiovascular system. Periodic monitoring of the vital signs is one of the best ways of identifying impending problems. Changes in heart rate and rhythm, in respiration, and in BP can provide clues to the need for further assessment. The nurse should validate vital signs and reinforce with the assistant nursing staff the importance of accurately assessing vital signs and weights. Staff should be properly educated in the importance of promptly reporting a change in vital signs or weight so that an additional assessment can be started. Mental status should also be monitored. A resident who is having an acute cardiovascular episode such as a myocardial infarction without complaints of chest pain may show signs of confusion or increased lethargy.

Effectiveness of drug therapy, as well as side effects of drugs, should be monitored. This is particularly important because the frail older person with cardiovascular problems will probably be taking at least one, if not more, medications.

In addition to the preceding therapies, encouraging the resident to elevate the legs if fluid accumulates and elevating the resident's head while the resident is in bed if breathing is a problem can ease the symptoms of cardiovascular and peripheral vascular disease. Teach the resident proper use of the emergency call system in the room, bathroom, and common area. The resident may also have periods of anxiety or depression about the effects of the diseases. Talking with the resident and understanding the basis of these feelings are important. When doing so, sit at eye level with the resident. Avoid the use of placating phrases such as "everything will be fine" or "you have nothing to worry about." Older adults have significant concerns that should never be discounted.

In the private or family home

A major consideration in the care of older adults at home is establishing a monitoring system to assess significant and possibly life-threatening changes. Many older adults live alone and have little in the way of home health services available. Because problems affecting the cardiovascular system may impair patients' ability to monitor and interpret changes in their own condition, it is helpful to identify a person who is willing to visit the patient on a regular basis or to call to see that the patient can at least answer the telephone. The person who will be monitoring the patient will need to know the signs that suggest a problem (Box 10-7).

In addition, a nurse may temporarily monitor the patient. The payment mechanism through Medicare for home health services allows only visits that can be justified on the basis of need for specific types of nursing services. Most older adults cannot afford to pay out of pocket for a nurse to provide monitoring services.

If the patient is living with a family member, that family member must also be clear about the

> ## BOX 10-7 CARDIOVASCULAR MONITORING PARAMETERS FOR HOME CARE PROVIDERS
>
> - Confusion
> - Lack of appetite
> - Pain or discomfort
> - Feelings of anxiety
> - Fatigue
> - Disheveled appearance
> - Hallucinations
> - Rapid breathing
> - Rapid pulse
> - Diaphoresis
> - Pallor
> - Edema

signs that suggest a deterioration in the older adult's status. It is also helpful to have patients be clear, if possible, about any advance directives they may want in writing, such as not wanting to be admitted to a hospital. Family members should be aware of these advance directives.

Arrangements may need to be made for items such as a hospital-type bed or commode to be brought to the home. Being able to raise the head of a bed may help a person who has orthopnea to sleep more easily. There may also be a need for oxygen. The nurse may need to make arrangements with a home care supply company to bring in oxygen equipment. There is a great variation in charges for this equipment. Knowing the costs may save the patient or family from considerable financial burden, because Medicare will only pay a specific amount for the equipment.

For older adults who have a high anxiety level about needing help and not being able to obtain it, such as may happen with a heart attack or stroke, establishing a link with emergency community services may alleviate some anxiety. Some communities have a lifeline program, in which a direct line is established with an emer-gency service. Contact can frequently be made simply by pushing a button that sets up an automatic response system at the emergency service site. For communities that do not have this sophisticated type of service, it may be desirable to establish linkages to a family member, friend, or volunteer service that can act on the patient's behalf in an emergency.

EVALUATION

Evaluation is an integral phase of the nursing process. Reassessment and replanning may be the result of an evaluation, if the patient's short-term goals are not met in a timely fashion. Interventions are evaluated in terms of their acceptance by patients and their families and in terms of their ability to assist in the accomplishment of the planned goals. Documentation and validation of goal attainment, including health promotion and education, is an essential component of the evaluation phase of the nursing process.

REFERENCES

Applegate, W.B., & Rutan, G.H. (1992). Advances in management of hypertension in older persons. *Progress in Geriatrics, 40,* 1164-1174.

Aronow, W. (1995). Treatment of ventricular arrhythmias in older adults. *Journal of the American Geriatrics Society, 43,* 688-695.

Bierman, E.G. (1994). Aging and atherosclerosis. In W.M. Hazzard, E. Bierman, J. Blass, W. Ettinger, & J. Halter (Eds.), *Principles of geriatric medicine and gerontology.* New York: McGraw-Hill.

Bruno, A. (1993a). Ischemic stroke: 1. Early, accurate diagnosis. *Geriatrics, 48*(3), 26-34.

Bruno, A. (1993b). Ischemic stroke: 2. Optimal treatment and prevention. *Geriatrics, 48*(3), 37-54.

Cohn, J. (1992). The prevention of heart failure—A new agenda. *New England Journal of Medicine, 327,* 725-727.

Dalen, J.E. (1994). Atrial fibrillation: Reducing stroke risk with low-dose anticoagulation. *Geriatrics, 49*(5), 24-32.

The fifth report of the Joint National Committee on detection, evaluation, and treatment of high blood pressure. (1993). *Archives of Internal Medicine, 153,* 154-183.

Gamble, C.L. (1994). Lipid disorders: When—and why— you should treat at-risk adults. *Geriatrics, 49*(10), 33-37.

Gawlinski, A., & Jensen, G.A. (1991, November). Cardiovascular aging. *American Journal of Nursing, 26-30.*

Giordano, J.M. (1983). A practical approach to peripheral vascular disease. *Modern Medicine, 51,* 105-116.

Juul-Möller, S., Edvardsson, N., & Rehnquist-Ahlberg, N. (1990). Sotalol versus quinidine for the maintenance of sinus rhythm after direct current conversion of atrial fibrillation. *Circulation, 82,* 1932-1939.

Kelley, W.N. (1989). *Textbooks of international medicine.* Philadelphia: J.B. Lippincott.

Laupacis, A., et al. (1992). Antithrombotic therapy in atrial fibrillation. *Chest, 102,* 426S-433S.

Luchi, R., Taffet, G., & Teasdale, T. (1991). Congestive heart failure in the elderly. *Journal of the American Geriatrics Society, 39,* 810-825.

Massie, B.M. (1994). First-line therapy for hypertension: Different patients, different needs. *Geriatrics, 49*(4), 22-30.

McFarland, G.K., & McFarlane, E.A. (1993). *Nursing diagnosis and intervention: Planning for patient care* (2nd ed.). St. Louis: Mosby.

Pearson T., et al. (1994). Primer in preventive cardiology. Dallas: American Heart Association.

1996 physicians genRx: The complete drug reference. (1996). St. Louis: Mosby.

Pritchett, E.L.C. (1992). Management of atrial fibrillation. *New England Journal of Medicine, 326,* 1264-1271.

Shephard, R.J. (1993). Exercise and aging: Extending independence in older adults. *Geriatrics, 48*(5), 61-64.

Thiele, B.L., & Strandness, D.E., Jr. (1994). Peripheral vascular disease. In W.M. Hazzard, E. Bierman, J. Blass, W. Ettinger, & J. Halter (Eds.), *Principles of geriatric medicine and gerontology.* New York: McGraw-Hill.

U.S. Department of Health and Human Services. (1994). *Clinicians handbook of preventive services.* Washington, DC: U.S. Government Printing Office.

Wenger, N.K. (1992). Cardiovascular disease in the elderly. *Current Problems in Cardiology, 17*(10), 609-690.

BIBLIOGRAPHY

Baer, M., & Goldschlager, N. (1995). Atrial fibrillation: An update on new management strategies. *Geriatrics, 50*(4), 22-29.

Cacciabaudo, J.M., & Pecker, M.S. (1995, May-June). Hypertension: Managing the silent killer. *Contemporary Nurse Practitioner,* 24-30.

Cannon, L.A., & Marshall, J.M. (1993). Cardiac disease in the elderly population. *Clinical Geriatric Medicine, 9*(3), 499-525.

Elnicki, M., & Kotchen, T.A. (1993). Hypertension: Patient evaluation, indications for treatment. *Geriatrics, 48*(4), 47-62.

Gamble, C.L. (1994). Lipid disorders: Tailoring diet and drug therapy for individual needs. *Geriatrics, 49*(11), 52-58.

Jensen, G.A. (1991). The complications of cardiovascular aging. *American Journal of Nursing, 91*(11), 26-30.

Kenney, R.A. (1989). Physiology of aging chicago: Year Book Medical Publishers.

Krumholz, H.M., et al. (1994). Lack of association between cholesterol and coronary heart disease mortality and morbidity and all-cause mortality in persons older than 70 years. *Journal of the American Medical Association, 272,* 1335-1340.

Larson, E.B., & Bruce, R.A. (1987). Health benefits of exercise in an aging society. *Archives of Internal Medicine, 147,* 353-356.

Leaf, D.A. (1994). Lipid disorders: Applying new guidelines to your older patients. *Geriatrics, 49*(5), 35-41.

Malasanos, L., et al. (1990). *Health assessment* (4th ed.). St. Louis: Mosby.

Masiello Miller, M. (1994). Current trends in the primary care management of chronic congestive heart failure. *Elsevier Science Inc., 19*(5), 64-70.

Poole, R.M., & Chimowitz, M.I. (1994). Ischemic stroke and TIA: Clinical clues to common causes. *Geriatrics, 49*(6), 37-42.

Silva-Smith, A. (1994). Reducing the risk of stroke in patients with chronic, nonvalvular atrial fibrillation. *Elsevier Science Inc., 19*(2), 38-44.

Thompson, J., et al. (1993). *Mosby's clinical nursing* (3rd ed.). St. Louis: Mosby.

U.S. Department of Health and Human Services. (1992). *Healthy People 2000: National health promotion and disease prevention objectives.* Washington, DC: Author.

U.S. Preventive Services Task Force. (1989). *Guide to clinical preventive services.* Williams & Wilkins.

Vogt, A.R., Funk, M., & Remetz, M. (1994). Comparison of symptoms, functional ability, and health perception of elderly patients with coronary artery disease managed with three different treatment modalities. *Cardiovascular Nursing, 30*(5), 33-38.

Wei, J.Y. (1992). Age and the cardiovascular system. *New England Journal of Medicine, 327*(24), 1735-1739.

Wei, J.Y. (1994). Disorders of the heart. In W.R. Hazzard, R. Andres, E.L. Bierman, & J.P. Blass (Eds.), *Principles of geriatric medicine and gerontology* (3rd ed.). New York: McGraw-Hill.

Weinberg, M. (1993). Renal effects of angiotensin converting enzyme inhibitors heart failure: A clinician's guide to minimizing azotemia and diuretic-induced electrolyte imbalances. *Clinical Therapeutics, 15,* 3-15.

Each step in the path oxygen takes from the air to the metabolizing cell is vulnerable to aging.

R.A. KENNEY, *Physiology of Aging*

Respiration

■ Learning Objectives

On completion of this chapter, the reader will be able to do the following:

1. Explain the normal structure and function of the respiratory tract.
2. Identify age-related physiologic changes of the respiratory system.
3. Identify and describe the common pathophysiologic changes that affect the respiratory system of older adults.
4. Assess the respiratory functioning of older adults.
5. Recognize the psychosocial and environmental factors that influence the nursing management of older adults with respiratory problems.
6. Develop nursing diagnoses and a plan of care for an older person with respiratory impairment.
7. Provide appropriate nursing interventions and evaluations for older adults with respiratory impairment.

The respiratory system stretches from the nasal cavity to the lungs. The system is divided into the upper and lower respiratory tracts. The normal structure and function of the respiratory system is reviewed here before addressing its age-related changes.

■ Normal Structure and Function

UPPER RESPIRATORY TRACT
The upper respiratory tract begins at the nasal cavity and extends to the vocal cords, which are located within the larynx (Figure 11-1).

Nasal cavity

When a person inhales, air passes through two openings, termed *external nares* or *nostrils.* A vertical partition, the *nasal septum,* divides the two nasal cavities, which have six main functions: conduction of air, filtration, temperature control, humidification of inhaled air, voice resonance, and olfaction.

Pharynx

Next the inhaled air passes through the pharynx. The *pharynx,* also known as the "throat," is

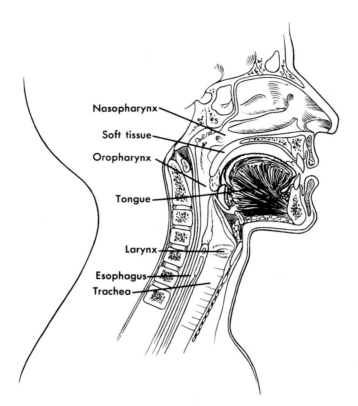

Nasopharynx

Soft tissue

Oropharynx

Tongue

Larynx

Esophagus

Trachea

FIGURE 11-1 Upper respiratory tract. (From Phipps, W., Cassmeyer, V., Sands, J., & Lehman, M.K. [1995]. *Medical-surgical nursing: Concepts and clinical practice* [5th ed.]. St. Louis: Mosby.)

divided into the following three sections: nasopharynx (upper section), oropharynx (middle section), and laryngopharynx (lower section). The pharynx is a long, tubelike structure with two main functions: (1) serving as a passageway for air to travel to the trachea and for food to travel to the esophagus and (2) aiding in the formation of vocal sound.

Larynx

The *larynx,* which connects the pharynx with the trachea and is known as the "voice box" because of its major role in the production of sounds, is a major structure of the upper respiratory tract.

LOWER RESPIRATORY TRACT
Trachea

The *trachea,* or the "windpipe," is a tubular passageway approximately 11 to 12 cm long and 2.5 cm in diameter, located in front of the esophagus. It extends from the cricoid cartilage of the larynx to about the seventh thoracic vertebra. It is here, at the carina, that the trachea divides into the left and right main bronchi.

Bronchi, bronchioles, and alveoli

The left and right main *bronchi,* which branch from the trachea, deliver the inhaled air to the lungs. Each main bronchus divides several times,

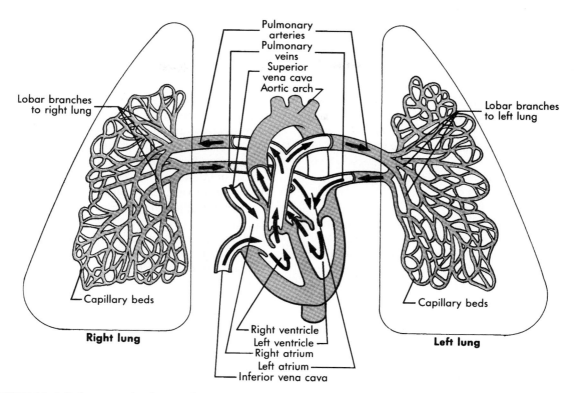

Lobar branches
to right lung

Pulmonary
arteries
Pulmonary
veins
Superior
vena cava
Aortic arch

Lobar branches
to left lung

Capillary beds

Right lung

Capillary beds

Left lung

Right ventricle
Left ventricle
Right atrium
Left atrium
Inferior vena cava

FIGURE 11-2 Pulmonary circulation, illustrating the right and left pulmonary veins and arteries and the branching capillaries. (From McCance K. & Huether, S. [1994]. *Pathophysiology: The biologic basis for disease in adults and children* [2nd ed.]. St. Louis: Mosby.)

ultimately giving rise to tiny *bronchioles.* These bronchioles subdivide many times, forming terminal and respiratory bronchioles. Each *respiratory bronchiole* subdivides into several alveolar ducts that end in clusters of small, thin-walled air sacs termed *alveoli.* Often, several alveoli open into a chamber termed an *alveolar sac.*

All structures distal to the terminal bronchiole make up the terminal respiratory unit (TRU), sometimes referred to as the *acinar unit,* or the *acinus.* This is considered the basic unit of the lung. The alveolus is the most distal structure within the TRU at which gas exchange occurs (Figure 11-2).

Lungs

The two lungs are elastic cone-shaped organs, with the apex of each lung fitting into the thoracic cavity behind the clavicle. The base of each lung rests on the surface of the diaphragm. The left lung has two lobes, as well as a concavity for the heart on its medial surface; the right lung has three lobes.

The space between the two lungs is termed the *mediastinum.* Besides separating the left and right lung, the mediastinum also accommodates several important structures: the heart, the aorta, the venae cavae, the pulmonary vessels, the esophagus, part of the trachea and bronchi, and the thymus gland.

Pleura

The *pleura* is a double-walled sac, one of which encloses each lung. It consists of two layers: the *visceral pleura* adheres firmly to the lungs, whereas the *parietal pleura* lines the walls of the thoracic cavity. The pleural cavity is the extremely narrow area between the two layers of the pleura. The pleural cavity is filled with pleural fluid, which is secreted by the pleura and acts as a lubricant, reducing friction between the two layers during respiratory movements.

Respiratory membrane

The very thin respiratory membrane separates the air in the alveoli from the circulating blood. Oxygen and carbon dioxide diffuse across this membrane during respiration, while maintaining the integrity of the vascular system.

PULMONARY CIRCULATION

For the deoxygenated blood to pass through the lungs, it must be pumped from the right ventricle, through the pulmonic valve, and into the *pulmonary artery,* also called the "pulmonary trunk." The pulmonary artery divides into two branches: (1) the right pulmonary artery, supplying the right lung, and (2) the left pulmonary artery, supplying the left lung (Figure 11-3).

Each pulmonary artery follows the bronchi to the terminal bronchioles, where the *arterioles,* small arteries, branch into capillaries in the alveolar walls. A vast and dense network of pulmonary capillaries, termed the *pulmonary capillary bed,* surrounds the alveoli and provides the contact necessary for gas exchange to occur between the alveoli and the blood.

Once gas exchange has occurred at the pulmonary membrane, oxygenated blood collects in small venules, which unite to form four large veins, termed the *pulmonary veins.* The pulmonary veins drain into the left atrium.

The most distinguishing features of the pulmonary circulation are its low pressure and its low resistance. These features result from the great distensibility of the vessels and from the low resistance to blood flow of the pulmonary vascular beds.

The pulmonary circulation connects with the bronchial circulation deep within the lung tissue; the bronchial circulation system is relatively small, receiving only 1% to 2% of the total cardiac output. Its primary function is to provide a continuous supply of nutrient blood to the conducting airways and terminal respiratory units so that the lungs can carry out their many functions.

Bronchial arteries follow the airways into the lung parenchyma, elaborately branching along the way and rejoining to form networks around the bronchi. Upon reaching the end of the conducting airways and the beginning of TRUs, these vessels anastomose with pulmonary artery capillaries from the pulmonary circulation. Blood returns to the heart via true bronchial veins, flowing into azygous veins, and eventually to the superior vena cava, and then the right atrium. Approximately 65% to 75% of the bronchial circulation flows into the pulmonary veins.

THE PROCESS OF RESPIRATION

The process of respiration can be defined in terms of three distinct events that occur with breathing: ventilation, diffusion or external respiration, and gas transport or internal respiration.

Ventilation

Ventilation is the mechanical movement of air into and out of the lungs, between the atmosphere and the lung alveoli. Ventilation involves two phases: *inspiration* (movement of air into the lungs) and *expiration* (movement of air out of the lungs). Ventilation is influenced by mechanical (muscular), neurologic, physical, and chemical events.

Muscles of respiration   The act of breathing occurs through muscular actions that change intrapulmonary and intrapleural pressures and result in air volume change within the lungs. Normal, quiet inspiration is accomplished almost entirely by the diaphragm, which is the major muscle of this phase of respiration.

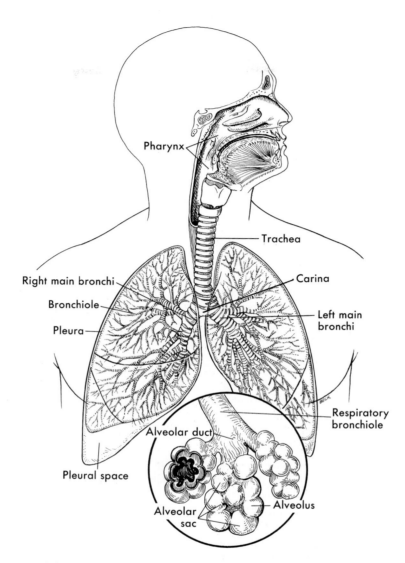

FIGURE 11-3 Structures of the pulmonary system. The circle denotes the acinus, in which oxygen and carbon dioxide are exchanged. (From Thibodeau G. [1990]. *Anthony's textbook of anatomy and physiology* [ed 13.]. St. Louis: Mosby.)

Other muscles involved in inspiration are the external intercostal muscles, which increase the anterior–posterior diameter of the thorax by elevating the ribs. The accessory muscles of inspiration include the scalene and sternocleidomastoid muscles in the neck and are responsible for raising the clavicles, upper ribs, and sternum. These muscle groups are not usually involved in normal, quiet respiration but are needed in some disease states.

Expiration is normally a passive action, resulting from the recoil tendency of the lungs through the relaxation of the inspiratory muscles. However, when increased levels of expiration are required, the abdominal and internal intercostal muscle groups are used (Levitzky, 1991).

Neurologic regulation   Breathing is regulated by the central nervous system. The respiratory centers are groups of neurons that function together as a unit to regulate inspiration and expiration. The medullary respiratory center is located in the medulla oblongata, and the apneustic and pneumotaxic centers are located in the pons. These centers are involved in the regulation of the respiratory rate and depth. Impulses travel down the phrenic nerves to the diaphragm, and then via the intercostal nerves to the intercostal muscles, where changes in the rate and depth of respiration occur.

Conscious control of breathing, through nerve impulses from the motor areas of the cerebral cortex, can override the involuntary respiratory centers. This mechanism adjusts voluntary breathing to meet increased oxygen needs that result from changes in activity.

Physical forces   The diaphragm and intercostal muscles contract as a result of stimulation from the central nervous system. Respiratory muscles alternately compress and distend the lungs, which causes the pressure in the alveoli to rise and fall. Gas moves from an area of greater pressure to one of lesser pressure. The pressure in the lungs and thorax must be less than atmospheric pressure for inspiration to occur. Expiration is passive, as muscles relax; intrathoracic pressures rise, and air moves out of the lungs to the atmosphere. Very little pressure change is required to move air into and out of the lungs.

Physical forces are also involved in effective gas movement. The elasticity of the lung tissue (i.e., *resistance*), the size of the large air passages, and the *compliance* of the chest wall affect respiration and can alter the work of breathing. *Surfactant,* a lipoprotein, is secreted by the epithelial cells in the alveoli. The presence of this substance contributes to lung elasticity, thereby increasing lung compliance (Levitzky,

1991). These factors are especially altered by the process of aging.

Chemical control   The chemical centers that influence respiration involve central and peripheral chemoreceptors that signal the respiratory centers to change the rate and depth of respiration. Central chemoreceptors are located in the medulla and are sensitive to changes in carbon dioxide and to the acid base balance in the blood and the cerebrospinal fluid. Peripheral chemoreceptors are located in the aortic bodies near the aortic arch and in the carotid bodies near the bifurcation of the common carotid arteries. These receptors are sensitive to changes in oxygen levels in the blood and in the interstitial fluid surrounding the receptors.

Alveolar ventilation

One of the most important factors in the respiratory process is alveolar ventilation. Air can travel through the large air passages, but if the alveoli are not open, as is the case in atelectasis or pneumonia, true ventilation does not take place. Respiratory rate and volumes are important in that they affect alveolar ventilation.

Diffusion or external respiration

Ventilation refers to the mechanical movement of air into and out of the lungs. *Diffusion,* the next step in the process of respiration, is the actual transfer of oxygen into and carbon dioxide out of the blood. It is also termed *external respiration.*

During normal inspiration the alveoli fill with air. The concentration of oxygen in the alveoli is higher than the concentration of oxygen in the blood. The concentration of carbon dioxide in the alveoli is lower than that in the blood. Oxygen diffuses into the blood and carbon dioxide diffuses out of the blood across the alveolar capillary membrane until equilibrium is reached. The rate of diffusion is altered in the presence of pathophysiology. Diffusion is altered in the aging lung as a result of a decrease in functional alveoli and a reduced pulmonary capillary blood flow (Timiras, 1994).

Gas transport or internal respiration

Oxygen transport, or *internal respiration,* the third event in the process of respiration, begins after diffusion takes place. During internal respiration, oxygen moves into the cells and carbon dioxide leaves the cells to enter the blood. Arterial blood transports oxygen to the tissues, either in plasma or bound to hemoglobin. Oxygen has an affinity for the iron molecules of hemoglobin. Approximately 97% of oxygen in the blood reaches the tissues bound to hemoglobin. This concentration is determined by the oxygen level of the inspired air and the hemoglobin level in the blood. Oxygen resists being dissolved in plasma, and only 3% is carried to the tissues by this method.

Carbon dioxide transport is more complicated. Carbon dioxide is released by the tissues into the bloodstream. It travels to the lungs in three ways: (1) as a gas, dissolved in plasma (7%), (2) combined with hemoglobin (23%), and (3) combined with water in the form of carbonic acid (70%). Blood moves through the capillaries into the venous system, where carbon dioxide is reformed. This gas is diffused into the alveoli (external respiration) and is excreted in the lungs.

When oxygen-rich arterial blood reaches the body tissue cells, internal respiration, or gas exchange between systemic capillaries and interstitial fluid, takes place. This involves pressure gradients, as is the case in the diffusion process. Oxygen is transported into the interstitial fluid to nourish the cells. Age-related changes or pathophysiology of the respiratory system can affect the rate of transfer and the amount of oxygen that is given off to the tissues by making the unloading of oxygen more difficult.

■ Age-Related Changes

It is difficult to differentiate among the effects of the aging process, the lifelong environment of the individual, and disease on the respiratory system. In healthy older adults, breathing is usually sufficient to supply oxygen for normal function (Hogstel, 1994). However, this supply- and-demand balance is frequently altered when stress or pathology increase oxygen need and consumption.

An understanding of the normal changes that can be expected to occur as the adult lung ages will provide the necessary framework for the nursing process as it develops into an individualized treatment plan for the patient with respiratory disorders. These age-related changes are classified as being either "structural" or "functional."

STRUCTURAL CHANGES

Structural or anatomic changes in the aging lung are described as being either *extrapulmonary* (of skeleton and muscle) or *intrapulmonary* (of the lung parenchyma). Both result in a decrease in potential expansion, which alters the flow of air into and out of the lungs (Timiras, 1994).

Skeletal changes

Osteoporosis of the ribs and the vertebrae and calcification of the costal cartilages cause increased stiffness or rigidity, decreased rib mobility, and reduced compliance of the chest wall. Degeneration of the intervertebral disks may be seen clinically in the development of kyphosis and scoliosis. These skeletal changes of the thoracic region of the spine produce a shorter thorax with an increased anterior–posterior diameter. In severe cases, the rib cage may rest on the pelvic bones and cause marked limitation of thoracic movement.

The trachea and large bronchi are also increased in diameter because of the calcified cartilage changes. These large airway structures serve as reservoirs to conduct air from the atmosphere to the alveoli. The overall effect is both an increase in "dead space," where no diffusion takes place, and a decrease in the volume of air that actually reaches the alveoli in the aged lung.

Muscular changes

The muscles involved in respiration, like other muscles in the body, weaken with age. The result is less forceful contraction, which decreases inspiratory and expiratory effort. Atrophy of the muscles supporting the rib cage is also involved in the development of kyphosis in older adults. The combination of increased stiffness of the chest wall and decreased muscle strength results in less efficient breathing. Older people may depend more on accessory abdominal muscles to compensate for weakened thoracic muscles.

The diaphragm does not appear to lose mass with aging. This muscle continues to contribute significantly to changes in thoracic cage volume. The breathing patterns of the older adult are even more dependent on changes in intra-abdominal pressure and may be greatly affected by increased abdominal pressure or body position.

Lung parenchyma changes

The age-related changes in the lung parenchyma, where gas exchange takes place, alter respiratory efficiency and have the greatest functional effect. The lung becomes less elastic as it ages, as a result of changes in the collagen substance surrounding the alveoli and alveolar ducts. This substance has a major role in the elastic recoil properties of the lungs. During aging, the collagen stiffens and forms cross-linkages that interfere with the lung's elastic ability to expand with inspiration and contract with expiration (Timiras, 1994). This actually increases lung tissue compliance, but the effect is outweighed by that of the decreased compliance of the rib cage. With advanced age the overall compliance of the respiratory system decreases.

Changes in the lung parenchyma are also seen in the terminal bronchioles, alveolar ducts, alveoli, and capillaries. These changes begin in the third decade and continue over the remaining years. The total number of alveoli remains constant throughout the life span, but there is a decrease in the number of functioning alveoli. There is a thinning of the walls, accompanied by a progressive loss of the interalveolar septum. This results in larger alveoli and dilated bronchioles, with a decreased air exchange surface for

external respiration to take place. The aged lung looks like an emphysematous lung on chest x-ray and is referred to as "senile lung."

Changes in pulmonary vessels

The process of aging also affects the pulmonary blood vessels. In the young adult, the thin-walled pulmonary vessels have relatively low pressure because of their high distensibility and low resistance. In older adults the vessels become more fibrous and less distensible. There is also an increase in the diameter and thickness of the pulmonary artery and a consequent increase in pressure and pulmonary vascular resistance.

The mucosal bed of the alveolar capillary membrane thickens which affects the surface area available for diffusion of gases to take place. The number of capillaries declines, resulting in decreased alveolar vascularity. This combines with a diminished cardiac output to cause a decrease in pulmonary capillary blood volume.

It is unclear whether the aging process affects pulmonary surfactant. Surfactant is a lipoprotein secreted by epithelial cells in the alveoli (type II alveolar cells). This substance increases the surface tension in the alveoli and reduces the alveoli's normal tendency to collapse. Many pulmonary disease processes interfere with surfactant production. Older adults have a higher incidence of lung disease than do other adults, and they are at a greater risk for alveolar collapse secondary to decreased surfactant than are their healthy peers.

FUNCTIONAL CHANGES

The structural changes previously discussed affect respiratory function by altering the volume of air conducted to the alveolar surface, and the rate at which it is conducted, consequently affecting the volume and rate of diffusion or gas exchange in the alveoli.

Lung volumes and rate of airflow

Older adults develop altered lung volumes secondary to changes in elastic recoil and musculoskeletal changes in the chest wall. Although the change in total lung capacity is minimal in the older adult, variations are seen in the specific components of lung volume. The decreased compliance of the bony thorax accounts for major differences in residual volume and expiratory reserve volume. Residual volume increases with age by as much as 50% as a result of loss of elastic recoil. However, vital capacity decreases by 25% as the chest wall becomes less mobile and the inspiratory-expiratory capabilities are decreased (Miller, 1994). Inspiratory capacity is reduced as the ability to deep breath decreases with age. The loss of elastic recoil tends to increase total lung volumes, but this gain is offset by reduced muscle power and increased stiffness of the chest wall.

The rate of airflow from the atmosphere to the alveoli is influenced by the size of the airways, the resistance in the airways, the muscle strength, and the elastic recoil. Although airway resistance is unchanged in the healthy older person, the decrease in efficiency of elastic recoil results in early closure of the small airways and accounts for reduced rate of airflow during expiration (Timiras, 1994). In addition, the reduced muscle strength and shallow breathing patterns that usually are seen in older adults result in an increased residual volume. This problem is intensified by the supine position. For this reason, nursing plans for older adults must include both deep breathing and activity in the upright position.

Pulmonary function tests

Pulmonary function tests measure these volumes and are useful in determining the presence and degree of lung impairment, especially in the absence of overt pulmonary symptoms. For example, these tests are useful in assessing lung function in older adults who need to undergo surgical or other invasive procedures that will increase stress on respiratory patterns. They are useful in developing a specific plan of activity according to the older person's functional ability. These tests require the use of a spirometer. Because of compromising musculoskeletal changes, not all functionally impaired older adults will be

able to participate in the testing methods. The older adult will also take longer to complete pulmonary function tests, even when free of lung disease.

Gas exchange

Gas exchange is the primary function of respiration, and it includes distribution of ventilation and blood flow to ventilated areas. Optimum gas exchange requires a closely matched balance of ventilation and perfusion (V-Q ratio). The shallow breathing pattern of an older person may result in hypoventilation, which decreases the V-Q ratio and is ineffective in achieving maximum gas exchange.

Measurements of partial pressure of oxygen in the arterial blood (PaO_2) and partial pressure of carbon dioxide in arterial blood ($PaCO_2$) are indicators of gas exchange adequacy in the adult. Research demonstrates a gradual decrease in arterial oxygen in the aging person, at the rate of 4 mm Hg per decade (Britt, 1993). A PaO_2 measurement of 90 would be normal in a healthy 20-year-old, whereas a value of 75 would be acceptable by age 70 (Timiras, 1994).

Several factors related to ventilation can be identified to account for the change in PaO_2: decreased areas of lung ventilation (dependent areas), early airway closure, and a decrease in functioning alveolar surface area. Other factors affect perfusion, such as decreased cardiac output and age-related hemoglobin reduction, which decreases the oxygen-carrying capacity of the blood.

Control of respiration

Central and peripheral chemoreceptors respond to hypoxemia and hypercapnia. The control of respiration by these receptors is markedly altered in older adults (Timiras, 1994). Responses to hypercapnia (increased PCO_2) and hypoxia (reduced PO_2) are reduced by 50% in the aged as compared to the young (Timiras, 1994). Normally the clinical response to hypoxemia is an increase in respiratory rate and depth. However, the older person may not exhibit the normal respiratory response to hypoxia because of age-related changes. Nursing assessment must include observation of other symptoms, such as mental confusion and restlessness. It is also important to remember that minor increases in oxygen demand will cause hypoxic symptoms more quickly in older adults and that older adults will respond more slowly to treatment for hypoxia.

Altered defense mechanisms

The older person is at increased risk for developing both upper and lower respiratory tract infections for several reasons. Both cough forcefulness and the number of cilia decrease with age. The so-called mucus escalator (which helps to move mucus and foreign materials up the respiratory tract and facilitates the coughing of mucus out through the oral cavity) is impaired. As a result, inhaled foreign material is not cleared as effectively from the large air passages. Mucus plugging of the small air ducts is also more common with aging. The alveolar macrophages, the final line of defense at the alveolar level, are less efficient (Britt, 1993). Another factor contributing to reduction of the body's defensive abilities is a decrease in IgA, the secretory immunoglobulin of nasal and respiratory mucosal surfaces, which normally neutralizes viruses (Britt, 1993).

■ Common Health Deviations

There are two types of pulmonary pathology: obstructive diseases and restrictive diseases. *Obstructive diseases* are characterized by increased resistance to airflow from one or more pathologic processes. These processes are either from inside the airway (lumenal obstruction), from outside the airway (peribronchial obstruction), or from within the wall of the airway (intrinsic airway narrowing).

Restrictive diseases are produced by a variety of disorders and diseases that affect the chest wall, pleural space, lung parenchyma, and other areas that are peripheral to the lungs. These diseases are characterized by a decrease in lung volume caused by limited lung expansion, as demonstrated by a pattern of abnormal function on the pulmonary function tests.

OBSTRUCTIVE PULMONARY DISEASES

The major obstructive pulmonary disease prominent in older adults is chronic obstructive pulmonary disease (COPD). *COPD* is an encompassing term applied to a group of pulmonary conditions that includes chronic bronchitis, pulmonary emphysema, and bronchial asthma. Usually, chronic bronchitis and pulmonary emphysema coexist in a patient, making differential diagnosis impossible. These disease entities are all of long duration and are characterized by increased resistance to or obstruction of airflow either entering or exiting the lungs as the main pathophysiologic feature.

The following facts about COPD were published by the U.S. Department of Health and Human Services (USDHHS) in a 1993 publication by the National Institutes of Health: More than 13.5 million Americans are thought to have COPD. It is the fifth leading cause of death in the United States. Between 1980 and 1990, the total death rate from COPD increased by 22%. In 1990, it was estimated that there were 84,000 deaths caused by COPD, approximately 34 per 100,000 people. Although COPD is still much more common in men than in women, the greatest increase in the COPD death rate between 1979 and 1989 occurred in women. These increases reflect the increased number of women who smoke cigarettes.

COPD attacks people at the height of their productive years, disabling them with constant shortness of breath. It destroys their ability to earn a living, causes frequent use of the health care system, and disrupts the lives of the victims' family members for as long as 20 years before death occurs. In 1990 COPD was the cause of approximately 16.2 million office visits to doctors and 1.9 million hospital days. The economic costs of this disease are enormous. In 1989 an estimated $7 billion was spent for care of people with COPD and another $8 billion was lost to the economy by lost productivity caused by morbidity and death from COPD.

Chronic bronchitis

Chronic bronchitis is defined as excessive production of mucus in the bronchi and is manifested by a chronic cough and production of mucoid or mucopurulent sputum for a minimum of 3 months per year for at least 2 consecutive years, or for 6 months during 1 year, in the absence of any other known conditions that could produce these symptoms. According to a 1993 publication by the National Institutes of Health, an estimated 12.1 million Americans have chronic bronchitis.

Middle-aged men are most often afflicted, and smoking is the most important etiologic factor. The prevalence of chronic bronchitis increases as the lifetime cigarette consumption increases beyond approximately 8 pack years of exposure, pack years being calculated by multiplying the number of packs/day times the number of years smoked (Cooper, 1993). However, environmental pollution and occupation may also play a role in the development of this disease.

The onset of bronchitis is generally insidious. It usually appears as a chronic cough that the patient, if a smoker, attributes to smoking. The course of the disease may be slow, with breathing problems not becoming apparent for many years.

Pathophysiologically, there is hypertrophy of the bronchial mucous glands and the goblet cells, and effective cilia are reduced. Death is generally due to bronchopneumonia, respiratory insufficiency, and right-sided heart failure, which occurs years after the onset of symptoms.

Pulmonary emphysema

Emphysema can only be diagnosed with certainty during a postmortem examination because it is defined morphologically as abnormal and permanent dilatation of the terminal air spaces of the lungs, combined with destruction of the alveolar wall (Cooper, 1993). The alveoli of the lungs become distended to the point of rupturing. Loss of lung elasticity accompanies this distention or rupture. The number of individuals with emphysema in the United States is estimated to be 2 million (National Institutes of Health, 1994).

On the basis of the patient's clinical picture and pulmonary function test results, a presumptive diagnosis can be made. The symptoms are slow in onset and resemble normal age-related changes in the respiratory system.

Clinically the patient develops chronic dyspnea on exertion, with or without cough. As the disease progresses, the patient demonstrates a look of anxiety, has a large hyperinflated chest, and is thin and often emaciated because of the inability to eat sufficient amounts related to the chronic dyspnea. The patient struggles to breathe, unconsciously utilizing pursed-lip breathing techniques in an effort to rid the lungs of excess trapped air. The expiratory phase of breathing is prolonged, often with wheezes (Cooper, 1993). If a cough is present, it is usually nonproductive.

Emphysema causes trapping of air in the lungs and decreases gas exchange. The trapping of air is caused by the loss of normal elastic recoil within the lungs. This loss of elasticity decreases the support and increases the collapsibility of the noncartilaginous terminal airways. This, in turn, regionally decreases lung ventilation. Decreased gas exchange leads to both pulmonary diffusion and pulmonary perfusion abnormalities.

Asthma

Asthma is a disease usually associated with childhood. However, in the older adult patient, asthma can either be of recent onset or a chronic disease from younger years. Data on the prevalence of asthma among older adults in the general population are available from several studies and are remarkably similar. Various estimates state that between 27% and 38% of adults with childhood remission of asthma have a recurrence of the disease after 45 years of age (Bardana, 1993).

There are two main types of asthma: (1) *Extrinsic,* or *IgE-triggered asthma* is primarily an allergic reaction mediated by antigen-antibody responses and is more common in the young. (2) *Intrinsic,* or *nonallergic, asthma* usually begins after the age of 35 years and may occur even later in life. This type is more commonly found in older adults. The common precipitating factor is respiratory infection. However, exposure to cigarette smoke, dust, polluted air, or just a change in temperature can precipitate an attack.

Acute exacerbation of the disease is characterized by bronchoconstriction, tracheobronchial mucosal edema, and increased secretion of thick, tenacious mucus. Local obstruction of airways can cause ventilation-perfusion mismatch. Large mucus plugs can cause complete airway obstruction.

As a result of the presence of other chronic problems, especially other cardiopulmonary disease, the older asthmatic patient has some special problems. Characteristic of moderate to severe asthma is hypoxemia. In the older adult, hypoxemia may exacerbate cardiac ischemia, as well as adversely affecting the patient's mental status.

Survival of patients with COPD is closely related to the level of their lung function at the time of diagnosis and the rate at which they lose this function. Overall, the median period of survival is about 10 years for patients with COPD who have lost approximately two thirds of the normally expected lung functioning capacity at diagnosis (National Institutes of Health, 1994). Although symptomatic relief may be obtained through pulmonary rehabilitation and education, progressive deterioration is inevitable in most patients.

RESTRICTIVE PULMONARY DISEASES

Restrictive pulmonary diseases are classified in terms of (1) whether they are acute or chronic and (2) where the pathology is located. If the primary etiologic or pathologic areas lie outside the lungs, peripheral to the visceral pleura, the disease is *extrapulmonary.*

Pulmonary restriction applies to those etiologies that lie within the lung tissue itself and that involve, to varying degrees, the alveolar and interstitial spaces, the capillary bed, or both. The major pathologic processes include loss of lung tissue, loss of functioning alveoli, and decreased lung and chest wall compliance.

Pneumonia

Pneumonia is an inflammatory process of the lung parenchyma, most commonly caused by infection. Infections of the lower respiratory tract, such as pneumonia and influenza, are a major cause of morbidity and death in older adults. The infectious agent is often present among the normal flora of the respiratory tract. Therefore the development of pneumonia can be attributed to an impaired immune system, which often occurs with aging (Timiras, 1994).

In fact, approximately 80% of deaths attributable to pneumonia and influenza occur in people older than 65 years (Fein et al., 1991). Pneumonia is the leading infectious cause of death and the fourth most common cause of death overall in older adults (Dobson & Ruben, 1993).

Sir William Osler (1892) summed things up well when he wrote that "pneumonia is the special enemy of old age. In the aged, chances are against recovery. So fatal is it in this group that it has been called the natural enemy of old man."

Today more than 800,000 hospital admissions are attributed to pneumonia each year, at a cost to the American health care system of about $1.5 billion. Approximately 37% of this figure is directed specifically at managing pneumonia in older adults (Lynch, 1992).

Pneumonia is second in frequency to urinary tract infections in older adults living in long-term care facilities. This high frequency is in part caused by the closed environment of a long-term care facility which can set the stage for periodic outbreaks of infection. Pneumonia accounts for 48% of institutionally acquired infections and is the leading cause of death from nosocomial infection in this population (Niederman, 1993).

Morbidity and mortality rates from pneumonia are also known to be higher in older individuals who have associated chronic diseases, a weakened cough reflex, a general debilitated condition, late diagnosis, and a decrease in mobility.

The events that lead to the development of pneumonia in older adults include colonization of bacteria on pharyngeal epithelial cells, aspiration, and subsequent lung infection (Wade, 1993). Aspiration has been cited as the single most important risk factor for pneumonia in the gerontologic patient. Aspiration is thought to occur during sleep in as many as 50% of all patients. Concomitant bacteremia is encountered in 25% to 40% of these patients; death occurs in more than 50% of older patients in this category (Wade, 1993).

It is important to the diagnosis and treatment of pneumonia to know where the patient acquired the infection. There are specific site-related pathogens responsible for pneumonia, resulting in its classification as long-term care pneumonia, nosocomial pneumonia, or community-acquired pneumonia.

Long-term care pneumonia The most commonly encountered pathogens in long-term care pneumonia include Staphylococcus aureus, streptococci groups A and B, gram-negative rods, and H. influenza. Infections caused by Pseudomonas species are rare. Viral diseases are also important, because they predispose patients to, and often precede or coexist with, bacterial infection (Wade, 1993).

Nosocomial pneumonia Nosocomial infections differ from institution to institution. Many cases of nosocomial pneumonia appear in the acute care setting, where the infectious organisms tend to be especially resistant to antimicrobial agents.

S. aureus and gram-negative bacilli are the two most important organisms causing nosoco-mial pneumonia. Death most often is associated with infections involving Pseudomonas and Klebsiella species. Escherichia coli and Serratia, Proteus, Enterobacter, and Acinetobacter species are common pathogens. Infections involving these organisms frequently occur when organisms colonized on the oropharynx are aspirated, or through aerosolization from respiratory equipment (Wade, 1993).

Patients being fed through small-bore feeding tubes and nasogastric tubes are at risk for aspiration pneumonia. The nurse must be careful to position the patient so that the head of the bed is elevated before initiating any type of feedings. When administering tube feedings, the nurse must check the position of the tube by aspirating the gastric contents and checking for residual volumes of feedings that have not been digested. Gastrostomy tubes should be considered for long-term feeding in this population.

Community-acquired pneumonia Streptococcus pneumonia, most often the causative organism for pneumonia in noninstitutionalized older patients, accounts for approximately 50% of all cases; H. influenza causes 2% to 20% of cases. Older patients are more susceptible to gram-negative organisms in the community; these infections account for 5% to 15% of cases (Wade, 1993). Other important pathogens include viruses, mixtures of bacteria, mixtures of bacteria and viruses, S. aureus, and organisms that produce atypical pneumonia (Chlamydia pneumoniae, Chlamydia psittaci and Mycoplasma, Legionella, and Coxiella species.) Although organisms that produce atypical pneumonia appear less frequently in older patients than in younger patients, morbidity and mortality from these organisms remain significant (Wade, 1993).

Diagnosis The diagnosis and treatment of pneumonia in older adults is a challenge because of the subtle nonspecific manifestations and insidious onset. These subtle and sometimes very confusing clinical manifestations are not those of the typical textbook picture of pneumonia.

Chills, fever, dyspnea, cough, and pleuritic pain are rarely seen in this patient population. Instead, lethargy, confusion, obtundation, tachypnea, mild fever, and possibly evidence of dehydration may be the initial cues. Sometimes the only sign is worsening of preexisting diseases, such as COPD, diabetes, and congestive heart failure (CHF) (Ely et al., 1994b).

On chest examination, the typical findings of pneumonia, such as bronchial breath sounds in the region of consolidation and dullness to percussion, may not be present or discernible because of the increase in the anterior–posterior diameter and the presence of underlying disease common in this population. Nonspecific signs, such as a decrease in the intensity of breath sounds, rales, or rhonchi, may be present. In some patients, tachypnea may be the only finding. In some older patients an early-developing infiltrate may not be visible on x-ray, making the diagnosis extremely difficult (Bartlett, 1994).

Tuberculosis

Presently there is a resurgence of tuberculosis (TB) is the United States. New cases have increased by 10% nationwide, and many are drug resistant (Richman, 1992). Experts believe that about 10 million Americans are infected with TB germs. Only about 10% of these people will develop TB disease in their lifetime. The other 90% will never get sick from the TB germs or be able to spread them to other people (American Lung Association, 1994).

TB is an infectious disease of the lungs caused by the tubercle bacillus *Mycobacterium tuberculosis*. This disease is transmitted by the airborne spread of droplet nuclei containing tubercle bacilli surrounded by respiratory tract secretions. Coughing and speaking make these droplets airborne and available for inhalation by others.

Many older people were exposed to TB as children, when the disease was much more prevalent. Because TB is a disease that can lie dormant for years with reactivation occurring later in life, over 90% of newly reported cases of active TB in the United States involve a reactivation of dormant disease.

Twenty-five percent to 30% of all newly diagnosed cases of TB are found in people over 65 (Yoshikawa, 1992). The higher incidence of this disease in the older age group is probably the result of immunologic changes that normally occur with aging. Susceptibility is also increased by conditions that commonly afflict older adults, such as malnutrition, diabetes, cancer, long-term use of steroids, and other disease entities (American Lung Association, 1994).

The clinical picture of TB is very familiar: fever and night sweats are the classic symptoms of this disease. However, these symptoms frequently do not occur among older adults, so TB is often overlooked in this population. The older patient with TB may only exhibit weight loss and anorexia or fever. Further constraining accurate diagnosis, skin tests generally are not helpful in older adults, who often show false negatives, again possibly because of their reduced immune system activity (Mangura & Reichman, 1994). Accurate diagnosis of TB in older people is based on chest x-rays and demonstration of acid-fast bacilli in the sputum or cultures of other body fluids.

TB must always be considered a possibility in any older person with a pulmonary infection, especially if the individual is already known to be tuberculin positive or a recent skin test converter (Stead & Dutt, 1994). Health care providers are now required by the Occupational Safety and Health Administration (OSHA) to wear special particulate masks when caring for patients suspected of or having TB infection.

Treatment with modern chemotherapy is very effective. If the disease is diagnosed and chemotherapy is correctly prescribed, and if the prescribed drugs are taken faithfully for the recommended 6 to 18 months, a cure rate of almost 100% can be achieved. Drug therapy has changed during the past several years, in part because of the increased incidence of multidrug-resistant (MDR) TB.

All of the recommended drugs may have significant toxic effects, especially in older adults. It is very important that the nurse caring for the older patient with TB assess patient compliance with the drug regimen. Although ensuring close adherence to the drug regimen for a long time is difficult, it is essential if this disease is to be cured.

Lung cancer

Lung cancer, also referred to as bronchogenic carcinoma, is a major disease in older adults. Peak incidence for this disease occurs in the population 55 to 65 years of age. Most cases of lung cancer are seen in patients between the ages of 35 and 75 years. Each year more than 170,000 people learn that they have lung cancer (National Cancer Institute, 1993). In 1993 it was estimated that 88% of patients with a diagnosis of lung cancer would ultimately die from this disease (Perry, 1994).

The incidence of lung cancer continues to rise at remarkable rates. This form of cancer continues to be the most common fatal malignancy in men. However, increased smoking among women has resulted in a predictable increase in lung cancer in the female population. The risk of death from lung cancer is related to the degree of cigarette abuse. Fifteen or more years must elapse after a person stops smoking for the risk to approach that of nonsmokers (Perry, 1994).

Although the exact etiology of lung cancer is unknown, it is believed that the disease process begins with inhalation of carcinogenic pollutants by a susceptible host. Inhalation of such carcinogenic agents as tobacco smoke, industrial hazards, and air pollution accounts for an increase in incidence. Of these agents, tobacco smoke appears to play the major role. Lung cancer is 10 times more common in smokers than in nonsmokers.

There are four types of lung cancer: (1) squamous cell carcinoma, (2) adenocarcinoma, (3) small cell (oat cell) carcinoma, and (4) large cell carcinoma. The most common type is squamous cell. Lung cancers are classified according to the tumor node metastasis (TNM) staging system. There are five stages, 0 through 4, reflecting increasing extent or dissemination of the disease. Generally, non–small cell carcinomas respond to surgery, and small cell carcinoma responds to chemotherapy and/or radiation therapy. For all types of lung cancer, metastasis may occur in multiple sites, but bone, bone marrow, the liver, the lymph nodes, and the brain are the most common sites (Perry, 1994). Particularly low survival rates occur with small cell cancer. Life expectancy for this type of carcinoma is often given in weeks or months rather than in years, depending on staging of the disease.

The onset of lung cancer is insidious, producing either no signs and symptoms or signs and symptoms resembling those of pneumonia or other respiratory diseases that are common in the older population. Therefore, it is not uncommon for such signs to be ignored or to be attributed to other causes—smoking or bronchitis, for example. The most common early signs are cough, chest pain, and streaky hemoptysis.

The disease is more likely to be localized at diagnosis in older patients than in middle-aged patients. Localized cancers are generally more readily resectable and thus potentially curable (Perry, 1994).

The older patient facing tumor resection surgery poses a challenge to nursing. The nurse must supplement and reinforce the patient's understanding of the disease and the surgical procedure, as told by the physician. Preoperative teaching of techniques to prevent postoperative complications, as well as explanation of expected postoperative care and side effects of radiation therapy and chemotherapy, is necessary.

PULMONARY VASCULAR DISORDERS

Pulmonary vascular disorders rank among the most serious complications of respiratory or cardiovascular disease. Left untreated, these disorders cause severe lung damage that can dramatically impair or threaten a patient's lifestyle. The disorders that are commonly seen in the older patient are pulmonary edema, which usually stems from cardiac disease, and pulmonary embolism, which is caused by thrombus formation originating in the venous system.

In pulmonary vascular disorders, the pressure within the pulmonary circulation must be great enough to overcome pulmonary vascular resistance, to ensure adequate lung perfusion for gas exchange to occur. The human body reacts with two mechanisms to compensate for pulmonary vascular resistance: tachycardia and tachypnea. However, if pulmonary vascular resistance becomes chronic, these two mechanisms lead to further complications.

Pulmonary embolism and infarction

Pulmonary embolism (PE) is an obstruction of the pulmonary arterial bed by a dislodged thrombus or by foreign matter. It is known to be a complication of venous thrombosis. Pulmonary embolism is a common pulmonary complication and an important cause of morbidity and death in the older population. Of people with deep vein thrombosis, 500,000, or 10%, develop PE; 50,000 of these cases prove fatal (Mosher, 1994). PE is difficult to diagnose clinically. Pulmonary angiography is the most definitive test used for diagnosis.

Pulmonary infarction (tissue death) results when the PE is extensive enough to produce necrosis or death of lung parenchyma. This occurs in about 10% to 30% of PE patients. Pulmonary infarction is most likely to occur in patients (1) of advanced age, (2) with septic embolism and the associated inflammatory process in the lungs, (3) with already diseased pulmonary arteries from conditions such as COPD and pulmonary vasculitis, and (4) with reduced blood flow to the bronchial arteries supplying the lungs, which occurs in CHF and prolonged shock. Pulmonary infarction may evolve from PE, especially in patients with chronic cardiac or pulmonary disease.

Three basic factors relate to the development of venous thrombosis and subsequent PE: (1) venous stasis or slowing of the blood flow, (2) injury to the vein wall, and (3) hypercoagulability (Hunninghake, 1994). Risk of thrombus formation is increased by (1) obesity, (2) heart failure, (3) varicose veins, (4) abdominal infection, (5) cancer, and (6) prolonged inactivity or immobility. PE occurs predominantly in bedridden patients because of their immobility. The single condition that most predisposes a person to venous thrombosis is CHF. This is important to keep in mind when caring for older people, who frequently have some form of CHF. Prophylaxis to prevent the development of venous thrombosis is especially important in the gerontologic population (Hunninghake, 1994).

The classic presentation of PE is dyspnea, apprehension, anginal or pleuritic chest pain, hemoptysis, and a pleural friction rub in the setting of thrombophlebitis (Hunninghake, 1994). The older patient may not be able to describe the type or intensity of pain being experienced. If the patient has underlying respiratory or cardiac disease, such symptoms could be common to those diseases. The older person might ignore the symptoms or attribute them to other pathologic conditions.

Pulmonary edema

Pulmonary edema refers to accumulation of serous fluid in extravascular lung spaces. It can occur as a chronic condition, or it can develop quickly with death rapidly ensuing. It is a common complication of many cardiopulmonary diseases. Pulmonary edema usually results from left ventricular failure (LVF). Common causes of LVF include arteriosclerotic, cardiomyopathic, hypertensive, and valvular cardiac diseases which result in increased pulmonary capillary hydrostatic pressure.

Pulmonary edema can also occur in diseases that result in decreased colloid osmotic pressure in the lungs. This type is commonly referred to as noncardiogenic pulmonary edema or adult respiratory distress syndrome (ARDS). This syndrome is associated with such clinical disorders as severe malnutrition, burns, trauma, pancreatic or hepatic disease, nephritis, hematologic disorders, inhalation of noxious gases, liquid aspiration, and inflammation or infection (Matthay & Hopewell, 1994). Any lung injury that interferes with the diffusion of oxygen consequently results in tissue hypoxia, which further increases the tendency toward pulmonary edema.

In the early stages of this process, evidence of pulmonary edema reflects interstitial and alveolar fluid accumulation and diminished lung compliance. Dyspnea on exertion, paroxysmal nocturnal dyspnea, and orthopnea are the usual presenting signs and symptoms. Respirations become labored and rapid, with coughing productive of the classic "frothy pink-tinged or bloody sputum." The patient may also start to show signs of a decreased level of consciousness and of confusion as gas exchange becomes increasingly impaired.

The treatment for pulmonary edema is diuretic therapy. Such therapy will improve gas exchange and myocardial function by reducing extravascular fluid. It is also important to correct the underlying pathologic process.

■ Nursing Process

ASSESSMENT

The multidimensional status of the older patient is the focus of assessment. Essential for conducting a successful assessment of the respiratory system is the development of a complete and accurate data base.

The nurse, as the examiner, must be able to set up effective communication with the patient to obtain a complete and accurate health history. When caring for the older adult, this may be very difficult to achieve because of other medical and possibly cognitive problems.

Should the older patient be a poor historian, it is important to seek other means of obtaining information. Information can be obtained from family members, friends, previous health records,

Aging Alert

- Efficiency in collecting patient data is enhanced by developing and maintaining trust between the patient and the nurse.
- Carefully listening to the patient's responses ensures the collection of complete and pertinent patient data.
- The nurse uses inspection, palpation, percussion, and auscultation to assess the patient's respiratory status.

or other health care professionals. Having family members describe the patient's condition is helpful because they may be able to provide needed information.

Often, older patients neglect to report symptoms because they believe that their symptoms are a result of aging and are not amenable to treatment. The nurse needs to be skillful in directing questions and in carefully listening to the older patient's responses.

History

A health history is the first element of the data base. It is the single most important element in establishing the patient's problems. A comprehensive health history gives the examiner a picture of the patient's past and current problems.

To adequately assess the respiratory status of the older person, the nurse must determine three important points: (1) the presence and extent of signs and symptoms that indicate pulmonary disease or impairment, (2) the presence of environmental factors (particularly smoking) that interfere with respiratory function, and (3) the extent to which the patient's normal lifestyle and activities of daily living (ADLS) have changed or have become limited as a result of impaired respiratory function.

Important questions when assessing overall respiratory functioning include the following:

1. Do you have a history of respiratory problems, such as asthma, pneumonia, chronic lung disease, influenza, or frequent colds?
2. Do you take any prescription medication for respiratory problems?
3. Do you take any over-the-counter (OTC) preparations for coughs, colds, or allergies?
4. Do you smoke now, or have you ever smoked? Do you live with a smoker?
5. Do you now live, or have you ever lived, in a neighborhood where there was a lot of pollution from traffic or industry?
6. Have you ever been employed where you were exposed to air pollutants, dust, or fumes?
7. Do you ever have difficulty breathing or get short of breath? Does this occur when doing particular activities, such as walking or climbing stairs?
8. Do you ever feel as though you can't catch your breath or you're not getting enough air?
9. Do you have trouble breathing that is related to changes in the weather or temperature?
10. Do you ever wheeze?
11. Do you have coughing spells? If so,
    a. When do they occur?
    b. How long do they last?
    c. What brings them on?
    d. Are they dry, or do they produce sputum?
    e. What does the sputum look like?
12. Do you use more than one pillow at night? Do you change your position frequently because of difficulty in breathing?
13. Do you get tired or fatigued easily?
14. Do you have any other chronic diseases, such as hypertension, arthritis, or cardiac disease?
15. Have you recently had a chest x-ray, arterial blood gas analysis, or any pulmonary function tests?
16. Have you ever had immunizations for pneumococcal pneumonia or influenza?
17. Have you ever had TB or contact with anyone with the disease?
18. Have you ever had a positive TB skin test?

Physical examination

When examining older people, it is important to properly and thoroughly prepare the patients. Explain your actions; help them to relax; answer any questions they may have; do not rush; make sure the examination room is well lighted, warm, and quiet; and provide privacy to the patients.

Examination of the respiratory function of the patient requires use of the four key techniques: inspection, palpation, percussion, and auscultation. Equipment necessary to evaluate the respiratory system in the older adult is a stethoscope. Using a tape measure to determine the diameter of chest expansion is a waste of time because of the normal age-related changes.

Inspection or observation To inspect the patient properly, observe everything, including the patient's behavior. The following areas should be included in the inspection phase of the physical examination.

Head and neck

1. Mental state—Delirium, confusion, or hallucinations may mean severe hypoxia or hypercarbia. With older patients, be cautious not to attribute disorientation to age. Fearfulness, restlessness, and an anxious facial expression are often seen in patients with acute respiratory distress.
2. Color—Observe for pallor, flushing, cyanosis of the buccal mucosa and lips, and extremely pink or ruddy skin.
3. Lips—Look for breathing out through pursed lips or circumoral cyanosis.
4. Nose—Look for nasal flaring.
5. Neck—Look for retraction of accessory muscles, vein engorgement, and trachea position.

Chest

1. Movement—Look for inspiratory intercostal retractions or bulges, use of accessory muscles during respiration, and abdominal breathing.
2. Sternal abnormalities—Look for pigeon, barrel, or funnel chest.
3. Spinal abnormalities—Look for kyphosis, scoliosis, or kyphoscoliosis.

Barrel chest and spinal abnormalities may be attributed to normal age-related changes. However, further investigation is warranted to make a differential diagnosis.

Extremities

1. Skin—Look for elevated temperature, diaphoresis, or clamminess.
2. Fingers and toes—Look for clubbing, asterixis, or nail bed cyanosis.
3. Legs—Look for signs of thrombophlebitis: Check the patient's calves for redness, swelling, warmth, and positive Homan's sign; check for ankle edema.

Palpation Inform the patient that you are about to put your hands on the patient's back. Be aware of the following areas: expect limited chest expansion in the older adult because of the normal age-related changes of stiffness of the rib cage and decreased muscle strength; check for increases or decreases in intensity of tactile fremitus, both anteriorly and posteriorly; palpate for abnormal masses or lumps; watch for tender areas, because rib fractures are common in older adults.

Percussion The lungs of the healthy older patient may sound resonant on percussion. Hyperresonance is usually a sign of an abnormal increase in the amount of air in the lungs, as in emphysema. Dull or flat sounds can be signs of areas of possible consolidation, tumor, or effusion.

Auscultation The older patient may not be able to take the deep and frequent breaths needed for auscultation of the lung fields. The nurse must remember that the sounds heard over normal lung tissue are no different in older versus younger adults. The breath sounds of older patients with scoliosis or kyphosis will sound distant in affected areas. All adventitious sounds—such as rales, rhonchi, wheezes, and rub—are abnormal and are heard only if disease is present.

Diagnostic studies

The complete patient data base also includes findings from diagnostic studies. Depending on the information obtained from the history and physical examination, some appropriate diagnostic studies are the following:

1. Arterial blood gas analysis
2. Pulmonary function test
3. Chest roentgenogram
4. TB skin test
5. Laboratory values
6. Sputum examination
7. Lung scan
8. Pulmonary angiography
9. Insertion of a Swan-Ganz catheter
10. Exercise tolerance test
11. Mental status examination (MSE)
12. Electrocardiogram (ECG)

Values assessment

The nurse's assessment should also help to identify the patient's values and should serve to assist the patient in providing advance health care directives on the basis of those values. If the patient is competent to make such decisions, it is important to have these stated directives put in a legal document, such as a living will or medical durable power of attorney. This is particularly important in the current age of modern technology, in which increasingly complex ethical dilemmas occur in hospitals and in long-term care facilities.

Older patients who are suffering from a chronic respiratory disease are faced with making decisions that will affect their quality and length of life, such as decisions regarding the following:

1. Resuscitation in the event of cardiopulmonary arrest
2. Performance of a tracheostomy in the event that the older patient cannot adequately clear the secretions from the lungs
3. Placement on a life-support system, such as a ventilator, because the older patient is unable to sustain adequate breathing because of a worsening disease process or patient fatigue
4. In the event of placement on such a life support system, determining whether the device should be maintained indefinitely or should be withdrawn when no clinical sings of improvement are demonstrated

Many individuals have very strong feelings about what they would and would not want to have done for them. It is clearly in the patient's best interest that these wishes be explored beforehand and that they be put in writing, as well as being discussed with family members who may be ultimately responsible for making such decisions about the patient's care.

Psychosocial assessment

Psychosocial assessment evaluates cognitive function, affective function, and the social support system. The psychosocial assessment can be focused to gather information pertinent to a specific area of nursing concern. One area to consider when caring for an older patient with a chronic respiratory condition is that person's ability to take prescribed medications correctly.

Older adults face specific risks in each area of psychosocial functioning. In the area of cognitive functioning, older adults are most likely to complain of or to experience memory impairments. It is difficult but crucial to differentiate between changes that are related to age and those that are related to respiratory disease.

Assessment of affective functioning is essential in planning appropriate interventions. If older patients are depressed, anxious, feeling hopeless, or otherwise psychosocially impaired, they will be unable to comply with the plan of care and many needed interventions.

The patient's social support system includes the social network of family and friends who are available to the patient for different types of support. Questions about economic resources and religious affiliation can be included in this section of the assessment. The purpose of a nursing assessment of the patient's social support system is to identify resources that are available to meet basic needs and to improve the quality of life for the patient.

The older individual with respiratory disease may need assistance in obtaining, as well as in correctly taking, medications. The nurse needs to consider the following:

1. Does the patient have the monetary resources or health insurance coverage to pay for the medications?
2. Does the patient have the transportation to get to a pharmacy?
3. Is the patient competent to take the medications as prescribed?
4. Is someone available to assist the patient in obtaining, taking, and monitoring the effects of medications?

Environmental assessment

The well-being of older adults is influenced by the environment, whether in the home, the hospital, or a long-term care facility. The environmental assessment specific to respiratory problems is presented in Box 11-1.

NURSING DIAGNOSES

Upon completion of a thorough history and physical examination, the nurse prepares to analyze the data and formulate appropriate nursing diagnoses. Following the nursing diagnoses, a plan of care with individualized interventions that best address the needs of the older person is developed. Input into the plan of care is elicited from the patient, family members, or significant others involved in caring for the patient.

BOX 11-1
ENVIRONMENTAL ASSESSMENT

1. What are the distances between the living areas where the patient spends most of the time (e.g., bedroom, bathroom, and kitchen)?
2. Are stairs present, and how often per day must the patient climb them?
3. Is the patient's environment safe and free of clutter, to promote ease of ambulation?
4. If the patient is dependent on oxygen, is there room for the equipment, and is the equipment portable?
5. Is the room temperature comfortable for the patient suffering with respiratory disease?
6. Does the patient at home need a hospital bed so that the head of the bed can be elevated to assist with effective breathing?

The following three North American Nursing Diagnosis Association (NANDA) diagnoses are the most applicable for respiratory problems:

1. Ineffective airway clearance related to presence of bronchial secretions, secondary to normal age-related decrease in cough forcefulness and mucociliary transport action and overall decrease in number of cilia
2. Ineffective breathing pattern related to decreased energy or fatigue, secondary to normal age-related musculoskeletal changes
3. Impaired gas exchange related to altered oxygen supply, secondary to normal age-related lung parenchyma and pulmonary vasculature changes

Ineffective airway clearance

The condition is evidenced by changes in the rate and depth of respirations, tachypnea, dysp- nea, choking or gasping, cyanosis, noisy respirations, nasal flaring, fever, anxiety, apprehension, cough (effective or ineffective, with or without sputum), or presence of adventitious breath sounds (e.g., rales, rhonchi, wheezes, or stridor).

Ineffective breathing pattern

The condition is evidenced by exertional dyspnea, shortness of breath, tachypnea, fremitus, abnormal arterial blood gases, cyanosis, cough, nasal flaring, respiratory depth changes, pursed-lip breathing and prolonged expiratory phase, increased anterior–posterior diameter of the chest wall, use of accessory muscles, altered chest excursion, verbal report of decreased energy or fatigue, or anxiety.

Impaired gas exchange

The condition is evidenced by dyspnea, confusion, somnolence, restlessness, irritability, inability to move secretions, hypercapnia, hypoxia, cyanosis, decreased mental acuity, tachycardia or arrhythmias, anxiety, or clinical evidence of abnormal blood oxygen levels.

PLANNING AND GOAL IDENTIFICATION

The planning for patient care involves analysis of data, prioritizing of problems, setting of goals, and deciding on appropriate nursing interventions.

Ineffective airway clearance

Short-term goals in achieving expected patient outcomes are the following:

1. Patient will be able to cough effectively and will have normal sputum production and expectoration of sputum.
2. After effective coughing, patient's lung fields will be clear of adventitious breath sounds upon auscultaton.
3. Patient's chest x-ray will be normal.
4. Patient will maintain adequate hydration.
5. Patient's arterial blood gases will return to the normal baseline level.
6. Patient will be able to maintain airway patency.

Long-term goals are the following:

1. Patient will understand and be able to explain the need for adequate hydration, for monitoring of sputum, and for taking medications as prescribed.
2. Patient will demonstrate controlled coughing techniques.
3. Patient or caregiver will be able to perform effective chest physiotherapy procedures, particularly postural drainage.
4. Patient or caregiver will know and report signs and symptoms that indicate the need for medical intervention.

Ineffective breathing pattern

Short-term goals in achieving expected patient outcomes are the following:

1. Patient will be able to establish a respiratory rate within five breaths per minute of the patient's normal baseline respiratory rate.
2. Patient's arterial blood gases will return to normal.
3. Patient will express a feeling of comfort in breathing.
4. Patient will be able to properly demonstrate diaphragmatic pursed-lip breathing.
5. Patient will achieve maximum lung expansion with adequate ventilation.

Long-term goal is that the patient will demonstrate skill in conserving energy while performing ADLs.

Impaired gas exchange

Short-term goals in achieving expected patient outcomes are the following:

1. Patient's respiratory rate will remain within five breaths per minute of normal baseline respiratory rate.
2. Patient will express a feeling of comfort in maintaining air exchange.
3. Patient will demonstrate the ability to cough effectively and to expectorate sputum.

4. Patient will maintain a PaO_2 value within the normal range.
5. Patient's fluid intake will be sufficient to prevent dehydration.
6. Patient will perform ADLs to the level of tolerance.

Long-term goals are the following:

1. Patient will have normal breath sounds upon auscultation.
2. Patient's arterial blood gases will return to normal baseline levels.
3. Patient will perform relaxation techniques every 4 hours during the daytime.
4. Patient will demonstrate correct bronchial hygiene practices.

IMPLEMENTATION

Nursing interventions define the actions necessary to help resolve the patient's health deviations and to achieve the desired patient outcomes. These activities should be individualized and written specifically for each patient. Nursing interventions include monitoring, educating, supporting, referring, and providing direct care for patients with respiratory diseases.

The following interventions are directed at maximizing breathing ability and are appropriate for all health care settings:

Relaxation exercises
Deep breathing and correct posture exercises
Pursed-lip breathing techniques
Therapeutic coughing and deep breathing
Incentive spirometry therapy
Pharmacologic therapy
Aerosol and humidification therapy
Hydration therapy, to keep secretions liquid
Nutritional intervention
Regular mobility program to prevent atelectasis and improve oxygenation
Oxygen therapy to supplement oxygen supply

Chest physical therapy techniques (positioning, percussion, vibration, and postural drainage) will need to be modified for the person who has other chronic illnesses. Patient with cardiovascu-

Aging Alert

- Nursing strategies are individualized to ensure effectiveness of patient care according to the patient's unique needs.
- High-quality nursing care of the older pulmonary patient includes emphasis on the prevention of infection.
- Careful planning of care and strict adherence to prescribed strategies are necessary to meet the respiratory needs of older patients.

Health Promotion
Components of a health promotion and education program

1. Smoking cessation
2. Preventive vaccines and skin testing
3. Prevention of infection
4. Maintaining adequate nutrition
5. Pulmonary rehabilitation
6. Pharmacologic management

lar diseases, arthritis, or back pain may not tolerate the Trendelenburg position and chest percussion and vibration. These treatments should not be performed on patients with osteoporosis or rib fractures because of the danger of lung punctures from skeletal fractures.

Health promotion and education are the cornerstones of chronic pulmonary disease management. It is essential that the patient understand the program and be committed to program compliance.

Smoking cessation

Tobacco use is responsible for more than one of every six deaths and is the single most important preventable cause of death and disease in our society. Cigarette smoking is a major risk factor for disease of the heart and blood vessels, chronic bronchitis, emphysema, and cancer. There is even evidence that smoking can be linked to an increased risk of osteoporosis. Cigarette smoking accounts for about 434,000 deaths annually, including 87% of all lung cancer deaths (USDHHS, 1992).

One of the primary goals of the Healthy People 2000 Public Health Service initiative for the United States is to reduce the use of tobacco by the year 2000 (see Healthy People 2000 Objectives, p. 304). Other objectives target re-

Tai chi at any age. *Courtesy Loy Ledbetter, St. Louis.*

ducing lung cancer and chronic obstructive pulmonary disease, placing restrictions on smoking in the workplace and public places, and encouraging provision of smoking cessation assistance by primary care providers (USDHHS, 1992).

Older adults took up smoking before its harmful effects were well understood. Surveys of members of the American Association of Retired Persons (AARP) show that older smokers (age 50 and older) are significantly less likely than younger smokers to believe that smoking harms health (Maloney, 1992).

Healthy People 2000 Objectives

3.4 Reduce cigarette smoking to a prevalence of no more than 15% among people aged 20 and older. (Baseline: 29% in 1987, 32% for men and 27% for women.)

From U.S. Department of Health and Human Services. (1992). *Healthy People 2000: National health promotion and disease prevention objectives* (DHHS Pub. No. [PHS] 91-50212). Washington, DC: U.S. Government Printing Office.

BOX 11-2 SMOKING CESSATION

By quitting smoking, I will gain these benefits:
1. I will greatly lessen my chances of getting cancer or having a heart attack.
2. I will have fewer colds or flu episodes each year.
3. I will have better-smelling clothes, hair, breath, and home.
4. I will climb stairs and walk without losing my breath.
5. I will have more money to spend on other things.
6. I will have fewer wrinkles.
7. I will be free of my morning cough.
8. I will increase my sense of control over my life.
9. I will _____
   (fill in personal benefit from smoking cessation)

I lose these benefits each day that I do not quit smoking.

From U.S. Department of Health and Human Services, 1993, January: *Nurses: Help your patient stop smoking* NIH Pub. No. 92-2962); Washington, DC: U.S. Government Printing Office.

Recent evidence shows that changing certain health behaviors, even in old age, can improve health and quality of life. Cigarette smoking is one of these habits. A report of the surgeon general outlined the health benefits of smoking cessation. Improved circulation is an almost immediate response. Coughing lessens, breathing is easier, and energy increases. The risks of heart disease, lung disease, cancer, and stroke diminish. Over time, the risk of cancer and heart disease diminish to the level of one who has never smoked (Health Benefits, 1990).

Smoking cessation and behavior modification programs may be successful with people of any age group. Patients need support from nursing personnel, as well as from significant others, as they try to alter the habitual, addictive behavior of smoking. Acknowledgement of the difficulty of stopping a lifelong habit will demonstrate the nurse's positive regard for the older person as an individual. Family and friends may feel that the patient is responsible for the illness and may not understand addiction principles or be therapeutic in helping patients to adjust. The objectivity of the nurse will support the patient in attempts to stop smoking. The nurse must continue to accept, support, and encourage patients in the difficult task of trying to change their smoking behavior (Box 11-2).

Preventive vaccines and skin testing

Influenza vaccine The influenza vaccine continues to be the most effective way of minimizing the morbidity and mortality associated with influenza. Approximately 80% to 90% of all influenza-associated deaths in the United States occur in people age 65 and older, the fastest growing age group of the population. Reduction of deaths in this age group has been hindered by low levels of vaccine utilization, as well as by the decreased immune response of older adults to the vaccines.

Healthy People 2000 Objectives

20.2 Reduce epidemic-related pneumonia and influenza deaths among people aged 65 and older to no more than 7.3 per 100,000. (Baseline: Average of 9.1 per 100,000 during 1980 through 1987.)

From U.S. Department of Health and Human Services. (1992). *Healthy People 2000: National health promotion and disease prevention objectives* (DHHS Pub. No. [PHS] 91-50212). Washington, DC: U.S. Government Printing Office.

BOX 11-3 CANDIDATES FOR INFLUENZA VACCINATION

1. People 65 years old and older
2. Residents of long-term care facilities
3. Patients with chronic cardiovascular or pulmonary disorders (including asthma)
4. Patients with chronic metabolic diseases, diabetes, chronic renal failure, hemoglobinopathies, or immunosuppressive diseases
5. Physicians, nurses, and other personnel in outpatient and inpatient settings
6. Employees of long-term care facilities who have direct patient contact
7. Providers of home care to people at high risk
8. Household members (including children of people at risk)

Adapted from Centers for Disease Control and Prevention. (1994). Prevention and control of influenza: 1. Vaccines. *MMWR, 43,* RR-9.

In response to this problem the U.S. Public Health Service has identified as part of the Healthy People 2000 initiative a primary objective of reducing pneumonia and influenza deaths (see Healthy People 2000 Objectives above). Other objectives target methods to increase vaccine utilization in the 65-and-older age group and to improve the match between vaccines and circulating influenza strains, thus reducing reactions to the vaccines.

Nurses can make a positive contribution by disseminating information regarding vaccination availability and infection control to high-risk groups. The individuals with the highest priority for receiving influenza vaccine are listed in Box 11-3.

New influenza vaccines are developed every year, based on information about the strains of viruses that are most likely to affect the population during the influenza season. Vaccines are made from inactivated viruses and should have minimal side effects. There is a 2- to 3-week delay in the development of antibody response, so vaccinations do not provide immediate protection. Although influenza vaccination is not 100% effective, it will help most older people. Because of the albumin in the influenza vaccine, it should

not be given to individuals who are allergic to eggs or to egg products ("Influenza 1994-95," 1994).

Current recommendations suggest that influenza vaccine be administered annually between mid-September and mid-November because exposure to the virus peaks between December and March. The timing of the vaccine is most important in high-risk groups. The period of maximum antibody titers should coincide with the time during which patients are most likely to be exposed to the virus. The vaccine can also be given during an influenza epidemic. During an outbreak of type A influenza, administration of a 2-week prophylaxis course of amantadine or rimantadine is recommended until protective antibody levels are reached or if the vaccine cannot be given. These antiviral agents are not effective against influenza type B ("Influenza 1994-95," 1994).

Pneumoccal vaccine Vaccination against pneumococcal infection is recommended for all people over the age of 65 and for patients of any age who have underlying pulmonary or cardiovascular disorders, alcoholism, cirrhosis, splenic dysfunction, diabetes, immunodeficiency, renal disease, or malignancy (Ely et al, 1994b) The vaccine protects against 88% of the bacteria that cause pneumonia (National Institute on Aging, 1994).

Most people only need to get the pneumonia vaccine once. However, the vaccine can be repeated every 6 years if necessary. Both the influenza vaccine and the pneumococcal vaccine may be administered at the same time at different sites without increased risk of side effects. Detailed immunization records must be kept because influenza vaccine is given annually, whereas pneumococcal vaccine is usually required only once in an adult.

Tuberculin skin testing Residents of long-term care facilities have a higher prevalence of tuberculosis than do older adults living in the community. Skin testing programs in these facilities are recommended by the Advisory Committee for the Elimination of Tuberculosis in the United States (McArthur et al, 1995). Indications for testing include the following: cough, hemoptysis, weight loss; laboratory or chest x-ray abnormalities suggesting TB; recent contact with a person with active TB; human immunodeficiency virus (HIV) infection; medical conditions that increase the risk of TB; and exposure to immigrants from areas with a high prevalence of TB.

The frequency of testing depends on the risk level. Residents of long-term care facilities should be tested for TB upon admission. It is important to remember that tuberculin skin test reactivity declines with advancing age (Mangura & Reichman, 1994). The two-step TB skin test is recommended for older patients. If the reaction to the first test is negative, a second test is done within 1 week of the first test. If the reaction to the second test is positive, the patient is considered infected and needs to be treated. If the second test is negative, the patient is considered uninfected (Couser, 1994).

Prevention of infection

Infection is a complication frequently encountered by patients with pulmonary disease. To prevent infection, patients should avoid crowds and particularly people known to have respiratory infections or influenza. Whether in the hospital, long-term care facility, or private or family home, clean respiratory equipment is essential to preventing the spread of infective organisms. Proper dental hygiene is also necessary because bacterial growth often begins in the mouth of patients with poor dental hygiene.

Early signs of respiratory infection are changes in the color, consistency, or volume of sputum, increased cough, increased dyspnea and/or chest tightness, decreased activity tolerance, and fever or chills. Patients should report any of these changes to the appropriate health care provider. Patient education should also cover signs and symptoms of other potential complications such as bronchospasm, fluid retention, and cardiac dysfunction.

Maintaining adequate nutrition

Dietary instruction is a necessary part of patient education. Maintaining adequate nutrition is frequently a problem for the older patient with lung disease. The process of eating requires energy expenditure, and it is difficult to eat when short of breath. Patients should be encouraged to ingest and chew food slowly, to eat smaller meals, to avoid gas-forming foods, to eat high-protein foods, and to avoid fatty foods that take longer to leave the stomach. Food ingestion increases mucus production, and patients with respiratory problems already have large volumes of mucus. Foul-tasting mucus may decrease appetite. In addition, medications prescribed for patients with lung disease, especially bronchodilators, may cause nausea. If appropriate, medications that might cause nausea should be taken with food.

Pulmonary rehabilitation

Older patients with lung disease who remain breathless despite therapy may experience a decrease in symptoms as a result of exercise training. A study by O'Donnell et al. (1993) evaluated breathlessness in older individuals. This research demonstrated significant reduction in breathlessness, increased activity tolerance, and overall improvements in psychosocial and functional abilities as a result of such training.

Pharmacologic management

A variety of medications are prescribed for patients who have altered respiratory function. The choice of drug depends on the primary pulmonary disease, as well as on the presence of other diseases and modifying factors in the patient's life.

Chronic obstructive pulmonary disease

The term *chronic obstructive pulmonary disease,* or *obstructive airway disease,* refers to a collection of disorders that have in common an airflow limitation during expiration. Emphysema and chronic bronchitis are the major disorders recognized under the umbrella of COPD. Asthma, technically defined as reversible airflow obstruction, is a type of reactive airway disease. The airflow obstruction of asthma is caused by the hyperresponsiveness of the tracheobronchial tree to a variety of stimuli (Adair, 1994). Clinical features depend on the extent of bronchospasm, mucosal inflammation with abnormal and excessive mucus production, and structural damage to the lungs (Poe & Israel, 1994). Although each disease has a different etiology and pathology, there is significant overlapping of symptoms. Similar medications are prescribed to treat all three of these diseases.

Medical management of COPD is becoming more complex, with the introduction of new pharmacologic agents and nicotine replacement products for smoking cessation. A therapeutic pharmocologic plan can only be developed after a comprehensive assessment of the older patient has been completed. Such a treatment plan is based on knowledge of the following overlapping factors and conditions:

1. Degree of pulmonary obstruction
2. Extent of pulmonary functional disability
3. Reversibility of the pulmonary obstruction process (pure asthma will respond to a different regimen than will emphysema)
4. Overlapping conditions that will affect medication absorption or excretion, such as nutritional, cardiac, renal, or metabolic dysfunction
5. Coexisting illnesses
6. Risk factors, such as smoking, obesity, or environmental air quality

Pharmacologic intervention for COPD is directed toward improving lung function and controlling symptoms with medications having the fewest side effects. The overall aim is to enhance the quality of life and to improve functional performance. Compliance with this complicated drug regimen will help to decrease the frequency of hospitalizations for exacerbation of lung diseases; therefore simplification of this program is essential. The following discussion highlights the most frequently prescribed medications for the treatment of COPD (Schapira & Reinke, 1995).

Bronchodilators Bronchodilators are one of the preferred medications for administration to patients with pulmonary disease. The principal action is to relax the smooth muscles surrounding the bronchial tree, thereby producing bronchial dilation. This action assists in preventing the accumulation of secretions in the dependent areas of the lungs.

Bronchodilators can be administered intravenously, subcutaneously, or orally in pill or liquid form. Aerosol and metered-dose aerosol preparations are available, which significantly decrease the incidence of side effects in the older patient.

Although there are numerous bronchodilator preparations available to treat COPD, several general types have proven effective. These are anticholinergic agents, beta-agonists, and xanthine derivative medications.

Anticholinergic bronchodilators antagonize the bronchoconstrictive effect of the parasympathetic nervous system, which is believed to be increased in COPD. Recent studies indicate that ipratropium (Atrovent) is more effective than inhaled beta-agonists as a bronchodilator in COPD (Schapire & Reinke, 1995). In addition, ipratropium carries minimal risk of adverse cardiovascular effects as compared with the older preparation atropine or with beta-agonists. Ipratropium has a gradual onset of action but longer duration than beta-agonists. Patients should be advised of these characteristics, so that they do not assume that the medication is ineffective. It is not a drug of choice for acute exacerbations of COPD. The dosage of ipratropium can be adjusted from 3 to 6 puffs 4 times a day for maximum bronchodilator effect (Ferguson & Cherniack, 1993).

Until the usefulness of ipratropium was demonstrated, *beta-adrenergic agonists* were the traditional cornerstone in the management of COPD. Currently, most authorities recommend that beta-agonists be used as a second line of therapy, either to replace ipratropium or to supplement iprotropium for patients who do not clinically benefit from this agent alone.

Many beta-agonist medications that are currently available in inhaled forms are selective for the beta-2 receptor sites on bronchial smooth muscle. Administration by the inhaled route helps to minimize the systemic effects, but beta-agonists may result in tachycardia, palpitations, tremors, and hypokalemia. Nonselective beta-stimulators that affect both beta-1 and beta-2 receptors (isoproterenol) may cause or aggravate CHF, hypotension, or arrhythmias, or they may potentiate existing muscle tremors. The most therapeutic adrenergic agonist bronchodilator is the one with the most beta-2 and the fewest beta-1 properties.

Recent studies have suggested that the combination of an inhaled anti-inflammatory corti-

Aging Alert

Over-the-counter bronchodilator inhalers and combination cold preparations that contain epinephrine and ephedrine may worsen hypertension and urinary retention or aggravate hyperglycemia in diabetic patients. Older adults must be cautioned about the use of these readily available products.

costeroid agent with an inhaled beta-agonist has long-term beneficial effects on outcome of pulmonary function, as compared with inhaled bronchodilator therapy alone. A combination beta-agonist and anticholinergic in a metered-dose inhaler (MDI) preparation is awaiting approval from the Food and Drug Administration (Schapira & Reinke, 1995).

None of the pharmacologic agents available for managing COPD has created more controversy in recent years than *theophylline*. This xanthine derivative was discovered in 1888 and first recognized as a bronchodilator in humans in 1922. For more than 60 years theophylline was one of the most frequently prescribed bronchodilators (Poe & Israel, 1994).

The potential benefits of theophylline include both bronchodilator and systemic effects. Advantages for patients with COPD include increased mucus clearance; improvement of contractility of the diaphragm, which reduces respiratory muscle fatigue; and stimulation of the central respiratory centers. In addition, increased cardiac contractility results in improved blood and oxygen supply to the lungs and other vital organs. Theophylline is also known to have a diuretic effect, an issue to be remembered with patients already undergoing diuretic therapy.

The benefits of theophylline therapy must be weighed against the well-known disadvantages. A number of drugs effect theophylline metabolism and clearance, resulting in increased blood concentration. These include erythromycin, cimetidine, propranolol, ciprofloxacin, corfloxacin, allopurinol, and the influenza vaccine (Adair, 1994). Newer H_2 blockers do not have this effect. Smoking is also thought to alter the metabolism of theophylline by increasing clearance, resulting in a need for increased dosage.

In addition, theophylline is known to have arrhythmogenic effects. Theophylline toxicity is common, and its symptoms include nausea, insomnia, nervousness and irritability, gastrointestinal distress, muscle twitching, tremors, and tachycardia. Seizures are known to occur with high serum drug levels, especially in older adults.

Because theophylline has a relatively narrow therapeutic range and its metabolism is affected by so many variables that may be present in the older patient, it is advised that therapeutic drug levels be monitored weekly in acute care settings, and at least every 6 months in the long-term care and home care environments. To avoid the potential for drug toxicity, the blood theophylline level in older patients should probably be maintained in the lower end of the commonly recommended range of 10 to 20 mg/100 ml (Adair, 1994).

Oral preparations are frequently in the form of timed-release tablets, which should not be crushed. Liquid preparations are available for those individuals who cannot swallow pills or are fed through a feeding tube; these are more rapidly absorbed and have greater side effects than the timed-release tablets.

The absorption and metabolism of theophylline preparations in the older patient are affected by the existence of other chronic illnesses and drug regimens. Food intake may alter the rate of absorption of some of the timed-release products. It is wise to consult manufacturers' information for specific drug interactions and administration guidelines. Recent literature recommends adding theophylline only when a patient with COPD has not responded to first-line therapy with ipratropium (Atrovent) and a beta-agonist (Poe & Israel, 1994).

Corticosteroids Corticosteroids have been proven useful in treatment regimens for asthma, but their role in the treatment of emphysema and chronic bronchitis is still evolving. Oral agents appear to benefit about 10% of patients with clinically stable COPD (Schapira & Reinke, 1995). They are thought to decrease airway inflammation and increase the response to beta-agonists and may be considered for COPD patients whose symptoms are not well controlled with ipratropium, beta-agonists, and theophylline. They are usually reserved for acute exacerbations of COPD.

Aerosol steroids inhaled into the lungs are used as maintenance regimens for patients with chronic lung disease. The addition of an inhaled corticosteroid may lessen the oral requirement by as much as 5 to 10 mg per day (Schapira & Reinke, 1995). Inhaled corticosteroids can produce local side effects. Oral candidiasis occurs in about one third of patients and is related to frequency of administration and to total dosage. Gargling with water after treatment, or the use of a spacer may decrease the incidence of yeast infections. Another side effect is hoarseness (Mathewson & Kovac, 1994).

Several side effects are commonly associated with oral or parenteral steroid administration, but not with inhalants. These include glucose intolerance (diabetes), fluid retention, and weight gain or osteoporosis secondary to calcium depletion in the bones. Mood swings, decreased healing of wounds, retinal changes, and decreased ability to fight infections are also common and must be monitored.

A nursing plan for patient education should incorporate realistic methods for the patient to use in evaluating, measuring, and reporting any decrease in symptoms or the occurrence of side effects of steroid therapy. Administration of these drugs should not be continued unless they are useful.

PATIENT'S INSTRUCTIONS FOR USE

Serevent®
(salmeterol xinafoate)
Inhalation Aerosol

Bronchodilator Aerosol For Oral Inhalation Only

Before using your Serevent® (salmeterol xinafoate) Inhalation Aerosol, read complete instructions carefully.

Allen & Hanburys

1. SHAKE THE INHALER WELL immediately before each use (see Figure 1).

2. REMOVE THE CAP FROM THE MOUTHPIECE (see Figure 2); the strap on the cap will stay attached to the actuator. If the strap is removed from the actuator and lost, the inhaler mouthpiece should be inspected for the presence of foreign objects before each use. Make sure the canister is fully and firmly inserted into the actuator.

As with all aerosol medications, it is recommended to "test spray" the inhaler. Do this by spraying four times into the air before using for the first time and when the inhaler has not been used for a prolonged period of time (i.e., more than 4 weeks).

3. BREATHE OUT THROUGH THE MOUTH (see Figure 3a). Place the mouthpiece in the mouth, holding the inhaler in the position shown in Figure 3a and closing the lips around it. Alternatively, the inhaler may be positioned 1 to 2 inches away from the open mouth (see Figure 3b).

4. WHILE BREATHING IN DEEPLY AND SLOWLY THROUGH THE MOUTH, PRESS DOWN FIRMLY AND FULLY ON THE TOP OF THE METAL CANISTER with your index finger (see Figure 4).

5. CONTINUE TO INHALE AND TRY TO HOLD YOUR BREATH FOR 5 TO 10 SECONDS. Before breathing out, remove the inhaler from your mouth and release your finger from the canister.

6. WAIT ABOUT 30 SECONDS AND SHAKE the inhaler again. Repeat steps 3 through 5 for each inhalation prescribed by your doctor.

7. REPLACE THE MOUTHPIECE CAP AFTER EACH USE.

8. CLEANSE THE INHALER THOROUGHLY AND FREQUENTLY. Remove the metal canister and cleanse the plastic case and cap by rinsing thoroughly in warm, running water at least once a day. After thoroughly drying the plastic case and cap, gently replace the canister into the case with a twisting motion and replace the cap.

9. DISCARD THE CANISTER AFTER YOU HAVE USED THE LABELED NUMBER OF INHALATIONS. The correct amount of medication in each inhalation cannot be assured after this point.

DOSAGE: Use only as directed by your doctor.

WARNINGS: Serevent® (salmeterol xinafoate) Inhalation Aerosol is different from your other asthma medications. Serevent Inhalation Aerosol provides a relatively longer duration of effect. The bronchodilation action of Serevent Inhalation Aerosol usually lasts for at least 12 hours. Therefore, it is important that you carefully read and understand the following information:
1. **Do not use Serevent Inhalation Aerosol more frequently than two times daily, morning and evening, approximately 12 hours apart, at the recommended dose of two inhalations each time.**
2. **Do not use Serevent Inhalation Aerosol to relieve sudden asthma symptoms** (e.g., sudden severe onset or worsening of wheezing, cough, chest tightness, and/or shortness of breath that has been diagnosed by your doctor as due to asthma). **If you experience sudden asthma symptoms while using Serevent Inhalation Aerosol, you should not take more Serevent Inhalation Aerosol to relieve these symptoms.** Instead, you should treat these sudden asthma symptoms with a different medication that has been prescribed by your doctor (e.g., an inhaled, short-acting bronchodilator such as albuterol). If you do not have an inhaled, short-acting bronchodilator, contact your doctor to have one prescribed for you.

3. While you are using Serevent Inhalation Aerosol, tell your doctor immediately if you are getting worse, as indicated by any of the following situations.
• Your short-acting, inhaled bronchodilator becomes less effective for treatment of sudden asthma symptoms.
• You need more inhalations than usual of your short-acting bronchodilator for treatment of sudden asthma symptoms.
• You are using four or more inhalations per day of your short-acting bronchodilator for 2 or more days consecutively.
• You use more than one canister of a short-acting bronchodilator in an 8-week period (i.e., there are 200 inhalations per canister).
4. Use other inhaled medications only as prescribed by your doctor.
5. **Do not use Serevent Inhalation Aerosol as a substitute for oral or inhaled corticosteroids.** If you have been prescribed corticosteroids, you should not change your dosage of these medications or stop taking these medications without talking to your doctor, even if you feel better.
6. If you are using Serevent Inhalation Aerosol to prevent exercise-induced bronchospasm, you should inhale the dose at least 30 to 60 minutes before exercise.

Avoid spraying in eyes. Contents under pressure. Do not puncture or incinerate. Protect from freezing temperatures and direct sunlight. Do not store at temperatures above 120°F. Keep out of reach of children.

Store between 2° and 30°C (36° and 86°F). As with most inhaled medications in aerosol canisters, the therapeutic effect of this medication may decrease when the canister is cold; for best results, the canister should be at room temperature before use. Shake well before using.

Store canister with nozzle end down.

For use with Serevent Inhalation Aerosol actuator only. The actuator should not be used with other aerosol medications.

Serevent Inhalation Aerosol is available from your pharmacist in a refill canister without the plastic actuator. By requesting the refill canister, you may reduce the cost of your prescription.

Note: The indented statement below is required by the Federal government's Clean Air Act for all products containing or manufactured with chlorofluorocarbons (CFCs).

This product contains trichlorofluoromethane and dichlorodifluoromethane, substances that harm the environment by depleting ozone in the upper atmosphere.

Your doctor has determined that this product is likely to help your personal health. **USE THIS PRODUCT AS DIRECTED, UNLESS INSTRUCTED TO DO OTHERWISE BY YOUR DOCTOR.** If you have any questions about alternatives, consult with your doctor.

Allen & Hanburys, Division of Glaxo Inc.
Research Triangle Park, NC 27709
December 1994
RL-164

FIGURE 11-4 Patient instruction: Inhalation aerosol.

Inhaler techniques The effectiveness of all inhaled agents depends on how much drug reaches the lungs. Metered-dose inhalers are one of the important adjuncts to drug management for pulmonary disease. When used properly, they deliver an automatic preset amount of medication. However, the therapeutic value of MDIs may be compromised by poor patient technique (Figure 11-4).

Two methods are currently recommended for inhaling drugs from an MDI. The closed-mouth technique is the most common, but the open-mouth technique has advantages. When used properly, the open-mouth technique results in increased drug delivery and a decrease in the gagging and nausea that some patients experience with the closed-mouth technique (Toogood, 1994).

Teaching proper use of an inhaler is one of the important responsibilities of nursing. Improper inhalation technique is a major problem. Poor coordination of MDI actuation and inspiration often prevents adequate medication from entering the lungs. This is especially true in older patients. A spacer (reservoir) can be adapted to the inhaler for those patients who have difficulty using the inhaler. Because this spacer holds the medication for a few seconds after the inhaler is triggered, the person does not have to coordinate the activation of the aerosol device with inhalation (Box 11-4).

A newer alternative is the use of breath-activated inhalers (BAIs). Data show that older patients handle a breath-actuated inhaler more successfully, regardless of previous MDI experience (Chapman et al, 1993). Another new product is the dry powder formulation. Because only a few bronchodilator and corticosteroid inhaled preparations are currently available in the dry powder BAI form, the spacer is more commonly used for older adults.

Patient education is paramount to the effectiveness of bronchial inhalants. The individual must understand that these devices deliver potent medication and should only be used as prescribed. The patient must be instructed to assemble the cartridge and the inhaler according to the manufacturer's directions. The mouthpiece should be cleansed in warm soapy water, rinsed, and allowed to air dry at least once a day. This may be convenient to do with the evening meal or at bedtime. Inhalation techniques are difficult for the older person but should be performed as efficiently as possible for the most therapeutic effect of the medication.

If corticosteroid metered-dose inhalers are used in conjunction with inhaled bronchodilators, the bronchodilator should be used first, to

BOX 11-4 HOW TO USE AN MDI PROPERLY

1. Predose stage
   a. Remove cap from MDI.
   b. Shake canister 3 or 4 times.
   c. Hold MDI upright and exhale normally (to functional residual capacity).
   d. Close lips around mouthpiece of MDI (closed-mouth technique), or hold mouthpiece two finger-breadths in front of open mouth (open-mouth technique).
2. Dosing stage
   a. Begin to inhale slowly. After 1 to 2 seconds, discharge one puff from the MDI.
   b. Continue to inhale slowly for 5 to 10 seconds. Count the seconds while inhaling.
   c. Hold breath for 5 to 10 seconds.
   d. Exhale.
3. Follow-up
   a. Wait 1 minute before inhaling the next puff (if prescribed). Then repeat steps 1b through 2d.
   b. If the inhaled drug is a corticosteroid, rinse mouth with tap water when finished. Spit the water out; do not swallow it.

From Toogood, J. H. (1994). Helping your patients make better use of MDIs and spacers. *Journal of Respiratory Diseases, 15*(2), 151-166.

facilitate maximum action of the corticosteroid and to prevent bronchospasm. The patient should wait 10 to 15 minutes before using the steroid inhaler, for maximum effect. If two puffs of the medication are ordered, the patient should be instructed to wait several minutes between inhaling subsequent puffs. Often the patient finds it beneficial to use bronchodilating inhalers before any activity that may cause shortness of breath. Patients should be cautioned not to overuse the inhaler.

The complexity of inhalers may prevent their practical use in some older patients. However, nursing intervention may help to facilitate their effectiveness. If used correctly, inhalers are very useful in reducing respiratory symptoms with minimal systemic absorption and side effects.

Mucolytic agents The benefit of mucolytic agents and expectorants in the control of secretions is not well documented (Schapira & Reinke, 1995). Acetylcysteine inhalation therapy may be useful in patients with excessive mucus. This drug should be used for mucus retention only when hydration and usual bronchial hygiene treatments are ineffective. Adverse effects include coughing and bronchospasm; therefore this agent should only be used in conjunction with a bronchodilating agent.

Expectorants and antitussive agents Oral expectorants such as guaifenesin may help to loosen bronchial secretions. They are not consistently effective, and their use should be reserved for acute exacerbation of COPD rather than for chronic disease treatment. Long-term use may result in toxic effects and increased mucus production.

Antitussive agents are not useful for COPD in the absence of a dry, hacking cough. They are not to be used to treat a cough arising from retained secretions.

Inhaled human recombinant deoxyribonuclease Inhaled human recombinant deoxyribonuclease (DNASE) is an enzyme currently used to treat patients with cystic fibrosis. It has also been shown to decrease the purulent sputum in patients with COPD (Schapira & Reinke, 1995).

Antibiotics Antibiotic therapy is usually reserved for acute lung infection in patients with COPD or for those older patients with symptoms of pneumonia. Antibiotics are effective against bacteria but not against viruses. Selection of appropriate antimicrobial therapy is dependent on the rapid determination of the organism, as well as the environmental influence (community-acquired or nosocomial infection).

Certain guidelines have been developed for antibiotic choice. For seriously ill patients with community-acquired pneumonia and no identified organism, erythromycin and cefuroxime or erythromycin and trimethoprim-sulfamethoxazole are recommended. Broad-spectrum antimicrobial therapy is usually indicated for the treatment of aspiration pneumonia until the specific organism is isolated on sputum culture.

Treatment of nosocomial pneumonia acquired in an extended care facility or a hospital is much more difficult because of the development of drug-resistant strains of bacteria. An aminoglycoside and a broad-spectrum agent are recommended (Bartlett, 1994). Caution must be used when administering aminoglycosides because they may be nephrotoxic and ototoxic. Dosages usually have to be adjusted in the older patient to minimize these detrimental effects. Baseline assessment of renal and hearing parameters should be determined before initiation of therapy.

Antitubercular therapy A positive TB test indicates that the tested person has TB infection. Presence of symptoms, a positive sputum for AFB, and a positive chest x-ray indicate that the person has the active disease. People with a TB infection but no active disease should undergo preventive therapy with a daily dose of isoniazid (INH) for up to 6 months. People who have the disease need to be treated with a combination of several drugs (American Lung Association, 1994).

A 9-month course of isoniazid and rifampin is indicated for newly diagnosed older patients. This is usually well tolerated by older adults. The Centers for Disease Control (CDC) guidelines recommend the addition of another agent (ethambutol or PZA). This may not be necessary in older adults whose infection was acquired many years ago and who probably do not have drug-resistant tuberculosis. However, multidrug-resistant TB (MRTB) should be suspected in patients who have a relapse of symptoms in spite of previous treatment for active TB. In addition to the previously mentioned anti-TB regimen, other drugs that may be included in treatment of MRTB include streptomycin, aminosalicylate sodium, and cycloserine (Stead & Dutt, 1994). The appropriate selection and combination depends on the severity and extent of the disease.

Some of these medications are potentially toxic to the liver, especially in older adults. Nursing assessment must include attention to skin tone, urine, and sclera for development of icteric signs of jaundice. Other symptoms that might alert the practitioner to impaired liver function include fatigue, anorexia, nausea, vomiting, malaise, and weakness. Liver function test results should be monitored to detect drug-induced hepatitis.

Peripheral neuropathy and retinal changes may develop in the patient undergoing treatment for tuberculosis, especially the frail, malnourished older patient. An ophthalmologic evaluation is recommended before treatment with ethambutol. Changes in hearing and disequilibrium may accompany treatment with streptomycin. These sensory changes need to be evaluated frequently during treatment in the older person with tuberculosis.

Lung cancer The use of chemotherapy treatment for lung cancer in older adults is dependent on the type of primary cancer and the extent of metastasis. Several combination therapy regimens have been promising for small-cell lung cancer (SCLC), but not for non–small cell lung cancer (NSCLC), which is relatively unresponsive to chemotherapy (Perry, 1994). Quality-of-life issues must be addressed with the older person, who may consider chemotherapy investigational protocols for lung cancer. The toxic effects on the frail older person may alter the person's functional abilities more quickly than the disease process. Informed consent is essential before such a decision is made.

Pulmonary embolism Drug treatment for pulmonary embolism includes intravenous administration of heparin for the acute event, followed by long-term oral anticoagulation therapy with warfarin. Use of thrombolytic therapy for pulmonary embolism continues to be individualized and usually reserved for massive embolism when cardiovascular hemodynamics are compromised. Because all of these agents increase the potential for bleeding, they may be contraindicated in the older person with a recent history of gastrointestinal or cerebrovascular bleeding. The inherent risks are weighed against the severity of the embolism before a choice is made. If anticoagulant therapy is absolutely contraindicated in the older patient, an inferior vena cava filter may be inserted to prevent clot movement through the circulatory system to a vital organ. Anticoagulants are always used cautiously in the older population.

Whatever the health care setting, patient education concerning the risks of anticoagulant therapy is an essential part of the nursing plan. Several principles guide the development of the care plan for patients being given anticoagulants:

1. Patients should be instructed to observe for signs of bleeding and to report the following: bleeding gums or wounds, nosebleeds, hematuria, headaches, vomiting of dark material, hemoptysis, or black or bloody stools. In addition, lethargy, fatigue, dizziness, chills, or tachycardia may indicate internal bleeding.
2. Vitamin K deficiency may increase the risk of bleeding. Nutritional instruction should cover foods that are high in vitamin K. Patients should also be advised that broccoli, turnip greens, cabbage, spinach, and liver are foods that interfere with the effectiveness of anticoagulants.
3. Any OTC medications containing aspirin or ibuprofen should be avoided, because these interfere with platelet adhesion and can increase the risk of bleeding.
4. Periodic coagulation laboratory tests must be performed, to determine the therapeutic effect of anticoagulants.

Pulmonary edema Diuretics are the main pharmacologic agents used in the acute phase treatment of pulmonary edema. Older adults undergoing diuretic therapy are at great risk for developing fluid and electrolyte imbalance. Signs and symptoms that might indicate the presence of these imbalances include dry mucous membranes, thirst, poor tissue turgor, confusion, weakness, lethargy, muscle cramps, restlessness, hypotension, oliguria, and cardiac arrhythmias. In addition, overzealous diuresis can place patients at risk for the development of renal failure.

The nurse is in a position to teach the patient how to recognize these side effects, as well as the importance of strict adherence to the prescribed diuretic schedule. Diuretics can be administered at a convenient time for the patient, as long as doses are not missed. The older person who wants to travel for the day must be reminded to take the diuretic before the end of the day to prevent exacerbation of CHF, which would contribute to pulmonary edema.

Compliance with prescribed medication regimens is a major problem facing the older patient, especially in the home care environment. Strategies to improve compliance are an essential part of patient education. The nurse is encouraged to incorporate the following principles in planning the older patient's medication regimen:

1. Medication instructions and regimens should be as simple as possible. As many medications as possible should be taken at the same time of day. This will decrease the number of times the older person has to remember to take medications.
2. Relatives, caregivers, and significant others should be instructed in the regimen. Written directions should be available. Memory aids such as drug calendars, pillboxes, or envelopes with a dose supply may be helpful.
3. Sensory aids may be helpful for those with visual impairment. Pasting a different fabric (with a distinctive texture) on the top of each pill bottle may help the older adult to identify the right bottle.

Devices such as these are only appropriate for the individual without mental impairment.
4. Regular review of instructions and evaluation of methods is essential to ensure compliance with multiple medication regimens.

In the acute care setting

The older patient in the hospital is frequently placed on mechanical ventilation as part of the treatment for an acute lung problem. The intention of such therapy is the temporary support of breathing until the patient can breathe sufficiently to meet the body oxygen requirements.

Complications from mechanical ventilation have a high incidence in the older, hospitalized patient population. The impaired ability to communicate and the painfulness of existence on mechanical ventilation, combined with the physical insults of barotrauma, pneumothorax, decreased venous return, oxygen toxicity, and infection, compromise the ability of the older individual to overcome the critical pulmonary condition.

Psychologic trauma, sensory deprivation, and poor quality of life are issues with which the nurse is confronted. Older patients often die while on a ventilator in the intensive care unit (ICU). Death in this way may be more painful for both the patient and the family than a peaceful death experienced in a more natural homelike environment.

Nursing interventions during this time focus on psychologic support for the individual and significant others, in addition to performance of technical tasks directed at care of the patient on ventilation. The nurse is sensitive to the patient's needs and is able to make the final days as comfortable as possible. Nurses are in a position to interpret and evaluate the patient's preferences because of their close contact with the patient and significant others.

As the patient advocate, the nurse has an opportunity and an obligation to contribute to the resolution of the ethical dilemma surrounding the question of discontinuing ventilator support. This costly treatment will maintain the individual but is not curative. It is hoped that in the future, medical and nursing interventions will emphasize education of the public about decisions regarding the use of mechanical ventilation when the result of treatment is not beneficial to the patient.

In the long-term care setting

Interventions in the long-term care setting focus on prevention of recurring respiratory infection and the promotion of respiratory well-being. Treatment is similar to that in other health care settings. However, nursing actions are expanded to include managing and coordinating the activities of other health care team members as they perform interventions to correct problems related to breathing. In addition to breathing exercises, regular schedules of activity—either ambulation or turning and position change—are necessary to prevent the development of pneumonia.

Frequently, older residents with chronic respiratory problems also suffer from impaired mobility. These two impairments may combine to put the resident at risk for aspiration pneumonia. The nurse must closely supervise the feeding of all debilitated long-term care facility residents, in an effort to negate the risk of aspiration pneumonia. Techniques to prevent aspiration of enteral tube feedings, such as elevating the head of the bed and administering feedings slowly, are integral parts of the care of the older person with impaired swallowing ability.

Increasingly, residents of long-term care facilities require highly technical pulmonary skills. Nursing interventions for these patients require advanced assessment skills, airway clearance techniques, tracheostomy care, sterile suctioning procedures, and ventilator care. A multidisciplinary team approach involving the nurse, physician, respiratory therapist, dietitian, physical and occupational therapist, and social worker is essential in achieving the best patient outcomes. Facilities that care for patients requiring long-term mechanical ventilation are supported around the clock by respiratory therapists practicing under specific written guidelines.

In the private or family home

When older patients with severe lung disorders return to their homes from either an acute care or a long-term care facility, they may need to be monitored by professional health care providers. Patients with chronic lung disease often adjust more readily to their disability through a comprehensive home care program. Nursing is a major component of such programs.

Few third-party players, including Medicare, pay for continuous 24-hour nursing coverage. However, most insurance companies, including Medicare, reimburse for intermittent nursing visits. The number and duration of nursing visits usually can be negotiated with a third-party payer, if a cost savings is realized (Dettenmeier, 1992).

Other health care providers, such as respiratory therapists, technicians from oxygen supply companies, and home health aides, are frequently part of the team that enables the patient to remain at home. Guidelines are needed to help determine eligibility for home care treatment. The American Thoracic Society has developed specific criteria for home care referral (Box 11-5).

The federal government has established guidelines to define eligibility for financial reimbursement for home care. They include consideration of homebound status, medical instability, and the need for skilled nursing care rather than custodial care. Other financial resources may be available for support in the home environment. Additional information is available from social services agencies in the community and from the American Lung Association.

Older patients with severe chronic lung disease may be able to live more comfortably at home if respiratory inhalation treatments and

---

BOX 11-5 CRITERIA FOR REFERRAL FOR HOME CARE

1. Patients with unstable cardiopulmonary status or complex treatment program
2. Patients who require only periodic medical supervision, not constant supervision
3. Patients with the "revolving door" syndrome (i.e., frequent hospitalizations)
4. Confused, highly anxious, or depressed patients
5. Patients whose behavior or care places an unusual burden on the family
6. Patients who do not have the support of family members or significant others
7. Patients with new equipment who are discharged from the hospital

From American Thoracic Society (1977). Home use of equipment for patients with respiratory disease. *American Association of Respiratory Disease, 115,* 893-895. (Currently under revision.)

---

oxygen are available to them. The benefits of therapy must be weighed against the risks and costs before making a decision to use home equipment. Once this decision is confirmed, the nurse may be the person responsible for helping the patient to select the oxygen therapy vendor.

It is necessary to consider the patient's medical insurance and financial capabilities. Medicare standards restrict reimbursement for home oxygen use to patients with a documented oxygen saturation of under 88% or a PaO_2 value under 55 mm Hg (Schapira & Reinke, 1995). However, if they have supplemental insurance or elect to pay for these services, many other patients can benefit from the oxygen therapy.

Oxygen is supplied to the home through oxygen concentrators, high-pressure cylinders, or liquid oxygen cylinders. Oxygen may be delivered by a variety of devices, including nasal cannulae and masks.

Regardless of which system is used in the home, the nursing intervention plan must stress safety factors. Smoking around oxygen is prohibited for both the patient and others. Patients who use gas stoves for cooking are advised to avoid cooking when oxygen is in the same room. Although oxygen itself is not *flammable*—that is, it will not ignite a fire—it is *combustible* and will make a fire burn hotter and faster. Vendors supplying respiratory equipment and oxygen are available to teach patients about these treatments.

The use of home mechanical ventilation is a rapidly growing intervention, especially for respiratory failure resulting from neurologic disorders. Although this technology is not yet prevalent in the treatment of lung diseases, especially in the older individual, it may develop in the future, because the cost of in-hospital treatment of pulmonary disease is escalating. However, most pulmonary specialists presently discourage home use of the high-cost, noncurative mechanical ventilation for chronic lung disease.

EVALUATION

Evaluation is the final step of the nursing process. Evaluation of the effectiveness of the nursing interventions and attainment of expected outcomes is ongoing. Each nursing intervention is continuously reevaluated, taking into consideration the needs of the individual patient and the realistic attainment of the desired outcomes.

REFERENCES

Adair, N. (1994). Chronic airflow obstruction and respiratory failure. In W. Hazzard, E. Bierman, J. Blass, W. Ettinger, & J. Halter (Eds.), *Principles of geriatric medicine and gerontology* (pp. 583-595). New York: McGraw-Hill.

American Lung Association. (1994). *Facts about tuberculosis* (Pamphlet No. 1091). Author.

Bardana, E. J. (1993). Is asthma really different in the elderly patient? *Journal of Asthma, 30,* 77-79.

Bartlett, J. (1994). Pneumonia. In W. Hazzard, E. Bierman, J. Blass, W. Ettinger, & J. Halter (Eds.), *Principles of geriatric medicine and gerontology* (pp. 565-573). New York: McGraw-Hill.

Britt, T. L. (1993). Elderly patients. In J. M. Clochesy, C. Breu, S. Cardin, E. B. Rudy, & A. A. Whittaker (Eds.), *Critical care nursing* (pp. 1351-1372). Philadelphia: W. B. Saunders.

Centers for Disease Control and Prevention. (1994). Prevention and control of influenza: 1. Vaccines. *Morbidity and Mortality Weekly Report, 43*, RR-9.

Chapman, K., Love, L., & Brubaker, H. (1993). A comparison of breath actuated and conventional metered-dose inhaler inhalation techniques in elderly subjects *Chest, 104*, 1332-1337.

Cooper, D. (1993). Patients with chronic obstructive pulmonary disease. In J. M. Clochesy, C. Breu, S. Cardin, E. B. Rudy, & A. A. Whittaker (Eds.), *Critical care nursing* (pp. 569-588). Philadelphia: W. B. Saunders.

Couser, J. (1994). Interpreting tuberculin skin tests in the elderly. *Journal of Respiratory Diseases, 15*, 869-870.

Dettenmeier, P. A. (1992). *Pulmonary nursing care* (pp. 385-439). St. Louis: Mosby.

Dobson, M. E., & Ruben, F. L. (1993). The special challenge of pneumonia in the elderly. *Journal of Respiratory Diseases, 14*, 1145-1164.

Ely, E. W., Pegram, P. S., & Haponik, E. F. (1994a). Managing and preventing pneumonia in the elderly. *Journal of Respiratory Diseases, 15*, 295-311.

Ely, E. W., Pegram, P. S., & Haponik, E. F. (1994b). Working up the elderly patient with pneumonia. *Journal of Respiratory Diseases, 15*, 222-234.

Fein, A. M., Feinsilver, S. H., & Niederman, M. S. (1991). Atypical manifestations of pneumonia in the elderly. *Clinical Chest Medicine, 12*, 319-336.

Ferguson, G. T., & Cherniack, R. M. (1993). Management of chronic obstructive pulmonary disease. *New England Journal of Medicine, 328*, 1017-1022.

Health benefits of smoking cessation: A report of the surgeon general. (1990).

Hogstel, M. O. (1994). *Nursing care of the older adult.* New York: Delmar.

Hunninghake, G. W. (1994). Interstitial lung disease, hypersensitivity pneumonitis, and pulmonary vascular disease. In W. Hazzard, E. Bierman, J. Blass, W. Ettinger, & J. Halter (Eds.), *Principles of geriatric medicine and gerontology* (pp. 597-606). New York: McGraw-Hill.

Influenza 1994-95: Now's the time to prepare. (1994). *Journal of Respiratory Diseases, 15*, 675-687.

Levitzky, M. G. (1991). *Pulmonary physiology* (3rd ed.). New York: McGraw-Hill.

Lynch, J. P. (1992). Community-acquired pneumonia: What new trends mean in practice. *Journal of Respiratory Diseases, 13*, 1619-1643.

Maloney, S. K. (1992). *Smoking among older adults: Findings from three surveys.* American Association of Retired Persons Health Advocacy Services.

Mangura, B. T., & Reichman, L. B. (1994). Tuberculosis: Guidelines for preventive therapy. *Journal of Respiratory Diseases, 15*, 109-121.

Mathewson, M. D., & Kovac, A. L. (1994). Update on inhaled steroids. *Respiratory Care, 39*, 837-839.

Matthay, M. A., & Hopewell, P. C. (1994). Critical care for acute respiratory failure. In G. Baum & E. Wolinsky (Eds.), *Textbook of pulmonary diseases* (5th ed., Vol. 2). Boston: Little, Brown and Company.

McArthur, M. A., Simor, A. E., Campbell, B., & McGeer, A. (1995). Influenza and pneumococcal vaccinations and tuberculin skin testing programs in long-term care facilities: Where do we stand? *Infection Control and Hospital Epidemiology, 16*(1), 18-24.

Miller, C. (1994). *Nursing care of older adults: Theory and practice* (2nd ed.). Philadelphia: J. B. Lippincott.

Mosher, K. M. (1994). Pulmonary embolism. In G. Baum & E. Wolinsky (Eds.), *Textbook of pulmonary diseases* (5th ed., Vol. 2). Boston: Little, Brown and Company.

National Cancer Institute. (1993, June). *What you need to know about lung cancer* (NIH Pub. No. 93-1553). Washington, DC: U.S. Department of Health and Human Services.

National Institute on Aging. (1994). *Pneumonia prevention: It's worth a shot* (AGE PAGE). Washington, DC: U.S. Department of Health and Human Services.

National Institutes of Health, National Heart, Lung, and Blood Institute. (1994, November). NIH Pub. No. 93-2020. Washington, DC: U.S. Department of Health and Human Services.

Niederman, M. S. (1993). Pneumonia in residents of long-term care facilities: A guide to diagnosis and management. *Long-term Care Forum, 3*(2), 1:12-15.

O'Donnell, D. E., Webb, K. A., & McGuire, M. A. (1993). Older patients with COPD: Benefits of exercise training. *Geriatrics, 48*(1), 59-66.

Osler, W. (1892). *Principles and practice of medicine.* New York: D. Appleton and Company.

Perry, M. C. (1994). Lung cancer. In W. Hazzard, E. Bierman, J. Blass, W. Ettinger, & J. Halter (Eds.), *Principles of geriatric medicine and gerontology* (pp. 607-613). New York: McGraw-Hill.

Poe, R. H., & Israel, R. H. (1994). Theophylline: Still a reasonable choice? *Journal of Respiratory Diseases, 15*(1), 19-30.

Richman, L. (1992). A looming public health nightmare. In *Lungs at work.* American Lung Association.

Schapira, R. M., & Reinke, L. (1995). The outpatient diagnosis and management of chronic obstructive pulmonary disease. *Journal of Geriatric Internal Medicine, 10,* 40-55.

Stead, W., & Dutt, A. (1994). Tuberculosis: A special problem in the elderly. In W. Hazzard, E. Bierman, J. Blass, W. Ettinger, & J. Halter (Eds.), *Principles of geriatric medicine and gerontology* (pp. 575-582). New York: McGraw-Hill.

Timiras, P. S. (1994). *Physiological basis of aging and geriatrics* (2nd ed.). Boca Raton, FL: CRC Press.

Toogood, J. H. (1994). Helping your patients make better use of MDIs and spacers. *Journal of Respiratory Diseases, 15,* 151-166.

U.S. Department of Health and Human Services. (1992). *Healthy People 2000: Public health service action* (DHHS Pub. No. [PHS] 91-50212). Washington, DC: U.S. Government Printing Office.

U.S. Department of Health and Human Services. (1993, January). *Nurses: Help your patient stop smoking* (NIH Pub. No. 92-2962). Washington, DC: U.S. Government Printing Office.

Wade, W. E. (1993). Managing pneumonia in the elderly. *Clinical Consult, 12*(1), 1-7.

Yoshikawa, T. (1992). Tuberculosis in aging adults. *Journal of the American Geriatrics Society, 40,* 178.

BIBLIOGRAPHY

Allen and Hanburys. (1994). *Patient's instructions for use of inhalation aerosol* (Pamphlet No. RL-164). Author.

Alspach, J. G. (1991). *Core curriculum for critical care nursing* (4th ed.). Philadelphia: W. B. Saunders.

Kenney, R. A. (1989). *Physiology of aging.* Chicago: Yearbook Medical.

McCance, K., & Huether, S. (1994). *Pathophysiology: The biologic basis for disease in adults and children* (2nd ed.). St. Louis: Mosby.

Phipps, W., Cassmeyer, V., Sands, J., & Lehman, M. K. (1995). *Medical-surgical nursing: Concepts and clinical practice* (5th ed.). St. Louis: Mosby.

Thibodeau, G. (1990). *Anthony's textbook of anatomy and physiology* (13th ed.). St. Louis: Mosby.

C H A P T E R   12

Give me a young man in whom there is something of the old, and an old man with something of the young: guided so, a man may grow old in body, but never in mind.

CICERO

Mobility

■ Learning Objectives

On completion of this chapter, the reader will be able to do the following:

1. Define mobility.
2. Understand the anatomy and physiology of the musculoskeletal system.
3. Know the physical and psychosocial aspects of mobility in the older adult.
4. Recognize normal age-related changes and common health deviations in the musculoskeletal system that affect mobility of the older adult.
5. Specify common psychosocial problems in relation to health deviations in mobility.
6. Assess functional mobility of the older adult.
7. Use the nursing process in determining the care of people with problems in mobility.
8. Develop methods for promoting healthy mobility throughout the adult life span.

The ability to move from one point to another without fear of pain or injury is one most adults take for granted. In the life of a small child the event of the first step is welcomed with a great deal of parental pride and trepidation. The parents' mixed feelings originate in the realization that the ability to stand and walk is the beginning of the child's ability to express free and independent action. This independent state and the freedom of choice is the hallmark of adult life. To be free to walk or run wherever you want, whenever you want, and at whatever speed you want is one of the unrecognized gifts of life. For the older adult, the ability to run is severely limited or nonexistent; the ability or the will to walk may be limited or just more difficult to initiate and to sustain.

Mobility is defined as the independent ability to move or to be moved—a body capable of locomotion. This definition does not preclude mobility achieved through assistive devices, such as a motorized wheelchair, specially equipped automobile, or artificial limbs. In a more traditional view, assessment of mobility both clinically and for research purposes may be achieved by measurement of three physical activities: walking, climbing stairs, and transferring (Ettinger, 1994).

At first the concept of mobility seems simple and uncomplicated. On further investigation, however, the complexity of mobility in the older adult becomes apparent. Necessary ingredients for mobility are (1) cognition and motivation, (2) a skeletal system that is capable of supporting the body's weight, (3) muscles with enough strength to move the body, and (4) a neurologic system that is capable of interaction with the musculoskeletal system (Figure 12-1).

Factors that impede mobility in the older adult can be physical, psychologic, social, or environmental. Myriad physical age-related changes, such as slowed neurologic response and decreased muscle strength, can make mobility a physical challenge for the older adult. Abnormal gait and poor balance increase the challenge of safe mobility in older adults.

A psychologic condition that affects some older adults is the fear of injury. Often the older adult makes a realistic appraisal of the physical and environmental conditions and concludes that there is an increased risk of injury. How the older adult accommodates for the increased risk is the paramount issue. If the response to the risk is not to walk, not to cross the street, or not to travel, thereby significantly diminishing the risk of injury, the older adult may no longer be mobile or independent.

Related to the fear of injury is the fear of embarrassment. Actually, it is difficult to separate the two emotional responses of older adults as

FIGURE 12-1 Mobility: A multifaceted human function.

they cope with the loss of physical vigor and agility. Planning for a day of shopping, which most people do with ease, is quite a different experience for older adults who have limited mobility. The difficulties encountered by older adults who are trying to maintain their independence and their pride in spite of impaired mobility relate to transportation, environmental obstacles, and public opinion.

Transportation is a major issue: Is there public transportation? If so, can the older adults step on and off the bus or van? Is there a relative or friend who will provide transportation and take them shopping? Can the older adults still safely drive or afford a taxi? Is there a local program that offers van transportation for people in wheelchairs?

Unexpected changes in the weather also may create a hazard for older adults, particularly those with limitations in mobility. Physically, older adults are more susceptible to the extremes of cold or heat and are at higher risk for falls during icy and rainy weather.

Other environmental factors encountered during a shopping trip are stores with difficult entrances, inclines that are slanted and poorly lighted, electric doors that are poorly marked, items that are on high shelves, fast-moving escalators, and corridors and shops that offer no place to sit and rest.

Many older adults find themselves embarrassed by either or both of the following extremes of public opinion: At one extreme is the clerk or fellow shopper who has little patience for the slow pace of the older adult shopper, or the clerk who is indifferent in providing the extra assistance needed to reach the items higher on the shelf. Either of these may cause the older adult to lose a sense of confidence. At the other extreme is the overprotective person who treats older adult shoppers as if they are 5-year-olds who have lost their mothers. As one older woman with limited mobility remarked, "Just because I've lost the ability to walk doesn't mean I've lost the ability to think." It is difficult to maintain mobility while overcoming the fear and embarrassment that result from everyday experiences.

As with many aspects of life, mobility becomes increasingly difficult for many older adults. It is a testimony to the unrecognized strengths of older adults that the majority remain mobile, active, and occupied with all aspects of living. Nurses have the opportunity and the responsibility to recognize the strengths of older adults, provide encouraging comments about their ability to meet the challenge of maintaining mobility, and contribute to increasing their self-esteem.

The next sections of this chapter present the normal musculoskeletal system, the normal age-related changes that occur in this system, and the common health deviations that affect the mobility of many older adults.

■ Normal Structure and Function

The musculoskeletal system consists of bones, muscles, tendons, ligaments, joints, and bursae. The contribution of the skeleton to mobility is to provide structure to the human form and to facilitate movement. The skeleton is made up of bone, which is continuously involved in the processes of formation and resorption throughout the life cycle. Bone growth is partially regulated by mechanical stimuli, such as physical activity and weight bearing. Diet and genetic factors also contribute to bone growth. Skeletal mass increases during the growth years, and a peak in bone mass usually is reached between the ages of 20 and 30 years. Bone formation is the major process that contributes to the growth of bone mass.

There are two significant types of bone tissue: (1) *Trabecular bone* forms the majority of bone in the vertebral body and in the flat bones. (2) *Cortical bone* forms most of the long bones. Bones are composed of an organic matrix, 95% of which is collagen fibers and ground substance (bone salts). The bone salts principally comprise calcium and phosphate, with smaller amounts of magnesium, sodium, potassium, and carbonate ions. Calcium provides bone with its great compressional strength.

Bone gives shape to the musculoskeletal system, but other structures supply connections, strength, and flexibility. *Ligaments* are flexible bands of strong connective tissue, which connect the articular extremities of bone and which allow freedom of movement. *Tendons* are fibrous cords of connective tissue that serve as the mechanism for connecting muscle to movable structures such as bone. *Joints* provide the point of articulation between bones. *Bursae* are small, fluid-filled sacs surrounding the points of friction in joints.

There are three identifiable types of skeletal muscle fibers: type I (slow-twitch, high-oxidative fiber), type II (fast-twitch, high-oxidative fiber), and type IIB (fast-twitch, slow-oxidative fiber). The slow-twitch muscle fibers can sustain tension for long periods, are slow to fatigue, and have high aerobic capacity (high oxidation). The fast-twitch fibers, on the other hand, develop high tension rapidly but with no endurance over time and have anaerobic capacity (slow oxidation) (Schwartz & Buchner, 1994).

In conjunction with the skeletal system, muscles interact with the neurologic system to produce body movements: flexion, extension, abduction, adduction, pronation, supination, and both internal and external rotation. Disuse of muscles leads to *atrophy,* which decreases both the size and the strength of muscles.

■ Age-Related Changes

The normal musculoskeletal system undergoes various age-related changes that affect mobility (Box 12-1). Between the ages of 30 and 50 years, an equilibrium is established, in which the processes of formation and resorption stabilize the amount of bone mass. After age 50 this equilibrium shifts, and an incremental process of bone resorption without the successful formation of new bone mass leads to a gradual bone loss. That is, from age 50 on, the resorption of bone gradually extracts calcium and destroys the bone's organic matrix, thereby diminishing bone mass.

Aging-changes in cortical bone, which accounts for 75% of the skeletal weight, leads

BOX 12-1 AGE-RELATED CHANGES IN THE MUSCULOSKELETAL SYSTEM AND MOBILITY

1. Gradual loss of bone mass
2. Diminished muscle strength
3. Decrease in reaction time
4. Decrease in speed of movement

to a reduction in cortical thickness and an increase in porosity resulting in progressive cortical thinning. Trabecular bone accounts for the remaining 25% of bone weight. Aging affects trabecular bone by thinning and destruction of the bone (Baylink & Jennings, 1994).

The initial, significant loss of bone mass occurs in trabecular bone, which leads to a susceptibility to compression fractures in the vertebral column. Cortical bone loss occurs later than trabecular bone loss, and this loss leads to a susceptibility to fractures of the femur.

In normal, healthy older adults the regulation of calcium blood levels remains in a normal range. The exchange of calcium is a complex interaction among the extracellular fluid, the intestine, the skeleton, and the kidney. Calcium metabolism is influenced by parathyroid hormone (PTH), phosphate, vitamin D, and calcitonin (a thyroid hormone). In older adults the PTH levels have shown an increase, and vitamin D and calcitonin levels a decrease. Because bone and calcium metabolism are highly integrated, the age-related calcium loss from bone results from the body's need to maintain normal calcium levels (Baylink & Jennings, 1994).

In women, major bone loss determinants are estrogen deficiency, calcium malabsorption, lifestyle factors, and genetic history. The first 5 to 8 years after menopause is when major bone loss occurs. Lifestyle factors that influence bone volume are calcium intake and exercise. Estrogen replacement therapy has risks and benefits, and each woman must make a decision based on accurate, individualized, and current information.

Aging brings a decline in numbers of muscle fibers, which results in a reduced muscle mass. As people age, there is a decrease in total muscle mass, a decrease in number and size of type II (fast-twitch) muscle fibers, and a decrease in the metabolic and oxidative capacity of muscle cells (Schwartz & Buchner, 1994). For many older adults there is a sequential loss in muscle strength. The degree of loss varies greatly among muscle groups, and changes attributed to the aging process are significantly less where the muscle group has been used. In different groups of older adults, studies have shown that regular exercise, especially resistance training (weight lifting), demonstrates a reduced rate of muscle strength decline (Buchner et al., 1992; Fiatrone et al., 1990). The decline in muscle function depends on other systems, such as the neurologic and the musculoskeletal systems. As a result of age-related changes in the neurologic system, there is a progressive decrease in reaction time and speed of movement, and this adversely affects muscle function.

The loss of muscle strength creates a cycle of debilitating events as people begin to think that, because they are older, they have lost strength and cannot exercise, when actually the loss of strength is compounded by a lack of exercise. The body's adaptability to exercise remains unimpaired with aging. Recent investigations support the proposition that much of what has been attributed to aging is a result of inactivity. Recovery from exercise may take longer for older adults, but under proper guidance, an effective exercise program can lead to increased muscle strength. The axiom "Use it or lose it" directly relates to aging muscle.

Many health professionals unquestioningly accept stereotypic descriptions of older adults, such as "kyphotic," and "having muscular rigidity," because of their experience with institutionalized, inactive older adults. They come to accept the debilitative condition of institutionalized older adults as a result of the aging process and

Aging Alert

1. Disuse of muscles leads to loss of muscle strength.
2. Physical inactivity is a major threat to health.
3. Exercise is a vital component of a healthy lifestyle.

chronic disease. This is a mistake. It would be more accurate to ascribe this condition at least partly to inactivity and inappropriate care. A treatment plan that does not provide for exercise or for activities for all older adults is neglectful. Lack of appropriate care contributes to the loss of strength and the loss of spirit that lead to a loss of mobility, a triple jeopardy for institutionalized older adults.

Inactivity, bed rest, and subsequent immobility lead to a rapid loss of muscle size and strength. To prevent this type of loss, the nurse, along with other members of the health care team, needs to be aware of the potential problems that can arise because of prolonged muscle disuse.

■ Common Health Deviations

OSTEOPOROSIS

Osteoporosis is a disease of multiple etiologies. A common element in all cases of the disease is reduction of bone mass to a level leading to fracture, especially of the vertebrae, distal radius, and femur. Skeletal osteopenia refers to bone mass reduction. Inasmuch as bone loss is universal, osteoporosis as a clinical entity occurs only if there is an associated fracture.

Osteoporosis is a common occurrence in the older population, leading to an estimated 1.5 million fractures per year. The cost and burden of suffering associated with this condition have

Dancers of the Third Age (DTA), a multigenerational modern dance company, is one of many programs sponsored by The Dance Exchange. The Dance Exchange, founded by dancer-choreographer Liz Lerman, is a nonprofit arts organization whose work is based on the inseparable concerns of artistic excellence and community involvement. By bringing dance to senior adults, people in hospitals, children, people without homes, and women in shelters, as well as concert stage audiences, The Dance Exchange demonstrates its philosophy that dance is for everyone. (Printed with permission of The Dance Exchange, Inc., 1746-B Kalorama Road, NW, Washington, DC 20009.) *Photo by Dennis Deloria.*

become a public health concern. Of women who are now 35 years of age, 8% will experience a hip fracture in their lifetime. The mortality rate for hip fractures is as high as 20%. Thirty percent of women and 15% of men over the age of 60 years have clinical osteoporosis. Risk factors that influ-ence the development of osteoporosis are the level of bone mass at maturity, gender, age, diet, disease, alcoholism, smoking, medications, and mobility (Chestnut, 1994) (Figure 12-2).

Skeletal mass at maturity is less for women than for men; 18-year-old women have 20% less

RISK FACTORS FOR OSTEOPOROSIS

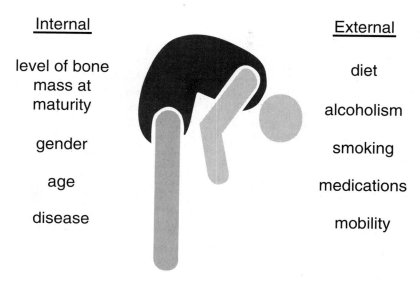

Internal	External
level of bone mass at maturity	diet
gender	alcoholism
age	smoking
disease	medications
	mobility

FIGURE 12-2 Risk factors for osteoporosis.

bone mass than 18-year-old men. Women lose bone mass more rapidly than men. Following the cessation of menses, the rate of bone loss is accelerated for approximately 5 to 8 years. The type of bone lost in this initial high-loss period is trabecular bone, the loss of which is associated with compression fractures of the spine. Cortical bone is lost at a slower rate, and its loss is more directly associated with fractures of the femur. With bone loss there is a decrease in bone strength, and there is a thinning of the vertebral body in the spine. For many older adults, this thinning process leads to decreased height and to increased vulnerability to compression fractures of the spine, caused by only minor degrees of trauma.

Estrogen deficiency in postmenopausal women is thought to be one cause of accelerated bone loss. Estrogen replacement therapy may be medically recommended in women who are not at risk for the detrimental side effects of such therapy, who have no contraindications, and who will adhere to a careful follow-up program that includes annual mammography (Culliton, 1987). The estrogen compounds prevent the loss of bone mass but do not restore previously lost bone mass. Their value seems to be prophylactic. Side effects of estrogen therapy include endometrial cancer and thromboembolic disease, and there is a possible association with gallbladder disease and breast cancer (Chestnut, 1994). The combined use of estrogen and a progestational agent decreases the risk of endometrial cancer but causes repeated episodes of uterine bleeding. The combination therapy of estrogen and progesterone also decreases the efficiency of estrogen in providing protection for the cardiovascular system.

Vitamin D levels have also been found to be lower in osteoporotic women than in nonosteoporotic women. A multivitamin with 400 to 800 IU of vitamin D is therapeutic for postmenopausal women (Chestnut, 1992). The pallor of many older adults is the result of a lack of exposure to sunshine. Vitamin D deficiency can be alleviated by encouraging and helping older adults to spend some time outdoors. When the individual is adequately dressed, exposure to fresh air and sunshine offers physical and psychologic benefits.

The demonstrated need for an increase in calcium in the diet of older adults, especially women, has created an increased awareness of this nutrient as a requirement. Calcium intake is deficient in teenage, perimenopausal, and postmenopausal American women. Although data are conflictual on the efficacy of increased calcium intake as a preventive measure against hip fractures, it is generally thought that perimenopausal and postmenopausal women need a minimum of 1000 to 1500 mg of calcium a day. Milk, dairy products, and calcium carbonate supplements are adequate, available, and reasonably priced sources of calcium.

Calcitonin is an anti–bone resorption agent that has been shown to slow bone loss and increase bone mass. Negative aspects of the drug are the expense, the route of administration (injection), and the short duration of efficacy (2 to 3 years). For some women calcitonin will be a safe prophylactic and a reasonable alternative to estrogen therapy until a more viable method of administration is developed. Recent development and use of a calcitonin nasal spray has shown encouraging results (Overgaard et al., 1992).

It is known that immobility leads to osteoporosis even in healthy young men. Inactivity is associated with a dramatic loss of strength. Studies in older adults have shown a consistent but variable gain in muscle strength through resistance exercise programs. Endurance training such as riding a stationary bike has resulted in a 10% to 25% functional improvement in arthritic patients (Minon et al., 1989). The need to avoid a sedentary lifestyle is an especially important factor to consider in the care of older adults. Prevention of osteoporosis should begin at an early age, with emphasis on lifestyle variables that may alleviate the progression of bone loss.

ARTHRITIS

Table 12-1 describes some of the data relevant to two common forms of arthritis—osteoarthritis (OA) and rheumatoid arthritis (RA).

TABLE 12-1 Osteoarthritis and rheumatoid arthritis differences

	Osteoarthritis	Rheumatoid arthritis
Morning stiffness	Lasts for a few minutes	Lasts for an hour or more
Pain	Usually follows activity	Occurs even at rest
Joint involvement	May be asymmetric; interphalangeal and metacarpophalangeal joints always involved	Symmetric; knees, hips
Synovial fluid	Viscosity decreased	Viscosity normal
Weakness	Usually follows activity	Often severe
Fatigue	Not usual	Usually pronounced
Emotional depression	Not usual	Common

Adapted from Calkins, E., Reinhard, J., & Vladutiu. (1994). Rheumatoid arthritis and the autoimmune rheumatic disease in the older patient. In W.M. Hazzard, E. Bierman, J. Blass, W. Ettinger, & J. Halter (Eds.), *Principles of geriatric medicine and gerontology*. New York: McGraw-Hill.

Osteoarthritis

The incidence of osteoarthritis (OA) increases with age; this condition affects up to 40 million Americans and is the second leading cause of disability (Fife, 1994). Osteoarthritis is a noninflammatory disease of movable joints, characterized by deterioration of articular cartilage and commonly known as "degenerative joint disease (DJD)." Although the definitive cause of OA is not known, there are a number of risk factors: obesity, repetitive mechanical overuse of a joint, and a familial tendency. Certainly nothing can be done concerning a person's genetic makeup, but health teaching concerning obesity and the need to protect joints used in work or sports is an area in need of nursing's input.

The clinical manifestations of OA are joint pain, swelling, decreased range of motion of the joint, and crepitus. Typically the large weight-bearing joints (hips and knees) are affected, as well as joints of the hand. Heberden's nodes, lateral enlargements at the distal interphalangeal joints, are diagnostic of osteoarthritis. The frequency and severity of the disease increase markedly with age, particularly in women. Osteoarthritis of the knee is 3 times more prevalent in older women than in older men, and hip involvement is twice as prevalent in older women as in older men. The progression of osteoarthritis does not follow a systematic, predictable pathway for all individuals afflicted with the disease. Different joints may be involved, which affects the pattern of response of the individual.

The cardinal symptom is pain, which at first occurs after movement of the joint and is relieved by rest. The pain is usually characterized as "aching" and is poorly localized. Stiffness on awakening in the morning or after inactivity is a common complaint, although it is of relatively short duration, rarely persisting for more than 15 minutes.

Medical treatment of osteoarthritis consists of symptomatic relief and minimizing further joint destruction. In addition, some environmental factors can be changed to slow the progress of joint degeneration. Weight-bearing joints such as the knee can be protected from further damage by not engaging in activities that produce large amounts of high impact, such as jogging or aerobic exercise. Swimming is an excellent form of exercise that produces only low impact on weight-bearing joints. Rest is an important aspect of treatment, in combination with exercise that minimizes impact on weight-bearing joints. People who have osteoarthritis and who are overweight should be encouraged to lose weight. Obesity has been found to be associated with some types of osteoarthritis.

A mainstay of treatment is early intervention with physical and occupational therapies. Maintaining muscle strength, improving posture, and protecting joints are invaluable functions that need to be incorporated into the lifestyle of the older adult suffering from osteoarthritis. For appropriate exercises to improve posture, see Figure 12-3. Arthroscopic surgery may produce results for certain older adults with severe knee involvement. If the progression of the disease severely limits mobility and the older person is healthy, surgical joint replacement may be recommended. Hip and knee replacement surgeries are usually very successful and alleviate pain and restore mobility.

Nonsteroidal anti-inflammatory drugs (NSAIDs) provide symptomatic relief because of their analgesic and anti-inflammatory properties, but they do not slow the progression of the osteoarthritis. NSAIDs account for 4% of all prescription drugs used in the United States and for 20% of the drugs used by adults over 60 years of age. This class of drugs has the potential to be life threatening without the ability to be life saving. In spite of the fact that NSAIDs are widely prescribed, it behooves the nurse to understand the potential harm of these drugs. Acetaminophen, a significant pain reliever that does not carry the potential for harm, has been shown to be at least as effective as NSAIDs (Bradley et al., 1991).

The most common adverse effects of NSAIDs are gastrointestinal (GI) symptoms, which have

Stretching Exercises to Improve Posture

A

Gently pull chin in lengthening back of neck. Hold this position for _____ seconds.

Repeat: _____ Times
_____ Times a day.

B

C

Continued

FIGURE 12-3 Exercises for improving posture. (From VHI Geriatric Exercise and Rehabilitation Exercise Kit. [1993]. *Visual health/stretching charts.* Tacoma, WA.)

Stretching Exercises to Improve Posture—cont'd

D Gently pull chin in while lengthening back of neck. Hold 10 seconds while counting out loud.

Repeat: _____ Times
_____ Times a day.

E Place hands behind your head and pull elbows back as far as possible. Hold 10 seconds while counting out loud.

Repeat: _____ Times
_____ Times a day.

F With feet 6 inches from wall, lean as much of back against the wall as possible. Gently squat down 5 inches, keeping back against wall. Hold 10 seconds, counting out loud.

Repeat: _____ Times
_____ Times a day.

G With arms behind doorjam, gently lean forward. Hold the position for ___ seconds. Stretch is felt across chest.

Repeat: ____ Times
____ Times a day.

H Bring arms straight up over head and back as far as possible, causing back to arch gently.

Repeat: _____ Times
_____ Times a day.

FIGURE 12-3, cont'd. For legend see opposite page.

BOX 12-2 ADVERSE DRUG REACTIONS FROM NONSTEROIDAL ANTI-INFLAMMATORY DRUGS

Gastrointestinal tract
  Gastric ulcer
  Duodenal ulcer
  Upper GI tract bleeding
  Gastritis
Kidney
  Acute renal failure
  Chronic renal failure
  Hyperkalemia
  Hyponatremia
  Acute flank pain syndrome
Liver
  Acute hepatitis
  Fulminant hepatitis
  Chronic hepatitis

Adapted from Carlson, J., & Strom, B. (1994). Nonsteroidal anti-inflammatory drugs. In W.M. Hazzard, E. Bierman, J. Blass, W. Ettinger, & J. Halter (Eds.), *Principles of geriatric medicine and gerontology.* New York: McGraw-Hill.

been reported in up to 61% of patients. The symptoms can range from mild upset to GI hemorrhage. The highest risk profile is that of people over 60 years of age, undergoing corticosteroid therapy and anticoagulant therapy, and indulging in heavy alcohol use (Gabriel et al., 1991). Nearly every NSAID has been associated with reports of liver disease, from mild elevation of liver enzymes to acute liver disease. Benoxaprofen, an NSAID, was withdrawn from the marketplace in the 1980s after a series of reports of fatal liver disease (Taggert & Alderice, 1982). Renal disease and interactions with other drugs are adverse effects to be mindful of when patients are taking NSAIDs. Certainly older adults who have a history of ulcers, liver disease, or renal disease, or who are taking anticoagulants or steroids should not be taking prescribed or over-the-counter NSAIDs (Carlson & Strom, 1994). The nurse must be aware of the potential adverse drug reactions for older adults associated with the use of NSAIDs (Box 12-2). The community nurse's challenge is to inform the patient of the risk without introducing unnecessary fear and to consult with the attending physician regarding whether there is any question concerning the appropriateness of a particular drug. Other health care providers, such as the dentist and the podiatrist, should be informed about the medications being taken by their older patients.

Rheumatoid arthritis

Rheumatoid arthritis (RA) is a chronic systemic inflammatory disease of movable joints. The course of the disease varies from individual to individual and is characterized by unexplained periods of remission and exacerbation. The frequency of RA increases with age, and for those over 65 years of age, 1.8% of men and 4.9% of women will have RA (Lawrence et al., 1989). Common complaints are fatigue and swollen, painful joints, with morning stiffness that lasts longer than 1 hour. Usually distribution of involved joints is bilateral and symmetric. Any joint may be affected, but the most frequently affected joints are those of the fingers, hand, wrist, shoulders, and knees. Laboratory tests may show mild anemia and an elevated sedimentation rate. Presence of a rheumatoid factor is important, although false positives are prevalent in older populations.

A significant area of concern is the difficulty in differentiating RA from OA in older adults. Many older adults will have grown old with RA, and others will have new-onset disease. In addition, some older adults will have both RA and OA, and others will have polymyalgia rheumatica. Diagnoses, whether by nurses or physicians, should never be made based on the evidence of one dimension; a cluster of data is necessary for reaching any clinical diagnosis (Box 12-3). Pharmacologic treatment of these diseases of similar presenting symptoms is guided by correct diagnosis and therefore a necessary

BOX 12-3 CRITERIA FOR DIAGNOSIS OF RHEUMATOID ARTHRITIS

1. Morning stiffness
2. Arthritis in three or more joints
3. Arthritis of hand joint
4. Symmetric arthritis
5. Rheumatoid nodules
6. Serum rheumatoid factor
7. Radiographic changes

element of care. See Table 12-1 for factors used in differentiation of RA from OA.

The treatment goals are to reduce inflammation, alleviate pain, preserve function, and prevent deformity. Conservative treatment includes rest, physical therapy, and drug therapy. Aspirin is the first drug used in the management of symptoms. If the patient's symptoms persist, NSAIDs may be prescribed. An additional drug class available for difficult-to-manage symptoms is the corticosteroids. It is always crucial to be aware of side effects, even of the most commonly used drugs, such as aspirin, which may cause gastric irritation, tinnitus, and hearing loss. There are no risk-free drugs.

Exercise has an important place in the treatment plan for older adults with all types of arthritis including RA. The toxic effects of drugs and the great possibility of their untoward interactions with other types of drugs increase the importance of alternative treatment modalities. It is of interest to note that a physician who was an early leader in the specialty of rheumatology is quoted as saying that effective treatment for arthritis "does not come out of a bottle" (Calkins et al., 1994). The reliance on drugs as the "magic bullet" cure for arthritis is not tenable. The patient must be committed to a lifelong program of rehabilitation that includes a daily exercise program that assists in maintaining mobility. It takes courage and perseverance to learn to live a

full and fruitful life despite living with disease, but it is possible. Older adults with RA need support in their efforts to sustain and maintain their treatment programs.

Gouty arthritis

Gout is a systemic disease caused by hyperuricemia (high uric acid), common in middle-aged men, and characterized by recurrent episodes of acute arthritis. Usually the first attack occurs at night, and the most frequently involved site is the great toe. The toe becomes reddish-purple, swollen, and extremely painful. Later attacks may be precipitated by stress or by overindulgence in food or alcoholic beverages. Medical treatment consists of drug therapy to control the uric acid level and a low-purine diet, although there is debate as to the benefits of the diet.

Drug therapy consists of three drugs: (1) colchicine, an anti-inflammatory drug specific in its response to gout; (2) allopurinol, which reduces uric acid formation; and (3) probenecid, a uricosuric drug.

Some aspects of the treatment for gout require nursing interventions. For one thing, the nurse must help the older adult who is taking these drugs to be aware of the possible side effects of each drug. The most frequent side effect of colchicine is gastrointestinal irritation. The patient is advised that diarrhea, nausea, vomiting, and abdominal pain may be side effects of this drug. The importance of weight control, the avoidance of excessive alcohol intake, and the need for good hydration—especially for those patients taking probenecid—should be emphasized in any patient education program. Fasting should be discouraged, because it may precipitate an attack of acute gout. There is an increased risk for the development of renal calculi. Therefore the nurse should advise people with gout to develop the habit of drinking 3 L of fluid (water) a day. The desired outcome for the treatment is to control symptoms without exposing the older adult to further physical harm from hyperuricemia and from side effects of the drugs that control the uric acid level.

POLYMYALGIA RHEUMATICA

Polymyalgia rheumatica is a well-defined syndrome occurring in both sexes after age 50. Symptoms include pain and stiffness in the muscles and an accompanying high sedimentation rate. Onset can be gradual or sudden and can be accompanied by fever, anorexia, weight loss, and apathy. Medical treatment is corticosteroid therapy, which yields a dramatic response. Patients vary in the amount of prednisone needed for a therapeutic effect and in the length of treatment required.

FIBROMYALGIA

Fibromyalgia, commonly called "fibrositis," is considered to be a non–joint-involving rheumatic condition that is characterized by chronic aching, pain, stiffness, and tenderness in the soft tissue of the musculoskeletal system. Symptoms of fibromyalgia include (1) widespread pain of at least 3 months' duration, with multiple tender points; (2) sleep disturbances, with morning fatigue; (3) normal laboratory study results; and (4) emotional distress.

Treatment includes alleviating any emotional distress, massaging affected areas, and locally applying heat; also, the affected person should be instructed to take hot showers, engage in only moderate activity, get appropriate rest, and avoid cold or wet weather (by staying inside except in warm and dry weather). It is important that the nurse understand the symptoms, the treatment, and the non–life-threatening nature of this mild but painful condition.

■ Foot Problems

Although congenital conditions can cause foot problems, most difficulties with feet in the older adult population are the result of footwear and habit. Women, especially, have been unsuspecting victims of the insidious process of causing harm to the basic structure of the foot. Shoes with high heels, pointed toes, and hard soles, as well as tight stockings, interfere with the normal mechanism of gait. Shortening of tendons, debili-

tation of intrinsic muscles, and shifting of ligaments result from shoes that pinch the toes and modify the angle of the foot. Corns, hammertoes, and halluces valgus (bunions) are examples of the results of harmful environmental processes, combined with genetic factors, that compound the efforts required of older adults to remain mobile and pain free (Figure 12-4).

A bunion is evidenced by (1) the big toe's overriding or underlying the second toe, which may be a hammertoe; (2) enlargement of the medial portion of the first metatarsal head; and (3) inflammation of the bursae over the medial aspect of the joint. Not all bunions are symptomatic, and many older adults may be free from pain despite having large bunions. An older adult who has a bunion that is symptomatic will experience both pain and difficulty in walking.

Treatment may consist of an interdisciplinary team effort that includes nursing, podiatry, medicine, and physical therapy. Shoes should be designed to eliminate stress on the inflamed area. This may require special shoes or modification of the patient's available footwear. Exercise and arch supports are appropriate interventions. The nurse may serve as an advocate for treatment. The rationale that the patient has had a bunion for a long time is not a contraindication to treatment.

Treatment of the various foot problems depends on their severity. Assessment of passive range of motion may be the first step in detecting the severity of the deficit. Prevention of further loss may be accomplished by encouraging both safe, appropriate footwear and foot exercises. If foot problems are severe, referral to a podiatrist or to an orthopedic surgeon may be the appropriate nursing intervention. Patients should be encouraged to acquire types of footwear that allow a healthy gait.

■ Falls

Falls are a frequent and important health problem that affects the mobility of many older

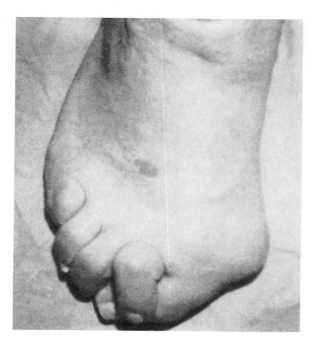

FIGURE 12-4 Hammertoe associated with hallux valgus. (From Crenshaw, A.H. [1992]. *Campbell's operative orthopaedics* [8th ed.]. St. Louis: Mosby.)

adults. Falls affect large numbers of older adults, with a significant increase in falls among those who are over 75 years of age. It is estimated that, yearly, 28% to 30% of the older adult population experiences a fall; however, most falls result only in minor physical injury. One half of those people who fall will experience recurrent falls (Tinetti, 1994).

Muscle weakness, a significant factor in older adult falls, is itself the result of four factors: aging changes in the musculoskeletal system, the effects of chronic disease and the medications used in the treatment of chronic disease, sedentary lifestyle, and undernutrition.

Although there has been a significant decline in death caused by falls, falling still accounts for a large degree of morbidity and is a prevalent form of serious injury that occurs in the older adult population. On a yearly basis, an estimated 1% of falls result in over 250,000 hip fractures. Within the first year following a hip fracture, approxi-

mately 23% of older adult patients will have died, and 50% or more will need nursing home care (Grisso & Kaplan, 1994).

The risk of falls is increased for women, especially women over the age of 75. Other significant risk factors for hip fracture are white race, prolonged immobility, thin body build, family history of osteoporosis, smoking, heavy alcohol use, use of psychotropic drugs, and visual impairment. Falls and their sequelae are significant health problems for many older adults, and their nursing care spans a continuum that encompasses primary, secondary, and tertiary care (prevention of falls, acute care after falls, and rehabilitation to restore function).

■ Health Promotion: Exercise

Exercise can help to change not only the stereotype, but also—more importantly—the health of older adults. Most older adults, regardless of physical condition and age, should be encouraged to

Health Promoting Behaviors

1. Exercise regularly.
2. Make sure shoes fit properly and are in good condition; avoid wearing high heels.
3. Be aware of environmental hazards, such as steep stairs, slippery roads and sidewalks, dimly lit hallways, lack of handrails, loose rugs, or items blocking walkways.
4. Use assistive devices if necessary.
5. Understand effects of medications on balance, coordination, and health conditions.
6. Limit alcohol intake.
7. Keep eyeglasses clean.

begin stretching exercises to promote greater flexibility, muscular coordination, balance, and mobility. The types of stretching exercises used should follow normal body movements (see Figure 12-3). Walking helps to build endurance and usually creates an optimistic view of life. Resistance training, otherwise known as weight lifting, has been shown to be successful in increasing skeletal muscle size in older nursing home residents. The importance of competent leg muscles for the task of walking cannot be overstated.

Participation in physical activity has been shown to be predictive of a high level of physical function, to increase strength in older women, to reduce adipose tissue, to increase bone mineral density in older women, and to improve health (Hunter et al., 1995; Morey et al., 1989; Treuth et al., 1995; Vico et al., 1995; Young et al., 1995).

■ Nursing Process

Previous sections of this chapter presented the physical health deviations that significantly affect the older adult's ability to remain mobile. As with all human function, mobility exists along a continuum that ranges from optimum mobility to complete immobility. The variability in the level of mobility is a function of multiple physical, psychologic, social, and environmental factors, and no single factor can predict the individual's level of mobility. Knowledge of the multiple factors that influence an older adult's mobility is fundamental to being able to provide appropriate nursing care. The challenge for nursing is to help older adults to reach and maintain their optimum potential for mobility along that continuum.

There are different terms used in the literature and throughout the health care field to describe physical impairment. The World Health Organization (1976) defines *impairment, disability,* and *handicap* as follows:

Impairment is any loss or abnormality of psychological, physiological, or anatomical structure or function . . . *Disability* is any restriction or lack (resulting from an impairment) of ability to perform an activity in the manner or within the range considered normal for a human being . . . *Handicap* is a disadvantage for a given individual, resulting from impairment or a disability, that limits or prevents the fulfillment of a role that is normal (depending on age, sex, and social and cultural factors) for that individual.

These definitions are valuable in that they may begin to standardize the use of these terms.

In the field of gerontologic nursing the diagnosis most often used to denote alteration in mobility is impaired physical mobility. The challenge for many nurses is to identify the interrelationship of multiple factors, to analyze the problem of comorbidity, and to cope with the overlapping of different diagnoses and etiologies. It is crucial to clarify the human response of the individual patient to the aging process or to a health deviation, and to emphasize the role of nursing in the patient's treatment. This emphasizes the appropriateness of the nursing focus on the functional state of the older adult. The following sections examine the use of the nursing process in the care of a patient with an impairment in mobility.

ASSESSMENT
History

The primary purpose of taking a history is to obtain accurate information that pertains to the past, present, and future health of the patient. The second purpose of taking a history is to establish a relationship with the patient. When obtaining the patient's history, there are five fundamental points to remember: (1) if the older adult is responding to the questions, allow ample time for the response; (2) ask only one question at a time; (3) do not anticipate or give the answer for the patient; (4) listen to the response; and (5) most importantly, validate the patient's response.

History taking is both a science and an art. Many diagnostic puzzles can be solved by carefully attending to the patient's description of symptoms and by establishing a nurse-patient relationship that is reciprocal and respectful. Direct questions concerning health habits, living arrangements, and abilities in activities of daily living are less threatening when this type of relationship exists.

If a family member accompanies the older adult patient to the history-taking session, note that there may be several reasons for this arrangement. The family member may always have accompanied the older adult to health care interviews, or this arrangement may be a result of the family member's assessment of the patient's declining ability to give an accurate history. A family member's assessment of the older adult's ability to give an accurate history may or may not be correct; it is the nurse's responsibility to make an independent judgment of the patient's abilities in this regard. During the interview, be alert to the patient's response. Does the family member correct the older adult, and if so, does the patient accept this? Be aware of the mood of the participants. Also remember that family members often are a significant source of support and may provide important information regarding the health of the older adult.

The participants may view the interview as stressful if the health care situation seems threatening. A history taking that is part of a normal, routine checkup for arthritis will elicit a different response than will a history taking in an emergency room after a fall or upon admission to a nursing home.

Assessment is the first phase of the nursing process, and it is usually the first interaction that occurs between the nurse and the older adult patient. It is important that the assessment yield accurate data that will assist in arriving at appropriate and timely diagnoses and treatments. Most important, it is the opportunity for an initial interaction with the older adult. The nurse must bring a sophisticated array of interpersonal skills to the interview.

During history taking, the questions that pertain exclusively to mobility are centered around the patient's present functional level:

1. Have you noticed any change in the way you are walking? (If the patient responds by asking for clarification, ask a more specific question.)
2. Have you noticed a change in your ability to walk up (or down) stairs?
3. Have you experienced a difference in your ability to walk a long distance?
4. Are you having any difficulty rising from a chair?
5. How do you manage your daily activities, such as dressing, bathing, and toileting?
6. Are you having any difficulty getting into and out of the bathtub?
7. Have you experienced any recent falls? If the answer is yes, please tell me about your fall.
8. Have you noticed any change in your sense of balance?
9. Are you able to go outside of your home?
10. Are you able to drive a car or to use public transportation?
11. Do you have difficulty stepping off a sidewalk curb?
12. Do you use any assistive devices, such as a cane or a walker? If an assistive device

is used, when did you first use it? How often is it used now? Can you demonstrate your use of the assistive device?

13. Has there been any change in your ability to clean your house, do your laundry, or shop for groceries?

14. Have changes in your ability to get around (move about) required any significant adjustment in how you live your everyday life?

15. Is there anything I have forgotten to ask or something more you would like to tell me?

In addition to information about the patient's present level of function, there is also concern about the patient's perceptions and experiences related to that level of function. For example, pain on movement may pose a psychologic problem, inability to walk quickly to a bathroom may be the cause of a new problem of incontinence, and feelings of isolation may result from no longer being able to drive a car. These few examples show the interdependence of functions. Often, a difficulty in one area of function, such as mobility, can precipitate a disturbance in another function, such as elimination.

Other aspects of the history that are important to consider when the patient exhibits an impairment in mobility include weight; pain related to movement; activity and rest patterns; type, purpose, and effectiveness of medications (prescription and over-the-counter); and an overview of physiologic systems (e.g., musculoskeletal and neurologic).

After completion of the history the nurse begins a physical assessment but remains alert to information the patient may volunteer throughout the physical examination. Often, an older adult's memory is stimulated, and significant history remembered during the physical exam. Also the nurse may have an additional question that emerges from some aspect of the physical exam, such as noticing a scar or bruise about which no mention was made during the initial history taking.

BOX 12-4 PHYSICAL ASSESSMENT PARAMETERS

1. Gait
2. Posture
3. Physical strength
4. Range of motion
5. Condition of joints
6. Balance and coordination
7. Cognitive ability

Physical examination

Physical examination includes the collection of relevant information for a nursing assessment of mobility. The two major systems that primarily influence mobility are the musculoskeletal system and the neurologic system.

The initial assessment of mobility is usually made by observation (Box 12-4). The gait and overall posture of the older adult patient are critical elements in the patient's general appearance and therefore should be systematically inspected during the first minutes of an assessment. To be able to walk across a room and respond appropriately to a normal greeting such as "Hello! How are you feeling today?" entails lower body muscle strength, a functioning neurologic system, cognitive ability, and an intact skeletal system. Health professionals process a great deal of pertinent information about the health status of patients from observing such normal patterns of function.

When assessing gait, the nurse should remember that improperly fitting shoes or high-heeled shoes, poor balance, lower extremity muscle weakness, and neurologic impairments such as Parkinson's disease can adversely affect gait.

Significant age-related changes can be observed in the posture of most older adults. Studies have demonstrated (1) significant decreases in hip flexion and extension; (2) a decrease in height, caused by the thinning of vertebrae; and (3) a widening of the bony pelvis, which causes a shift in the center of gravity. Because of the shortened spine, older adults often may develop a degree of kyphosis. As a result of these postural changes and other changes, such as a neurologic slowing of response time, many older adults demonstrate a slow, deliberate, short-stepped gait. These changes may affect the health and well-being of some older adults, but it is important to consider that most older adults are not adversely affected by these changes. Also, a lifestyle that includes physical exercise may alleviate or delay some of these changes.

After gait and posture have been assessed, the nurse systematically assesses the muscle strength, range of motion, and condition of each joint. If the patient is not ambulatory, an assessment of muscle strength may be obtained by shaking the patient's hand. This is an appropriate action to convey your interest in and regard for the individual, and it allows an initial assessment. Despite the fact that cultural factors may influence the manner in which a handshake is given, the examiner can palpate the hand and assess strength, joint condition, skin turgor, and social response. It is best to use two hands when greeting older adult patients, because this allows more opportunity for tactile stimulation and conveys an aspect of caring.

Muscle mass usually decreases as a function of the aging process, and atrophy of some muscle groups may give the appearance of disease or may cause certain joints to appear larger than normal. Muscle strength is tested by resistance, with the knowledge that there will be a wide range of normal strength. The condition of the joints and the range of motion may also be affected by physical changes that accompany the aging process and by common conditions, such as osteoarthritis. Each individual joint should be palpated for tenderness, warmth, crepitus, and range of motion. The importance of history taking and the emphasis on functional level are critical to remember when assessing mobility.

Balance, coordination, and cognitive ability are assessed during the neurologic examination. These are important factors that contribute to an individual's ability to sustain mobility, although they are often not critically examined when dealing with an older adult. Also, the normal slowing of neurologic response time is a factor contributing to changes in mobility and should be considered in the assessment.

Although the two major systems related to mobility are the musculoskeletal and neurologic systems, the nurse should always be alert to the complexity and interdependence of body systems in relation to mobility. If a patient has a deficit in the ability to maintain adequate ventilation, then the mobility function will be adversely affected. The same is true if tissue perfusion is not adequately maintained. Psychologic status, such as depression, is often detrimental to the patient's attempts to maintain physical mobility.

After data have been gathered from the history and the physical examination, the medical record, if available, should be reviewed. It usually is a source of valuable information.

To ensure a systematic approach to the assessment of mobility, a specific amount of time should be provided at the end of the examination to review and to verify that all the necessary and pertinent data have been collected.

Psychosocial assessment

Successful adaptation to limitations can be considered one of the developmental tasks of older adults. The variability across older adult individuals in meeting this developmental task is noteworthy. Therefore it is critical that a wholistic assessment be performed for every patient who has a limitation in mobility.

The psychosocial assessment concentrates on people's subjective appraisal of their mobility, their feelings, and their behavior related to this very important function. Motivation—or the will to remain mobile in spite of limitations—is of paramount importance to the older adult's ability to maintain mobility.

Assessment of this aspect of the human spirit can first be inferred from the physical assessment. If the older adult has multiple decrements in the musculoskeletal and neurologic systems but is living independently or semi-independently, then it is rather safe to infer a strong motivation to sustain and maintain mobility. Older adults may manage the psychologic aspect of their limitations through a rational appraisal of their strengths and limitations or through a denial of limitations. Denial may serve a useful purpose in allowing the individual to continue to be mobile and independent and is often the choice of the older adult.

An incremental loss of some facets of mobility is the most frequent experience. An example of the incremental change is the loss of the ability to climb stairs, which then interferes with social engagements, such as visiting friends and relatives whose homes have many stairs. How the individual adapts to this incremental loss is the focus of the psychosocial assessment.

Questions that help older adults to talk about their adaptations to changes in mobility are either open ended or direct. The nurse conducting the assessment must determine the types of questions to use; the goal should be to gather information that gives an accurate picture of how the patient is adapting to the functional changes and how the patient feels about the current level of mobility. The following examples show both types of questions:

1. How do you rate your overall health? *(direct)*
2. Compared to other people your age, how do you rate your ability to accomplish on a daily basis what you want to do? *(direct)*
3. Can you tell me about the changes you have had to make in your life since your change in mobility? *(open ended)*
4. Is there someone whom you can count on for assistance when you need it? *(direct)*
5. It must be difficult. How do you manage? *(open ended)*

6. When you feel discouraged, is there someone to whom you can freely talk about your feelings? *(direct)*

During the psychosocial assessment the nurse should be alert to signs of depression, because this may influence the patient's level of mobility; depression is a treatable condition that is not a normal part of aging. Depression may be a significant factor in problems associated with mobility. Because mood affects physical function, it should always be part of a wholistic assessment. Loss of self-esteem or of self-confidence may accompany a decrease in mobility.

Another important psychologic factor that significantly impedes mobility is fear of falling. This can severely limit the ability of the older individual to adapt to physical limitations. It may be especially relevant for people who have suffered a fractured hip as a result of a fall. By limiting mobility, these older adults may reduce their fear, but they also reduce their level of function.

Fear is not to be confused with anxiety. *Anxiety* is a vague uneasiness related to unidentifiable threats, whereas *fear* is a protective mechanism mobilized against a real threat to the individual (McFarland & McFarlane, 1993). If the nurse thinks that the patient has a fear of falling, it is crucial for the nurse to validate this with the patient.

The psychosocial assessment should provide an insight into the level of ability and the skills that the older adult is using to adapt to the limitation in mobility. Also included in the psychosocial assessment is a determination of the patient's social support system, which includes family and friends, as well as formal and informal resources on which the patient can rely to enable continued function in the area of mobility.

Environmental assessment

Assessment of an older adult's living arrangement is a purposeful and goal-directed undertaking. When the care of a patient with a limitation in mobility necessitates a home visit by the nurse, it is within the realm of nursing to consider the appropriateness of assessing the home for safety hazards. Before doing so, the nurse must obtain the permission of the older adult to do a room-by-room safety assessment of the home; as with all nursing care, inclusion of the patient in the planning and implementation of the care is essential. The goal is not only assessment, but also implementation of recommendations.

Most people do not make major adjustments in their way of living unless they come to value, accept, and understand the reason for the change. Spending time explaining things and getting to know the patient and family is of primary importance in any home visit. It is important to involve the older adult and the caregiver in the process of assessment. Equally important is clarification of particular recommendations, such as removal of obstacles in the traffic pattern or the installation of grab rails in the bathroom.

One of the major risks for older adults with limitations in mobility is the risk of serious injury from a fall. Therefore the environmental assessment focuses on the reduction of risk from the physical hazards of the home environment. Prevention of falls is multifaceted, and the environment is not the only factor that contributes to the large number of falls experienced by older adults. Gaining knowledge concerning what constitutes a home hazard and assisting the patient in taking steps that reduce the environmental risks are nursing responsibilities (Box 12-5). Respecting the autonomy and dignity of the older adult and the family members while conducting a hazards assessment of the home is a delicate task. Recommendations may be viewed as criticism if care has not been taken to include and to value the input of the older adult patient and the family.

NURSING DIAGNOSES

After completion of the history, the physical examination, and the psychosocial and environmental assessment, the nurse has collected all

BOX 12-5 ASSESSMENT FOR HOME HAZARDS

OUTSIDE OF HOME

1. Location of mailbox
2. Parking space for automobile
3. Entrance to significant door
4. Condition of walkway, steps, and railing
5. Location of trash receptacle
6. Ability to manage results of weather conditions, such as icy stairs or wet leaves
7. Crime rate in the community

IN APARTMENT BUILDING

1. Condition of lobby
2. Condition of elevator
3. Condition of significant hallway

INSIDE OF HOME

1. Traffic pattern
2. Use of extension cords
3. Telephone location
4. Use of scatter rugs
5. Availability of lighting
6. Use of night-lights
7. Broken pieces of furniture
8. Stairs (worn rugs)
9. Inadequate bannisters on stairs
10. Bathroom: need for grab bars, raised toilet seat, shower stool, hand-held shower, or rubber bath mat

the pertinent data concerning the status of the older adult's mobility. The next step in the nursing process is to cluster the data and synthesize the information gleaned from the assessment. The goal is to formulate nursing diagnoses that are specific to the individual and that can be validated by the data collected.

Nursing diagnoses to be considered when caring for a patient with an impairment in mobility include the following:

1. Impaired physical mobility
2. Risk for injury

The following potential diagnoses may be secondary to impaired physical mobility:

1. Activity intolerance
2. Fatigue
3. Impaired home maintenance management
4. Self-esteem disturbance
5. Body image disturbance
6. Fear

The following are examples of nursing diagnoses that relate to mobility:

1. Impaired physical mobility related to condition of knee joint, as evidenced by
   a. Pain when bearing weight
   b. Range-of-motion limitation
   c. Lower extremity weakness
   d. Change in gait
   e. Inability to use stairs
   f. Decreased social involvement
2. Risk for injury from fall, related to physical impairment and hazardous behaviors, as evidenced by
   a. Range-of-motion limitation
   b. Lower extremity weakness
   c. Change in gait
   d. Poor or no use of assistive devices
   e. Home hazards
   f. Inappropriate use of alcohol

PLANNING AND GOAL IDENTIFICATION

The planning component of the nursing process consists of setting priorities for interventions and establishing both short- and long-term goals. The stated goals are specific to each diagnosis, definite in their expectations of patient behavioral outcomes, exact in specifying time for their achievement, and precise in establishing accountability for implementation of a plan (Yura & Walsh, 1988).

A short-term goal associated with a diagnosis of impaired physical mobility could be the following: with the supervision of a nurse, the patient will walk with the assistance of a cane twice a day for periods of 15 minutes. A long-term goal for the same diagnosis may be as follows: the patient will be able to walk independently for a distance of 200 yards.

The most difficult aspect of planning for nursing care of the older adult patient with a limitation in mobility is the setting of priorities. The complexity of multiple limitations and conditions can overwhelm a novice nurse. It is imperative that an orderly, systematic, comprehensive, and wholistic assessment be conducted by the nurse, with input from all members of the health care team. This team includes not only health care professionals, but also the patient and the family and significant others in the patient's life.

Life-threatening problems are given the highest priority in planning for the nursing care of an older adult patient. As these problems are resolved, the more difficult daily aspects of maintaining the integrity and dignity of an older patient challenge the skill and resources of the nurse. The goal of maintaining mobility, if appropriate for the patient, should be accorded a high priority in planning care.

IMPLEMENTATION

Nursing interventions are specific to the diagnoses and address the developed goals. Often, interventions that are specific to a diagnosis in the area of mobility deal with the defining characteristics and the causes of the problem. It is important to make use of interpersonal skills that help to motivate and to ensure the dignity and personhood of the older adult patient in carrying out crucial goal-oriented interventions. Purposeful and goal-directed nursing interventions seek

Aging Alert
Goals of mobility-related nursing care

- Prevent further loss of mobility.
- Believe in the possibility of rehabilitation.
- Emphasize and offer encouragement for small gains.
- Coordinate and/or foster wholistic interdisciplinary care.
- Preserve the dignity of the patient.

to improve the quality of life for those patients entrusted to care.

In the next section, nursing interventions related to improvement of mobility are discussed in reference to three types of settings: an acute care setting, a nursing home, and a private or family home.

In the acute care setting

Older adults usually experience joint replacement surgery in one of two ways: (1) in response to an emergency or (2) as elective surgery.

Often, the unexpected, traumatic occurrence of a fracture that leads to a sudden, unplanned hospital admission and an unanticipated surgical procedure may threaten not only the physical well-being but also the psychologic and spiritual well-being of the older adult. On the other hand, the patient who has made a conscious decision to have elective joint replacement. surgery is usually anticipating pain relief and is exercising freedom of choice. The scenario of elective surgery is less of a threat to the older adult's psychologic well-being. By having had time to prepare for surgery, the older adult has had time to seek medical care for any coex-

isting health problems and can devote full attention to assisting in the recovery and rehabilitative phases of surgery.

Often, an older adult may experience a fracture of the hip that results from a fall. When this occurs, the classic picture is that of a patient with complaints of pain in the hip or thigh, external rotation and adduction of the affected leg, and an inability to bear weight. Another, less common, type of hip fracture results from minor, unnoticed trauma, and the only evidence may be discomfort and minimal shortening of the leg.

Advanced age is not a contraindication to surgical interventions in hip fractures, because outcomes are favorable for older adult patients (Peterson et al., 1989). If surgical intervention is the medical treatment of choice, the nurse will be involved in the preoperative and postoperative care of the patient.

If the surgery is not done as an emergency procedure, there is time for preoperative teaching. A comprehensive nursing assessment is necessary. Patients may not understand what is happening, and it is often necessary for the nurse to answer questions and to offer explanations of all procedures. By attentively listening and expressing appropriate reassurance, the nurse can alleviate some of the fears that the patients and their families may have.

During the preoperative period, functional aspects not related to the immediate preoperative phase may go unnoticed by the surgical team. Areas on which the nurse should focus attention are the patient's use of over-the-counter and prescription drugs, including eyedrops, and either normal or unusual alcohol intake. The patient's vision and hearing level, nutritional status, smoking history, prior reaction to analgesic drugs, and mental status are areas about which the nurse should obtain information, because these will affect the postoperative course.

Postoperatively, the short-term goals are (1) management of pain without compromising the physical or mental status, (2) prevention of infection, and (3) avoidance of complications that accompany immobility. The long-term goal is to return the patient to at least the preoperative level of functioning. Treatment for an older adult who experiences a hip fracture usually entails a period of hospitalization, with an accompanying period of inpatient rehabilitation that may last from 2 to 3 months. Many older adults who sustain a hip fracture are able to return to their prior functional level, but for many others, nursing home care is the only feasible alternative.

Other features of nursing care of the older adult during hospitalization that pertain to mobility are in the realm of prevention of falls during the hospital stay. A patient falling in a hospital is an area of concern, and the prevention of falls is a major task. Data from several studies report that the number of patient falls ranges from 62 to 238 per 10,000 admissions. Age is a significant factor in all studies. In a study of older hospitalized patients who had experienced an in-hospital fall, the investigators found five significant risk factors: confusion, cardiovascular diagnosis, decreased mobility of lower extremities, general weakness, and elimination needs (Kippenbrock & Soja, 1993). The use of benzodiazepine sedatives has been shown to be associated with an increased risk of falls both in institutions and in private or family homes (Sorock, 1988). The nurse should be especially alert when older adult patients receive any type of sedative, narcotic, or hypnotic.

Patients should be instructed to sit on the side of the bed with legs dangling for a few minutes before they get out of bed, to prevent orthostatic hypotension. The greatest risk is at night, when the older adult patient may waken in an unfamiliar environment, a bed with side rails, and experience the need to urinate. Slowly getting out of bed may not be a natural response. To alleviate this hazardous situation, the call light should be attached where the patient can see it at night and use it easily, so that the nurse can immediately respond to the call for help. Night-

lights also help to orient the older adult patient to the environment and to decrease the amount of confusion experienced during hospitalization. These measures contribute to decreasing the likelihood of falls.

In the nursing home

Most older adults who reside in nursing homes are highly dependent. The 1985 National Nursing Home Survey showed that over 60% of the residents had a limitation in mobility (National Center for Health Statistics, 1987). Glick and Swanson (1995) found that motor performance was a discriminating factor that differentiated residents who were in a dependent state from those who were functioning more independently. The ability to turn while walking, an action that requires balance, upper body strength, ability to change direction, and skill in locomotion, was a significant predictor for independence. This study reinforces nursing knowledge of the importance of gait training to improving the quality of life for nursing home residents.

Assistive devices are considered important resources for older adult individuals who have a physical impairment that affects their mobility. It is the nurse's role to observe whether the assistive device is being used correctly. If it is not, the nurse must teach correct usage, to help older adult patients to increase their level of mobility (Figure 12-5).

Many nursing home residents rely on wheelchairs to enable them to get around in the nursing home. One way to view this phenomenon is to regard the wheelchair as either a bicycle or a small automobile. It facilitates the transportation of the resident from one area to another. The risk is not in the use of the wheelchair itself but in the total reliance on the wheelchair, which may bring a lack of motivation to continue using the skill of walking. Thus in spite of the benefits of wheelchair use, the nurse should be alert to signs of further loss in mobility. One potential hazard is the overreliance on the wheelchair by the staff and by the older adult

FIGURE 12-5 Assistive devices. *A,* Ortho cane with wrist strap. *B,* A forearm crutch stabilizes your elbow while you walk. *C,* New "rolling" crutch provides smoother contact with the ground. *D,* Walker with front wheels allows constant contact with the ground. *E,* Quad cane offers more support than a single-stem walker. *Courtesy Lumex, Inc., New York.*

as the only form of mobility. This will lead to a decrease in physical strength, and in turn to a loss of the ability to walk. Loss of the strength that is necessary for walking is one of the greatest risks faced by institutionalized older adults.

The nurse must recognize both the risks and the benefits of wheelchair use and be able to arrange a plan of care that maximizes all aspects of the patient's health. A plan that allows an element of choice in activities and freedom of movement is essential to preserving the dignity and well-being of the older adult. The plan should also include time for staff to walk and exercise with the older adult, to ensure that muscle strength will be maintained.

Another feature of the standard wheelchair that presents a potential hazard is the design. Footrests on the wheelchair may cause the older adult to trip and stumble, especially when trying to get out of the chair. The brakes may be difficult for the older adult to lock because of lack of hand strength and the placement of the hand brake. Special care must be taken in teaching the older adult how to dismount from a wheelchair. The position of an older adult resident sitting in a wheelchair needs to be monitored and changed regularly.

It is also critical to verify whether the individual is consistently using the device. Often the older adult considers the cane or walker a stigma and will refuse to use it. Validating the patient's feelings concerning the use of a cane or walker is part of intervening. The nurse respects and tries to understand how the patient perceives the situation. Accepting small gains is one of the principles of care when the patients are older adults who are struggling to maintain positive self-images and self-respect. Allowing the patient to express negative feelings without judging those feelings may help to speed the patient's acceptance of the cane or walker, or it may just make the patient feel better. The nurse can express concern and discuss the reality of a decrease in function and in mobility that results from not using the cane or walker. Over time, allowing expression of feelings and providing a reality orientation will facilitate an acceptance of the assistive device for most patients.

Some residents who are afflicted with severe dementia still have a high level of mobility; this can be detrimental, as in the case of the older adult with dementia who is agitated and who wanders or paces constantly. Other residents may have limited mobility yet may be cognitively alert, so they may continue to function because of their use of assistive devices and assistance from nursing staff. Still other residents may be immobile and dependent on nursing staff to assist them in many aspects of life, as a result of the sequelae of stroke or other debilitating conditions. Recognition of the wide variations in mobility of nursing home residents is an important consideration in providing individualized nursing care.

Many aspects of care for older adult patients are guided by standards and principles of practice that pertain to all adults or to other selected patient groups. For example, the principles of nursing care for an immobile patient may be highly applicable to the care of many older adult patients. The complexity of nursing care is predicated on the knowledge of the effects of multiple confounding conditions that are so often apparent when caring for older adults. For example, care of the immobile older adult patient may be made more complex by the fact that the patient is hard-of-hearing; this condition interferes with the patient's understanding of the instructions for assisting with movement and transfers.

This level of complexity occurs very often in the care of the nursing home resident who has limited mobility. Nursing care of older adults requires the most sophisticated level of nursing judgment, and nursing interventions in this context demand a high level of interpersonal and technical skill.

In the private or family home

Many older adults living in private or family homes have functional dependencies. Three times as many people who are in the 85-and-older age group as in the 65- to 75-year age group report the need for assistance with activities of daily living (National Center for Health Statistics, 1991). Because of this preponderance of functional dependencies in the older population, many of the patients encountered during home care visits may exhibit limitations in mobility. Sometimes the home visit may be directly related to the physical impairment that results from a loss of mobility, but at other times the limitation in mobility may become evident only after a thorough assessment.

Hazards The nurse caring for the older adult patient in the home must be alert to the potential for home hazards (see Box 12-5). Often, older adults and their family members have been living with these hazards for many years and have difficulty in regarding such things as stairs as a hazard. The addition of a safety mechanism is one way to minimize a hazard—for example, adding a bannister to a staircase or a grab bar in the bathroom. For some older adults, the expense of a safety mechanism may be beyond their financial resources; referral to social services may be an appropriate intervention.

Another nursing intervention to promote the health of the patient is to explain the importance of restoring mobility. The patient can be encouraged to ambulate in a safe manner when it is appropriate. Stretching exercises that improve posture should be part of the nursing interventions for every older adult (Lewis and Campanelli, 1993) (see Figure 12-3). Health practices that protect joints and improve the mobility function should be encouraged.

Foot care The importance of foot care cannot be overemphasized. An assessment of the condition of the patient's feet can be included in the early stage of planning interventions to promote good health practices that contribute to the mobility function (Box 12-6).

During the assessment of the patient's feet, the nurse elicits complaints of any problems (such as itching or pain on walking) that the patient may be experiencing. If shoes do not fit properly, the nurse should determine the ability and the willingness of the patient to buy new

---

BOX 12-6 FOOT ASSESSMENT

1. Appropriateness of types of shoes
2. Condition of shoes
3. Fit of shoes
4. Condition of socks
5. Patient's ability to remove socks and shoes without assistance
6. Condition of feet
   a. Cleanliness
   b. Condition of skin
   c. Edema
   d. Dry, scaly skin
   e. Color
7. Condition of toes
   a. Infection
   b. Fungus
   c. Toenails
   d. Ingrown toenails
   e. Nail thickening
8. Abnormal features
   a. Hammertoe
   b. Bunion
   c. Calluses
   d. Corns
   e. Other

---

shoes. One problem may be transportation to a shopping area where shoes can be purchased. Often, alerting family members to the need may be sufficient to solve the problem; at other times it may be necessary to involve social services.

Medications The nurse reviews with the patient and family members all of the older adult patient's medications and the side effects of each medication. The potential for injury for adults of advanced age who are taking multiple medications and living in private or family homes is high. Two methods of prevention are to increase the patient's awareness of the combined effects of drugs and to teach behaviors that will diminish the risk of injury.

Exercise A program of exercise is an essential interdisciplinary intervention for older adult patients who have limitations in mobility and who are physically able to participate in a prescribed program (Galindo-Ciocon et al., 1995). Many older adults lead a sedentary life that is detrimental to their health. Walking on a regular basis can play an important role in the maintenance of physical and psychologic health. Before suggesting a program of exercise for an older adult home care patient, it is important to consult with the physician to ascertain the type and amount of exercise prescribed.

During the assessment phase, some older adults may be identified as being at high risk for falling. There are times when well-meaning health care professionals restrict mobility because of a perceived need to protect the older adult from the risk of a fall. The paradox in this treatment is that mobility may be lost through the treatment. However, a fractured hip does introduce a significant risk to the life of many older adults, so caution is certainly appropriate. Clinical decisions regarding an older adult's mobility are to be guided by ethical principles of autonomy and beneficence. The clinical dilemma between doing good (beneficence) and providing for choice (autonomy) may be described as a conflict between protection from injury and the risk to the spirit when choice is lost.

Realizing the importance of individualized care and inclusion of the patient in the planning of care is paramount because of the large degree of physical, psychologic, and social variability in the population of older adults.

EVALUATION

The final phase of the nursing process is the evaluation of the results of the plan in terms of accomplishment of the delineated goals. A criterion method that deals with measurable and observable outcomes is employed to validate the effectiveness of the nursing interventions. Also, using qualitative measures to evaluate the patient's perception of outcomes and the acceptance of the nursing care is an important evaluative function. Documentation of evaluation is critical and fundamental to nursing science.

REFERENCES

Baylink, D. & Jennings, J. (1994). Calcium and bone homeostasis and changes with aging. In W.M. Hazzard, E. Bierman, J. Blass, W. Ettinger, & J. Halter (Eds.), *Principles of geriatric medicine and gerontology.* New York: McGraw-Hill.

Bradley, J.D. et al. (1991). Comparison of an antiinflammatory dose of ibuprofen, an analgesic dose of ibuprofen and acetaminophen in the treatment of patients with osteoarthritis of the knee. *New England Journal of Medicine, 325,* 87.

Buchner, et al. (1992). Effects of physical activity on health status in older adults: 2. Intervention studies. *Annual Review Public Health, 13,* 469.

Calkins, E., Reinhard, J., & Vladuitiu. (1994). Rheumatoid arthritis and the autoimmune rheumatic disease in the older patient. In W.M. Hazzard, E. Bierman, J. Blass, W. Ettinger, & J. Halter (Eds.), *Principles of geriatric medicine and gerontology.* New York: McGraw-Hill.

Carlson, J., & Strom, B. (1994). Nonsteroidal antiinflammatory drugs. In W.M. Hazzard, E. Bierman, J. Blass, W. Ettinger, & J. Halter (Eds.), *Principles of geriatric medicine and gerontology.* New York: McGraw-Hill.

Chestnut, C.H. (1992). Osteoporosis and its treatment. *New England Journal of Medicine, 326,* 402.

Chestnut, C.H. (1994). Osteoporosis. In W.M. Hazzard, E. Bierman, J. Blass, W. Ettinger, & J. Halter (Eds.), *Principles of geriatric medicine and gerontology.* New York: McGraw-Hill.

Culliton, B.J. (1987). Osteoporosis reexamined: Complexity of bone biology is a challenge. *Science, 235*(4791), 833-834.

Ettinger, W. (1994). Immobility. In W.M. Hazzard, E. Bierman, J. Blass, W. Ettinger, & J. Halter (Eds.), *Principles of geriatric medicine and gerontology.* New York: McGraw-Hill.

Fiatrone, et al. (1990). High intensity strength training in nonagenarians. *Journal of the American Medical Association,* 263-3029.

Fife, R. (1994). Osteoarthritis. In W.M. Hazzard, E. Bierman, J. Blass, W. Ettinger, & J. Halter (Eds.), *Principles of geriatric medicine and gerontology.* New York: McGraw-Hill.

Gabriel, S.E., et al. (1991). Risk of serious gastrointestinal complications related to use of nonsteroidal antiinflammatory drugs: A meta-analysis. *Annals of Internal Medicine, 115,* 787.

Galindo-Ciocon, D., Ciocon, J., & Galindo, D. (1995). Gait training and falls in the elderly. *Journal of Gerontological Nursing, 21*(6), 10-17.

Glick, O., & Swanson, E. (1995). Motor performance correlates of functional dependence in long term care residents. *Nursing Research, 44*(1), 4-8.

Grisso, J.A., & Kaplan, F. (1994). Hip fractures. In W.M. Hazzard, E. Bierman, J. Blass, W. Ettinger, & J. Halter (Eds.), *Principles of geriatric medicine and gerontology*. New York: McGraw-Hill.

Hunter, G., Treuth, M., Weinsier, R., Kekes-Szabo, T., Kell, S.H., Roth, D.L., & Nicholson, C. (1995). The effects of strength conditioning on older women's ability to perform daily tasks. *Journal of the American Geriatric Society, 43*(7), 756-760.

Kippenbrock, & Soja. (1993). Preventing falls in the elderly: Interviewing patients who have fallen. *Geriatric Nursing, 14*, 205-209.

Lawrence, R.C., et al. (1989). Estimates of the prevalence of selected arthritic and musculoskeletal disease in the United States. *Journal of Rheumatology, 16*, 873.

Lewis, C. & Campanelli, L. (1993). VHI Geriatric Exercise and Rehabilitation Exercise Kit. *Visual health/stretching charts*. Tacoma, WA.

McFarland, G., & McFarlane, E. (1993). *Nursing diagnosis and intervention: Planning for patient care*. St. Louis: Mosby.

Minon, M.A., Hewett, J.E., & Webel, R.R. (1989). Efficacy of physical conditioning exercise in patients with rheumatoid arthritis and osteoarthritis. *Arthritis Rheumatoid, 32*, 1396.

Morey, et al. (1989). Evaluation of a supervised exercise program in a geriatric population. *Journal of the American Geriatric Society, 37*, 348-354.

National Center for Health Statistics. (1987). Preliminary data from the 1985 National Nursing Home Survey (Advance data 135). Washington, DC: Government Printing Office.

National Center for Health Statistics. (1991). *Current estimates from the National Health Interview Survey Series 10: Data from the National Health Survey No. 184* (Vital and Health Statistics, DHHS Pub. No. [PHS] 93-1512). Hyattsville, MD: U.S. Department of Health and Human Services, Public Health Service, Centers for Disease Control, National Center for Health Statistics.

Overgaard, K., et al. (1992). Effect of calcitonin given intranasally on bone mass and fracture rates in established osteoporosis: A close-response study. *British Medicine Journal, 305*, 556.

Peterson, V.S., Solgaard, S., & Simonsen, B. (1989). Total hip replacement in patients aged 80 years and older. *Journal of the American Geriatric Association, 37*(3), 219-222.

Schwartz, R.S., & Buchner, D.M. (1994). Exercise in the elderly: Physiologic and functional effects. In W.M. Hazzard, E. Bierman, J. Blass, W. Ettinger, & J. Halter (Eds.), *Principles of geriatric medicine and gerontology*. New York: McGraw-Hill.

Sorock, G. (1988). Falls among the elderly: Epidemiology and prevention. *American Journal of Preventative Medicine, 4*(5), 282-288.

Taggert, H.M., & Alderice, J.M. (1982). Fatal cholestatic jaundice in elderly patients taking benoxaprofen. *British Medical Journal, 285*, 1372.

Tinetti, M.E. (1994). Falls. In W.M. Hazzard, E. Bierman, J. Blass, W. Ettinger, & J. Halter (Eds.), *Principles of geriatric medicine and gerontology*. New York: McGraw-Hill.

Treuth, M.S., Hunter, G.R., Kekes-Szabo, T., Weinsier, R.L., Goran, M.I., & Berland, L. (1995). Reduction in intra-abdominal adipose tissue after strength training in older women. *Journal of Applied Physiology, 78*(4), 1425-1431.

Vico, L., Pouget, J.F., Calmels, P., Chatard, J.C., Rehailia, M., Minaire, P., Geyssant, A., & Alexandre, C. (1995). The relations between physical ability and bone mass in women aged over 65 years. *Journal of Bone Mineral Research, 10*(3), 374-383.

World Health Organization. (1976). *International classification of impairment, disabilities, and handicaps* (WHA 29, 35). Geneva, Switzerland: Author.

Young, D.R., Masaki, K.H., & Curb, J.D. (1995). Associations of physical activity with performance-based and self-reported physical functioning in older men: The Honolulu Heart Program. *Journal of the American Geriatric Society, 43*(8), 845-854.

Yura, H., & Walsh, M.B. (1988). *The nursing process*. East Norwalk, CT: Appleton and Lange.

BIBLIOGRAPHY

Arnett, F.C. (1989). The 1987 revised American Rheumatism Association criteria for classification of rheumatoid arthritis. In D.J. McCarthy (Ed.), *Arthritis and allied conditions: A textbook of rheumatology* (p. 20). Philadelphia: Lea and Febiger.

Grob, D. (1989). Common disorders of muscles in the aged. In W. Reichel (Ed.), *Clinical aspects of aging* (pp. 296-313). Baltimore: Williams & Wilkins.

Tinetti, M.E. (1987). Factors associated with serious injury during falls by ambulatory nursing home residents. *Journal of the American Geriatric Society, 35*(3), 644-648.

Aging is not for sissies.

TERRY SCHUCKMAN, 1975

Urinary Incontinence

■ Learning Objectives

On completion of this chapter, the reader will be able to do the following:

1. Identify and describe the types and causes of urinary incontinence experienced by older adults.
2. Describe and/or perform history taking, and physical and functional assessments for patients with urinary incontinence.
3. Describe urodynamic assessment.
4. Recognize the psychosocial consequences of urinary incontinence for older adults and their families.
5. Identify and describe behavioral therapies for urinary incontinence.
6. Provide appropriate nursing interventions, patient education, and advocacy for older adults with urinary incontinence.

Urinary incontinence (UI), the involuntary loss of urine, is a troublesome health problem among older adults, with an incidence of 37.7% in women and 18.9% in men who reside in private or family homes (Diokno et al., 1986). It is more common in nursing homes, where approximately 50% of the residents experience incontinence (Mohide, 1986; Ouslander, 1992). Research indicates that this condition often contributes to the decision to place homebound individuals in long-term care facilities (Johnson & Warner, 1982; Noelker, 1987; Smallegan, 1985). In acute care settings the rate of incontinence in older patients is estimated to range from 15% to 35%,

although these episodes may be transitory and related to acute illnesses (Mohide, 1986; Ouslander, 1992).

Although incontinence increases with age, it is not a part of the normal aging process; neither is it untreatable. During the past decade, advances in the assessment and treatment of urinary incontinence have shown that urinary incontinence can be successfully diagnosed and treated in even the oldest of individuals (Ouslander, 1986; Ouslander, 1992; Resnick et al., 1989). Still, a large number of older people do not seek help for this condition (National Institutes of Health [NIH], 1988). Some fear surgical intervention and are not aware that nonsurgical approaches are available. Others are unaware that treatment of any form is available. Many health care providers lack information about incontinence and hold negative attitudes about the problem. Too often, patients are told, "It is something you will have to learn to live with," when in fact, incontinence can be significantly improved or cured in nine out of ten (NIH, 1988). In many communities there is a scarcity of nurses, physicians, and other health care providers who have the knowledge and skills to apply nonsurgical approaches to the problem of incontinence. As more health care providers become educated in this specialty, the problem of incontinence in older people should decrease considerably.

■ Normal Structure and Function

Normal micturition is a complex process that involves the lower urinary tract, the spinal cord (T11 to S4), the brain, and the autonomic and somatic nervous systems. The bladder, the detrusor muscles surrounding the bladder, the urethra, and the internal and external sphincters make up the lower urinary tract (Figure 13-1). Bladder relaxation and urethral contraction, which are important in the maintenance of continence, are controlled by the sympathetic nervous system. Bladder contraction, essential for the expulsion of urine, is stimulated by the parasympathetic nervous system. The bladder and the urethra are supported by pelvic floor muscles, which are important in bladder control. The pelvic floor, including the external sphincter, is controlled by the somatic nervous system, specifically the pudendal nerve.

Micturition is mediated by the brain. The cerebral cortex appears to inhibit the loss of urine, whereas the brainstem facilitates urination (Ouslander, 1994a, 1994b). Maintenance of continence requires the coordination of all these systems. During bladder filling, stretch receptors in the bladder wall signal the sacral spinal cord. Once a critical volume is reached, approximately 300 ml, a spinal reflex stimulates the bladder to empty. At the same time, bladder sensory nerves transmit signals via the spinal cord to the brain. Although the neurophysiology of urination is still under investigation, it appears that the cerebral cortex sends inhibitory messages to delay urination. Thus continence is maintained. Any disorder that affects the normal physiologic function of any of these systems may cause incontinence to occur.

■ Age-Related Changes

A variety of pathologic and functional factors that are frequently seen in older adults may predispose them to loss of bladder control. For example, benign prostatic hypertrophy (BPH) increases with age in men and often leads to urinary incontinence, urinary frequency, urgency, decreased force of the urinary system, and hesitancy in initiating urine flow. Similarly, normal age-related estrogen loss in women causes changes in the squamous epithelium of the distal urethral and vaginal wall, a decrease in vaginal muscular tone, and vascular profusion. These physiologic and anatomic changes contribute to urinary incontinence in older women and may be accompanied by urgency or frequency of urination.

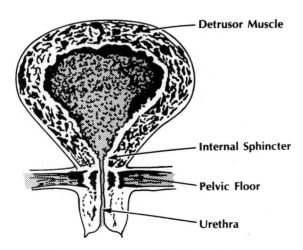

— Detrusor Muscle

— Internal Sphincter

— Pelvic Floor

— Urethra

FIGURE 13-1 The urinary bladder.

Increasing age is also associated with an increase in involuntary bladder contractions, a reduction in bladder capacity, and an increase in residual volume (Leach & Yip, 1986; Staskin, 1986). These alterations in bladder function, especially involuntary contractions, may contribute to the development of urinary incontinence in older adults.

The complex nature of urination, combined with age-related physiologic changes, underscores the importance of comprehensive assessment to discover the underlying cause of urinary incontinence in older adults. Only after the mechanism of the incontinence has been identified can appropriate treatments be applied with success.

■ Types of Urinary Incontinence

Urinary incontinence (UI) is typically categorized as acute (transient) or persistent (established) (Box 13-1). Acute alterations in urinary elimination are associated with acute illness, which may either be systemic or involve the urinary tract specifically. Many illnesses, such as hip fracture, congestive heart failure, pneumonia, and delirium, can upset the homeostatic balance of the older adult sufficiently to affect urinary control. Factors associated with acute health breakdown, such as bed rest, inability to toilet independently, or lack of staff or caregivers to assist in toileting, also affect the patient's ability to maintain urinary control. Continence is usually restored once the acute illness, immobility, and resulting dependency are resolved. Conditions such as acute urinary tract infection, urethritis, or vaginitis cause irritation and inflammation of the bladder and urethral squamous epithelium, resulting in involuntary urine loss. Appropriate treatment of these conditions will result in a return to normal bladder function in most instances. Fecal impaction can result in urinary incontinence, either by causing obstruction of the urethra and occluding urine flow or by inducing bladder spasms by means of pressure from the distended bowel. Removal of fecal impaction and institution of a bowel regimen

---

BOX 13-1 TYPES OF URINARY INCONTINENCE

Acute (transient)
Persistent (established)
  Stress
  Urge
  Overflow
  Functional

---

often result in a reduction or elimination of urinary incontinence in affected individuals.

Medications often result in underreported side effects in older adults. Antidepressants, antipsychotics, and narcotic analgesics have an anticholinergic effect, which can inhibit or diminish bladder contractions, resulting in inadequate bladder emptying and overflow incontinence. Alpha- and beta-adrenergic agonists and calcium channel blocker agents are used in the treatment of cardiovascular disease and have also been implicated in causing urinary retention, with resulting overflow incontinence (Ouslander, 1994a, 1994b).

Incontinence that has been present over a period of months and is not the result of acute illness or effects of medication is called persistent incontinence. Major types of persistent incontinence include stress, urge, overflow, and functional incontinence (NIH, 1988).

STRESS INCONTINENCE

Stress incontinence, one of the most common forms of incontinence in women, is the involuntary leakage of urine that occurs with physical exertion, such as coughing, sneezing, laughing, lifting, or exercising. These activities cause a rise in intraabdominal pressure, which results in increased bladder pressure. If the urethra is competent and pelvic floor muscle tone is adequate, continence is maintained. However, increased intra-abdominal pressure in people with incompetent urethras or weak pelvic floor muscles can result in accidental urine loss. Stress incontinence in women is associated with damage to the pelvic musculature during pregnancy, vaginal delivery, or trauma during gynecologic or urologic surgery. Men rarely experience stress incontinence, except as the result of urethral injury, such as injury that occurs during prostatectomy (Hadley et al., 1986).

URGE INCONTINENCE

Urge incontinence is also seen frequently in older adults. In this condition the bladder escapes central nervous system inhibition and contracts spontaneously, resulting in leakage of small to large amounts of urine. Uninhibited detrusor spasms are commonly referred to as "bladder instability" or "detrusor instability." Typically, patients experience an urgent sensation to void followed quickly by involuntary loss of urine. Frequent urination and nocturia are commonly associated with this condition. Patients often complain of not being able to get to the bathroom in time, or of inability to control the bladder when putting the key in the door to a locked bathroom or when washing their hands. Urge incontinence is seen in patients with spinal cord damage or central nervous system problems—for example, Parkinson's disease, strokes, dementia, bladder or urethral irritation and/or infection, fecal impaction, uterine prolapse, prostatic hypertrophy, or radiation damage to the bladder or urethra (Ouslander, 1994a, 1994b). It has also been asserted that the habit of frequent urination can contribute to development of bladder instability and incontinence (Frewen, 1978, 1980). Frequently, however, none of these conditions exists in patients experiencing this form of incontinence. Urge incontinence often coexists with stress incontinence in older adults. In such mixed cases of incontinence, one form usually predominates.

OVERFLOW INCONTINENCE

Overflow incontinence is caused by incomplete bladder emptying that results in urinary reten-

tion. Leakage of urine occurs when pressure resulting from a chronically full bladder exceeds urethral pressure. Frequent leakage of small amounts of urine, with or without urgency, is noted. Patients may also describe an inability to empty the bladder. Causative factors include atonic bladder, side effects of medication, mechanical obstruction, detrusor hyperactivity with incomplete bladder contraction (DHIC), and dyssynergia of sphincter and bladder contraction.

Atonic bladder is characterized by failure of the detrusor muscle to contract adequately and to expel the total volume of urine. This condition typically results from spinal cord injury or diabetes mellitus. Also, side effects of medications, such as muscle relaxants, antidepressants, or antipsychotics, can reduce the force of detrusor muscle contraction, resulting in incomplete bladder emptying.

Mechanical obstruction caused by an enlarged prostate, uterine prolapse, a large cystocele, or fecal impaction can cause urinary retention through partial or complete occlusion of the urethra. Dyssynergia and DHIC are more complex and less common. In dyssynergia, the urinary sphincter and bladder contract simultaneously. Normally the muscles surrounding the urethra relax as the bladder contracts, permitting micturition to occur. Dyssynergia is most often seen in patients with suprasacral neurologic impairment.

FUNCTIONAL INCONTINENCE

Functional incontinence is caused not by bladder or sphincter dysfunction, but by physical, mental, psychologic, or environmental factors. Physical disabilities that interfere with gait and ambulation can impair a patient's ability to reach the toilet in a timely fashion. Patients with cognitive disabilities have difficulty remembering the location of the bathroom or recognizing the need to void. Other patients may be acutely depressed and lack motivation to attend to personal habits. Environmental barriers can also play an important role in the inability to toilet properly. People confined to bed or physically restrained cannot be expected to remain continent if regular toileting is not provided by their caregivers. Bathrooms located at a great distance from the patient with gait problems and slowed ambulation can create an obstacle beyond the person's ability to overcome. Similarly, inadequate toilet facilities in public or private buildings put even the most agile and continent older individuals to the test.

■ Nursing Process

ASSESSMENT

The purpose of assessing the patient who is experiencing urinary incontinence is to discover any altered mechanism that underlies the condition, so that appropriate therapies can be initiated. The assessment includes a history; physical examination; psychosocial, functional, and environmental assessments; urodynamic evaluation; and a daily diary of bladder habits and incontinent episodes. The subjective reports and objective observations are important data that assist the nurse in arriving at an accurate nursing diagnosis.

History

The incontinence history covers the onset, progression, characteristics, and circumstances of the patient's urinary incontinence. It also contains information regarding the patient's bladder habits, and the signs and symptoms of urinary pathology (Box 13-2). The patient's description of the problem is one of the most important aspects of the assessment. Ideally this information will be provided by the patient. However, if the patient is cognitively impaired, family care providers and nursing records are valuable resources that the nurse can utilize to obtain relevant data.

Through a comprehensive health history (Box 13-3), the nurse seeks to discover the patient's perceptions of the continence problem, and to determine general health and functional

---

BOX 13-2
HISTORY OF INCONTINENCE

1. Characteristics of incontinence: onset, clinical course, frequency and volume of urine loss
2. Circumstances associated with urine loss: coughing, sneezing, laughing, lifting, stooping, walking, climbing stairs, sleeping, urgency, running water, cold weather, caffeine, alcohol, fluid intake, medications, postvoid dribbling, urine loss without sensation, continual leakage
3. Bladder habits: frequency and volume of daytime urination, frequency and volume of nocturia, methods of management (e.g., frequent voiding, pads, diapers, or urine collection device), fluid intake
4. Other signs and symptoms: urgency, burning, pain, hematuria, weakness of urinary stream, hesitancy, intermittent stream, constipation, bowel incontinence

---

status. Careful history taking should reveal current medical problems, current medications, and past medical, surgical, urologic, and obstetric events that may impinge on the current situation.

The nurse should always ask specifically about current or past diagnoses of diabetes mellitus, congestive heart failure, bladder infections, kidney infections, stroke, Parkinson's disease, depression, memory problems, and other neurologic conditions or injuries, because any of these conditions can affect bladder function. (Box 13-3 lists general areas of health history that should be included as part of the assessment of urinary incontinence.) The history taking should determine whether the patient has undergone urologic evaluation, urologic surgery, or other treatments for incontinence. Women should be asked

---

BOX 13-3
GENERAL HEALTH HISTORY

- Current medical problems
- Current medications and treatments
- History of diabetes mellitus, congestive heart failure, stroke, Parkinson's disease, other neurologic conditions of trauma, depression, dementia
- Previous urologic evaluations and treatments for incontinence
- Number of pregnancies, number of births, birth weights, types of delivery
- Number of years since menopause
- History of urinary tract infections, prostate disease, prostate surgery, kidney stones, gynecologic surgery

---

about their obstetric history, especially the types of delivery, weights of the infants, and trauma during delivery. Questions regarding previous gynecologic surgeries (e.g., repair of a cystocele or prolapsed uterus) are helpful in establishing a profile of factors that may affect the patient's current continence status.

Functional assessment

The functional assessment is one of the most important aspects of any examination of the gerontologic patient. In spite of existing health problems, many older adults are independent and able to perform usual activities of daily living (ADLs). Others are proficient in some aspects of daily life, but not in others. The patient's ability to function is not always clear on casual observation. Only by asking the appropriate questions and observing activities will the nurse know whether impairment in functional ability is a factor in the continence status of the patient. Functional status can be assessed through unstructured inquiry or by using established instru-

ments, such as the OARS physical activities of daily living (Duke University Center for the Study of Aging and Human Development, 1978) or the Katz index of activities of daily living (Katz et al., 1963). Questions about the patient's ability to ambulate, to dress and undress, to sit on a commode, and to perform personal hygiene are helpful in establishing the patient's functional capacity to toilet appropriately. The patient should also be asked about coordination difficulties and visual deficits that may impede adequate toileting.

Direct observation of mobility and toileting skills will provide the most useful information. The following observation is a guide:

1. The patients are placed 15 feet from the toilet.
2. The patients are asked to walk or propel their wheelchairs to the toilet.
3. When the patients reach the toilet, they are observed for their ability to undress and position themselves for voiding.
4. If the patients cannot complete the toileting sequence independently and a nurse or caregiver regularly provides assistance, then the toileting procedures should be observed with the nurse or caregiver assisting.

Mental status should be assessed using a standardized instrument such as the Folstein Mini–Mental State Examination (Folstein et al., 1975). Decline in cognitive ability can affect the patient's ability to recognize the need to urinate or to locate the toilet and can affect the patient's ability to remove clothing before voiding. In addition, the patient's ability to recall and learn new skills will play an important role in planning and implementing urinary incontinence interventions.

The diagnosis of dementia or cognitive deficits alone should not result in the conclusion that UI is caused by dementia, nor should physical impairment be identified as the cause of incontinence in patients with physical deficits, without ruling out other potential causes. Urge UI is common in people with dementia and incontinent individuals who ambulate slowly. Therefore, complete assessment of urinary incontinence is required in even the most severely disabled, because many patients will have bladder pathology that can be corrected regardless of cognitive or functional status.

Environmental assessment

Environmental factors may present barriers to toileting. The bathroom may be at a considerable distance from the patient, the height of the toilet may be too low for the patient, or the patient may need bars to assist in positioning. The bathroom may not be large enough to accommodate a patient using a wheelchair, or a bedside commode may not be available for patients who cannot reach the toilet. In the hospital or nursing home, the lack of privacy may inhibit toileting. Call bells may not be available to call for assistance. Staff may be unavailable or unwilling to take the patient to the toilet or to provide a bedpan or urinal. Box 13-4 presents important components of environmental assessment.

Psychosocial assessment

Assessment of psychologic and social factors focuses on the consequences of incontinence in the patient's life. Patients should be asked whether being incontinent (1) restricts activities (such as attending social functions, going to church, or visiting friends and family); (2) affects their self-esteem, mood, or sexual activity; or (3) affects family relationships. It is also important to assess the patient's desire and willingness to participate in treatment for incontinence. If the patient does not desire treatment, the nurse should explore the reasons for this lack of motivation, such as lack of knowledge, depression, or an overwhelming social, psychologic, or physical problem.

Older adults with physical or mental disabilities who live at home may be dependent on family or other caregivers to assist in toileting.

BOX 13-4
ENVIRONMENTAL ASSESSMENT

- What is the distance between the patient and the toilet facilities?
- Is the height of the toilet appropriate for the patient?
- Are toilet facilities large enough to accommodate both patient and wheelchair?
- Are grab bars present if needed?
- Do physical barriers such as poor lighting or furniture or other objects obstruct the path to the toilet?
- Are caregivers or nursing staff available if needed?
- Is the call bell available to the patient if needed?

The family members or caregivers may have physical disabilities themselves that prevent them from providing assistance. They may also feel burdened in caring for the incontinent individual or lack knowledge about incontinence and therapies that are available. Consequently, assessment of family and caregivers should determine (1) whether a caregiver is available and capable of assisting the patient; (2) whether the caregiver is willing to assist the patient; (3) the caregiver's attitude toward the patient and toward incontinence; and (4) the caregiver's knowledge about behavioral and other strategies to decrease or eliminate episodes of incontinence.

Physical examination

A physical examination should be performed that includes the following:

1. General inspection of gait and balance, and the presence or absence of tremors
2. Neurologic assessment of deep tendon reflexes, sensation of pain and light touch, and vibratory sensation of the

lower extremities (these assessments ascertain the presence or absence of a neurologic deficit, such as that caused by stroke, peripheral neuropathy, or spinal cord injury)

3. Abdominal examination, to determine the presence or absence of bladder distention, of suprapubic tenderness (present in bladder infections), and of costa vertebral tenderness (a sign of kidney infection)

4. Rectal examination, to note the presence or absence of fecal impaction, rectal sensation, and tone (also, in men, it is important to evaluate the size, shape, and consistency of the prostate gland, because prostatic obstruction may be the cause of urinary incontinence)

5. Two-position blood pressure measurement and examination of the heart and lungs, to reveal a cardiovascular process, such as postural hypotension, congestive heart failure, or severe arrhythmia, that may impair the patient's overall functional status

6. A pelvic examination, essential in women with complaints of involuntary loss of urine, which includes inspection of the vagina for conditions that may contribute to urinary incontinence, such as the presence of atrophic changes, vaginitis, a cystocele, rectocele, or uterine prolapse

Urodynamic assessment

Postvoid catheterization for residual urine is an essential component of urodynamic assessment that can be performed by the nurse. Residual volume of 100 ml or greater indicates urinary retention, whereas postvoid residual volume below 100 ml is usually considered normal in older adults and indicates adequate bladder emptying. In addition to the postvoid assessment of residual volume, a simplified urodynamic assessment, including cystometrogram, can be performed by a nurse practitioner or clinical specialist who has learned to perform and interpret the test. Box 13-5 describes the procedure for urodynamic assessment, which may be used at the bedside (McDowell & Burgio; 1990; McDowell et al., 1989; Ouslander, 1986).

Stress or urge incontinence can be assessed by means of a pad test when patients have a full bladder. Instruct patients to notify you when they perceive the need to urinate or to refrain from voiding for at least 3 hours before the appointment. In a private room, such as the bathroom, ask the patient to stand on an absorbent pad, or to wear a pad. Instruct the patient to cough 3 times, and note any involuntary leakage of urine. Also, observe for leakage of urine on the patient's standing or walking. Leakage of urine during these maneuvers is indicative of stress urinary incontinence. Next, have the patient listen to running water and then wash his or her hands. Leakage that occurs under these circumstances signals the presence of urge incontinence.

Bladder records

One of the most beneficial assessment tools is the bladder diary. Bladder diaries are used to determine the frequency of urination and incontinent episodes, the approximate volume of accidents, and the circumstances of involuntary urine loss, such as coughing, position change, urgency, or inability to reach the toilet in time. Wyman and colleagues (1988) examined the test-retest reliability of a 1-week bladder diary and reported that it is a reliable method of evaluating frequency of incontinent episodes and voluntary urination. A sample bladder record is shown in Figure 13-2 (Wyman et al., 1988). Patients and caregivers need careful instruction in the proper use of the form if it is to accurately reflect the patient's bladder habits.

The diaries can be used in the home, hospital, or nursing home, by the patient, nurses, nurse aides, or other care providers. These diaries provide a more objective and accurate record of the patient's bladder habits than can be recalled from memory. Records should be kept for

---

BOX 13-5 BEDSIDE URODYNAMIC ASSESSMENT

Step 1. Have patient void. Observe voiding; note slowed or interrupted urinary stream, and record. Measure and record amount voided.

Step 2. Catheterize with a 14 French catheter; measure and record postvoid residual urine. With catheter in place, attach a 50-ml bulb syringe (without the bulb attached).

Step 3. Instill sterile water or normal saline into the syringe, allowing gravity to fill the bladder, while maintaining syringe at 15 ml above the pubis area.

Step 4. While instilling the solution, ask patient to report (1) first urge to void, (2) when the patient would normally void, (3) when the patient is comfortably full, and (4) when the patient can hold no more. Record the amount of solution instilled in each instance.

Step 5. Observe for the occurrence of fluid rising in the syringe and whether it is associated with the patient's report of an urge to void.

Step 6. Continue to fill bladder until patient reports being uncomfortable or filling stops. Note total amount instilled. (Do not fill beyond 500 ml.)

Step 7. Remove the catheter, but do not drain the sterile solution from the bladder. Ask patient to cough 3 times, and observe for leakage.

Step 8. Ask patient to sit and then stand. Observe for leakage. If no leakage has occurred in 15 to 30 seconds, ask patient to cough 3 times, and observe for leakage. Note whether leakage occurs during coughing or begins after coughing has ceased. Note whether leakage stops when the coughing stops or persists afterward. Have the patient void, and measure the amount.

Reprinted with permission, McDowell, Burgio, and Candib. (1989). Assessment of Urinary Incontinence in the Elderly. *Journal of the American Academy of Nurse Practitioners, 1*(1), 24-29.

---

1 to 2 weeks for accurate assessment of urinary incontinence and urinary frequency.

Bladder records are also essential during treatment to document progress and to evaluate the effectiveness of the intervention. It is imperative that the nurse review the record carefully with the patient, caregiver, or nurse aide. Careful review is necessary for accurate interpretation of the records, as well as to indicate to the patient or caregiver that their efforts in accurate recording are important.

Other assessment

Routine and microscopic assessment of the patient's urine is required to rule out urinary tract infection or hematuria. The findings of this test should be reported to the patient's physician or nurse practitioner. Other routine laboratory tests include assessment of blood glucose, blood urea nitrogen (BUN), and creatinine, to identify conditions such as diabetes mellitus or renal disease, which will require medical intervention and which may affect bladder control.

NURSING DIAGNOSES

The history, physical examination, functional assessment, and recorded report of the patient's bladder habits are all necessary to arrive at an accurate diagnosis of the type of incontinence the patient is experiencing. In some cases, complex urodynamic testing or simplified tests performed by the nurse are needed to identify the dysfunction that results in incontinence. Acute urinary incontinence must be ruled out or treated. If the problem is not acute but chronic in nature, then the diagnosis of persistent incontinence

NAME: _____ DATE:

Instructions:
1. In the 1st column, mark the time every time you void.
2. In the 2nd or 3rd column, mark every time you accidently leaked urine.
3. In the 4th column, enter the event that caused the accident, or the circumstances of the accident.

URINATED IN TOILET	SMALL ACCIDENT	LARGE ACCIDENT	REASON FOR ACCIDENT

No. of Pads Used Today: _____ No. of Accidents: _____

Comments: _____

_____

FIGURE 13-2 Bladder diary. *Courtesy of the Benedum Geriatric Continence Program, Pittsburgh, Pennsylvania.*

must be considered. Persistent incontinence is characterized as the involuntary loss of urine that has continued over a period of months and is not the result of acute illness, delirium, urinary tract infection, or vaginitis. A nurse in advanced practice in urinary incontinence can synthesize the assessment information and identify the underlying etiology of the problem so that appropriate treatment can be applied.

The following four nursing diagnoses are used to classify the types of persistent incontinence experienced by older adults:

1. Stress incontinence
2. Urge incontinence
3. Overflow incontinence
4. Functional incontinence

The next sections describe the pertinent findings that characterize each of these diagnoses.

Stress incontinence

History Involuntary leakage of urine is reported during periods of increased intra-abdominal pressure (e.g., coughing, sneezing, lifting, walking, or rising from a chair).

Objective findings There is leakage of urine from a full bladder during stress maneuvers such as coughing. Signs of pelvic relaxation or weakened pelvic floor muscles are often observed on pelvic examination.

Bladder records There is documented loss of urine during physical activities that increase intra-abdominal pressure, such as coughing or lifting.

Urge incontinence

History An urgent sensation to urinate, followed quickly by involuntary loss of urine, is reported. Symptoms of frequency of urination or nocturia may also be noted.

Objective findings The cystometrogram may reveal small bladder capacity (less than 300 ml) and/or detrusor contraction during bladder filling. (Symptoms of urge incontinence may be present, however, without objective urodynamic evidence of bladder dysfunction.) Involuntary leakage of urine with hand washing or with the sound of running water is common. The patient usually has difficulty stopping the stream of urine once it has started. Fecal impaction or severe atrophic vaginitis may also be seen in patients with urge incontinence.

Bladder records There is documentation of urine loss associated with urgency. Frequency of urination and nocturia are also often noted.

Note that many patients will experience a combination of stress and urge incontinence, as evidenced by history and objective tests; however, one type is usually predominant.

Overflow incontinence

History The patient reports frequent involuntary leakage of small amounts of urine, often with physical exertion. A decreased force of urinary stream and a sensation of not emptying the bladder completely are often present. Other symptoms may include hesitancy or frequent voiding of small amounts of urine. Patients with overflow incontinence may report taking antidepressant or other medications with anticholinergic properties, which may impede adequate bladder contractions during normal voiding.

Objective findings There is a large residual volume (greater than 100 ml) of postvoid urine—the hallmark of overflow incontinence with retention. A palpable distended bladder may be noted on examination of the abdomen. Impaired perineal sensation may be present, indicating neurologic disease. A large prostate in men, or cystocele in women, may be noted and suggests that the problem may be caused by obstruction.

Bladder records Frequent leakage of small amounts of urine is documented.

Functional incontinence

History Voiding in places other than a toilet, commode, bedpan, or urinal is reported, despite an absence of symptoms of urge, stress, or overflow incontinence. The patient may be unaware of the need to void or may report inability to toilet appropriately because of physical disabilities.

Objective findings There is no involuntary loss of urine with urge or stress maneuvers. The postvoid residual urine volume and cystometrogram are normal. A mental status examination score indicating cognitive impairment or impairment of mobility or toileting skills is noted during functional assessment.

Bladder records There is documentation of urinary accidents of large amounts of urine without symptoms of urgency or stress incontinence.

PLANNING AND GOAL IDENTIFICATION
Stress incontinence

A long-term goal would be to have the patient reduce or eliminate stress accidents. Short-term goals would include the following:

1. Patient will recognize activity that precipitates involuntary urine loss.
2. Patient will learn behavioral interventions that will help to avoid stress accidents.
3. Patient will practice exercises to strengthen the pelvic floor muscles and strategies to avoid involuntary leakage of urine.

Urge incontinence

The long-term goal might be that the patient will reduce or eliminate urge accidents. Short-term goals might include the following:

1. Patient will learn to recognize situations in which urge incontinence is likely to occur.
2. Patient will learn behavioral interventions that will help to prevent urge accidents.
3. Patient will practice the use of behavioral strategies to prevent involuntary urine loss.

4. Patient will practice strategies to suppress urge sensations and to expand time intervals between voiding.

Overflow incontinence

A long-term goal would be to have the patient reduce incontinence caused by urinary retention and overflow leakage. Short-term goals would include the following:

1. Patient will seek urologic examination.
2. Patients who are found to have obstructive uropathy will seek surgical correction of this problem.
3. Patients who have atonic bladders will learn and practice strategies to completely empty the bladder.

Functional incontinence

A long-term goal would be to have the caregivers help the patient through specific behavioral strategies to reduce or eliminate urinary accidents. Short-term goals would include the following:

1. Caregiver will recognize the patient's voiding pattern and will learn to assist the patient in toileting appropriately.
2. Caregiver will remove environmental barriers to proper toileting.
3. Caregiver will learn behavioral strategies to help patients with impaired mental status to avoid episodes of incontinence.
4. Caregiver will provide assistance and will encourage appropriate toileting and continence for patients with physical disabilities.

IMPLEMENTATION
Overview of nursing interventions

Nursing interventions for persistent urinary incontinence focus on behavior therapies. Research has shown that behavioral interventions can be helpful in eliminating or decreasing persistent involuntary urine loss in older patients residing in long-term care institutions or in the community (Burgio et al., 1985; Burgio et al., 1988; Fantl et al., 1990; Rose et al., 1990; Smith et al., 1989). Nurses play a major role in the implementation of behavioral interventions for urinary incontinence (Brink et al., 1983; Dougherty et al., 1989; McDowell et al., 1989; Morishita, 1988; Newman & Smith, 1989; Smith, 1988). However, many nurses have little formal preparation for these therapies. Behavior therapies should be an important part of nursing practice in a variety of situations, such as in the management of behavioral problems seen in patients with dementia and with personality disorders, as well as noncompliant patients and patients with UI. The following presentation addresses the various interventions used to treat urinary incontinence. The types of interventions appropriate for each individual depend on (1) the type of incontinence, (2) the cognitive and physical status of the patient, and (3) the setting in which the older person resides (Table 13-1).

Before initiation of specific therapies, the patient must be examined for acute urinary incontinence and treated appropriately. If UI is chronic or persistent, the treatment of choice is often behavioral intervention. The 1988 NIH Consensus Development Conference on Urinary Incontinence in Adults resulted in the following guideline: "As a general rule, the least invasive or dangerous procedures should be tried first. For many forms of incontinence, behavioral techniques meet this criterion" (NIH, 1988). Behavior therapies (described next) include (1) scheduled voiding (bladder retraining and habit training), (2) prompted voiding, (3) pelvic floor muscle training, and (4) biofeedback training.

Scheduled voiding

Scheduled voiding encompasses a group of treatments for which temporal voiding schedules are the common denominator. The type of scheduled voiding procedure varies, depending on the patient's level of independence and the goals of therapy (i.e., avoiding incontinent episodes versus altering bladder capacity and function). For

Health Promoting Behaviors
- Accept the need for early screening.
- Drink adequate amount of fluids.
- Avoid drinking caffeinated beverages, such as coffee, tea, or soda, and alcohol, because these have a diuretic effect.
- Drink fluids and eat foods that acidify the urine and decrease the risk of bladder infections.
- Void every 3 to 4 hours. Do not ignore the urge to void.
- For older women, perform exercises to strengthen pelvic muscles.
- Assess the environment for factors that may contribute to incontinence, such as distance from the bathroom or toilet, or inadequate lighting in the bathroom.
- Report any difficulty with bladder control to the nurse or other health care provider.

example, cognitively intact, motivated individuals are most responsive to a procedure such as bladder retraining, which requires active patient participation in a self-managed treatment. For dementia patients who are caregiver dependent, treatment of incontinence requires that the caregiver implement either habit training or prompted voiding, both of which involve the control of environmental factors (Burgio & Burgio, 1986).

Bladder retraining Bladder retraining, also called "bladder drill," encourages patients to adopt an expanded voiding interval in order to correct the habit of frequent voiding, to suppress bladder instability, and to diminish urgency. The patient is asked to postpone voiding in spite of a sensation of urgency and instead to void by the clock (Burgio & Burgio, 1986; McDowell et al.,

TABLE 13-1 Nursing interventions

Type of incontinence	Cognitively intact patient	Cognitively impaired patient
Urge	Pelvic floor muscle training Biofeedback Bladder retraining Urge strategies	Habit training Prompted voiding
Stress	Pelvic floor muscle training Biofeedback Stress strategies	Habit training Prompted voiding
Mixed	Pelvic floor muscle training Biofeedback Bladder retraining Urge and stress strategies	Habit training Prompted voiding
Overflow	Regular voiding schedule Crede maneuvers Intermittent self-catheterization	Habit training Prompted voiding Crede maneuvers applied by the nurse Intermittent catheterization
Functional	Habit training Environmental adjustments Caregiver assistance Bladder retraining	Prompted voiding Environmental adjustments Caregiver assistance

1989). This procedure is most useful for patients experiencing urge incontinence.

Habit training Habit training consists of timed voiding every 2 to 4 hours, whether or not a sensation of need to void is present. The objective is to keep the patient dry, not to modify bladder function. Voiding schedules may be fixed, or they may be flexible, in which case the voiding interval may be varied and tailored to the patient's needs. Habit training has been the most frequently used behavioral method of managing incontinence among cognitively impaired patients (Burgio & Burgio, 1986; McDowell & Burgio, 1990).

Prompted voiding

Prompted voiding is a multicomponent approach in which scheduled prompts to void (habit training) are supplemented with physical assistance, encouragement of self-initiated toileting, and positive reinforcement (i.e., caregiver attention)

for appropriate voiding and periods of dryness. Prompted voiding procedures have been utilized in nursing home populations with positive results. A prompted voiding program with adjusted intervals depending on the patient's dryness or wetness was conducted by Burgio and colleagues (1988) with four subjects who had varying levels of incontinence at baseline. All four subjects improved, with the average percentage of dry checks increasing from 30% at baseline to 62% during treatment (Burgio et al., 1988). However, the difficulties in training staff, as well as the problems inherent in the ability of staff to monitor and keep up with the prompted voiding schedules, were also noted.

In another study of prompted voiding, this one involving female nursing home residents, Kaltreider et al. (1990) noted that women who were most incontinent at baseline and who were the most cognitively intact showed the greatest reduction in wet episodes.

Pelvic floor muscle training

Pelvic floor muscle training was first reported by A.H. Kegel in 1948 as a method of increasing intraurethral pressure and decreasing urinary incontinence through increased strength and coordination of the circumvaginal muscles (Kegel, 1948). Contraction of these muscles exerts a closing force in the urethra, thus reducing or preventing leakage of urine during periods of increased intraabdominal pressure, such as coughing, bending, or changing positions. Patients with urge incontinence also benefit by learning to contract periurethral muscles, thereby facilitating bladder inhibition or reducing the loss of urine during uninhibited bladder contraction (McDowell et al., 1990).

Many clinicians use verbal feedback based on vaginal or anal palpation. In this procedure the nurse inserts one or two fingers into the vagina or anus and instructs the patient to contract the pelvic floor muscles. When the patient performs this maneuver, the nurse provides verbal feedback regarding the correctness of the contraction.

Biofeedback training

Biofeedback is a form of behavioral training that reverses incontinence by altering physiologic responses of the bladder and pelvic floor muscles, specifically the striated muscles of the pelvic floor and abdominal wall and the smooth detrusor muscle, which mediate bladder emptying. Both sphincter contraction and bladder inhibition are acquired physiologic responses that preserve continence. With biofeedback, oriented, motivated patients can learn these responses through operant conditioning by observing the results of their attempts to control bladder and sphincter responses voluntarily (Burgio & Burgio, 1986).

Furthermore, benefit from the pelvic muscle exercise therapy can be facilitated by using biofeedback to assist in teaching the pelvic muscle exercise (McDowell et al., 1992). Burgio et al. (1986) compared the effectiveness of teaching pelvic floor muscle exercises with bladder-sphincter biofeedback and muscle training with verbal feedback based on vaginal palpation in 24 women with stress incontinence. An average 75.9% reduction in incontinence was noted in the biofeedback group, significantly higher than the 51.0% reduction shown by the verbal feedback group.

Burgio et al. (1985) used bladder and sphincter biofeedback combined with toileting skills training in 39 older outpatients—19 who had stress incontinence, 12 with detrusor instability and urge incontinence, and 8 with urge incontinence without bladder instability. Patients with stress incontinence showed an average of 82% improvement; patients with detrusor instability showed an average of 85% improvement; and patients with urge incontinence with stable bladders showed an average of 94% reduction in incontinence. Thirteen patients achieved total continence, and 19 had fewer than one accident per week after treatment. The results of this study illustrate the effectiveness of biofeedback-assisted behavioral interventions for urge and stress urinary incontinence in older adults.

Anorectal biofeedback provides patients with simultaneous feedback on rectal sphincter activity and pelvic floor muscles, as well as abdominal pressure, by the use of a rectal probe. Patients can learn selective responses of pelvic and abdominal musculature by viewing their muscle activity on a computer monitor. Patients are typically unable to contract pelvic floor muscles without using abdominal muscles on initial attempts. Visual and auditory biofeedback using this procedure can assist patients in learning to contract pelvic floor muscles selectively while keeping abdominal muscles relaxed.

Home practice

After training with biofeedback or verbal feedback, patients are instructed to practice contracting and relaxing the pelvic floor muscles 45 times or more each day, divided into three practice sessions. The patient is asked to exercise

BOX 13-6 PELVIC FLOOR MUSCLE EXERCISES

1. Continue to keep your bladder diary.
2. Do 45 pelvic floor exercises *every day.*
   - 15 at a time
   - 3 times a day
   - 15 lying down
   - 15 sitting
   - 15 standing up
3. For each exercise,
   - Squeeze for _____seconds
   - Relax for _____seconds
4. Remember to *relax* all the muscles in your abdomen when you do these exercises, and continue to breathe normally.
5. Practice slowing or stopping the stream of urine when you void.

lying down, sitting, and standing, to learn to control the muscles in any position. Patients should also be reminded to avoid the use of abdominal muscles during exercise, because this increases intraabdominal pressure. Patients are also asked to practice slowing or stopping the urinary stream while voiding. This procedure helps them to check their use of the proper muscles during exercise and to evaluate their progress. Box 13-6 gives instructions for practice of pelvic floor muscle exercises.

In addition to daily exercises, patients benefit from active use of pelvic floor muscles to prevent urine loss. Patients with stress incontinence should be instructed to contract the pelvic floor muscles before and during activities that result in the leakage of urine, such as bending, standing, sitting, or coughing. Muscle contraction helps to occlude the urethra and to prevent leakage of urine.

Patients with urge incontinence should be taught to contract the pelvic floor muscles when they note a sensation of urgency to inhibit invol-

untary bladder contractions and incontinent episodes. Specifically, when the patients note a sensation to void, they are instructed to sit or stand quietly and to relax while contracting only pelvic floor muscles. After the urgency has subsided, the patients should proceed at a normal pace to the toilet to void.

Patients with urge incontinence often experience frequent urination. In this situation it is beneficial to combine the preceding procedure with bladder retraining to expand the intervals between voids. Time between voids should be extended in a stepwise manner, using ½-hour increments. The goal should be to void no more frequently than every 3 hours.

Other nursing interventions

Patients with overflow incontinence should be examined by a urologist for treatable causes of overflow incontinence. If the condition is not treatable, nursing measures, such as Crede maneuvers, may be helpful. This method of expelling urine from the bladder is accomplished by applying pressure over the suprapubic area. Intermittent catheterization performed several times a day by the patient or caregiver is another procedure that can be used for patients with overflow incontinence. The use of intermittent catheterization in older adults has not been well studied, although this method has been used safely in younger patients with neurologic disease.

The nurse must be alert to medications that cause urinary retention or bladder contractions and consult with the patient's physician about adjustment of dosage or medication change.

Older patients are prone to developing constipation and fecal impaction, which can cause or exacerbate urinary incontinence. Nurses should observe and assess the patient regularly for this problem and institute dietary measures, such as increased fiber, use of fruits such as prunes, and adequate hydration, to enhance regular bowel movements. If the problem persists, the nurse and the patient's physician should collaborate to determine other interventions.

Many older people with urinary incontinence decrease their fluid intake, expecting that if they drink less they will have fewer accidents. This self-management technique is not helpful and can result in dehydration, as well as a compromised health state. The nurse should encourage adequate fluid intake and educate the patient and caregiver regarding the health risks encountered by patients who do not receive adequate hydration.

In the acute care setting

Often, older patients in acute care settings who are incontinent are not examined to determine the cause of the problem. Sier et al. (1987) found, in a study of 363 patients 65 years of age and older in a university hospital medical-surgical unit, that 35% were incontinent of urine. Indwelling catheters were used in 50% of the incontinent patients studied. The complications of chronic catheterization, particularly urinary tract infections, are well documented (Ouslander et al., 1987; Platt et al., 1983; Warren et al., 1981). Although external catheters are often used in men instead of indwelling catheters, they are not without side effects. Ouslander et al. (1987) found an increased incidence of bacteriuria among male patients with external catheters. Only recently have external devices been studied for use in women, and little is known about their safety.

The use of indwelling and external catheters should be discouraged in acute care settings. Other measures, such as regular toileting procedures or frequent changes of pads and undergarments, should be instituted to keep the patients dry.

Older patients with acute illness frequently become dehydrated, resulting in concentrated urine. The nurse should discuss the problem with the patient's physician, and fluids can then be increased if this is not specifically contraindicated. Intake and output must be accurately recorded to help ensure adequate fluid intake.

The nurse should inquire about the patient's bladder function before the illness. Family and friends may be able to provide the needed information if the patient is confused. It is important to remember that patients may have hidden their incontinence from their family, friends, or doctors. Thus the family may not always be aware of the patient's prior incontinence. Frequently the patient is too ill for complete assessment of incontinence while in the hospital. Incontinence should be noted in the discharge information given to the patient, family, long-term care facility, or visiting nurse, so that adequate assessment of the problem can be made after the acute illness has abated.

Principles guiding care of incontinence in acutely ill, hospitalized older patients include the following: (1) Patients should be toileted every 2 to 3 hours if their condition permits. (2) If toileting is not possible, frequent changes of pads and undergarments are important to prevent skin breakdown. (3) Adequate hydration must be maintained. (4) Indwelling and external catheters are to be avoided.

In the nursing home

Older patients in long-term care facilities are often frail and suffer from physical and/or cognitive disabilities. Certainly one of the greatest nursing challenges is the management of incontinent patients in a long-term care setting, where the number of staff members is limited and most of the direct care is provided by nurse aides.

Upon admission to the nursing home, all residents are assessed for the causes of incontinence. Were the residents incontinent before their last acute illnesses? If the answer is yes, persistent incontinence is considered. If the answer is no, then acute causes of incontinence are considered and treated. Pad or underwear checks should be performed every 2 hours for the first 2 weeks after admission to determine the presence or absence of urinary incontinence. All residents should then be prompted to void at the time of each underwear or pad check. Often, after admission to the nursing home, residents are inaccurately assumed to be incontinent and are placed on pads, which may discourage proper toileting and may encourage incontinence. These negative cues may send a signal to the resident that incontinence is expected and/or accepted. The nurse must ensure that an assessment is made on each nursing home resident before any type of incontinence care is instituted.

Dehydration is not unusual among nursing home residents, and this compounds the problem of urge incontinence. Adequate fluid intake must be a priority for all residents, with or without involuntary urine loss, to maintain and enhance an optimal state of health.

Research indicates that the most frequent type of involuntary urine loss in nursing home residents is urge incontinence, with spontaneous detrusor (bladder) contractions seen in patients with functional impairment caused by cognitive or physical disabilities (Pannill et al., 1988; Resnick et al., 1989).

The two behavioral methods most often used in long-term care settings are habit training and prompted voiding. Habit training consists of toileting patients at regular intervals, ideally, every 2 hours. In situations where there is adequate staffing for a more individualized approach, it is beneficial first to document the resident's pattern of voiding and urine loss over 7 to 14 days. Then a voiding schedule can be developed and adjusted to meet the individual needs of a specific resident. These forms of therapy have been a part of nursing care of older adults in nursing homes for many years. Their success depends on nursing leadership and commitment to reducing the prevalence and severity of incontinence.

Prompted voiding, on the other hand, is relatively new. Research suggests that some nursing home residents will respond well to prompted voiding. Nursing personnel who use this treatment method should follow certain guidelines: (1) approach the resident at established intervals, usually upon the resident's arising in the morning, every 2 hours during the waking day, and just before bedtime; (2) encourage the resident to void; (3) provide assistance in

toileting, as needed; and (4) provide praise (positive reinforcement) for appropriate toileting, for requests for assistance in toileting, and for periods of dryness (Creason et al., 1989). When residents have incontinent episodes, their clothing should be changed in a timely manner but without the positive reinforcement of praise or socialization. Nursing staff members should never use any form of punishment, including verbal admonishment, for episodes of urine loss. Ensuring a constructive approach to the incontinent resident by each member of the nursing staff is the responsibility of the professional nurse.

Although many episodes of incontinence can be avoided by using therapies such as prompted voiding and habit training, some residents will continue to have incontinent episodes. This problem is most evident among the cognitively impaired residents who experience frequent spontaneous detrusor (bladder) contractions with involuntary emptying of the bladder. Frequent changes of pads or undergarments and scrupulous skin care are the nursing interventions of choice in these cases. Because indwelling or external catheters carry a high propensity for bladder infections and for urinary sepsis, which can result in death, these catheters should be considered an appropriate measure only in carefully selected situations. These situations include (1) management of decubiti, (2) severe urinary retention, with resulting infections or renal dysfunction, and (3) providing comfort for the terminally ill.

In the private or family home

Patients with adequate mental status who have urge or stress incontinence or a combination of the two, should be taught pelvic floor muscle exercises and strategies to prevent urge or stress accidents. This instruction can be provided in the home by specially prepared nurses.

Nurses have become specialized in the management of urinary incontinence. They have described methods for assessing the patient and for providing treatments such as pelvic floor muscle exercises, biofeedback, and habit training for homebound individuals (McDowell et al., 1994; Newman & Smith, 1989; Rose et al., 1990; Smith, 1988). Adjustment of environmental barriers to toileting and soliciting the cooperation of caregivers in assisting the patient are equally important treatment modalities. The treatment of urinary incontinence for the homebound older adult is one way of preventing or delaying institutionalization.

Nurses should be aware of the resources available in the community. If no continence programs are available, nurses should actively seek education in the treatment of incontinence so that untreated incontinence in older patients can be reduced. Patients should be educated about incontinence and reassured with the knowledge that it is a treatable condition that seldom requires high-risk surgical procedures.

Other treatments

When behavioral interventions do not yield satisfactory results, it is appropriate to consider pharmacologic and surgical options.

Pharmacologic therapy Several medications are currently in use for treatment of urinary incontinence. Drug therapy can reduce urge incontinence, stress incontinence, mixed incontinence, and overflow incontinence.

Drugs prescribed for urge incontinence are antispasmodic agents and estrogens. Antispasmodics such as oxybutynin, propantheline, dicyclomine, flavoxate, and imipramine inhibit detrusor contractions, which contribute to urgency, frequency, and urge incontinence. Estrogens relieve urge incontinence by relieving irritation and inflammation that contribute to urgency and detrusor contraction.

Potential side effects of these antispasmodic drugs include dry mouth, constipation, blurred vision, elevated intraocular pressure, confusion, depression, and precipitation of urinary retention. These drugs are contraindicated in patients with glaucoma. Dry mouth and constipation can usually be managed by ordinary measures; the

other side effects are rarely encountered. In older patients it is advisable to begin with small doses of the medications and to increase the dosage only as needed. Many older people respond well to small doses and consequently can avoid potential side effects.

Drugs for stress incontinence reduce leakage of urine by stimulating urethral smooth muscle to contract, increasing pressure in the urethra. Agents such as imipramine, phenylpropanolamine, and pseudoephedrine can prevent incontinence in this way. Potential side effects are headache, tachycardia, and hypotension. Estrogen is also used for women to help maintain the strength and tone of the pelvic floor muscles.

Surgery For some types of incontinence, surgery is the only appropriate treatment. For example, surgery is usually necessary to remove an obstruction of the urethra that prevents bladder emptying. In most cases this will be a form of prostatectomy. In addition, there are a number of other conditions, such as a bladder fistula, tumor, stone, diverticulum, or ectopic ureter, for which surgery is the best treatment.

Surgery for stress incontinence is an elective procedure. There are a variety of surgical approaches that have the same goal: to lift the urethra into its proper position in the pelvis, where it is effectively compressed during physical activities that increase abdominal pressure. When pressure from a cough is transmitted equally to the bladder and to the urethra, stress incontinence does not occur.

In very severe cases of stress incontinence, an artificial sphincter may be surgically placed, or a periurethral injection may be performed. Various substances, such as polytetrafluoroethylene or collagen, have been used for injection into the tissues around the urethra. This adds bulk and helps to keep the urethra closed.

EVALUATION

As part of a continuous process, evaluation is an integral component of the nurse's responsibility in ensuring appropriate and quality nursing care.

The focus of evaluation centers around the stated short- and long-term patient-centered goals. The patient's stated satisfaction with care is of paramount importance to the process of evaluation. Documentation of all parameters of the evaluative process must be recorded in formal health care records.

REFERENCES

Brink, C., Wells, T., & Diokno, A. (1983). A continence clinic for the aged. *Journal of Gerontological Nursing, 9*(12), 651-655.

Burgio, K.L., & Burgio, L.D. (1986). Behavior therapies for urinary incontinence in the elderly. *Clinics in Geriatric Medicine, 2*(4), 809-827.

Burgio, K.L., Robinson, J.C., & Engel, B.T. (1986). The role of biofeedback in Kegel exercise training for stress urinary incontinence. *American Journal of Obstetrics and Gynecology, 154,* 58-64.

Burgio, K.L., Whitehead, W.E., & Engel, B.T. (1985). Urinary incontinence in the elderly: Bladder-sphincter biofeedback and toileting skills training. *Annals of Internal Medicine, 103*(4), 507-515.

Burgio, L., Engel, B.T., McCormick, K., Hawkins, A., & Scheve, A. (1988). Behavioral treatment for urinary incontinence in elderly inpatients: Initial attempts to modify prompted voiding and toileting procedures. *Behavior Therapy, 19*(3), 345-357.

Creason, N.S., Glybowski, J.A., Burgene, L.S., Whippo, C., Yeo, S., & Richardson, B. (1989). Prompted voiding therapy for urinary incontinence in aged female nursing home residents. *Journal of Advanced Nursing, 14,* 120-126.

Diokno, A.C., Brock, B.M., Brown, M.B., & Herzog, A.R. (1986). Prevalence of urinary incontinence and other urological symptoms in the non-institutionalized elderly. *Journal of Urology, 136,* 1022-1025.

Dougherty, M., Bishop, K., Mooney, R., & Gimotty, P. (1989). The effect of circumvaginal muscle (CVM) exercise. *Nursing Research, 38*(6), 331-335.

Duke University Center for the Study of Aging and Human Development. (1978). *Multidimensional functional assessment: The OARS methodology.* Durham, NC: Duke University.

Fantl, J.A., Wyman, J.F., Harkins, S.W., & Hadely, E.C. (1990). Bladder training in the management of lower urinary tract dysfunction in women: A review. *Journal of the American Geriatric Society, 38*(3), 329-332.

Folstein, M.F., Folstein, S., & McHugh, P.R. (1975). Mini-mental state: A practical method for grading the cognitive state of patients for the clinician. *Journal of Psychiatric Research, 12,* 189-198.

Frewen, W.K. (1978). An objective assessment of the unstable bladder of psychosomatic origin. *British Journal of Urology, 50,* 246-249.

Frewen, W.K. (1980). The management of urgency and frequency of micturition. *British Journal of Urology, 52,* 367-369.

Hadley, H.R., Zimmern, P.E., & Raz, S. (1986). The treatment of male urinary incontinence. In P.C. Walsh, R.F. Gittes, A.D. Perlmutter, & T.A. Stamey (Eds.), *Campbell's urology* (5th ed., pp. 2658-2679).

Johnson, M.J., & Warner, C. (1982). We had no choice—A study of familial guilt feelings surrounding nursing home care. *Journal of Gerontological Nursing, 8,* 641-645, 654.

Kaltreider, D.L., Wei, H., Iqou, J.F., Yu, L.C., & Craighead, W.E. (1990, January-February). Can reminders curb incontinence? *Geriatric Nursing,* pp. 17-19.

Katz, S., Ford, A.B., Moskowitz, R.W., Jackson, B.A., & Jaffee, M.W. (1963). Studies of illness in the aged: The index of ADL—A standardized measure of biological and psychosocial function. *Journal of the American Medical Association, 185,* 94ff.

Kegel, A.H. (1948). Progressive resistance exercise in the functional restoration of the perineal muscles. *American Journal of Obstetrics and Gynecology, 56*(2), 242-245.

Leach, G.E., & Yip, C.M. (1986). Urologic and urodynamic evaluation of the elderly population. *Clinics in Geriatric Medicine, 2*(4), 731-756.

McDowell, B.J., & Burgio, K.L. (1990). Urinary incontinence. In A.S. Staab & M.F. Lyles (Eds.), *Manual of geriatric nursing* (pp. 432-456). Glenview, IL: Scott, Foresman/Little Brown Higher Education.

McDowell, B.J., Burgio, K.L., & Candib, D. (1989). Assessment of urinary incontinence in the elderly. *Journal of the American Academy of Nurse Practitioners, 1*(1), 24-29.

McDowell, B.J., Burgio, K.L., & Candib, D. (1990). Behavioral and pharmacological treatment of persistent urinary incontinence in the elderly. *Journal of the American Academy of Nurse Practitioners, 2*(1), 17-23.

McDowell, B.J., Burgio, K.L., Dombrowski, M., Locher, J., & Rodriguez, E. (1992). An interdisciplinary approach to the assessment and behavioral treatment of urinary incontinence in geriatric outpatients. *Journal of the American Geriatric Society, 40,* 370-374.

McDowell, B.J., Engberg, S., Weber, E., Brodak, I., & Engberg, R. (1994). Successful treatment using behavioral interventions for urinary incontinence for homebound older adults. *Geriatric Nursing, 15*(6), 303-307.

Mohide, E.A. (1986). The prevalence and scope of urinary incontinence. *Clinics in Geriatric Medicine, 2*(4), 639-655.

Morishita, L. (1988). Nursing evaluation and treatment of geriatric outpatients with urinary incontinence. *Nursing Clinics of North America, 23*(1), 189-206.

National Institutes of Health. (1988). *Urinary incontinence in adults: Consensus development conference* (Office of Medical Applications of Research, NIH Vol. 7, No. 5). Bethesda, MD: Author.

Newman, D.K., & Smith, D.A. (1989). Incontinence in elderly homebound patients. *Holistic Nursing Practice, 4*(1), 52-60.

Noelker, L.S. (1987). Incontinence in elderly cared for by family. *Gerontologist, 27,* 194-200.

Ouslander, J.G. (1986). Diagnostic evaluation of geriatric urinary incontinence. *Clinics in Geriatric Medicine, 2*(4), 715-730.

Ouslander, J.G. (1992). Geriatric urinary incontinence. *Disease of the Month, 38*(2), 71-149.

Ouslander, J.G. (1994a). Incontinence. In R.L. Kane, J.G. Ouslander, & I.B. Abrass (Eds.), *Essentials of clinical geriatrics* (2nd ed., pp. 139-189). New York: McGraw-Hill Health Professions Division.

Ouslander, J.G. (1994b). Urinary incontinence. In W.R. Hazzard, R. Andres, E.L. Bierman, & J.P. Blass (Eds.), *Principles of geriatric medicine and gerontology* (pp. 1123-1142). New York: McGraw-Hill.

Ouslander, J.G., Greengold, B., & Chen, S. (1987). Complications of chronic indwelling urinary catheters among male nursing home patients: A prospective study. *Journal of Urology, 138,* 1191-1195.

Pannill, F.C., Williams, F.T., & Davis, R. (1988). Evaluation and treatment of urinary incontinence in long-term care. *Journal of the American Geriatric Society, 36,* 902-910.

Platt, R., Polk, B.F., & Murdock, B. (1983). Reduction of mortality associated with nosocomial urinary infections. *Lancet, 1,* 893-897.

Resnick, N.M., Yalla, S.V., & Lawrence, E. (1989). The pathophysiology of urinary incontinence among institutionalized elderly persons. *New England Journal of Medicine, 320,* 1-7.

Rose, M.A., Smith, J.B., Smith, D., & Newman, D. (1990). Behavioral management of urinary incontinence in homebound older adults. *Home Health Care Nurse, 8* (5), 10-15.

Sier, H., Ouslander, J., & Orzek, S. (1987). Urinary incontinence among geriatric patients in an acute-care hospital. *Journal of the American Medical Association, 257*(13), 1767-1771.

Smallegan, M. (1985). There is nothing else to do: Needs for care before nursing home admission. *Journal of Gerontology, 25*(4), 364-369.

Smith, D.A. (1988). Continence restoration in the homebound patient. *Nursing Clinics of North America, 23*(1), 207-218.

Smith, J.B., Smith, D.A., Rose, M., & Newman, D.K. (1989). Managing urinary incontinence in community-residing elderly persons. *Gerontologist, 29*(2), 229-233.

Staskin, D.R. (1986). Age-related physiologic and pathological changes affecting lower urinary tract function. *Clinics in Geriatric Medicine, 2*(4), 701-710.

Warren, J.W., Muncel, H.L., & Berquist, E.J. (1981). Sequelae and management of urinary infection in the patient requiring chronic catheterization. *Journal of Urology, 125,* 1-7.

Wyman, J.F., Choi Sung, C., Harkins, S.W., Walson, M., & Fantl, A. (1988). The urinary diary in evaluation of incontinent women: A test-retest analysis. *Obstetrics and Gynecology, 71*(6), 812-817.

C H A P T E R 14

So here I sit in the early candle-light of old age—I and my book—casting backward glances over our travel'd road.

WALT WHITMAN

Bowel Elimination

■ Learning Objectives

On completion of this chapter, the reader will be able to do the following:

1. Explain the normal structure and function of the gastrointestinal (GI) system and identify age-related changes that influence bowel elimination.
2. Recognize the significance and prevalence of constipation in older adults.
3. Identify the contributing factors that cause constipation.
4. Assess patients for actual or potential constipation.
5. Develop a plan of care to manage constipation.
6. Discuss appropriate nursing interventions for patients with constipation.
7. Promote normal bowel elimination for older adults.
8. Evaluate the effectiveness of a plan of care for constipation.

■ Constipation

Constipation is the most common chronic digestive complaint among all age groups in the United States, affecting approximately 4.5 million people per year and causing considerable morbidity, physical discomfort, and emotional distress (Donatelle, 1990). Two and one-half million physician visits per year are made to manage this common complaint. As people age, the prevalence of constipation increases, with 4% of those age 65 to 74 years old experiencing constipation, and 10.2% of those over 75 years of age experiencing constipation. Women are twice as likely as men to complain of constipation, and

it is 1.3 times more common in nonwhite people than in white people (Goldstein & Oliveira, 1993).

Bowel elimination is highly subjective, and individuals have differing ideas about what constitutes normalcy. A standard definition of constipation is difficult to apply to all individuals, however, the literature for the United States demonstrates an objective consensus as to when constipation can be diagnosed. It is defined as being present when any of the following are described or observed in relation to the individual's elimination pattern: passage of stools fewer than 3 to 5 times per week; deficient quantity of stool; incomplete passage of stool; abnormally hard and dry stool; or straining at stools more than 25% of the time (Camilleri et al., 1994; Chenitz et al., 1991; Donatelle, 1990; Merkel et al., 1993). Constipation is considered a chronic condition when these characteristics last longer than 6 weeks (Castle, 1989). However, it must be noted that the preceding definitions are not accepted worldwide. In many different cultures and in different parts of the world, a normal elimination pattern of passage of stool 3 times a day is common.

Constipation can be classified into three broad categories according to its causes: (1) constipation that is caused by physiologic changes at a level that affects bowel function, including colorectal diseases (e.g. tumors and diverticular disease), metabolic and endocrine disorders, and neurologic disorders; (2) constipation that is caused by the administration of pharmacologic agents or other medical therapeutics; and (3) constipation resulting from extrinsic factors such as age-related changes in physical activity, the inadequate ingestion of fluids and fiber, and unfavorable environmental conditions such as lack of privacy or access to a toilet (Cameron, 1992; Donatelle, 1990; McMillan & Williams, 1989). Over 90% of complaints of constipation are attributed to nonpathologic factors (Camilleri et al., 1994). The patient and/or family members need to be educated about the contributing factors for constipation and therapeutic interventions that will enhance a routine bowel elimination pattern. The purpose of this chapter is to focus on the management of the clinical problem of constipation in older adults.

■ Normal Structure and Function

Bowel elimination is achieved as a result of the physiologic functions of motility and innervation of the gastrointestinal tract. The digestive tract is a muscular tube that extends from the mouth to the anus with the primary functions of storing, digesting, and absorbing nutrients, and eliminating waste (Figure 14-1). The primary areas related to bowel elimination are the small and large intestines, the rectum, and the anus. The structure of the intestinal wall is similar in both the large and small intestine and consists of five layers: the serosa, a longitudinal muscle layer, a circular muscle layer, the submucosa, and the mucosa. The motor functions of the gut are performed by layers of smooth muscle that lie in the deep layers of the mucosa (Guyton, 1991; Luckman & Sorensen, 1993).

There are two types of movement in the GI tract: mixing and propulsive. These movements are produced by rhythmic contractions of the smooth muscle fibers. Mixing movements occur when a portion of the small intestine becomes distended with gastric content, followed by contractions spaced at intervals along the intestine. As one set of contractions relaxes, a new set begins. Peristalsis is a propulsive contraction that forces the contents of the GI tract to move forward. Peristaltic waves occur much faster in the proximal intestine and much slower in the large intestine, and are greatly increased after meals (Guyton, 1991; Luckman & Sorensen, 1993). The gastrointestinal tract has an intrinsic nervous system that begins at the esophagus and extends all the way to the anus. This system is composed of two layers of neurons, the myenteric plexus and the submucosal plexus, and is responsible for coordination of movements of the intestine. The parasympathetic nervous system stimulates the plexuses, resulting in increased tone of the gut, decreased tone of the sphincters, and increased frequency, volume, and velocity of gut contractions. The actual urge to defecate results when feces enter the rectum. Distention of the rectal wall sends signals throughout the neural plexuses, initiating peristaltic waves in the descending colon, sigmoid, and rectum and forcing fecal matter toward the anus. The internal and external sphincters, via the defecation reflex, become relaxed, and fecal matter may then be passed. The individual may voluntarily suppress this urge by contracting the muscles of the pelvic floor (Guyton, 1991).

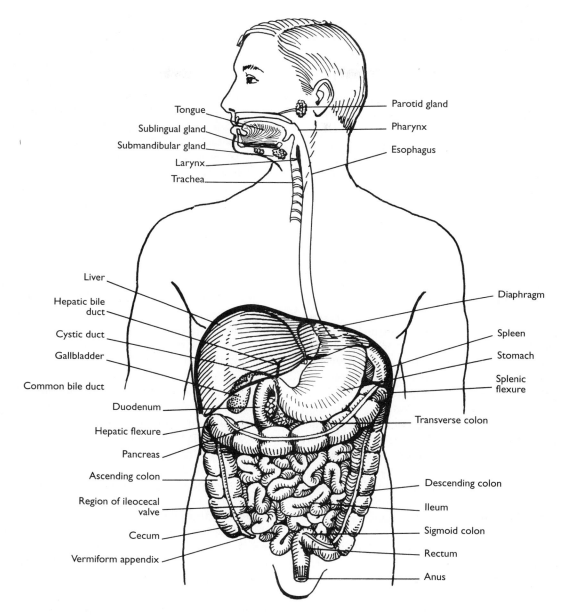

FIGURE 14-1 The organs of the GI system and related structures. (From Phipps, W.J. et al. [1995]. *Medical-surgical nursing: Concepts and clinical practice* [5th ed.]. St. Louis: Mosby.)

■ Physical Age-Related Changes Affecting Bowel Elimination

A variety of structural and functional changes in the GI system can be seen in older adults, although the incidence and significance of GI changes are not universal among them. Changes of the GI system begin with decreased saliva production after the age of 50, and altered taste and smell. These changes, combined with impaired mastication or swallowing, can affect the ability to eat foods high in fiber and roughage or to consume adequate fluid intake (Kallman, 1983). Throughout the small intestine there is little change in structure or transit time. In the large intestine there is a weakening of the colonic wall, which, in association with high lumenal pressures, leads to the development of muscular atrophy, abnormalities of the mucosal glands, and hypertrophy of the muscularis mucosa. A significant effect of aging on the GI tract is the loss of neurons from the intrinsic nervous system (Kenney, 1989). Colonic transit time can be decreased because of a deficit in innervation and decreased responsiveness of neurotransmitters (Hazzard et al., 1990; Kenney, 1989).

Changes in sensory mechanisms related to the urge to defecate may also occur. The inability to recognize the urge to defecate, repeatedly ignoring the call to defecate, and/or having physical limitations in toileting oneself appropriately can lead to a deterioration of the sensory mechanisms that stimulate the urge to have a bowel movement. When this occurs, as more stool arrives in the rectum, a reverse peristalsis occurs into the proximal parts of the colon, which may result in constipation and megarectum (Barnes, 1987). Constipation occurs when stool is delayed in the colon and water continues to be absorbed from the fecal matter. Stool becomes harder and drier and subsequently more difficult to pass (Guyton, 1991).

Constipation can lead to abdominal distention, which in turn can result in decreased oral intake, further resulting in dehydration and malnutrition. Hemorrhoids and anal fissures may result when excessive straining at stool produces

Aging Alert
Change in bowel habits

A sudden change in bowel habits could indicate an acute functional, metabolic, or neurologic condition that warrants referral to a gastroenterologist for a full medical physical examination and GI workup.

From Wong, R.D., Gold, S., & Blanchette, P.A. (1991, January-February). Correcting constipation: A regimen that works. *Senior Patient*, pp. 37-41.

tears or passive congestion of tissues near the rectum (Cheskin & Schuster, 1994). Hemorrhoids themselves cause pain, bleeding, and possible need for surgery (Chenitz et al., 1991).

A serious result of constipation is fecal impaction (Wrenn, 1989). Typical symptoms associated with impaction are anorexia, nausea, vomiting, abdominal distention, and abdominal pain. Paradoxic diarrhea and incontinence of urine and stool may be present. Continuous seepage of moist bacteria-laden mucus and stool may cause the development of decubitus. In the bowel itself, obstruction of the large bowel can occur. Continued pressure and ischemic necrosis on the wall of the colon may cause stercoral ulceration. Perforation of diverticula caused by increased intralumenal pressure may also occur. Fecal impactions need to be removed either with an enema or by gentle digital removal (Wrenn, 1989). Bladder elimination may also become affected when an impaction exists. Urinary problems of frequency, retention, overflow incontinence, and urinary tract infection are conditions commonly caused by impaction (Wrenn, 1989).

The complexity and sequelae of constipation, which occur as a result of the many associated physical and environmental factors, may be prevented through early detection and management of the problem.

■ Factors Influencing Bowel Elimination

The factors that contribute to the development of constipation in older adults are the following: (1) structural and functional changes of the GI tract resulting from aging; (2) diet; (3) activity; (4) medical conditions; (5) common medications taken by older adults; and (6) the environment. Many of these factors may overlap and contribute to the development or severity of constipation.

DIET

The two dietary factors that influence bowel elimination the most are fiber and fluid consumption.

Fiber

Dietary fiber is a term used for a diverse group of complex carbohydrates, found in plant structure, of differing chemical structure and physical properties that are not digestible by human intestinal enzymes (Taylor, 1990). In the colon, fiber increases stool bulk by holding water and acting as a substrate for colonic microflora. This process further increases stool bulk by increasing bacterial, water, and salt content and producing gases that augment the bulking effect. As a result of these properties, fiber exerts a laxative effect, accelerates intestinal transit, increases fecal weight, and reduces gastrointestinal pressure (Gorman & Bowman, 1993).

Over the last century in most Western countries there has been a steady decline in the consumption of fiber, from about 40 gm per day 100 years ago to a current value of 15 to 20 gm per day (Taylor, 1990; Cheskin & Schuster, 1990). The decreased intake can be attributed to the refinement of food that began in the industrial revolution. Since then, there has been a steady fall in the consumption of fiber, with a corresponding increase in the intake of sugar, fat, and protein (Taylor, 1990).

Consumption of fiber by older adults may be limited by the following:

1. Lack of knowledge of foods high in fiber
2. Inability to read food labels for fiber content
3. Intolerance of foods high in fiber as a result of dental or digestive disorders
4. Inability to purchase and prepare their own food
5. Institutional diets low in fiber
6. Poor appetite
7. Lack of interest in eating

Fluid

Fluid is needed in the gut to keep fecal matter soft and moving. An average of eight glasses of fluid per day should be consumed to promote normal bowel absorption in the small intestine and colon (Cameron, 1992). Absorption through the GI tract decreases this amount resulting in a daily stool volume of approximately 150 cc. A change of intake or absorption of even 100 cc can lead to harder, drier stools (Canty, 1994; Castle, 1989).

Consumption of fluid by older adults may be limited by the following:

1. Decreased thirst mechanism
2. Limited access to fluids
3. Therapeutic fluid restriction
4. Difficulty swallowing
5. Increased voiding

ACTIVITY

Propulsion of mass in the colon is correlated with physical activity. GI motility increases during and after ingestion of food; however, this propulsive movement is found only in physically active people. With inactivity there is slowed movement of feces into the descending colon and rectum (Harper & Lyles, 1988). The lack of propulsive movement in resting individuals has been shown to increase the occurrence of constipation (Barnes, 1987).

Physical activity in older adults may be limited by the following:

1. Decreased cognition and lack of motivation
2. Poor vision
3. Skeletal changes
4. Neuromuscular impairments
5. Poor environment

6. Lack of available assistance or assistive devices
7. Fear of personal safety in the neighborhood

MEDICAL CONDITIONS

Many older adults have at least one chronic medical condition, often treated with medication. Disease processes may directly alter bowel elimination, and the GI system is vulnerable to the effects of medication because of the nervous system control of GI motility. The effects of the medical condition and its treatment, and the impact on lifestyle need to be analyzed for factors that increase the risk for development of constipation (Chenitz et al., 1991; Donatelle, 1990; Kopac, 1993; Merkel et al., 1993; Wrenn, 1989).

Medical conditions that can affect bowel elimination in older adults include the following:

1. GI disorders
2. Endocrine and metabolic disorders (hypothyroidism, diabetes mellitus)
3. Neurologic impairments (Parkinson's disease, stroke)
4. Depression
5. Dementia
6. Anxiety

LAXATIVE USE

In the United States, cathartics are prescribed for more than 3 million people annually, and as many as 78% of patients in long-term care are dependent on laxatives for routine bowel evacuation (Donatelle, 1990; Rodrigues-Fisher et al., 1993). There are over 700 different laxative products on the market—the majority of which are available without a prescription. Annual expenditures on laxatives are between $250 and $400 million per year (Cerrato, 1989).

A review of commonly used laxatives follows.

Bulk-forming products

Bulk-forming products (e.g., bran and psyllium mucilloid [Metamucil]) provide a more concentrated form of fiber than can be obtained from most food sources. The dose needs to be adjusted so that the patient is ingesting up to 15 gm of dietary fiber a day. Each dose must be taken with 8 oz of fluids. Bulk laxatives usually work within 24 hours by absorbing water, swelling, and then stimulating peristalsis (Cerrato, 1989). Side effects include flatus, cramping, bloating, and obstruction if the laxatives are taken without adequate fluid (Allison et al., 1994; Tedesco, 1985). A positive effect can be the lowering of serum lipid levels (Melmon et al. 1992).

Stool softeners

Stool softeners (e.g., dioctyl sodium succinate, or docusate) facilitate the mixture of aqueous and fatty substances in the fecal mass. This mechanism softens the stool and increases water secretion in the small and large intestines. Peristalsis is not promoted, but the process makes hard stools easier to pass, either by breaking the fecal mass into smaller particles or by lubricating a dry stool. Stool softeners may take up to 72 hours to work (Cerrato, 1989) and are useful for short-term therapy, but have little value for the treatment of long-term constipation. They will not prevent constipation caused by major contributing factors (Tedesco, 1985).

Lubricants

Lubricants (a major lubricating laxative is mineral oil [Haley's M-O]) coat fecal contents and decrease colonic absorption of water, thus making stools easier to pass within 8 hours. Use of mineral oil should be avoided in debilitated patients or those at risk for aspiration pneumonia because toxic effects can occur in lung tissue if the mineral oil is aspirated (Castle, 1989; Tedesco, 1985).

Osmotic laxatives

Osmotic laxatives (e.g., Golytely and Colyte) pull fluids into the intestinal lumen, producing increased intralumenal volume that stimulates intestinal motility. They usually act within ½ hour to 3 hours when taken orally or within 15 to 30 minutes when taken rectally and can be given on a scheduled basis 2 to 3 times a week when all other measures have failed. Active agents in these laxatives include magnesium citrate, magnesium hydroxide, magnesium sulfate, and sodium phosphates (Tedesco, 1985). These laxatives are rarely used for treatment of common constipation; rather, they are used frequently in preparation for GI diagnostic testing.

Lactulose, sorbitol, and glycerin suppositories are sometimes used for treating constipation in older adults. Glycerin has an irritant, as well as osmotic, effect on the distal portion of the colon and on the rectum, and usually works in 30 to 60 minutes. Lactulose has an osmotic effect and is metabolized by bacteria in the colon, thus lowering the pH of the colon and increasing peristalsis. Lactulose usually requires 24 to 48 hours to work, and may cause flatulence, cramps, diarrhea, and electrolyte imbalances (Allison et al., 1994).

Stimulant laxatives

Stimulant laxatives (e.g., cascara or senna, castor oil, and bisacodyl) promote peristalsis by irritating the colon wall and nerves that feed it. They are more likely to work by increasing fluid secretion in the small intestine and colon (Melmon et al., 1992). A bowel movement can be anticipated within 6 to 8 hours after administration of an oral preparation and within 15 to 60 minutes after rectal insertion. These drugs should not be used over a long period because of potential severe abdominal cramping, nerve damage to the myenteric plexus, acid base disorders, and chronic long-term effects (atonic colon) (Cerrato, 1989; Melmon et al., 1992).

Laxative use should be discouraged, because many toxic effects are related to long-term use. Health-promoting behaviors such as appropriate food and fluid intake and regular exercise will help many older adults to develop regular patterns of bowel elimination without reliance on laxatives.

Aging Alert
Laxative abuse

Laxatives can contribute to constipation when abused or used on a long-term basis. Stimulant laxatives such as bisacodyl are the most commonly abused. Long-term use can cause damage to the neural fibers that regulate the movements of the colon, thereby causing motility dysfunction. Bulk-forming laxatives or fiber supplements taken without adequate hydration cause hard stools and may lead to development of fecal impaction.

From Castle, S.C. (1989). Constipation: Endemic in the elderly? Gerontopathophysiology, evaluation, and management. *Medical Clinics of North America, 73* (6), 1497-1509. Wrenn, K. (1989). Fecal impaction. *New England Journal of Medicine, 321*(10), 658-662.

MEDICATION USE

Common potentially constipating drugs taken by older adults include the following (Castle, 1989; Wrenn, 1989):

1. Minerals (aluminum-containing antacids)
2. Narcotics and opiates
3. Antihypertensives
4. Antiarrhythmics
5. Anticholinergics
6. Sympathomimetics
7. Nonsteroidal anti-inflammatory agents
8. Diuretics

ENVIRONMENT

Older adults are faced daily with multiple factors in the environment that may adversely affect their ability to maintain a regular bowel elimination pattern. The physical layout for toileting may be a huge deterrent in that the bathroom may be too small to accommodate a wheelchair. Older adults may be unable to lift their own weight off the toilet, and there may be a lack of assistive devices such as side bars. Shared bathrooms in institutions may be the cause of constipation because the need for privacy is not met. Other environmental constraints exist in all types of settings—home, acute care, and long-term care.

Environmental factors that may influence bowel elimination include the following:

1. Access to a toilet
2. Privacy
3. Available assistance for toileting
4. Caregiver embarrassment or repulsion regarding bowel elimination
5. Ability to maintain physical activity

■ Nursing Process

The literature presents strong evidence that most cases of constipation are not caused by underlying pathologic conditions of the GI system; thus constipation is primarily an issue that nursing can manage independently (Camilleri et al., 1994). In all settings of practice, the focus of management should be on *screening* and *prevention of constipation*. Promotion of routine bowel elimination should be the goal of those who are working with older patients in any setting or through community-based health promotion programs for independent older adults. Identification of those at risk for becoming constipated and prevention of constipation should be the focus of the health care provider. A thorough screening for the contributing factors for constipation provides the base from which the health care provider delivers care and teaches the patient and family healthy bowel elimination habits.

ASSESSMENT

The purpose of assessment is to discover contributing factors that cause or may cause constipation. The assessment should include the following areas: health history, bowel history, dietary history, medications, environment, and a physical examination. The patient, family member, caregiver, and medical record are all sources of data

---

BOX 14-1 BOWEL HISTORY

1. Do you have a set time for bowel elimination?
2. How many times a week do you have a bowel movement?
3. What is the consistency of your stool?
4. Do you have to strain to have a bowel movement?
5. Have you ever had a fecal impaction?
6. Do you ever delay having a bowel movement after you feel the urge to defecate?
7. Do you have a current ritual, including laxative use, for moving your bowels?
8. Are you able to get to a toilet when you feel the urge to defecate?
9. Do you ever have diarrhea accompanied by the feeling of incomplete evacuation?

---

utilized to complete the assessment of bowel elimination.

Health history

Begin the health history with a review of systems and include any surgical procedures, particularly oral and abdominal procedures. Recent weight gain or loss should also be documented.

Bowel history

The bowel history includes the patient's definition of normalcy and constipation. The terminology for bowel elimination may vary with patients. It is important for the nurse to speak in terms with which the patient is familiar regarding bowel elimination. If the patient is cognitively impaired or unable to give information, data are gathered from other sources. Specific questions about bowel elimination are listed in Box 14-1.

Diet history

Diet history is an important component of the assessment and is especially pertinent when a patient has a complaint of constipation. Begin the diet history with the type of diet, including any restrictions currently prescribed for the patient. An average 24-hour recall of food consumed is reviewed and analyzed for fiber content. Food frequently eaten, as well as food likes and dislikes, should also be reviewed. Other considerations in the diet history are religious or ethnic food restrictions and the effects of lifestyle variables such as food purchasing, preparation, and consumption habits (Seidel et al., 1995). A review of fluid intake must also be conducted, including type, frequency, quantity of fluid consumed per serving, and total 24-hour intake.

Medications

A review of medications must include prescribed medications, all over-the-counter medications, laxatives, and nondietary fiber supplements. It is important to ascertain the amount of liquids that the older adult takes with the medications and throughout the day. The use of any alternative cultural or herbal remedy for constipation should be assessed. The nurse should be sensitive to the cultural importance that the patient places on bowel elimination. This will ensure that the physical and cultural needs of the older adult are respected.

Environment and functional ability

Assessment of the environment includes the patient's ability to function in the environment to meet toileting needs, and the assistance of a caregiver if the patient is unable to meet these needs alone. Questions to include in assessing the environment are listed in Box 14-2.

Physical examination

For the physical examination, see Box 14-3.

Conclusion

A comprehensive assessment form is presented in Figure 14-2. The assessment form can be used in any setting of practice to determine the risk factors a patient has for potential or actual constipation.

BOX 14-2 ENVIRONMENTAL AND FUNCTIONAL ABILITY ASSESSMENT

1. What is the layout of your living arrangement?
2. Do you have access to a toilet when the urge to defecate is felt?
3. What type of device do you usually use for bowel elimination—toilet, bedside commode, bedpan, or incontinence brief?
4. Are you able to remove your clothing in time to have a bowel movement?
5. Is there a caregiver present who is able and willing to assist with toileting for bowel elimination?
6. Is there enough privacy to provide a relaxed atmosphere for elimination?
7. Is there enough time provided to have a bowel movement?

NURSING DIAGNOSIS

After a comprehensive assessment of the patient is completed, a diagnosis can be made based on the subjective and objective data that have been collected through the process of history taking and physical examination. In the case of constipation, the individual is experiencing inadequate bowel elimination. The defining characteristics associated with this diagnosis are the following:

1. Passage of stool less than 3 to 5 times per week
2. Insufficient quantity of stool to cause feeling of complete evacuation
3. Incomplete passage of stool
4. Passage of hard and dry stool
5. Straining at evacuation more than 25% of the time

The major factors contributing to constipation in older adults are the following:

1. Inadequate intake of dietary fiber and/or fluid
2. Limited physical mobility

BOX 14-3 PHYSICAL EXAMINATION

1. Cognition assessment—Mental status must be assessed, with attention focused on the older adult's ability to recognize the urge to defecate, the ability to request assistance if needed, the ability to find a toilet when the urge to defecate is felt, and memory retention of instructions on how to call for assistance.
2. Functional status assessment—Functional status includes the older person's ability to perform self-toileting. Older adults with arthritis or debilitating diseases may recognize the urge to defecate, but may move too slowly to toilet independently. One way to collect this data is to directly observe the patients toileting.
3. Physical endurance assessment—It is important to observe gait and strength, and to discuss with the patient average daily exercise and endurance for physical activity. It is important to assess the minimum activity level a patient can tolerate. This would include amount of exercise, distance for walking, ability to get up independently, ability to get up with assistance, or the inability to get out of bed.
4. Oral examination—The oral examination should include evaluation of dentition; mucous membranes; presence of lesions, sores, or tumors; gag reflex; swallowing; and taste sensation.
5. Abdominal examination—The abdominal examination should include the following: inspection—for contour, visible peristalsis, or visible bulges; auscultation—frequency and character of bowel sounds; percussion—for tympanic or dull sounds; palpation—tenderness or firmness over lower abdomen.
6. Rectal examination—A rectal examination should be done at the conclusion of the assessment. The following should be noted: hemorrhoids (external and/or internal), anal sphincter tone, presence of stool in the rectal vault, or presence of an impaction indicated by dry, hard stool.

From Allison, O.C., Porter, M.E., & Briggs, G.C. (1994). Chronic constipation: Assessment and management in the elderly. *Journal of the American Academy of Nurse Practitioners*, 6(7), 311-317; Bates, B. (1995). *A guide to physical examination* (6th ed.). Philadelphia: J.B. Lippincott; Seidel, H., et al. (1995). *Mosby's guide to physical examination* (3rd ed.). St. Louis: Mosby.

---

3. Environmental impediments to toileting
4. Medications that affect GI motility, hydration, or appetite
5. Cognitive impairment that affects independence in relation to defecation
6. Medical illness

The defining characteristics and contributing factors may vary from patient to patient; however, both components need to be included in the diagnosis. For example, the diagnosis might be as follows: alteration in bowel elimination: constipation—as defined by bowel movement less than 3 times a week associated with straining at

stool 25% of the time; related to activity intolerance (arthritis) and pain medication.

PLANNING AND GOAL IDENTIFICATION

The goal is to establish a bowel elimination regimen that facilitates normal bowel function that is appropriate and adequate for the patient's physical and emotional well-being. The patient's definition of normalcy must be considered when establishing the desired outcome. Intervention for maintaining bowel elimination must be based on the assessment data collected.

A common goal for bowel elimination can be stated as follows: *a soft-formed bowel movement*

ASSESSMENT OF CONTRIBUTING FACTORS FOR ALTERED BOWEL ELIMINATION

Name: _____ Date: _____

Medical History

- Hypothyroidism
- Hyperparathyroidism
- Hypercalcemia
- Hypokalemia
- Dehydration
- Diverticulosis
- Cancer
- Tumors
- Enlarged prostate
- Intestinal stricture
- Uremia
- Hemorrhoids

- Obstruction
- Diabetes
- Multiple sclerosis
- Parkinson's disease
- Paralysis
  - hemiplegia
  - paraplegia
  - quadriplegia
- Dysphagia
- Dementia

Medications

- Aluminum-containing antacids
- Anticholinergics
- Calcium channel blockers
- Calcium carbonate
- Iron salts
- Opiates
- Phenothiazines
- Sedatives
- Diuretics
- Anticonvulsants
- Antidepressants

- Laxative overuse
- NSAIDs
- Sympathomimetics

- Over-the-counter medications/diet supplements
  _____
  _____
  _____
  _____

Diet

Average fiber grams/day

- 0-10
- 11-15
- 16-20
- 21-30

Average fluid intake/day

- 0-500 cc
- 500-1000 cc
- 1000-1500 cc
- 1500-2000 cc
- >2000 cc

Type of Diet

- Regular/soft
- Mechanical/soft
- Pureed
- Low-fiber formula
- High-fiber formula

- Full liquid
- Clear liquid
- Fluid restriction
  _____cc/day

Continued

FIGURE 14-2 Assessment form for contributing factors for altered bowel elimination.

Activity

- Exercise 2-3x/week
- Walking 20-30 minutes QD
- Ambulating 50' TID
- Stationary exercises
- Up in chair TID
- Bedfast

Physical Exam

Bowel sounds

- Hypoactive
- Normal
- Hyperactive
- Absent

Inspection/palpation/percussion

- Flat
- Round/soft
- Distended/soft
- Distended/firm
- Tympanic
- Dull

Rectal Exam

Sphincter tone

- Present
- Absent

Stool in vault

- None
- Soft—small amount
- Soft—large amount
- Hard dry stool
- Impaction

Cognition/Function

- Recognize urge to defecate—toilet self
- Recognize urge to defecate-needs assistance
- Unable to recognize urge to defecate
- Unable to communicate need to defecate

Iatrogenic Factors

- NPO for medical or surgical reasons
- Radiologic studies with barium
- Reduction in activity
- Pain management with narcotics
- Impaired communication ⁒ interventions
- Impaired communication ⁒ call light use
- Low-fiber diet

FIGURE 14-2, cont'd. For legend see p. 379.

to be passed without straining at least once every 3 days.

IMPLEMENTATION

In addition to setting goal outcomes, the planning phase includes establishing appropriate nursing interventions. Implementation of these should start with the simplest interventions targeted at diet, activity, and habit training. Laxative use should be considered only after other measures are found to be ineffective or impossible to implement (Tedesco, 1985).

Factors for consideration in establishing nursing actions

Diet The most important factor in regulating bowel elimination is dietary intake of fiber and fluid. An adequate intake of both dietary fiber and fluid is physiologically important for normal bowel function (Camilleri et al., 1994).

Fiber Dietary fiber plays a therapeutic and preventive role in the management of gastrointestinal diseases and is used extensively in clinical practice to treat constipation. The American Dietetic Association recommends 20 to 35 gm of fiber per day for healthy adults from a variety of food sources for health promotion and disease reduction. Food, not dietary supplements, should be the primary source of fiber intake (Gorman & Bowman, 1993).

The goal for fiber consumption in the older adult is as follows: the older person should receive at least 20 gm of fiber per day (Gorman & Bowman, 1993).

There are a variety of ways to include fiber in the diet. Fiber is primarily available in grains and cereals, but is also present in fruits and vegetables, and cereals and breads made from whole grain. Foods high in fiber are presented in Table 14-1. High-fiber formula supplements for enteral feeding or nutritional supplements are also available. When advising an increase in fiber, it is important to warn the individual not to increase the amount too quickly because this may result in flatulence and cramping (Castle, 1989; Cerrato, 1989).

In addition to food that is high in fiber, natural dietary supplements or "natural laxatives" have been developed, tested, and shown to be very effective for maintaining bowel elimination (Battle & Hanna, 1980; Behm, 1985; Brown & Everett, 1990; Hall et al., 1994; Hope, 1983; Hope & Down, 1986; Miller, 1985). Examples of natural dietary supplements are as follows:

1. 2 cups miller's bran, 2 cups applesauce, and 1 cup unsweetened prune juice; the mixture should be refrigerated and served in 2 to 3 1-tbsp portions a day (Wong et al., 1991)
2. 15 gm bran flour (3 tbsp) in hot cereal every morning, with 120 cc prune juice with breakfast and 120 cc prune juice with lunch or dinner (Miller, 1985)
3. 2 lb raisins, 2 lb currants, 2 lb prunes, 2 lb figs, and 2 lb dates, ground together, then mixed with 2 28-oz containers undiluted prune juice concentrate; 30 ml per day up to 3 doses a day may be administered to achieve bowel elimination (Beverley & Travis, 1992)

Recipes using fiber supplements as an ingredient can also be used as a source of increased fiber (Box 14-4).

Fluid To ensure the success of increasing fiber intake as a method of managing constipation, it is imperative that patients maintain adequate fluid intake. Increasing fiber intake without maintaining adequate fluid intake may worsen the problem of constipation (Gorman & Bowman, 1993).

The goal for fluid consumption in the older adult is as follows: the older adult should receive between 1800 and 2000 ml of fluid per day unless restrictions are imposed because of a medical condition. This is the equivalent of eight 8-oz glasses per day.

The nurse must take an active role in maintaining fluid intake with two special groups of patients: those with physical or cognitive impairments severe enough to limit independent fluid maintenance and those who are fed via feeding tubes.

TABLE 14-1 Approximate fiber content of selected foods

	Grams of dietary fiber per serving	Size of serving
Grains and cereals		
White rice	1	½ cup
White bread	1	1 slice
Cornflakes	1	1 cup
Whole wheat bread	1	1 slice
Brown rice	2	½ cup
Instant oatmeal	3	1 cup
Rye bread	3	1 slice
Raisin Bran	7	1 cup
Vegetables		
Raw celery	1	½ cup
String beans	2	½ cup
New potatoes, canned	2	1 cup
Corn	3	½ cup
Broccoli	4	½ cup
Peas, canned	7	½ cup
Baked beans	7	½ cup
Kidney beans	10	½ cup
Fruits		
Grapefruit	1	½
Apples	2	½ large
Bananas	3	1 medium
Strawberries	3	1 cup
Raspberries	9	1 cup
Other		
Strawberry jam	1	3 tbsp
Peanut butter	3	3 tbsp
Popcorn	3	1 cup
Peanuts	4	2 tbsp

Interventions for meeting fluid requirements should include the following: (1) always having fluids within reach; (2) offering fluid every 2 to 3 hours while the patient is awake; and (3) implementing a fluid schedule of 1 to 2 8-oz glasses of fluid given upon rising, at each meal, and 2 to 3 hours before bedtime.

Activity Regular exercise is an important component of a bowel management program. Activity is necessary to promote bowel motility (Ellickson, 1988). Twenty to 30 minutes of walking per day can be effective for maintaining bowel elimination (Cheskin & Schuster, 1990).

Upright posture, abdominal exercises, and simple exercise such as walking have been shown to promote GI motility (Wrenn, 1989).

The goal for daily activity of the older adult is as follows: the older adult should achieve maximum mobility based on the individual's level of endurance and physical function.

Walking for 20 to 30 minutes per day is an excellent form of nonstrenuous exercise that should be encouraged in older adults who are physically able to do so. An exercise program for patients with limited endurance or mobility could include the following: ambulating 50 feet 2

BOX 14-4 HIGH-FIBER RECIPES

OATMEAL RAISIN HIGH-FIBER COOKIES

(Makes 12, 2.2 oz. cookies with 5.2 g fiber per cookie)

2.5 oz. white granulated sugar
5 oz. margarine
3.5 oz. molasses
2.5 oz. cholesterol-free egg substitute
4.25 oz. skim milk (fluid)
3 g cinnamon

2 g ground cloves
4 g baking powder
5.5 oz. all purpose flour
3.5 oz. old fashioned oatmeal
4.25 oz. powdered fiber supplement
3 oz. raisins

Cover raisins with tap water and let sit for 10 minutes.
Cream sugar and margarine. Add molasses and egg substitutes and cream for 4 minutes.
Mix in milk.
Add spices, flour, oats, and fiber supplement. Mix on low speed until blended.
Mix in raisins.
Dip with #16 scoop onto baking sheet spaced 3 × 5. Press cookies flat with gloved hand.
Bake at 350 degrees for 11 minutes.

BLUEBERRY HIGH-FIBER MUFFINS

(Makes 12, 3 oz. muffins with 4.2 g fiber per muffin)

4.75 oz. powdered fiber supplement
6.5 oz. all-purpose flour
8.5 oz. white granulated sugar
14 g baking soda
7 g baking powder

5 g table salt
12.5 oz. skim milk (fluid)
2.25 oz. cholesterol-free egg substitutes
5.75 oz. frozen blueberries

Combine powdered fiber supplement, flour, sugar, baking soda, baking powder, and salt in a mixing bowl.
In a separate bowl, mix milk, egg substitutes, and corn oil.
Add liquids to dry ingredients and stir until dry ingredients are moistened.
Mix in blueberries.
Spoon into paper-lined muffin tins with #12 scoop.
Bake at 350 degrees for 20-25 minutes.

From Hall, G.R., et al. (1995). Managing constipation using a research-based protocol, *Medsurg Nursing*, 4(1), 15.

to 3 times per day, leg kicks, abduction, trunk rotation, Kegel exercises, stomach pulls, and stationary bicycling (Karam & Nies, 1994). Abdominal and pelvic exercises should be taught to all cognitively able patients (Brown & Everett, 1990). In debilitated or bedfast patients, mobility must also be maximized. Turning the patient from side to side 2 or 3 times in a row, 3 to 4 times a day, followed by a lower abdominal massage, can be helpful in increasing GI motility.

Habit training The goal for bowel elimination habits of the older adult is as follows: the older person should establish a daily ritual for elimination.

Aging Alert
Caffeine
Fluids high in caffeine should be used cautiously and not counted in the total fluid volume. Caffeine has a diuretic effect and thus enhances fluid excretion from the body.

For patients who already have a regular time of day when they attempt to pass stools, it is best to allow the patient to continue on this schedule. When a regular schedule has not been established by the patient, the best times to recommend are after breakfast and after the evening meal, thus taking advantage of the postprandial gastrologic response. In the cognitively impaired it is worthwhile to impose a regular schedule for defecation. Providing 10 to 20 minutes of undistracted time after a meal will help establish a routine for elimination (Brown & Everett, 1990; Cheskin & Schuster, 1990).

In the acute care setting

Common reasons for which older adults are admitted to the hospital include the following: congestive heart failure, dehydration, mental status changes, cerebral vascular accidents, pneumonia, surgery, GI bleeding, and sepsis. Treatment of these conditions imposes many iatrogenic risks that may lead to the development of constipation.

Iatrogenic factors are especially significant in an acute care setting, where older adults often come in with medical conditions that exacerbate the risk of becoming constipated. The health care provider must be particularly astute regarding the greatest risk factors, which include the following:

1. The prescription of "nothing by mouth" for medical or surgical reasons
2. Radiologic studies using barium
3. Reduction in activity or mobility
4. Treatment with narcotics for pain from medical or surgical conditions
5. Inability to communicate the need to defecate related to therapeutic interventions, strange surroundings and unfamiliarity with the nurse call light, or medical condition or sedation

Constipation in the acute care setting is a significant problem, with at least 15% to 27% of acutely ill and chronically hospitalized gerontologic patients becoming constipated (Hall et al., 1995). The problem of constipation is costly in terms of discomfort and morbidity for the patient and in a financial sense for medical treatment of the problem.

The nurse plays a key role in the acute care setting in maintaining bowel elimination in older adults. Nursing management begins with realizing that older adults are at risk for constipation from the minute they come into the hospital. Prevention and early intervention need to be the focus of managing constipation. Bowel elimination must be considered an important part of the patient's well-being and should be considered as important as other body functions. Assessment of bowel movements and accurate charting must become an integral part of nursing care on a *daily* basis. A standard of care for bowel elimination for all patients over the age of 65 should be implemented on the patient's admission to the hospital.

Components to be included in a standard of care are as follows:

- Within 24 hours of the patient's admission to the hospital, a comprehensive assessment for constipation needs to be completed.
- The assessment is to be updated as indicated by changes in patient condition or medical management.
- An individualized plan of care should be implemented based on the causative factors.

> ### BOX 14-5 ELEMENTS FOR MANAGING BOWEL ELIMINATION IN AN ACUTE CARE SETTING
>
> 1. Think prevention and intervention.
> 2. Identify iatrogenic risk factors.
> 3. Utilize interdisciplinary approach.
>   - With dietitian—provide fiber foods and supplements
>   - With physical therapist—maximize physical activity
>   - With social worker—assist with home needs
>   - With occupational therapist—provide assistive devices for eating or preparing foods
>   - With physician—order laxative if needed
> 4. Set standards for bowel elimination for all patients over 65.
> 5. Use protocols for identified populations with known high-risk factors.

> ### BOX 14-6 ELEMENTS FOR HOME MANAGEMENT OF BOWEL ELIMINATION
>
> 1. Review recent hospitalization.
> 2. Identify causative factors.
> 3. Develop a plan based on environment and caregiver.
> 4. Assess caregiver attitude regarding managing bowel elimination.
> 5. Review food purchasing and preparation procedures.

- Protocols for treatment may be utilized in certain populations based on research specific to identified risk factors.
- Discharge planning needs to address factors that will influence bowel elimination.

Collaboration with representatives of other disciplines will assist the nurse in implementing a comprehensive plan for bowel elimination. Box 14-5 describes elements for managing bowel elimination in acute care settings.

In the long-term care setting

Patients in long-term care facilities have multiple problems that have led to their functional decline (Hope & Downs, 1986). Many of these conditions compound the complexity of constipation. The nurse in long-term care needs to focus on the nursing process and nursing interventions that address the cause of constipation. All members of the health care team, especially nonprofessionals, need to be educated regarding the factors that contribute to constipation. The bowel program for each patient needs to be followed on a daily basis. Assessment of bowel movements and accurate charting must become an integral part of the nursing care. The use of laxatives or enemas is sometimes necessary in patients with severe constipation. These should always be used judiciously, and alternative interventions should be tried periodically to avoid unnecessary long-term use. Long-term enema use can lead to poor rectal tone and can increase the risk of fecal impaction (Castle, 1989). Monitoring and follow-up of the bowel regimen must also be carried out on a regular basis.

In the home

Management of a bowel regimen at home begins with teaching the patient and/or caregiver about causative factors for constipation, then planning a bowel regimen based on the causative factors and environmental issues. If home care is a follow-up from a recent hospitalization, it is important to review the hospital course for any factors that contributed to constipation and interventions that were utilized for managing elimination. Teaching about the contributing factors for constipation should be addressed on the first home visit whether the patient is an independent

BOWEL ELIMINATION DOCUMENTATION RECORD (see KEY at bottom of page)

Name: ....

Date Assessed for Constipation:							
Time:							
ABDOMINAL ASSESSMENT							
Bowel Sounds							
normal							
hypoactive							
hyperactive							
Inspection/Palpation/Percussion							
round/soft							
distended/soft							
distended/firm							
tympanic							
dull							
Rectal Exam							
impaction							
manual removal							
INTERVENTION							
activity							
toileting							
fiber							
fluid / juices							
softener / laxative							
suppository / enema							
BOWEL MOVEMENT STATUS							
b.m. today							
frequency							
quantity							
consistency							
continent / incontinent							

ABDOMINAL ASSESSMENT....   place a check mark in box where condition noted.

INTERVENTION....
    activity –   ambulation (AMB), up in chair (↑/CH), turn (S-S), physical therapy (PT)
    toileting –   bathroom (BR), bedside commode (BSC), bedpan (BP), Attends
    fluids/juices –   quantity on the I & O, indicate if special juices are given
    dietary –   indicate if special foods are given
    softener / laxative –   specify which one is given, or none
    suppository / enema   specify which one is given, or none

BOWEL MOVEMENT STATUS...
    b.m. today –   yes or no (**if this changes within 24 hours, a new column needs to be completed)
    frequency –   indicate with a slash mark number of stools (**if number only increases on a
                subsequent shift, add slash marks to existing column)
    quantity –   none, smear, small, moderate, large
    consistency –   liquid, loose, semi-formed, formed-soft, formed-hard
    continent / incontinent –   indicate which route of elimination

FIGURE 14-3 Example of bowel elimination documentation record.

older adult or totally dependent on a caregiver. Environmental assessment, including the issues of food purchasing and preparation, needs to be addressed with the patient more thoroughly than in an environment where the health care provider has control over these areas. Easy access to toileting facilities, privacy, and comfortableness with the home care provider are important elements in establishing a bowel regimen in the home.

Also important in the home setting are the attitudes of the patient and caregiver regarding elimination. Bowel elimination is a very personal and potentially embarrassing occurrence for many individuals. This is true for the caregiver as well as the patient. The caregiver, patient, and health care worker need to establish a comfortable relationship for discussing and dealing with bowel elimination. Time should be allotted for discussing feelings about elimination and for establishing a comfortable relationship between all those involved with helping the older adult to achieve a bowel regimen. Feelings of apprehension, embarrassment, or repulsion need to be identified and discussed. Box 14-6, on page 385, describes elements for home management of bowel elimination.

EVALUATION

An integral part of the success of the plan for managing constipation is frequent and thorough evaluation of interventions related to the objective. Achievement of the patient's satisfaction and achievement of the objective are both vital components of the nursing process.

A centralized documentation record will assist in the evaluative process. (A sample documentation record is shown in Figure 14-3.) The record should include all components of the nursing process and results of interventions. Patients at home should be instructed in keeping a bowel elimination diary until a satisfactory management program is achieved.

REFERENCES

Allison, O.C., Porter, M.E., & Briggs, G.C. (1994). Chronic constipation: Assessment and management in the elderly. *Journal of the American Academy of Nurse Practitioners, 6*(7), 311-317.

Barnes, K.E. (1987). Monitoring bowel habit in elderly people. In P. Fielding (Ed.), *Research in the nursing care of elderly people* (pp. 27-46). Chichester, United Kingdom: John Wiley and Sons.

Battle, E., & Hanna, C. (1980). Evaluation of a dietary regimen for chronic constipation. *Journal of Gerontological Nursing, 6*(9), 527-532.

Behm, R. (1985). A special recipe to banish constipation. *Geriatric Nursing, 6,* 216-217.

Beverley, L., & Travis, I. (1992). Constipation: Proposed natural laxative mixtures. *Journal of Gerontological Nursing, 18*(10), 5-12.

Brown, M.K., & Everett, I. (1990). Gentler bowel fitness with fiber. *Geriatric Nursing, 11*(1), 26-27.

Cameron, J. (1992). Constipation related to narcotic therapy—A protocol for nurses and patients. *Cancer Nursing, 15*(5), 372-377.

Camilleri, M., et al. (1994). Clinical management of intractable constipation. *Annals of Internal Medicine, 121*(7), 520-528.

Canty, S. (1994). Constipation as a side effect of opioids. *Oncology Nursing Forum, 21*(4), 739-745.

Castle, S.C. (1989). Constipation: Endemic in the elderly? Gerontopathophysiology, evaluation, and management. *Medical Clinics of North America, 73*(6), 1497-1509.

Cerrato, P.L. (1989). Is America really constipated? *RN, 52*(5), 81-86.

Chenitz, W.C., Stone, J.T., & Salisbury, S.A. (1991). *Clinical gerontological nursing.* Philadelphia: W.B. Saunders.

Cheskin, L.J., & Schuster, M.M. (1990). Constipation. In W.R. Hazzard, et al. (Eds.), *Principles of geriatric medicine and gerontology* (2nd ed., pp. 1161-1167). New York: McGraw-Hill.

Donatelle, E.P. (1990). Constipation: Pathophysiology and treatment. *American Family Physician, 42*(5), 1335-1342.

Ellickson, E. (1988). Bowel management plan for the homebound elderly. *Journal of Gerontological Nursing, 14*(1), 16-19.

Goldstein, M., & Oliveira, J. (1993). Constipation and diarrhea. In T.T. Yoshikawa, E.L. Cobbs, & K. Brummel-Smith (Eds.), *Ambulatory Geriatric Care.* St. Louis: Mosby.

Gorman, M.A., & Bowman, C. (1993). Position of the American Dietetic Association: Health implications of dietary fiber. *Journal of the American Dietetic Association, 93*(12), 1446-1447.

Guyton, A. (1991). *Textbook of medical physiology* (8th ed.). Philadelphia: W.B. Saunders.

Hall, G., et al. (1995). Managing constipation using a research based protocol. *Medsurg Nursing, 4*(1), 11-20.

Harper, C.M., & Lyles, Y.M. (1988). Physiology and complications of bed rest. *Journal of the American Geriatrics Society, 36*(11), 1047-1054.

Hazzard, W.R., et al. (Eds.) (1990). *Principles of geriatric medicine and gerontology* (2nd ed.). New York: McGraw-Hill.

Hope, A. (1983). The relief of constipation in the elderly. *Australian Nurses Journal, 12*(10), 45-48.

Hope, A.K., & Downs, E.C. (1986). Dietary fibre and fluid in the control of constipation in a nursing home population. *Medical Journal of Australia, 144*(6), 3306-3307.

Kallman, H. (1983). Constipation in the elderly. *American Family Practice, 27*(17), 179-184.

Karam, S. E., & Nies, D.M. (1994). Student/staff collaboration: A pilot bowel management program. *Journal of Gerontological Nursing, 20*(3), 32-40.

Kenney, R. (1989). *Physiology of aging: A synopsis* (2nd ed.). Chicago: Year Book Medical.

Kopac, C. (1993). Demographics, theories and nursing process. In C.A. Kopac & V.L. Millonig (Eds.), *Gerontological nursing certification review guide for the generalist clinical specialist nurse practitioner.* Potomac, MD: Health Leadership Associates.

Luckman, J., & Sorensen, K. (1993). *Medical-surgical nursing: A psychophysiologic approach* (2nd ed.). Philadelphia: W.B. Saunders.

McMillan, S.C., & Williams, F.A. (1989). Validity and reliability of the constipation assessment scale, *Cancer Nursing, 12*(3), 183-188.

Melmon, K., et al. (1992). *Clinical pharmacology: Basic principles in therapeutics* (3rd ed.). New York: McGraw-Hill.

Merkel, I.S., et al. (1993). Physiologic and psychologic characteristics of an elderly population with chronic constipation. *American Journal of Gastroenterology, 88*(1), 1854-1859.

Miller, J. (1985). Helping the aged manage bowel function. *Journal of Gerontological Nursing, 11*(2), 37-41.

Rodrigues-Fisher, L., Bourguignon, C., & Good, B. (1993). Dietary fiber nursing intervention: Prevention of constipation in older adults. *Clinical Nursing Research, 2*(4), 464-477.

Seidel, H., et al. (1995). *Mosby's guide to physical examination* (3rd ed.). St. Louis: Mosby.

Taylor, R. (1990). Management of constipation: High fiber diets work. *British Medical Journal, 300*(6731), 1063-1064.

Tedesco, F.J. (1985). Laxative use in constipation. *American Journal of Gastroenterology, 80*(4), 303-309.

Wong, R.D., Gold, S., & Blanchette, P.A. (1991, January-February). Correcting constipation: A regimen that works. *Senior Patient,* pp. 37-41.

Wrenn, K. (1989). Fecal impaction. *New England Journal of Medicine, 321*(10), 658-662.

BIBLIOGRAPHY

Bassotti, G., & Whitehead, W. (1994). Biofeedback as a treatment approach to gastrointestinal tract disorders. *American Journal of Gastroenterology, 89*(2), 158-164.

Bates, B. (1995). *A guide to physical examination* (6th ed.). Philadelphia: J.B. Lippincott.

Campbell, A.J., Busby, W., & Horwath, C. (1993). Factors associated with constipation in a community based sample of people aged 70 years and over. *Journal of Epidemiol Community Health, 47*(1), 23-26.

Cristofalo, V.J. (1988). An overview of the theories of biological aging. In J.E. Birren & V.L. Bengtson (Eds.), *Emergent theories of aging* (pp. 118-127). New York: Springer.

Hogstel, M., & Nelson, M. (1992). Anticipation and early detection can reduce bowel elimination complications. *Geriatric Nursing, 34*(1), 28-33.

Lennard-Jones, J. (1985). Pathophysiology of constipation. *British Journal of Surgery, 72*(Suppl.), S7-S13.

Lennard-Jones, J.E. (1993). Clinical management of constipation. *Pharmacology, 47*(Suppl. 1), 216-223.

Marshall, J.B. (1990). Chronic constipation in adults: How far should evaluation and treatment go? *Postgraduate Medicine, 88*(3), 49-63.

Monane, M., et al. (1993). Anticholinergic drug use and bowel function in nursing home patients. *Archives of Internal Medicine, 153*(5), 633-638.

Muller-Lissner, S.A. (1993). *Adverse effects of laxatives: Fact and fiction.*

Murray, F.E., & Bliss, C.M. (1991). Geriatric constipation: Brief update on a common problem. *Geriatrics, 46*(3), 64-68.

Pharmacology, 47(Suppl.), 138-145.

Shafik, A. (1993). Constipation: Pathogenesis and management. *Drugs, 45*(4), 528-540.

Stewart, R., et al. (1992). Correlates of constipation in an ambulatory elderly population. *American Journal of Gastroenterology, 87*(7), 859-864.

U.S. Department of Health and Human Services. (1990). *Healthy People 2000: National health promotion and disease prevention objectives* (DHHS Pub. No. [PHS] 91-50212). Washington, DC: U.S. Government Printing Office.

Wingard, L., et al. (1991). *Human pharmacology—Molecular to clinical.* St. Louis: Mosby.

C H A P T E R 15

There is an appointed time for every thing,
and a time for every affair under the heavens.
A time to be born, and a time to die;
a time to plant, and a time to uproot.

ECCLESIASTES 3:2-3

Nutrition and Digestive Function

■ Learning Objectives

On completion of this chapter, the reader will be able to do the following:

1. Discuss nutritional requirements for the older adult.
2. Explain the use of the food guide pyramid and food labels.
3. Describe age-related changes in the digestive system of the older adult.
4. Recognize the physiologic, psychosocial, and environmental factors that influence the maintenance of the nutritional status of the older adult.
5. Discuss drug-nutrient interactions and their effect on older adults.
6. Discuss pathologic conditions that affect the nutritional status of the older adult.
7. Describe the components of nutritional assessment for the older adult.
8. Develop a plan of care for the older adult with an alteration in nutrition.
9. Design appropriate nursing interventions for older adults with alterations in nutrition.
10. Describe strategies for promoting optimum nutrition in the older adult.

As people go about their daily activities, whether at play, work, or rest, or even in sleep, their bodies need energy. Nutrition is one of the basic human needs that supplies this energy and sustains life. "Nutrition thus concerns the food people eat and how their bodies use it. Nutritional science comprises the body of scientific knowledge governing the nutritional requirements of humans for maintenance, growth, activ- ity, and reproduction" (Williams, 1989). Sound nutrition is considered to be a primary basis for promoting health and preventing disease throughout the life span.

Food provides the essential nutrients the body requires for its vital processes. A wide variety of foods provide important ingredients that sustain physiologic processes. Personal choice and food availability govern the selection

389

of nutrients. The major nutrients essential for healthy aging include protein, carbohydrates, fat, minerals, vitamins, and water.

Food plays a vital role in family life and is a part of many rituals and ceremonies in the larger society. Thus motivation for eating may spring from the need for love, belonging, or meeting the expectations of others. Furthermore, religious practices, as well as personal preferences, may dictate what older adults will eat and what they will refuse to eat. As with all of the important processes of life, meeting the nutritional requirements for a healthy life is neither simple nor easy.

■ Nutritional Requirements in Older Adults

The nutrient needs and nutrition status of older adults are becoming increasingly important, not only because of the unprecedented increase in the number of older people in the population, but also because of the high cost of nutrition-related chronic diseases. Good nutrition and adequate exercise can improve the quality of life and the health of older adults. Concern has been expressed in the literature regarding the adequacy of the available research data for guiding accurate recommendations for dietary intake, especially for older adults over 75 to 80 years of age (Brookbank, 1990). Many of the studies group all people age 65 and older in one category and do not differentiate among those in their later years.

The National Health and Nutrition Examination Survey provides needed information about the diet of Americans and is of major importance in establishing specific nutrient recommendations for groups of people over 50 years of age (1989). The tenth and most current edition of the recommended dietary allowances (RDAs) continues to use a category of 51+ years because the subcommittee of the National Research Council did not consider the data adequate to establish separate RDAs for people 70 years and older (National Research Council, 1989) (Table 15-1).

TABLE 15-1 Recommended dietary allowances for older adults (1989)

Characteristic or dietary element	Value	
	Male	**Female**
Age	51+	51+
Weight (kg)	77	65
Weight (lb)	170	143
Height (cm)	173	160
Height (in)	68	63
Protein (gm)	63	50
Vitamin A (µg, RE*)	1000	600
Vitamin D (µg)	5	5
Vitamin E (mg)	10	8
Vitamin K (µg)	80	65
Vitamin C (mg)	60	60
Thiamin (mg)	1.2	1.0
Riboflavin (mg)	1.4	1.2
Niacin (mg)	15	13
Vitamin B_6 (mg)	2.0	1.6
Folate (µg)	200	180
Vitamin B_{12} (µg)	2.0	2.0
Calcium (mg)	800	800
Phosphorus (mg)	800	800
Magnesium (mg)	350	280
Iron (mg)	10	10
Zinc (mg)	15	12
Iodine (µg)	150	150
Selenium (µg)	70	55
Copper (mg)	1.5-3.0	1.5-3.0
Manganese (mg)	2.0-5.0	2.0-5.0
Fluoride (mg)	1.5-4	1.5-4
Chromium (µg)	50-200	50-200
Molybdenum (µg)	75-250	75-250
Sodium (mg) minimum	500	500
Chloride (mg) minimum	750	750
Potassium (mg) minimum	2000	2000

Adapted from National Research Council. (1989). *Recommended dietary allowances.* Washington, DC: National Academy of Sciences.
*µg = microgram, one millionth of a gram. RE = retinol equivalent, which is the vitamin A activity in foods.

The RDAs have been called "the Gold Standard for evaluating nutritional adequacy in the United States" (Sutnick, 1988, p. 193). They are defined as "the levels of intake of essential nutrients that, on the basis of scientific knowledge, are judged by the Food and Nutrition Board to be adequate to meet the known needs of practically all healthy persons" (National Research Council, 1989, p. 1). The RDAs are extrapolated from the measurements made on young adults. The National Research Council (1989) has noted the wide variations in health with advancing age and stated, "there is some evidence that the elderly have altered requirements for some nutrients" (p. 19). It must be stressed that the RDAs are not designed to account for changes resulting from disease, drug interactions, or psychosocial factors that affect food intake.

Data from the National Council of Aging indicate that undernutrition and malnutrition affect between 15% and 50% of the population of older adults, with signs and symptoms that are not always recognized by health care givers.

OVERVIEW OF BASIC NUTRIENTS
Protein

Protein is an essential nutrient for growth and tissue repair. Proteins are made up of carbon, hydrogen, oxygen, and nitrogen. When protein is used for energy, most of the nitrogen becomes a waste product and must be converted to urea and excreted. All living cells, including muscle, bone, lymph, blood, enzymes, and brain tissue, contain protein. For cellular synthesis to occur, protein must first be broken down to amino acids. These amino acids are classified as essential and nonessential.

Nonessential amino acids are synthesized by the liver from other amino acids, whereas the body relies on dietary sources for the essential amino acids. It is generally believed that essential amino acids must all be present in the right quantity and at the right time in order to facilitate their maximum efficient use for cellular metabolism. A food that contains adequate amounts of essential amino acids is classified as a complete protein of high biologic value. Animal proteins

such as eggs, milk and milk products, meats, poultry, and fish fall into this category. An incomplete protein of low biologic value is a food that is lacking in one or more of the essential amino acids. These foods (cereal, vegetables, and legumes), although lacking in some essential amino acids, may be combined with other non-animal proteins. If the right combination of non-animal proteins is consumed at the same meal, it will provide a protein quality equal to that of an animal protein.

Many older adults may have an inadequate intake of protein; attention should be given to encouraging them to eat foods that are good sources of protein. In spite of the wide acceptance of the RDAs as the standard of diet adequacy, there has been considerable discussion and disagreement in the literature concerning the recommended levels of protein for older adults.

The National Research Council (1989) continues to recommend the same level of protein for older adults as for young adults (0.8 gm/kg body weight). The council explains that because of the difference in body composition, this is actually a higher allowance per unit of lean body mass and should compensate for the lessened efficiency of older adults in utilizing protein. The daily requirement of protein for women can be met with 4 oz of fish, meat, or poultry, plus 2 oz of milk or 3 oz of cheese. For men, an additional 2 oz of meat will provide the required daily supply of protein. Usually, if 12% to 15% of total calories come from protein, this is enough to meet daily needs.

Carbohydrates

There are indications that carbohydrate absorption may be slightly decreased in older adults (Ausman & Russell, 1990). There are no RDAs for carbohydrate intake in older adults, but the U.S. Department of Agriculture, the American Cancer Society, and the American Heart Association have endorsed the suggestion that 55% to 60% of total calories be composed of carbohydrates. The carbohydrates in the diet should be primarily complex, with few simple sugars. Four or more servings of fresh or cooked fruits and vegetables incorporated into the diet will meet the standard recommended percentage.

Complex carbohydrate foods rich in fiber should make up at least 55% of the total intake of calories. When eating breads, pasta, and potatoes, the older adult must limit the amount of fats in the form of butter, margarine, and sour cream used to complement foods high in complex carbohydrates. Simple carbohydrates come mainly from sugars in fresh fruit and from low-fat milk and milk products.

Lipids

Lipids include fats and oils and are made up of carbon, hydrogen, and oxygen. They provide 9 calories per gram, with excesses stored mainly in adipose tissue. Lipids (1) provide linoleic and linolenic acids, essential fatty acids; (2) add taste and satiety value to foods; and (3) aid in the absorption of fat-soluble vitamins. The classification system for lipids contains three major branches: simple, compound, and derived. Simple lipids are made up of glycerol and fatty acids, which are further designated as monoglycerides, diglycerides, and triglycerides. The triglycerides make up over 90% of the lipids in food and in the body. Compound lipids are simple lipids with the addition of a nonlipid fraction like protein (lipoprotein), phospholipids, and glycolipids (glucose and lipid). Derived lipids such as cholesterol result from the breakdown of compound and simple lipids.

Saturated fats are found mostly in animal fats and in coconut and palm oil. These fats are thought to raise cholesterol levels and to contribute to the development of atherosclerosis. Unsaturated fats are classified as monosaturated or polyunsaturated fat. Hydrogenated fats, created by a commercial process with polyunsaturated fats, are saturated fats that seem to be as atherogenic as the naturally occurring saturated fat. Examples of hydrogenated fats are margarine and vegetable shortening, with the soft, tub margarine being less saturated than the hard, stick margarine. Plant lipids are mostly polyunsaturated. Olive oil, a monosaturated lipid, is thought to lower serum cholesterol.

Most lipid metabolism occurs in the liver, where lipids are released into the bloodstream as very low-, low-, and high-density lipoprotein (VLDL, LDL, and HDL) cholesterol. HDLs carry a higher proportion of protein to lipid than do the LDLs, and are believed to have a serum cholesterol lowering effect. The VLDLs have a higher proportion of triglycerides, which the cells use for energy.

The guidelines recommend that dietary fat should make up no more than 30% of the total caloric intake, with a daily cholesterol intake not to exceed 300 mg. The diet health guidelines also suggest limiting saturated fat intake to no more than 10% of the total fat intake, with 10% of the total fat intake being from monosaturated and the remaining from polyunsaturated fatty acid (National Research Council, 1989). This can be done by avoiding fried and fatty foods, trimming visible fat from meat, using low-fat milk, and reducing the amount of fats used as salad dressings and spreads. The amount of fat in the average American diet has usually exceeded the recommended percentage of 20% to 30% and is estimated to be in the range of 38% to 42% of total calories.

Minerals

Calcium, iron, and zinc are three of the minerals that are important dietary elements.

Calcium Discussions regarding calcium intake in older people, particularly in women, center around a concern about the prevention and treatment of osteoporosis, a condition of reduced bone mass that occurs after menopause. As they age, both men and women experience a reduction in bone mass, which is much more pronounced in women. The 1994 National Institutes of Health (NIH) consensus conference reported that both older men and older women average a daily intake of only 600 mg of calcium. The National Research Council (1989) recommends for older adults a daily intake of 800 mg of calcium, usually obtained in a balanced diet. This is the level recommended for healthy people and does not address the special needs of people with osteoporosis. Based on the high incidence of osteoporosis in women, the NIH conference recommended that postmenopausal women on estrogen consume 1000 mg/day and those not on estrogen consume 1500 mg/day. It was also recommended that the increases should come from dietary sources rather than from calcium supplements. The National Research Council emphasized that, besides calcium, other nutrients are necessary for bone health.

Some of the risks of a high intake of calcium were noted by the National Research Council, such as increased risk of urinary tract stones, especially in hypercalciuric men, and potential decreased absorption of iron, zinc, and other essential minerals. Constipation may also result. In addition to hypercalciuria, amounts of calcium higher than those recommended may cause hypercalcemia and deterioration in renal function. Because of the antacid effects of calcium, calcium supplementation at mealtimes can cause a reduction in dietary folate and iron absorption (Roe, 1987). For these reasons the National Research Council (1989) does not recommend supplementing calcium to a level much above the RDA for the average person.

Besides their calcium intake in later years, other factors that influence the rate and amount of bone mass loss in older women are exercise and the adequacy of calcium taken in during the peak years of bone mass development—the late teens and early 20s. For women ages 80 years and older, the RDA of 800 mg appears to be adequate (Anderson, 1990).

An increase in calcium intake for postmenopausal women needs to be encouraged. The best way to achieve this increase is through dietary means, such as low-fat milk, cheese, and yogurt. Some experts recommend calcium supplement

---

BOX 15-1 CALCIUM-RICH FOODS AND CALCIUM SUPPLEMENTS

CALCIUM IN THE KITCHEN

Tofu (8 oz): 280 mg calcium
Canned salmon, with bones (1 oz): 60 mg
Canned sardines, with bones (1 oz): 125 mg
Whole milk (8 oz): 290 mg
Low-fat milk (8 oz): 298 mg
Skim milk (8 oz): 300 mg
Yogurt (8 oz): 400 mg
Cottage cheese (8 oz): 170 mg
Mozzarella cheese, skim (1 oz): 183 mg
American cheese (1 oz): 170 mg
Parmesan cheese (2 tbsp): 140 mg
Green leafy vegetables (8 oz): 400 mg
Ice cream, vanilla (8 oz): 208 mg

. . . IN THE MEDICINE CHEST

Calcium carbonate (40% calcium)
Calcium sulfate (36.1%)
Dibasic calcium phosphate (29.5%)
Tribasic calcium phosphate (38.8%)
Calcium lactate (13%)
Calcium citrate (21%)
Calcium gluconate (9.3%)
Calcium glubionate (6.5%)

From Holm, K., & Walker, J. (1990). Osteoporosis: Treatment and prevention update. *Geriatric Nursing, 11*(3), 142.

---

administration with food. The addition of calcium supplements to the normal diet can be suggested along with dietary recommendations (see Box 15-1 for typical calcium supplements).

Iron There may be impaired iron absorption in older adults as a result of decreased secretion of hydrochloric acid, which is needed to convert the iron into a usable form for the body. Although this represents a potential risk of iron deficiency, there has been little evidence that decreased iron intake or absorption is a frequent cause of anemia in older adults. When iron deficiency does occur in older people, it is more often the result of bleeding from a variety of causes, such as chronic use of aspirin or similar drugs, peptic ulcer, esophageal varices, cancer, or inflammatory disease of the bowel (National Research Council, 1989).

There is a tendency for iron stores to increase with age, and the American diet, including that of older men and women, usually supplies more than the current RDA of 10 mg/day (Roe, 1987). Nonetheless, there is a risk of iron deficiency among poor older adults and those with mobility problems who are unable to acquire or prepare foods, such as meat and green leafy vegetables, that contain adequate sources of iron.

Zinc There is some evidence that the daily intake of zinc by older people is less than the recommended amounts of 15 mg for men and 12 mg for women. However, it is difficult to determine anyone's exact zinc status because of a lack of sensitive indicators (National Research Council, 1989). Suggestions have been made that deficiency of zinc may be responsible for the delay in wound healing and the decline in immune function that have been noted in older adults (National Research Council, 1989; Roe, 1987). There is also some suggestion that the loss of taste and smell may be related to low zinc levels. There is a need to reexamine the zinc requirements of older adults and to inform older adults regarding good dietary sources of zinc, such as selected seafoods and meats.

Vitamins

Vitamins are essential nutrients that perform special metabolic functions. Most vitamins are not produced by the body and must be obtained from dietary sources. They are required in small amounts for various physiologic functions including regulating metabolism and functioning as catalysts. They are generally classified as being either fat soluble or water soluble. The RDAs of vitamins for people over 50 years of age do not differ greatly from the RDAs for 25- to 50-year-

olds. Niacin, riboflavin, and thiamin requirements are slightly reduced. A number of studies indicate that the vitamin levels most likely to be low in older men and women are those of vitamin A, thiamin, riboflavin, and pyridoxine (vitamin B_6) (Yearick et al., 1980). Factors influencing adequate intake of vitamins are nutrient quality of the diet in view of reduced caloric intake; medication and alcohol use that could interfere with absorption; and socioeconomic and cultural factors.

The recommended adult dietary allowance of vitamin C is 60 mg/day. Adequate dietary intake of vitamin C is essential for the healthy nutrition of the aging person. Because vitamin C, along with the B-complex vitamins, is water soluble, it is not stored in the body's tissues as are fat-soluble vitamins. This storage incapability makes the water-soluble vitamins less apt to become toxic but more likely to be deficient.

Studies have shown that levels of vitamin C are lower in older men than in older women who eat the same diet (VanderJagt et al., 1987). Studies also indicate that smokers need a higher intake of vitamin C to reach required levels (Viteri, 1988).

There is some evidence that the onset of cataracts can be retarded with behavioral and nutritional modifications (Rosenberg, 1994). There seems to be a protective effect with increasing levels of vitamin C, vitamin E, and beta-carotene. This is an area in which health care professionals need to be involved, in research and in advancing sound, evidence-based health promotion activities.

Supplemental use of vitamin C and the clinical significance of high doses are controversial. No clinical benefits have been reported from taking high doses of vitamin C. In the 1970s, Nobel Laureate Linus Pauling popularized the notion that large doses of vitamin C would prevent or cure colds; this claim has not been substantiated (Dykes & Meier, 1975; Levine, 1986). (See Tables 15-2 and 15-3 for a summary of water- and fat-soluble vitamins.)

Water

Water functions as a medium for cell metabolism; it provides structure and form to the body by the turgor it gives to the tissue; and it helps to maintain body temperature. Water provides the aqueous medium necessary for many chemical and physical processes to take place. It helps to dilute water-soluble medications, aids in excretion of body wastes, and provides for the transport of nutrients. There is general agreement that the water content of the body decreases with age. The body of a mature adult is composed of about 70% water; at age 65, water content is about 60%. Recent findings indicate that people older than 80 years of age (late senescence) have body water content of less than 60% (Reif, 1987). The physiologic consequences of the decrease in body water in older adults can be far reaching. Concentrations of water-soluble drugs in the body are higher, and thermoregulation is less stable. There is an increased susceptibility to both dehydration and overhydration with a reduced water compartment. This risk of dehydration or overhydration is a significant physiologic threat to the health of the older adult. (For a summary of water and other minerals, see Table 15-4.)

DIETARY RECOMMENDATIONS

The food guide pyramid replaces the basic four food groups and reflects the current health recommendations with respect to food groupings and numbers of servings (U.S. Department of Health and Human Services [USDHHS], 1992). These recommendations, in turn, achieve the recommended dietary allowances when a variety of foods are selected from the groups with serving sizes adjusted according to individual caloric needs. (Recommendations for daily intake are seen in Figure 15-1.)

New food labels, legislated by the Food and Drug Administration (FDA), allow older adults to make informed, healthier food choices. The new food labels must follow strict guidelines in regard to serving sizes, nutritional content, and health claims. The daily values (DVs) replace the RDAs for protein, vitamins, and minerals and provide recommendations for total fat, saturated fat, cholesterol, and sodium. Maximum DVs are established for nutrients of fat, sodium, and cholesterol because of their linkages to the development of chronic diseases. However, maximum DVs for fiber, calcium, iron, and vitamins A and C are included because surveys reflect inadequate intake. The percent daily values show how the nutritional content of a particular food fits into a 2000-calorie diet. For an explanation of food labels, refer to Figure 15-2.

■ Age-Related Changes That Affect Nutrient Needs

METABOLISM

Total energy expenditure is composed of energy used at rest, in activity, and in thermogenesis. These components are affected by age, body size and composition, intake of energy, genetics, physiologic and pathologic conditions, and ambient temperature. Lean body mass declines, and as the muscle mass of the older person declines, energy requirements diminish. This makes it a challenge for older people to satisfy all of their micronutrient requirements through diet alone. Most health care providers ask older people to supplement their diet with at least one multivitamin on a daily basis.

Peripheral tissues of older people take up fat-soluble vitamins at slower rates; thus vitamin A and vitamin E intake results in higher circulating levels of vitamins A and E.

There is a decline in the immune function with age that may be responsible in part for the increased susceptibility to conditions such as infection and malignancy. There is some evidence that increased vitamin and mineral intake, including that of zinc, may counteract this age-related change (Chandra, 1992).

Metabolic utilization of vitamin B_6 is less efficient in older people. This in turn affects the immune system. Twenty percent of the older

TABLE 15-2 Summary of water-soluble vitamins

Name and coenzyme	Major functions	Deficiency symptoms
Thiamin; TPP	Glycolysis, citric acid cycle, and hexosemonophosphate shunt activity; nerve function	Beriberi: nervous tingling, poor coordination, edema, heart changes, weakness
Riboflavin; FAD and FMN	Citric acid cycle and electron transport chain activity; fat breakdown	Ariboflavinosis: inflammation of mouth and tongue, cracks at corners of mouth, eye disorders
Niacin; NAD and NADP	Glycolysis, citric acid cycle, and electron transport chain activity; fat synthesis, fat breakdown	Pellagra: diarrhea, bilateral dermatitis, dementia
Pantothenic acid; coenzyme A, acyl carrier protein	Citric acid cycle; fat synthesis, fat breakdown	Tingling in hands, fatigue, headache, nausea
Biotin; biocytin	Glucose production; fat synthesis; purine (part of DNA, RNA) synthesis	Dermatitis, tongue soreness, anemia, depression
Vitamin B_6, pyridoxine and other forms; PLP	Protein metabolism; neurotransmitter synthesis; many other functions	Headache, anemia, convulsions, nausea, vomiting, dermatitis, sore tongue
Folate; THFA	DNA and RNA synthesis; amino acid synthesis; red blood cell maturation	Megaloblastic anemia, inflammation of tongue, diarrhea, poor growth, mental disorders, birth defects
Vitamin B_{12} (cobalamin, methylcobalamin)	Folate metabolism; nerve function	Megaloblastic anemia, poor nerve function
Vitamin C (ascorbic acid)	Collagen synthesis; hormone and neurotransmitter synthesis	Scurvy: poor wound healing, pinpoint hemorrhages, bleeding gums

From Wardlaw, G.M., & Insel, P.M. (1996). *Perspectives in nutrition* (3rd ed.). St. Louis: Mosby.

TABLE 15-2 Summary of water-soluble vitamins—cont'd

Deficiency risk conditions	Adult RDA or ESADDI	Dietary sources	Toxicity
Alcoholism, poverty	1.1-1.5 mg	Sunflower seeds, pork, whole and enriched grains, dried beans, peas, brewer's yeast	None possible from food
Possibly use of certain medications if no dairy products consumed	1.2-1.7 mg	Milk, mushrooms, spinach, liver, enriched grains	None reported
Severe poverty where corn is the dominant food; alcoholism	15-19 mg NE	Mushrooms, bran, tuna, salmon, chicken, beef, liver, peanuts, enriched grains	Flushing of skin at intake levels >100 mg
Alcoholism	4-7 mg	Mushrooms, liver, broccoli, eggs (most foods have some)	None
Alcoholism	30-100 µg	Cheese, egg yolks, cauliflower, peanuts, liver	Unknown
Being female adolescent or adult; use of certain medications; alcoholism	1.6-2 mg	Animal protein foods, spinach, broccoli, bananas, salmon, sunflower seeds	Nerve destruction at doses of 2 gm/day or more for a few months or 500 mg/day for long-term use
Alcoholism; pregnancy; use of certain medications	180-200 µg	Green leafy vegetables, orange juice, organ meats, sprouts, sunflower seeds	None; nonprescription vitamin dosage is controlled by FDA
Being older, because of poor absorption; veganism	2 µg	Animal foods, especially organ meats; oysters; clams (not natural in plants)	None
Alcoholism; being older, male, and living alone	60 mg	Citrus fruits, strawberries, broccoli, greens	Doses >1-2 gm cause diarrhea and can alter some diagnostic tests; increased iron absorption can induce iron toxicity in some people

TABLE 15-3 Summary of fat-soluble vitamins

Vitamin	Major functions	Deficiency symptoms
A (retinoids) and provitamin A (carotenoids)	Promote vision, night and color; promote growth; prevent drying of skin and eyes; promote resistance to bacterial infection	Night blindness; xerophthalmia; poor growth; dry skin (keratinization)
D (cholecalciferol and ergocalciferol)	Facilitate absorption of calcium and phosphorus; maintain optimum calcification of bone	Rickets; osteomalacia
E (tocopherols, tocotrienols)	Antioxidant: prevent breakdown of vitamin A and unsaturated fatty acids	Destruction of red blood cells (hemolysis): nerve destruction
K (phylloquinone and menaquinone)	Help form prothrombin and other blood-clotting factors	Hemorrhage

Americans most at risk	Dietary sources	RDA	Toxicity symptoms
People in poverty, especially preschool children (still very rare)	Vitamin A: liver, fortified milk; provitamin A: sweet potatoes, spinach, greens, carrots, cantaloupe, apricots, broccoli	Women: 800 RE (4000 IU); men: 1000 RE (5000 IU)	Fetal malformations, hair loss, skin changes, pain in bones
Breastfed infants, older shut-ins	Fortified milk, fish oils, sardines, salmon	5-10 μg (200-400 IU)	Growth retardation, kidney damage, calcium deposits in soft tissue
People with poor fat absorption (still very rare)	Vegetable oils, some greens, some fruits	Women: 8 mg (alpha-tocopherol equivalents); men: 10 mg (alpha-tocopherol equivalents)	Muscle weakness, headaches, fatigue, nausea, inhibition of vitamin K metabolism
People taking antibiotics for months at a time (still quite rare)	Green vegetables, liver	60-80 μg	Anemia, jaundice

From Wardlaw, G.M., & Insel, P.M. (1996). *Perspectives in nutrition* (3rd ed.). St. Louis: Mosby.

TABLE 15-4 Summary of water and the major minerals

Name	Major functions	Deficiency symptoms	People most at risk
Water	Medium for chemical reactions, removal of waste products, perspiration to cool the body	Thirst, muscle weakness, poor endurance	Infants with fever; older persons especially those in nursing homes; endurance athletes
Sodium	A major electrolyte of extracellular fluid; nerve impulse conduction	Muscle cramps	People who severely restrict sodium to lower blood pressure (250-500 mg/day)
Potassium	A major electrolyte of intracellular fluid; nerve impulse conduction	Irregular heartbeat, loss of appetite, muscle cramps	People who use potassium-wasting diuretics or have poor diets, as seen in poverty and alcoholism
Chloride	A major electrolyte of extracellular fluid; acid production in stomach; nerve impulse conduction	Convulsions in infants	No one probably, as long as infant formula manufacturers control product quality adequately
Calcium	Bone and tooth strength; blood clotting; nerve impulse transmission; muscle contraction; cell regulation	Increased risk of osteoporosis	Women in general, especially those who constantly restrict their energy intake and consume few dairy products
Phosphorus	Bone and tooth strength; part of various metabolic compounds; major ion of intracellular fluid	Probably none; poor bone maintenance is a possibility	Older persons consuming very nutrient-poor diets; possibly vegans and people with alcoholism
Magnesium	Bone strength; enzyme function; nerve and heart function	Weakness, muscle pain, poor heart function	Women in general; people on thiazide diuretics
Sulfur	Part of vitamins and amino acids; drug detoxification; acid base balance	None has been described	No one who meets his or her protein needs

Continued

From Wardlaw, G.M., & Insel, P.M. (1996). *Perspectives in nutrition* (3rd ed.). St. Louis: Mosby.

*Values for calcium, potassium, and magnesium are RDAs. Values for other minerals are minimum requirements for health in adults.

†Just an approximation. It is best to keep urine volume greater than 1 L (4 cups) per day.

TABLE 15-4 Summary of water and the major minerals—cont'd

RDA or minimum requirement*	Nutrient-dense dietary sources	Toxicity
1 ml per kcal expended†	Water as such and in foods	Probably occurs only in those with mental disorders: headache, blurred vision, convulsions
500 mg	Table salt, processed foods, condiments, sauces, soups, chips	Causes hypertension in susceptible individuals, some increase in calcium loss in the urine
2000 mg	Spinach, squash, bananas, orange juice, other vegetables and fruits, milk, meat, legumes, whole grains	Causes slowing of the heartbeat; seen in kidney failure
700 mg	Table salt, processed foods, some vegetables	Causes hypertension in susceptible people when combined with sodium
800 mg (age >24 years); 1200 mg (age 11-24 years)	Dairy products, canned fish, leafy vegetables, tofu, fortified orange juice and other beverages, fortified bread and cereals	Very high intake may cause kidney stones in susceptible people and reduce mineral absorption in general
800 mg (age >24 years); 1200 mg (age 11-24 years)	Dairy products, processed foods, meats, fish, soft drinks, bakery products	Hampers bone health in people with kidney failure; causes poor bone mineralization if calcium intake is low
Men: 350 mg; women: 280 mg	Wheat bran, green vegetables, nuts, chocolate, legumes	Causes weakness in people with kidney failure
None	Protein foods	None likely

FIGURE 15-1 Food guide pyramid. *Courtesy U.S. Department of Agriculture.*

subjects in the Framingham heart study have reported low circulating levels of vitamins B$_6$ and B$_{12}$, along with low levels of folate (Rosenberg, 1994). It is thought that mild subclinical vitamin and mineral deficiencies play a part in declining neurocognitive function (Rosenberg & Miller, 1992).

DIGESTIVE SYSTEM

Many physiologic changes that occur with aging affect the digestive tract, but it is often difficult to separate these from pathologic or disease states. Age-related changes are presented in the following structures of the digestive system: oral cavity, esophagus, stomach, small intestine, colon, gallbladder, liver, and pancreas.

Oral cavity

As people age, there is an atrophy of the oral mucosa and underlying connective tissue and a resultant reduced ability to masticate (Baum & Ship, 1994). In some individuals, teeth become

more brittle, and there is a resorption of bone in the jaw, leading to loosening of teeth, increased infections in teeth and gums, and eventual loss of teeth. Some of these oral changes become evident as early as the fourth decade. Many older adults are edentulous and are faced with the challenge of wearing and caring for dentures. Ill-fitting dentures resulting from a change in gum structure may cause discomfort, which can result in poor nutrition.

Although in 1957, 55% of adults in the United States over 65 years of age were edentulous, in 1986 the percentage was down to 37% (Miller et al., 1987). Better nutrition, increased availability of dental care, advances in the prevention of dental diseases, and increased awareness of good dental health practices have contributed to the dramatic improvement of the dental health of older adults.

In the past it was thought that saliva production diminished with age. However, recent studies demonstrate that there is no change in saliva

Chili with Beans

Nutrition Facts

Serving Size 1 cup (253 g)
Servings Per Container 4

Amount Per Serving

Calories 260   **Calories from Fat** 70

	% Daily Value*
Total Fat 8g	13%
Saturated Fat 3g	17%
Cholesterol 130mb	44%
Sodium 1010mg	42%
Total Carbohydrate 22g	7%
Dietary Fiber 9g	36%
Sugars 4g	
Protein 25g	

Vitamin A 35%	•	Vitamin c 2%
Calcium 6%	•	Iron 30%

* Percent Daily Values are based on a 2,000 calorie diet. Your daily values may be higher or lower depending on your calorie needs:

	Calories:	2,000	2,500
Total Fat	Less than	65g	80g
Sat Fat	Less than	20g	25g
Cholesterol	Less than	300mg	300mg
Sodium	Less than	2,400mg	2,400mg
Total Carbohydrate		300g	375g
Dietary Fiber		25g	30g

Calories per gram:
Fat 9 • Carbohydrate 4 • Protein 4

Ingredients: kidney beans, water, tomato paste, butter, onions, salt, peppers, sugar, U.S. certified food color, and sodium nitrate

One serving of this food has 3 grams of a total of 20 grams of fat allowed on a 2,000 calorie diet. At 17% of the daily value it is moderately low in saturated fat.

At 42% DV one serving of this food is high in sodium.

% DVs for Calcium and Iron are for all calorie levels.

This information may be seen on larger labels and does not change from product to product.

FIGURE 15-2 Explanation of food label.

production in healthy older adults (Baum & Ship, 1994). The frequent reports of salivary loss mostly result from the fact that many older adults are taking medications that reduce salivary gland function. Oral complaints may be common, but age-related changes are not the cause. Although there seems to be less satisfaction with food, there is little to no evidence to suggest that taste buds are significantly altered by age alone (Weiffenbach, 1990). There does seem to be a slight decrease in an older person's ability to detect the taste of salt; otherwise, no significant change in taste ability has been shown to be age-related (Baum & Ship, 1994). Many older adults are at increased risk for inadequate food intake and poor nutrition because of multiple problems, both iatrogenic and physical, that lead to a loss of appetite.

Esophagus

The major age-related change in the esophagus is a smooth muscle weakness, which can result in delayed emptying and possible esophageal dilation. The lower esophageal sphincter may become incompetent, allowing a reflux of secretions from the stomach and therefore causing esophagitis. Gastroesophageal reflux disease is common in the U.S. population, and the prevalence increases after the age of 50 (Wu, 1994). The delayed emptying of the esophagus caused by the weakened muscle may give some people an unpleasant feeling of fullness in their chest under the sternum. The result can be diminished pleasure in eating meals (Brookbank, 1990).

Stomach

There is some controversy regarding whether or not gastric motility and emptying are affected by age. Some studies suggest a decrease in gastric mobility and emptying, whereas other studies do not. However, there is general agreement on the decrease in gastric acid secretion and the presence of some atrophic gastritis (Baime et al., 1994).

Small intestine

Although most of the essential nutrients are absorbed in the small intestine, few studies in human subjects have identified the effects of age on this organ. Changes associated with decreased function and atrophy of the small intestine may affect protein and fat absorption, as well as resulting in potential malabsorption of other nutrients, such as water-soluble vitamins, folate or vitamin B_{12}, iron, calcium, and vitamin D (Baime et al., 1994).

Colon

The colon plays a role in the digestive process and also plays a primary role as a storage organ. Age brings atrophy of the mucosa and a decrease in the musculature. Anorectal changes are caused by a loss of muscle elasticity.

It is difficult to differentiate changes in function that are the result of aging from those that are the result of decreased activity levels, long-term dietary habits, and side effects of medications (Sodeman, 1989). Nonetheless, it is gener-

ally recognized that many older people express concern about bowel function. Changes in bowel patterns are significant signals that call for prompt investigation of the possibility of abnormalities of the colon.

Gallbladder

The functions of the gallbladder include the concentration of bile and the delivery of bile to the small intestine. Studies have demonstrated that the common bile duct undergoes a progressive dilation with age, but at present, whatever changes may occur in the gallbladder are unknown. It is undisputed that the presence of gallstones increases with age, but advances in endoscopic therapy, lithotripsy, and dissolution therapy have improved management of biliary stones in older adults (Gilliam, 1994).

Liver

There is a substantial weight and size reduction in the liver in people between the ages of 60 and 90 years, as well as a decline in function. There is a decrease in the number of hepatic cells and, as a result, a diminished capacity for metabolism of drugs and hormones and a marked decrease in alcohol tolerance (Brookbank, 1990). Although there are structural and functional changes in the liver as people age, in the absence of disease, the liver usually retains an adequate level of reserve function in the healthy older adult.

Pancreas

Healthy older people who have no history of digestive diseases, alcoholism, or diabetes will have normal pancreatic exocrine function (Gilliam, 1994). Modern techniques, such as endoscopic retrograde cholangiopancreatography, have provided a more exact means of studying the effects of age on the pancreas. Special types of x-rays, computerized tomography, and ultrasound-guided needle biopsy have made it possible to examine this previously inaccessible gland.

In older adults, the pancreas is displaced to a lower position in the body, and there is dilation of the pancreatic ducts at the head, body, and tail of the pancreas. Fatty infiltration, fibrosis, and arteriolar sclerosis, as well as other abnormal changes, are frequent in the aged pancreas but do not seem to affect function to any great extent (Gilliam, 1994).

■ Psychosocial Factors Related to Nutrition

A number of factors other than physiologic changes affect older adults in meeting their nutritional needs. There are dynamic interrelationships among nutrition, aging, and health, which can only be understood in the context of the whole person. In addressing the care of older individuals, it is important to consider personal, cultural, socioeconomic, and psychologic influences. These are discussed in the following sections as they apply to the older adult.

PERSONAL FACTORS

People eat for many reasons other than to supply their bodies with essential nutrients. Food has multiple meanings for individuals and is linked with a person's way of life. There are personal beliefs about what is good food and what is not, which are associated with early conditioning, family tradition, and emotional satisfaction. These dimensions should be explored and analyzed before recommending changes in the eating behavior of older adults.

CULTURAL FACTORS

Perhaps the oldest and strongest aspects of a culture are the food habits of its people. Cultural background determines what is eaten, when it is eaten, and how it is eaten. Ultimately, food habits are based on availability, economics, and personal beliefs, but history and tradition play a part in the selection of foods. In many cultures, some foods and food practices have symbolic meanings. Ceremonies and religious rites, as well as major life experiences from birth to death, are closely related to gathering, preparing, serving, and consuming food. In many cases, older adults are the repositories of cultural traditions. They need to feel respected and to have their cultural heritage recognized. Dietary modifications should accommodate cultural habits whenever possible.

SOCIAL FACTORS

There are many social influences that affect older individuals in meeting their nutritional needs. Food is a symbol of sociability, warmth, and acceptance. Advice concerning food tends to be accepted from people who are deemed friendly and who are respected and trusted. The most long lasting and stable of food habits are those associated with family sentiments. Some foods have strong emotional ties related to family memories, which have little to do with their nutritional value. In addition, family income, community sources of food, availability of markets, availability of transportation, and ease of food preparation all play a part in food choices and intake. Limited sociability can lead to compromised nutrition. Older adults who live alone often skip meals or give food only cursory attention because it does not seem important enough to prepare food for one person. For those on fixed incomes, the expense of food can be an inhibiting factor in maintaining a balanced diet. Individuals may be unaware of or unaccepting of assistance programs such as food stamps and Meals on Wheels. These options should be explored with those older adults who could benefit from such support.

PSYCHOLOGIC FACTORS

A number of subjective elements condition the reaction to food. These elements are usually perceived as basic human drives and emotions, such as hunger, thirst, love, hate, fear, and joy. Other psychologic needs that can condition food reactions may include a sense of belonging, a need for adequacy, and a motivation to remain healthy.

In addition, the older person may be vulnerable to food fads. Misinformation about healthy foods and proper nutrition can lead to harmful food habits in all age groups. These practices are especially injurious to older people because they have less reserve on which to rely when they become malnourished. A number of food fads have existed in this country at various times and have gained many followers for short periods. Most of these fads are not based on scientific information, and even if they do not cause harm, they often fail to promote sound nutrition. They can result in disillusionment, and they are expensive. Older people may be easy prey to advertisers who promise relief from or a sure cure for a number of chronic problems with the use of a nutritional supplement. Lonely and ill people may be especially susceptible to some of these exaggerated claims for restoring health, vigor, or youth.

An example of a harmful food fad is the low-acid diet for arthritis. This diet excludes vinegar, additives, and preservatives. The harmful aspect of the diet is the exclusion of milk products, fruit, meat, and egg yolks, making it exceedingly difficult for the dieter to meet the requirements for a healthy diet.

ALCOHOL USE

It is estimated that over 15% of older adults over the age of 65 are problem drinkers. The experience of widowhood is identified as a risk factor in the development of problem drinking at an older age. Because alcohol is a depressant, it exacerbates not only loneliness but also any chronic disease the older adult may have. Tolerance to alcohol diminishes with age, and many times, its use leads to high-cost injuries such as falls.

■ Common Health Deviations

NUTRITIONAL DEFICIENCIES

Nutritional deficiencies or malnutrition in older adults can be caused by short- or long-term inadequacies in diets, such as deficiencies in specific nutrients or overall caloric energy. A diet is usually considered to be inadequate if it does not meet the needs of most healthy people in a particular age group. Dietary adequacy for older individuals should be individually determined.

In addition, a number of acute and chronic conditions can lead to nutritional inadequacies as a result of interference with food intake or retention, which may cause poor digestion, malabsorption, or loss of nutrients through excretion (Roe, 1987). Acute conditions tend to cause a reduction in food intake as a consequence of anorexia and an increase in metabolic demands. Chronic conditions are the most frequent type of disorders found in older adults, and they may manifest themselves with more subtle signs of malnutrition.

Protein calorie malnutrition

Acute protein calorie malnutrition Protein calorie malnutrition is a deficiency state that is most apt to be caused by acute and chronic disease but may be multifactorial in origin. This syndrome may develop in previously well-nourished or obese people who may be undergoing severe physiologic stress, such as that resulting from a starvation diet, severe infection, injury, or surgery. Signs of acute protein caloric malnutrition are apathy, weakness, edema, delayed wound healing, intolerance of anesthesia, susceptibility to adverse drug reactions, and impaired immune function (Roe, 1987). The condition can be reversed if diagnosed early enough and if prompt nutritional support is instituted. The oral route for nourishment is preferred if tolerated by the patient. In extreme situations, *enteral* (digestive tract) or *parenteral* (vascular system) feedings may be necessary. Diagnosis of this condition can be made by determining a clear history, carrying out a physical examination, identifying edema, and obtaining hematologic and biochemical studies showing lymphocytopenia and hypoalbuminemia, as well as deficient responses to skin tests.

Chronic protein calorie malnutrition Chronic protein calorie malnutrition is also termed *cachexia.* The most frequent etiologic factors in the development of cachexia are cancer, end-stage renal or hepatic disease, chronic neurologic disease associated with paralysis, and high-dose digitalis therapy. Cachexia is the result of severe wasting of the body over an extended period. It is caused by reduced energy and protein intake, combined with the catabolic effects of disease and excessive loss of nutrients by malabsorption or through protein-losing enteropathy. Manifestations of cachexia are emaciation, loss of subcutaneous fat, loss of lean body mass, brittleness of hair, ridged or banded nails, and a dermatosis of the lower area of the legs (Roe, 1987). Cachexia and acute protein calorie malnutrition may occur simultaneously. It may not be possible to reverse the course of cachexia, depending on the status of the chronic condition or disease that is the underlying cause. Aggressive nutritional support may be necessary, using total parenteral nutrition (TPN).

Protein malnutrition

Protein malnutrition differs from protein calorie malnutrition in that it is primarily the result of protein losses and not reduced intake. Specific causes are extensive burns, cancer, a blistering dermatosis (pemphigus), or severe renal disease with albuminuria. Treatment involves nutritional support and treatment of the underlying cause.

Vitamin deficiencies

Fat-soluble vitamin deficiencies Most often, the fat-soluble vitamin deficiencies found in older adults are in vitamins D, A, and K. Vitamin D deficiency results in *osteomalacia,* a condition in which there is a demineralization of the bone matrix, causing a generalized softening of bone (Porth, 1990). Vitamin A deficiency is not common in the older population as a whole, but some subgroups may be at risk, such as alcoholic individuals or people who have malabsorption syndrome.

Vitamin K deficiency can be caused by drugs or disease. Liver disease (such as cirrhosis or hepatitis) and drugs (such as anticoagulants or broad-spectrum antibiotics) can deplete vitamin K. Hemorrhage is the main sign of this deficiency, and it may be manifested as purpura or as bleeding from wound sites, from the gastrointestinal tract, or from body orifices. Vitamin K deficiency can be diagnosed when testing reveals a prolonged prothrombin time. It is treated by removing the cause and administering vitamin K.

Water-soluble vitamin deficiencies The water-soluble vitamin deficiencies of concern in older adults are those of vitamin B_{12}, folate, riboflavin, thiamin, vitamin B_6, and vitamin C. New data from the Framingham heart study suggest that the risk of folate and vitamin B_{12} deficiency increases with age and that as many as 20% of older adults may have low levels of vitamin B_{12}. Many of these vitamin deficiencies are often related to inadequate dietary intake, malabsorption caused by disease states, or adverse reactions to drugs. Deficiencies of thiamin and of vitamin B_6 are also related to alcohol abuse. In most cases these deficiencies can be treated successfully by replacement of the necessary vitamin. Full recovery is usual, except in instances where there has been long-standing neurologic damage, as in alcohol abuse or in undiagnosed pernicious anemia (Porth, 1990).

Findings from the Framingham heart study show that older adults with the highest blood levels of folic acid and vitamins B_6 and B_{12} have a significantly decreased risk of stroke (Lindenbaum et al., 1988). Some evidence exists to suggest that riboflavin requirements may be increased among people who have insufficient intakes of milk and milk products, as well as those who consume alcohol. In addition, it is known that there is a need to increase vitamin C intake, because surveys indicate that as much as 42% of the older population receives only half of the required amount of this important vitamin (Dwyer, 1991; USDHHS, 1989).

The importance of appraising the level of intake of vitamin D, especially in women at risk for osteoporosis, must be realized by health care providers. Particularly at risk are women living in the northern United States in the winter, because sunlight-generated vitamin D will be in scarce supply for them. It is recommended that dietary daily intake of vitamin D be kept at 400 IU (10 µg).

Mineral deficiencies

Usually, the intake of minerals, especially in the American diet, tends to be adequate, because the required amounts of minerals are relatively small (Roe, 1987). Malabsorption syndromes and drug reactions are causative factors in mineral deficiencies, which may include the following deficiencies in older adults: phosphate, potassium, magnesium, zinc, and iron.

DRUG-NUTRIENT INTERACTIONS

A number of drugs can cause malnutrition, especially when consumed by older adults, for whom multiple drug regimens are often prescribed. Sometimes more than one prescribed drug may deplete the same nutrient, which can result in a serious deficiency. An example of this is potassium depletion caused by use of both diuretics and laxatives. See Table 15-5 for drugs that may cause nutritional deficiencies.

Selected food-drug interactions can alter absorption, distribution, metabolism, and excretion of drugs. More drugs are prescribed for older adults than for any other age group in the United States. The practice of taking medications with very little fluid is not uncommon among older adults. In the presence of such a practice, the absorption of medications may be delayed. Fluids play an important role in drug absorption. Paradoxically, ice water, which is available to patients in the hospital or to residents in nursing homes, delays the dissolution of capsules.

Both food and food components may interact with drugs, and this can affect the drug's bioavailability. Food also may act as a mechanical barrier to medication, preventing the drug's access to the mucosal surface of the gastrointestinal tract. The

potential interaction of the following drugs with food should be considered. Acetaminophen is absorbed 5 times faster in fasting people than in people who have consumed a high-carbohydrate meal. Carbohydrates, particularly *pectin*

TABLE 15-5 Common drugs causing nutritional deficiencies in older adults

Drug group and drug	Deficiency
1. Cardiac glycosides	
Digitalis	Anorexia→protein energy malnutrition
	Zinc and magnesium deficiency
2. Diuretics	
Thiazides→	Potassium, zinc, and magnesium depletion
Furosemide	
Ethacrynic acid	
Triamterene→	Folacin deficiency
3. Anti-inflammatory drugs	
Aspirin	
Indomethacin→	Gastrointestinal blood loss→iron deficiency
Colchicine→	Malabsorption of fat- and water-soluble vitamins
4. Antacids (antacid abuse)	Phosphate depletion; osteomalacia
5. Laxatives (laxative abuse)	
Mineral oil→	Deficiency of vitamins A, D, and K
	Phenolphthalein (potassium deficiency)
	Multiple nutrient deficiencies due to malabsorption
	Folacin and vitamin D deficiency

From Roe, D. (1992). *Geriatric nutrition* (3rd ed., pp. 148-150, 167). Englewood Cliffs, NJ: Prentice-Hall. Reprinted with permission.

(an indigestible fiber), delay the absorption of acetaminophen (an analgesic), whereas proteins and lipids do not. Fasting causes a sevenfold increase in absorption of tetracycline (an antibiotic), and food intake reduces the absorption of tetracycline, ampicillin (an antibiotic), and hydrocortisone (a steroid hormone) (Barcheiya & Welling, 1982).

The age-related decrease in hydrochloric acid secretion that occurs in older adults can impair the absorption of calcium and iron and can delay the absorption of some drugs, such as amitriptyline (Elavil), diazepam (Valium), and some analgesics such as pentazocine (Talwin).

Emotional stress can delay gastric emptying. A decrease in gastric emptying in itself may create problems with the metabolism of medications such as penicillin, levodopa, and digoxin, making them less available for absorption in the small intestine (Evans et al., 1981). Alterations in circulation and body composition may have an effect on drug distribution. Total body weight may decrease in the very old, but the ratio of fat to lean tissue is usually greater than in younger years. Adipose tissue increases by about 18% to 30% in men and 35% to 48% in women (Rosenberg, 1994), which may cause an increase in the volume of lipid-soluble drugs such as diazepam and a decrease in the volume of water-soluble drugs such as acetaminophen. In addition, the plasma concentration may be decreased, and this may result in an elevated concentration of drugs such as warfarin (an anticoagulant).

In protein calorie malnutrition the albumin levels may fall. A decrease in the serum level of albumin will also decrease the duration of the action of medications that are bound to protein.

The oxidative capacity of the body also declines with age, and this decline is even greater among older adults who smoke cigarettes. This may affect the function of hepatic enzymes in detoxifying drugs.

High-protein diets can produce an acid urine (pH 5.9), whereas low-protein diets can produce alkaline urine (pH 7.5). If the urine is acidic, weakly alkaline drugs such as amitriptyline are excreted because they form water-soluble salts. Conversely, if the urine is alkaline, the drugs will be reabsorbed (Lamy, 1990a). Thus continued use of such drugs could lead to toxicity if older adults are regularly consuming low-protein diets. The dosage of drugs should be prescribed carefully, individually adjusted for older patients, and strictly monitored.

Drug-nutrient interactions are important to consider when caring for older adults, and identification of any over-the-counter vitamin, mineral, and amino acid supplements that an older adult may have purchased should always be included in a dietary assessment. Many health care professionals are unaware of the potential problems that can be averted by careful consideration of the older adult's dietary and medication habits.

■ Chronic Conditions Influenced by Nutrition

OBESITY

Obesity is a frequent nutritional problem among U.S. citizens and is very often found in the over-65 age group. *Obesity* is defined as being 20% or more over the ideal weight. The importance of body fat composition has also been a focus of recent research, because people with a greater muscle mass–to–fat ratio are not considered overweight, even if they are 20% over ideal body weight.

Problems arise in the understanding of what is the ideal weight and other individual variables because normal values in healthy people vary over a wide range. Two tables have been developed, one to demonstrate the range of normal weights and the other to highlight the difficulties in promoting one normal weight for individuals based only on height. The first table was developed in 1983 by the Metropolitan Life Insurance Company and the second was developed by the Gerontology Research Center. A comparison of these tables is seen in Table 15-6. Recent studies have shed new light on the interesting contro-

TABLE 15-6 Comparison of weights from Gerontology Research Center with those of Metropolitan Life Insurance tables*

Height (ft and in)	Metropolitan 1983 weights* (25-59 yr)		Gerontology Research Center age-specific weight ranges for men and women				
	Men	Women	20-29 yr	30-39 yr	40-49 yr	50-59 yr	60-69 yr
4 10	—	100-131	84-111	92-119	99-127	107-135	115-142
4 11	—	101-134	87-115	95-123	103-131	111-139	119-147
5 0	—	103-137	90-119	98-127	106-135	114-143	123-152
5 1	123-145	105-140	93-123	101-131	110-140	118-148	127-157
5 2	125-148	108-144	96-127	105-136	113-144	122-153	131-163
5 3	127-151	111-148	99-131	108-140	117-149	126-158	135-168
5 4	129-155	114-152	102-135	112-145	121-154	130-163	140-173
5 5	131-159	117-156	106-140	115-149	125-159	134-168	144-179
5 6	133-163	120-160	109-144	119-154	129-164	138-174	148-184
5 7	135-167	123-164	112-148	122-159	133-169	143-179	153-190
5 8	137-171	126-167	116-153	126-163	137-174	147-184	158-196
5 9	139-175	129-170	119-157	130-168	141-179	151-190	162-201
5 10	141-179	132-173	122-162	134-173	145-184	156-195	167-207
5 11	144-183	135-176	126-167	137-178	149-190	160-201	172-213
6 0	147-187	—	129-171	141-183	153-195	165-207	177-219
6 1	150-192	—	133-176	145-188	157-200	169-213	182-225
6 2	153-197	—	137-181	149-194	162-206	174-219	187-232
6 3	157-202	—	141-186	153-199	166-212	179-225	192-238
6 4	—	—	144-191	157-205	171-218	184-231	197-244

From Andres, R. (1990). Mortality and obesity: The rationale for height-weight age-specific tables. In W.R. Hazzard, R. Andres, E.I. Bierman, & J.P. Blass (Eds.), *Principles of geriatric medicine and gerontology* (2nd ed., p. 764). New York: McGraw-Hill.
*Values are for height without shoes and weight without clothes.

versy over what is a healthy weight for an older person. The review by Andres (1994) of weight, age, and mortality presents evidence that older people with the lowest weight and those with the highest weight are apt to die earlier than their peers. An American Cancer Society study suggests that men and women in their 70s should be permitted weight gain and it should be maintained into very old age (Lew & Garfinkel, 1979). Furthermore, studies have suggested that older people with weights that are relatively high have the lowest mortality (Andres, 1994).

The best approaches to the control of frank obesity include calorie restriction, modifications in behavior (eating patterns), and exercise. Older

people who are overweight do not necessarily overeat; rather, in many cases, it is just that they have a lower basal metabolic rate (BMR), and their energy expenditure is lower. Their caloric intake should be in the form of nutrient-rich foods, with avoidance of high-calorie, low-nutrient foods. Changes in lifestyle, well-defined eating schedules, activities that do not include high-calorie snacks, and eating companions who are following the same regimen help promote compliance with a lower-calorie diet. Principles of sound eating are based on a balance of energy needs with food intake. Special consideration should be given to ensuring that older dieters receive the recommended amounts of essential nutrients, because they are more subject to developing deficiencies than are younger people. In general, a food plan utilizing the food groups, with exchange lists, can be adapted for use with older adults.

ANEMIA

Anemia is a condition in which there is an abnormally low number of red blood cells, or abnormally low hemoglobin, or both. Some clinical and pathologic signs of anemia include excessive bleeding; destruction of red blood cells (hemolysis) or deficient red cell production caused by nutritional deficiency; lack of iron, folic acid, or vitamin B_{12}; and bone marrow failure (Porth, 1990). Anemia can be a health problem of all age groups, including older adults. In both men and women the incidence of anemia increases significantly with each decade. Based on 14 gm/100 ml as the normal level for hemoglobin, the second National Health and Nutrition Education Survey found a large percentage of older men to be anemic. A high prevalence of anemia also has been noted in older individuals in a variety of settings, such as hospitals, long-term care institutions, and geriatric clinics (Lipschitz, 1994).

There is some question regarding a reduction of hemoglobin levels as a result of the aging process in otherwise healthy people, but evidence does not totally support this concept. A longitudinal 5-year study of healthy, affluent older adults living in New Mexico failed to show any increased prevalence of anemia; in fact, none of the subjects at the first testing was anemic (Garry et al., 1983).

The most common causes of anemia in older adults appear to be inflammatory or chronic diseases, especially those of the intestinal tract, and nutritional deficiencies (Lipschitz, 1994). There is some debate regarding the limits of normal findings for hemoglobin and hematocrit levels in older adults. The normal adult mean levels routinely used in hematology for hemoglobin are 15.5 gm/100 ml for men and 13.6 gm/100 ml for women. Lipschitz (1994) recommended a level of 12 gm/100 ml as a lower normal limit for older men and women.

Treatment of anemia always depends on the cause. Nutritional deficiencies are treated with replacement of the missing nutrient; chronic illness or bleeding is investigated, and appropriate measures taken. In the case of drug-induced anemia, medication use is reexamined. In some cases, despite adequate intake of nutrients, additional nutritional supplements may be required. Nutritional deficiency anemia in older people usually results in normocyctic, normochromic anemia. Many times there is a history of weight loss, and there is most likely a reduced serum albumin level. This type of anemia is correctable with improved nutrition (Lipschitz, 1994).

DYSPHAGIA

Dysphagia is derived from the Greek words *dys,* meaning with difficulty, and *phagia,* meaning to eat. Dysphagia can occur in all age groups, but is associated with a poor prognosis in older adults. There are multiple causes of dysphagia in older adults that include not only physical, pathologic conditions, but also cognitive problems and use of certain medications. Dysphagia may occur with stroke, Parkinson's disease, multiple sclerosis, myasthenia gravis, esophageal cancer, peptic stricture, and gastroesophageal reflux. Drugs that injure the older adult's esophagus are most notably potassium chloride and quinidine. It is most important that older adults taking medication do so with at least 8 oz of water. The nurse should obtain information on history in regard to voice changes, sleep disorders, changes in eating habits, and effects of medication on swallowing (Castell, 1994).

DISORDERS OF THE ORAL CAVITY

Diseases of the oral cavity include yeast infections (candidiasis), leukoplakia, glossitis, and cancer. Candidiasis is treated with oral nystatin, an antifungal agent. Possible predisposing causes such as systemic infections, diabetes, or long-standing antibiotic administration are also examined. *Leukoplakia* are white patches that appear in the mouth and on the tongue and may be either benign or malignant. The majority of these lesions have no abnormal tissue and will clear up with careful oral hygiene, avoidance of irritants such as smoking and spicy food, and the treatment of carious teeth or infected areas. *Glossitis* is an inflammation of the tongue, which can be caused by nutritional deficiencies such as inadequate amounts of iron, riboflavin, and folacin. Cancer of the oral cavity can occur on the lips, tongue, mouth, and pharynx and may be cured if discovered early. Oral mucosa cancer rates rise with age, and 95% of all oral cancers occur after age 40, with the average age of 60 years at diagnosis (Baum & Ship, 1994). All conditions affecting the mouth can impair appetite and food intake and should receive close attention.

DISORDER OF THE ESOPHAGUS: GASTROESOPHAGEAL REFLUX

Symptoms of gastroesophageal reflux include substernal burning, dysphagia, and regurgitation and can be described in lay terms as "heartburn." Symptoms usually occur after meals and with postural changes. This is a problem experienced by many older adults, and studies have shown that the prevalence increases after the age of 50. A medical examination is necessary to exclude life-threatening conditions such as myocardial infarction.

Lifestyle modification is a necessary aspect of treatment for this chronic condition (Wu, 1994). Elevation of the head of the bed by 6 inches for night sleeping is recommended. Dietary modifications are aimed at decreasing consumption of foods that irritate the esophagus and impair esophageal sphincter function, such as fats, chocolates, alcohol, and carminatives. Other lifestyle modifications include decreasing smoking, refraining from eating before reclining, and weight loss for the overweight person. Medications should be reviewed, because many prescribed medications, such as anticholinergics, calcium channel blockers, theophylline, diazepam, and beta-adrenergic agonists, lower sphincter pressure.

The use of antacids is widespread and seems to be effective in 60% to 70% of people afflicted with esophageal reflux (Wu, 1994). Omeprazole is more effective in abolishing gastric acid secretions, and has been shown to be the most effective agent for medical treatment of gastric reflux disease. At this time the FDA recommends use for only 2 to 3 months because the drug has been reported to cause carcinoid-like tumors in rats. However, these tumors have not been reported in patients after long-term use of the drug (Wu, 1994).

DISORDERS OF THE STOMACH
Helicobacter pylori

Helicobacter pylori is an important human pathogen associated with chronic gastritis, peptic ulcer disease, and gastric cancer. This organism may remain in the stomach for many years and cause continuous inflammation. It is not an invasive pathogen and is amenable to treatment. A triple-pronged therapy consisting of bismuth, metronidazole, and amoxicillin or tetracycline is effective in up to 80% of cases (Logan et al., 1991).

Gastritis

Gastritis, a frequent condition of older people, occurs both as an acute and a chronic condition. Gastric and duodenal ulcers occur in the aging population in greater numbers than in younger age groups, with more older people having gastric than duodenal ulcers (Kerr, 1994). Age-related changes and long histories of normal use and abuse of substances such as alcohol are factors that contribute to the frequency of disorders of the stomach in the older adult population. Many older adults are affected by musculoskeletal problems such as osteoarthritis and make long-term use of salicylate or nonsteroidal anti-inflammatory drugs (NSAIDs). These drugs are often associated with a drug-induced gastritis (Lamy, 1990b).

With increasing age, people with ulcers are more apt to suffer serious complications. There is a risk of gastrointestinal blood loss in the older adult with gastric disorders. Early detection is important. Symptoms may be vague and easily dismissed by many older adults or even by those health care professionals who provide their care in nursing homes or in ambulatory settings. Abdominal pain, bloating after meals, dyspepsia, weight loss, and bleeding may be important clinical manifestations that call for a medical consultation. Bleeding is a major problem, and the mortality rate of the older person is 4% to 10% higher than that of younger people. Eighty percent of those who die from ulcer disease are over 65 years of age (Gilinsky, 1990).

Medical treatment often includes histamine$_2$ (H$_2$) blockers and antacids. These drugs also have some adverse effects that the nurse must know about when caring for an older patient. Many antacids are high in sodium content and may cause problems for those patients who should observe a low-sodium diet. Cimetidine (Tagamet), an H$_2$ blocker, can cause mental confusion or arrhythmias in some older patients; ranitidine (Zantac), another H$_2$ blocker, seems to have fewer adverse effects on older people than does cimetidine (Dawson, 1984).

HEPATIC AND PANCREATIC DISEASE

The most frequent causes of intrinsic liver disease are drug-induced hepatitis, post-transfusion hepatitis, and various types of cirrhosis. Hepatitis, regardless of etiology, has a serious prognosis in older adults because of their debility and the presence of concomitant diseases. One cause of cirrhosis is alcohol abuse.

Drugs that may cause liver injury include antihypertensives (alpha-methyldopa), antibiotics (nitrofurantoin, sulfonamide, ketoconazole, penicillin, erythromycin, and tetracycline), psychotropics (chlorpromazine and imipramine), hormones (estrogen and anabolic steroids), and anesthetic agents (Gilliam, 1994).

Metastatic cancer is the most common type of malignancy to affect the liver, and it may be evidenced by elevated levels of the enzymes aminotransferase and alkaline phosphatase and by an enlarged, irregular liver. Hepatic imaging techniques reveal an abnormal liver, and liver biopsy confirms the diagnosis. Treatment is supportive and palliative, and generally the course of the disease is not long.

Carcinoma of the pancreas has a poor prognosis (Gilliam, 1994). Although diagnosis has improved considerably in recent years with advanced imaging techniques and ultrasonography, there has been little progress toward definitive treatment. Palliative surgery may be done to bypass an obstructed common duct, but radiation therapy and chemotherapy have not shown any useful results. Performing a radical pancreatectomy is not recommended for an older patient. Pain relief and supportive care are the primary approaches to care for these individuals.

DEHYDRATION

Water depletion, or dehydration, is a serious health problem in the older population. It is responsible for a large number of hospital admissions and a significant morbidity and mortality rate among older people (Kositzke, 1990). Nurses need to be aware of and knowledgeable about the aspects of water balance, to be able to recognize disturbances and intervene appropriately when these disturbances occur in older patients. Both hydration and concentration of various body fluids are controlled by fluid intake and renal excretion. Ordinarily, water balance is maintained through thirst, fluid intake, and urinary fluid loss. A number of body mechanisms are operative in the function of thirst and urinary loss, such as the kidneys, the adrenal glands, and the endocrine system.

Four major age-related changes play a part in predisposing older adults to dehydration and hypernatremia (high blood sodium): a decrease in total body water, an altered sense of thirst, a lowered ability of the kidneys to concentrate urine, and a decrease in the effectiveness of the antidiuretic hormone (ADH) that helps the body to conserve water. Although these changes by themselves do not cause dehydration, they do contribute to an increased vulnerability in aged individuals and add to the risk of fluid balance problems. A number of acute and chronic diseases prevalent in the older population can inhibit renal function and increase the potential for dehydration. Conditions such as hypertension, congestive heart failure, renal disease, infections, fever, diarrhea, and central nervous system disorders that diminish the thirst sensation are among the many disorders that can affect fluid balance in older people.

Sometimes, diagnostic tests requiring fluid restriction or the use of hypertonic dyes can overtax the older adult's system and can lead to dehydration. A variety of drugs, including diuretics and laxatives, also can alter fluid and electrolyte balance (Todd, 1989). In addition to diseases that directly affect the renal system and fluid balance, other conditions (physical, mental, and psychosocial) may indirectly contribute to water depletion. For example, people with mobility problems might have difficulty obtaining adequate fluids if liquids are not readily accessible. People who are confused and have diminished cognitive ability may not be aware of the need to drink or of the sensation of thirst. Some older people, particularly women who have problems with incontinence, may deliberately restrict their fluid intake to avoid events of incontinence. Unfortunately, this practice adds to their difficulties by facilitating the development of infections and may actually increase the number of episodes of incontinence.

Symptoms associated with fluid and electrolyte imbalance may be attributed to other conditions or to old age if a careful assessment is not done. A fluid balance history is an important component of assessment. Dehydration may be manifested by the following (Kositzke, 1990):

Skin—dry, warm skin; dry oral mucosa; altered tongue turgor
Neurologic symptoms—confusion, disorientation, pathologic reflexes (seizures), change in affect
Cardiopulmonary symptoms—weak rapid pulse, altered respirations, orthostatic hypotension
Genitourinary symptoms—scanty or concentrated urine, with marked ammonia odor
Laboratory values—elevations in sodium, hematocrit, and blood urea nitrogen

Treatment is directed toward reestablishing a normal fluid balance as quickly and safely as possible, before serious complications, such as renal damage, occur. The oral route for fluids is preferred whenever possible. Water is the fluid that is best for patients, although a choice of fluids is important also, especially fruit juices. Tea, coffee, cola, and sweetened beverages are diuretic in nature and should be avoided if possible. For very ill patients, parenteral fluids may be necessary until their condition stabilizes. Careful monitoring assessment of the patient's physical and mental condition and careful monitoring of intake and output are important parts of the treatment regimen. The best treatment for dehydration is prevention. The watchful vigilance of nurses caring for vulnerable older patients may avert this all-too-common disorder, or at least may provide early detection and avoidance of complications (Reedy, 1988).

■ Nursing Process

ASSESSMENT
Nutritional assessment includes the following components:

1. Clinical assessment
2. Dietary assessment
3. Anthropometric assessment
4. Hematologic assessment
5. Biochemical assessment
6. Immunologic assessment
7. Diagnostic assessment

Clinical assessment

Clinical assessment employs the health history, the psychosocial history, and the physical examination to identify signs of nutritional deficiency.

Health history The health history records the patient's or significant other's description of the problems related to nutritional status, such as weight loss or gain, loss of appetite, nausea or vomiting, food intolerance, difficulty in swallowing, drugs being taken, digestive disturbances (e.g., heartburn, bowel problems), sore mouth or tongue, anemia, bleeding problems, and any disabilities that might prevent adequate nutrition.

It is of critical importance to get an accurate history concerning the older person's usual 24-hour intake of food and fluids. A 24-hour dietary diary is an excellent assessment tool if the older person or a caregiver is able and willing to provide the necessary information.

Other pertinent questions to ask about nutritional status are the following:

1. Have you noticed any weight gain?
2. Have you noticed any weight loss?
3. Have you been trying to gain or lose weight?
4. Have you noticed a change in your appetite?
5. Have you had any nausea or vomiting?
6. Have you had any difficulty in swallowing solids or liquids?
7. Have you had any heartburn?
8. Have you had any change in your pattern of bowel movements?
9. Have you noticed any sores in your mouth?
10. Have you had any unexplained bruising?
11. What medications do you take regularly, both prescription and over-the-counter?
12. Are you having any difficulties with nutrition that you would like to tell me about?

Psychosocial history The psychosocial history is concerned with age, sex, lifestyle, activities of daily living, and characteristics that relate to the ability to obtain and prepare food and to live independently, as well as food habits and fads, motivation, job skills, family support, and social skills.

Suggested lifestyle questions concerning nutritional status are the following:

1. How do you obtain your groceries?
2. Do you have anyone to assist you in obtaining groceries?
3. Do you have anyone assisting you in preparing your meals?
4. How many meals do you eat each day?
5. Do you eat alone?
6. How much of your meal do you usually eat?
7. Are you using Meals on Wheels?
8. Do you eat any meals outside of your home?
9. Do you have adequate finances to cover the cost of your food?
10. Is there anything about your food habits that you would like to tell me or that you think I should know?

Physical examination The physical examination includes the measurement of height and weight and the inspection and palpation of the skin and mucous membranes, primarily for signs of dryness, ecchymosis (bruising), and edema. Extremities are examined for weakness or tremor. Mental status is checked for signs of confusion, disorientation, memory loss, or mood disturbances.

The clinical assessment of an older adult can be especially challenging because of the multifactorial etiologies involved and also because the signs and symptoms are more vague and general in older adults and less specific to particular organs and functions. For instance, easy bruising can be the result of vitamin K deficiency, anticoagulant therapy, or simply the increased fragility of aging skin which results in spontaneous bruising. Another possible problem in performing clinical assessment of older adults is the tendency of health care professionals to minimize symptoms or to explain them away as signs of aging.

Dietary assessment

Dietary assessment is done for a number of reasons: to obtain data on food consumption patterns of individuals and groups over a period of time; to obtain actual food energy and nutrient intake information for each individual; to investigate episodes of food poisoning; and to assess the feeding practices of institutions where older adults are housed.

There are a number of methods of obtaining a dietary history, depending on the purpose for which the information is being obtained. In a history interview of an older patient, a record of food intake can be obtained by using a short questionnaire about food items, frequency of intake, methods of preparation, and amounts eaten.

Records of food purchases may also be obtained to determine the adequacy of diet indirectly. If a limited selection is being purchased repeatedly, this could reflect potential deficiencies. Another method of obtaining information from alert people without memory deficits is the 24-hour dietary recall. A food diary may be used with patients who have received complete instructions and understand what they are to record. This has the advantage of reducing dependence on unassisted recall.

The nurse's direct observation at mealtime can also help to assess food intake. This method can be used readily in hospitals and nursing homes.

Anthropometric assessment

Anthropometric assessment includes measurement of height, weight, midarm circumference, and skin folds; these measurements should be as accurate as possible. Special problems with these measurements in older adults are related to change in height caused by aging and the increased compressibility of the fat folds on the older adult's arm (Roe, 1987). In spite of these difficulties, anthropometric measurements can be useful in the initial assessment of nutritional status and in determining therapeutic progress. Combined with other types of assessment, such as gathering dietary and biochemical information, these measurements can be helpful as screening tools.

Hematologic assessment

Hematologic assessment serves as a screen for malnutrition. Determination of a complete blood count (CBC) with differential is needed to diagnose nutritional anemia, as well as to provide supporting evidence for the biochemical status and clinical assessment of the patient. Characteristic changes occur in the structure of the red and white cells, in the hemoglobin level, in the computed red cell indices, and in the packed red cell mass in nutritional anemias (Roe, 1987).

Biochemical assessment

Biochemical assessment can identify recent intake of nutrients, estimate nutrient stores in the body, and yield measures of nutritional adequacy and risk. Levels of albumin, transferrin, and a number of vitamins and minerals can be measured to assess clinical signs of deficiency. Serum albumin levels below 3.5 gm/100 ml may indicate protein malnutrition, although there is evidence of a decline in albumin levels related to age (Rosenberg, 1994). Biochemical measures should always be used in combination with other assessment tools because there are some limitations to these data taken alone (Roe, 1987). These factors, coupled with logistic difficulties in collecting samples and with the inadequate laboratory facilities in some long-term care institutions, should promote conservative interpretations of biochemical findings in older adults.

Immunologic assessment

This assessment involves the use of skin tests to identify delayed reactions to microbial and fungal antigens. Other indications of immune function are lymphocyte and differential white cell counts and albumin levels. Negative reactions on skin tests suggest serious protein energy malnutrition. Positive reactions can be interpreted as positive response to nutritional intervention, but negative findings do not necessarily solely indicate malnutrition. Age-related changes and cancer can also result in a diminished response to antigens.

Diagnostic studies

Diagnostic studies are often made by administration of the suspected deficient nutrient (or nutrients). It is important to consider safety in this type of diagnostic intervention and to avoid obscuring an accurate assessment. For example, administration of folic acid could mask the presence of pernicious anemia, with resultant neurologic damage. Other factors, such as response to treatment, could be the reason for positive outcomes, as well as the administration of a particular nutrient (Roe, 1987).

NURSING DIAGNOSES

Several nursing diagnoses have been identified by the North American Nursing Diagnosis Association (NANDA) for nutrition problems; those with particular relevance for older adults are listed here:

1. Altered nutrition: less than body requirements
2. Altered nutrition: more than body requirements
3. Altered nutrition: potential for more than body requirements

The nursing diagnosis most frequently encountered in older adults, and one of great concern to nurses caring for them, is altered nutrition: less than body requirements. In this state, an individual experiences an intake of nutrients insufficient to meet metabolic needs.

Defining characteristics

Weight loss to a weight 20% or more under ideal weight
Reported food intake less than RDA
Evidence of lack of food intake
Lack of interest in food
Aversion to eating
Reported altered taste sensation
Satiety immediately after ingesting food

Related factors

Advanced age
Depression
Stress in response to living alone
Societal influences

PLANNING AND GOAL IDENTIFICATION

A long-term goal would be that the patient will regain lost weight up to within 10% of ideal weight. A short-term goal would be to have the patient increase intake of nutrients, especially carbohydrates and proteins. Another goal, relating to socioeconomic factors, would be to have the patient gain knowledge about and use resources available in the community.

IMPLEMENTATION
In the acute care setting

There is a high prevalence of malnutrition in hospitalized older patients (Lipkin, 1990). Studies have shown that many older adults have severe protein calorie malnutrition at the time of admission to the hospital (Katz et al., 1986). The method of nutrient administration for the hospitalized older patient depends on the patient's nutritional status, the expected length of illness, the ability to swallow, the available gastrointestinal tract, and the metabolic response to illness (Goodwin & Wilmore, 1988). Nutritional requirements can change over the course of a hospitalization. As the patient recovers from a serious condition, metabolic needs decrease and the role of diet may change from that of restoring health to that of maintaining health.

Normal, oral self-feeding is the desired method for the older adult's obtaining nutritional requirements. Hogstel and Robinson (1989) emphasize the special importance of safety in feeding the hospitalized older adult, as well as the need for meeting essential nutrient requirements. They identify selection and consistency of foods, timing of meals, and the portions of food as considerations in providing safe nutrition for older patients. If the patient has impaired swallowing ability, the nurse assesses for gag and cough reflexes before the patient eats or drinks; these reflexes protect the person from aspiration (Thompson et al., 1989). It is also important for the nurse to ensure that the patient is in an appropriate sitting position while eating to avoid choking and/or aspiration.

Most older adults have increased energy needs while hospitalized. The food provided by the hospital may not be appealing to the older adult patient. The nurse is responsible for monitoring the older adult's response to the food that is served; the patient's intake at all meals should be recorded, and if adequate amounts of nutritious food are not being eaten, dietary adjustments should be considered.

If the patient is depressed or oversedated at mealtimes, the nurse should review the medications and consult with the physician. Reviewing an existing problem and making recommendations for change may increase the older patient's abilities to maintain oral feedings during hospitalization. Changes in medication schedules or discontinuation of some medications may be an appropriate intervention, depending on the particular situation. The nurse initiates appropriate consultation to determine ways to maintain the patient's oral nutrition while hospitalized.

The nurse employed in the hospital is one of the health care professionals whose responsibility it is to see that the nutritional requirements of patients are met. Preparation of meals and tray delivery are usually the role of the dietary department. The nurse is responsible for the care of the patient, however, and the nutritional status of the patient is an important component of that care. The nurse is a member of the health care team and practices on the basis of a team concept. Consultation with the dietitian and with members of the dietary staff is an essential role of the nurse in maintaining the older patient's nutritional state.

One intervention frequently used to meet the nutritional requirements of hospitalized patients who are admitted with weight loss, anorexia, or dehydration is a dietary or nutritional supplement. High-calorie, high-protein milk shakes are commercially available and are widely used to augment hospital diets. These liquid supplements replace fruit juices and soft drinks. They are given at scheduled times and may require the physician's, the dietitian's, or the nurse's order, depending on hospital policies. The role of the nurse is to provide comfort, restore and preserve function, manage symptoms, and prevent complications (Osato et al., 1993). With respect to diet, the nurse must acknowledge responsibility for monitoring nutritional requirements and for recommending interventions concerning those requirements within the context of consultation with other health care professionals.

Enteral feedings are necessary for many hospitalized older patients. Physical conditions that may prompt this type of nutritional support are anorexia, central nervous system disorders, head and neck surgery, stricture or resection of the esophagus, malabsorption syndromes, and trauma (Hatchett-Cohen, 1988). The route, location, and type of nutrient used in tube feedings can vary, according to the advantages and disadvantages for the individual patient. The choice of route is between the nasogastric and gastrostomy routes.

Nasogastric tubes are the most common. Silicone tubes are of small caliber, cause little patient discomfort, and are easily placed. There is a significant risk of aspiration pneumonia associated with improper placement of the tube. Agitation caused by the discomfort of the tube has led to patients extubating themselves (Ciocon et al., 1992). Many times this begins a downward cascade of events resulting in physical restraints that only make the agitation worse.

Gastrostomy can now be accomplished by percutaneous endoscopic tube placement, and patients who were poor surgical risks are now able to receive enteral nutritional support (Shuster & Mancino, 1994). This method may lessen the risk of aspiration that accompanies nasogastric tube feedings. A significant complication encountered with tube feedings is diarrhea (Galindo-Ciocon, 1993). The role of the nurse is to monitor the patient's condition in order to prevent complications, promote adequate nutrition, and maintain the dignity and emotional stability of the older adult. The wishes of the patient regarding the appropriateness of this type of feeding arrangement must be considered in the decision-making process.

Mechanical aspects of the tube used for feeding and its functioning need to be monitored. The tube may become clogged unless it is irrigated after every feeding and after medications are administered. Placement of the tube must be checked before each feeding, and the patient should be monitored for signs of aspiration. Precautions must be taken during and after feeding to ensure that the position of the patient helps to prevent aspiration. During feeding, the patient's position should be at least at a 45-degree angle. Mouth care should be frequent to meet the patient's oral hygiene needs.

The patient who is receiving tube feedings may experience diarrhea. Although not all patients experience this problem, it is not an unusual complication. The nurse should monitor the feeding, to be sure that it has not been contaminated by inappropriate handling or inadequate storage, then should check to be sure that the feeding has been administered correctly. To prevent further loss of fluid and nutrient requirements when any type of complication occurs, the nurse must consult with the physician and the dietitian regarding adjusting the feeding substance, the route of delivery, or the schedule. Nutritional care for the older hospitalized patient involves a joint effort by the patient, the family, the nurse, the dietitian, and the physician.

In the nursing home

The nursing home setting presents distinctive challenges to providing adequate palatable nutrition for older adults. Undernutrition of residents in nursing homes is characterized by eating dependency (being fed by someone), poor intake, depression, and oral-dental problems (Blaum et al., 1995).

Assessing the nutrient needs of nursing home residents, as well as planning and serving nutritious meals, is the responsibility of professional dietitians and professional nurses. Close collaboration and communication between these two disciplines is essential if the nutrition needs of older adults are to be met.

Observations about nutrition and older adults in nursing homes present several stark realities. At the outset it is important to consider that the nursing home is not the same as the resident's own home; it usually requires time for residents to adapt to the differences. In terms of food and meals, no facility or institution, no matter how good, can meet the expectations of "home cooking" often held by the nursing home resident. Having recognized this fact, and having provided time for the resident to adapt to a different environment, diligent efforts can be directed toward providing nutritious meals in a timely fashion, with a high degree of personal attention and concern for safety, and in a pleasant, sociable, supportive environment.

The dietitians plan the food to be served in the nursing home. Consideration is given to the selection of food from the six food groups to ensure variety, as well as adequate calorie, mineral, and vitamin consumption. Once the dietitian has planned the regular menu, special needs are considered. For example, special diets are defined for diabetic, obese, or underweight residents, or residents with special ethnic or religious food preferences; menus may be defined according to these needs. Other residents also require mandated menu or dietary adjustments, and these are defined regularly.

When the dietary personnel have fulfilled their responsibilities, nursing personnel engage in providing the nutrient care of the older adult. Nursing and dietary personnel collaborate in the serving of food, according to the system followed in the facility. Once the food is served, nursing personnel become responsible for the following:

- Arranging the food on the tray and placing the tray so that the older adult can reach the food
- Providing utensils that the resident can handle, such as specially designed utensils for arthritic and poststroke patients

- Cutting those foods that are larger than bite size to enable the older adult to consume the food without choking
- Informing the resident about the type of food on the tray and where it is placed; this is especially important for blind or other visually impaired residents
- Monitoring the consumption of food and providing support and assistance in eating when necessary (this may be periodic or continuous throughout the meal)

Self-feeding interventions for cognitively impaired nursing home residents have demonstrated marked improvement with cues both nonverbal and verbal (Osborn & Marshall, 1993). One case study of feeding accompanied by touching showed a marked increase in the amount of food ingested by residents with severe dementia (Singer, 1992). The nurse instructs and monitors the nursing assistants in the appropriate manner for accomplishing optimal food intake in cognitively impaired nursing home residents.

The environment of the dining area is a significant factor in promoting a positive response to mealtime in the nursing home. In addition to ensuring that the main dining area, satellite dining areas, or the resident's own room are physically conducive to a positive dining experience, attention to the social atmosphere of the dining area is important. The residents should be free to choose their own seating arrangements. If the arrangements are defined by the staff, eating partners or associates should be selected with attention to placing those with similar interests and abilities together. Staff should make their presence in the dining areas a positive addition, encouraging and stimulating conversation and socialization during the mealtime. Usually this type of pleasant surrounding results in the residents' eating more of the available food and enjoying the process of eating as well.

Mealtimes often become very important events for older adults. It is not unusual to see residents wending their way to dining areas well in advance of the time for a meal. Dining can be a positive experience for the resident if the delivery and serving of meals is accomplished in a timely manner. If meal delivery is delayed, residents can become annoyed and irritable, which negatively colors the experience of mealtime and eating. Staff members should make every effort to provide nutritious meals in a timely fashion and in a pleasant atmosphere, to stimulate appetite and ensure good nutrition for the older adults in a nursing home.

In the private or family home

The oft-repeated adage "There is no place like home" is probably more true for older adults than for members of other age groups. The mere number of years that older adults have lived puts them in a position to have become quite accustomed to the environs of their own home and their own routines and comforts, including food selection, acquisition, preparation, serving, and consumption. Health care professionals usually are diligent in planning and providing care for older adults that will enable their return to their home environment as quickly as possible, if appropriate care can be provided in the home.

In this era of cost containment efforts, an increasing number of therapy programs are being implemented in the home, thereby reducing the cost of care. The goal of home enteral feeding is to meet the patient's nutrient requirements without limiting the quality or the functional ability of the person (Shuster & Mancino, 1994). Criteria necessary for older people to successfully engage in home enteral feeding include the following:

1. Medical indications for enteral nutrition
2. Adequate financial and psychosocial resources
3. Cognitive ability and manual dexterity provided either by self or by a competent caregiver

Monitoring the patient's physiologic state is an important consideration for the community nurse. Weights, laboratory assessments such as

Shopping for produce. *Courtesy Loy Ledbetter, St. Louis.*

albumin, hydration signs, condition of the skin, and electrolytes are just a few of the items the nurse must continuously assess to ensure the health of the older home enteral feeding patient. The amount and type of formula delivered every day is an important element in the care of this patient. There are different methods for figuring caloric needs; one rule of thumb frequently used is as follows:

Weight maintenance	25 kcal/kg
Weight gain	35 kcal/kg
Weight loss	20 kcal/kg

The nurse works closely with a clinical dietitian and the physician to develop appropriate feeding amounts and schedules.

As the number of older adults is growing, so also is the number of services that are or that can be provided within and by communities. Increasing numbers of communities offer various options for older adults through a continuum of services specifically directed toward helping them meet their nutritional needs. Some of the programs are authorized by the Older Americans' Act, Title VII and Title III (Williams, 1989). These programs include food assistance, food stamps, and distribution of surplus agricultural commodities.

Under Title VII of the Older Americans' Act, services made available include outreach and referral, health services and counseling, nutrition and consumer education, and transportation. The program was developed to meet the social and nutritional needs of older people who could not afford adequate meals at home, were isolated, or lacked incentive to prepare and eat their meals alone. In 1978 the Act (Title III) was amended to coordinate other services with the nutrition services. Congregate and home-delivered meals, as well as related nutrition services and education, were funded under this amendment.

Congregate meals are provided in senior centers and other public or private community buildings where older people can gather for socializing and for eating a hot, nutritionally sound meal. The delivered meals are brought by couriers to the older person's home; this pro-

Healthy People 2000 Objectives

2.3 Reduce overweight to a prevalence of no more than 20% among people aged 20 and older and no more than 15% among adolescents aged 12 through 19. (Baseline: 26% for people aged 20 through 74 in 1976-80, 24% for men and 27% for women; 15% for adolescents aged 12 through 19 in 1976-80.)

2.5 Reduce dietary fat intake to an average of 30% of calories or less and average saturated fat intake to less than 10% of calories among people aged 2 and older. (Baseline: 36% of calories from total fat and 13% from saturated fat for people aged 20 through 74 in 1976-80; 36% and 13% for women aged 19 through 50 in 1985.)

2.6 Increase complex carbohydrate and fiber-containing foods in the diets of adults to 5 or more daily servings for vegetables (including legumes) and fruits, and 6 or more daily servings for grain products. (Baseline: 2½ servings of vegetables and fruits and 3 servings of grain products for women aged 19 through 50 in 1985.)

2.7 Increase to at least 50% the proportion of overweight people aged 12 and older who have adopted sound dietary practices combined with regular physical activity to attain an appropriate body weight. (Baseline: 30% of overweight women and 25% of overweight men for people aged 18 and older in 1985.)

2.8 Increase calcium intake so . . . at least 50% of people aged 25 and older consume 2 or more servings daily. (Baseline: 7% of women and 14% of men aged 19 through 24 and 24% of pregnant and lactating women consumed 3 or more servings, and 15% of women and 23% of men aged 25 through 50 consumed 2 or more servings in 1985-86.)

2.9 Decrease salt and sodium intake so at least 65% of home meal preparers prepare foods without adding salt, at least 80% of people avoid using salt at the table, and at least 40% of adults regularly purchase foods modified or lower in sodium. (Baseline: 54% of women aged 19 through 50 who served as the main meal preparer did not use salt in food preparation, and 68% of women aged 19 through 50 did not use salt at the table in 1985; 20% of all people aged 18 and older regularly purchased foods with reduced salt and sodium content in 1988.)

2.13 Increase to at least 85% the proportion of people aged 18 and older who use food labels to make nutritious food selections. (Baseline: 74% used labels to make food selections in 1988.)

2.18 Increase to at least 80% the receipt of home food services by people aged 65 and older who have difficulty in preparing their own meals or are otherwise in need of home-delivered meals.

2.21 Increase to at least 75% the proportion of primary care providers who provide nutrition assessment and counseling and/or referral to qualified nutritionists or dietitians.

From U.S. Department of Health and Human Services. (1990). *Healthy People 2000: National health promotion and disease prevention objectives* (DHHS Pub. No. [PHS] 91-50212). Washington, DC: U.S. Government Printing Office.

vides the meal and some human contact for the older adult. A public health nutritionist is available in some communities to provide counseling and nutrition education, as well as community program planning.

As the community health nurse establishes a liaison with older adults in their own homes, a different kind of responsibility is assumed for their care than the responsibility that is experienced by the nurse in the hospital or the nursing home. The nurse should be keenly aware of entry into the patients' territory. There should be conscious concern on the nurse's part that the space and privacy of the patient not be needlessly invaded. A fine line exists between intrusion and provision of assistance; mutual respect and trust can be established between patients in their homes and the nurse only through the nurse's appreciation of the dignity of the patient and with clear communication of intent. Initial visits might not yield accurate data about the patient. Only after trust has been established can the nurse expect to obtain the information necessary to help and to support the patient. Once a feeling of respect has been established, the nurse will set patient goals dependent on the situation that is encountered. Some of the nurse's concerns include the following:

- How does the patient obtain groceries? Are there family members nearby who can and will regularly do the grocery shopping? Will the family member and patient be able to select a balanced diet and nutritious foods?
- Who is available to prepare food? Can the patient prepare meals without assistance? Should plans be made for home health aides to provide assistance with meal preparation daily? Every other day? Three or 4 times a week? Weekly?
- Are the appliances (stove, refrigerator) safe for use by the older person? Is the patient reliable in the use of the stove? Is the patient reliable in the storage of food? Is the food in the refrigerator regularly sorted to ensure freshness?
- Can the older adult care for the dishes and utensils following a meal? Can the garbage and trash be disposed of appropriately by the patient, or is assistance needed in this activity?

The nurse must regularly monitor these aspects of nutrition and food provision. When other people such as home health aides or family members enter the picture, the nurse is responsible for supervising these people, as well as for regularly supervising or monitoring the patient's status and activities. With adequate support from

people and services, older adults usually are happier in their own private or family homes. Their quality of life is usually improved, and their life is often prolonged.

See the Healthy People 2000 Objectives box on page 421 for further nutrition indications.

EVALUATION

Evaluation of the effectiveness of nursing interventions and of the plan of care is based on achievement of desired patient outcomes, as stated in terms of long- and short-range goals. All goals in nutrition therapy may take considerable time to achieve. Expected outcomes are related to improving the health of and preventing complications in the older population.

REFERENCES

Anderson, J.J. (1990). Dietary calcium and bone mass through the lifecycle. *Nutrition Today, 25*(2), 9-14.

Andres, R. (1994). Mortality and obesity: The rationale for height-weight tables. In W.R. Hazzard, et al. (Eds.), *Principles of geriatric medicine and gerontology* (3rd ed., pp. 847-853). New York: McGraw-Hill.

Ausman, L.M., & Russell, R.M. (1990). Nutrition and aging. In E.L. Schneider & J.W. Rowe (Eds.), *Handbook of the biology of aging* (3rd ed., pp. 384-406). San Diego: Academic Press.

Baime, M.J., Nelson, J.B., & Castell, D.O. (1994). Aging of the gastrointestinal system. In W.R. Hazzard, et al. (Eds.), *Principles of geriatric medicine and gerontology* (3rd ed., pp. 683-692). New York: McGraw-Hill.

Barcheiya, R.H., & Welling, P.G. (1982). Influence of food on the absorption of hydrocortisone from the gastrointestinal tract. *Drug-Nutrient Interaction, 1,* 103.

Baum, B.J., & Ship, J. (1994). The oral cavity. In W.R. Hazzard, et al. (Eds.), *Principles of geriatric medicine and gerontology* (3rd ed., pp. 431-440). New York: McGraw-Hill.

Blaum, C., Fries, B., & Fiatrone, M. (1995). Factors associated with low body mass index and weight loss in nursing home residents. *Journal of Gerontology: Medical Sciences, 50*(3), 162-168.

Brookbank, J.W. (1990). *The biology of aging.* New York: Harper and Row.

Castell, D. (1994). Eating and swallowing disorders. In W.R. Hazzard, et al. (Eds.), *Principles of geriatric medi-*

cine and gerontology (3rd ed., pp. 1259-1268). New York: McGraw-Hill.

Chandra, R.K. (1992). Effect of vitamin and trace-element supplementation on immune responses and infection in elderly subjects. *Lancet, 340*(2), 1124.

Ciocon, J., et al. (1992). Comparison of intermittent vs. continuous tube feeding among elderly. *Journal of Parenteral Enteral Nutrition, 16*(6), 525-528.

Dawson, J. (1984). Effect of ranitidine on gastric ulcer healing and recurrence. *Scandinavian Journal of Gastroenterology, 19,* 665.

Dykes, M.H.M., & Meier, P. (1975). Ascorbic acid and the common cold: Evaluation of its efficacy and toxicity. *Journal of the American Medical Association, 231,* 1073-1079.

Evans, M.A., et al. (1981). Gastric emptying in the elderly: Implications for drug therapy. *Journal of the American Geriatrics Society, 29,* 201.

Galindo-Ciocon, D. (1993). Tube feeding: Complications among the elderly. *Journal of Gerontological Nursing, 14,* 17-21.

Garry, P.J., et al. (1983). Iron status and anemia in the elderly. *Journal of the American Geriatrics Society, 31,* 389.

Gilinsky, N.H. (1990). Peptic ulcer disease in the elderly. *Gastroenterology Clinics of North America, 19,* 255.

Gilliam, J. (1994). Hepatobiliary disorders. In W.R. Hazzard, et al. (Eds.), *Principles of geriatric medicine and gerontology* (3rd ed., pp. 683-692). New York: McGraw-Hill.

Goodwin, C., & Wilmore, D. (1988). Enteral and parenteral nutrition. In D. Page (Ed.), *Clinical nutrition* (pp. 476-503). St. Louis: Mosby.

Hatchett-Cohen, L. (1988). Nasogastric tube feeding. *Geriatric Nursing, 9*(4), 88-91.

Hogstel, M., & Robinson, N. (1989). Feeding the frail elderly. *Journal of Gerontological Nursing, 15*(3), 16-20.

Katz, P., Dube, D., & Calkins, E. (1986). Special issues in malnutritional therapy. In E. Calkins, P. Davis, & A. Ford (Eds.), *The practice of geriatrics* (pp. 145-148). Philadelphia: W.B. Saunders.

Kerr, R. (1994). Disorders of the stomach and duodenum. In W.R. Hazzard, et al. (Eds.), *Principles of geriatric medicine and gerontology* (3rd ed., pp. 693-705). New York: McGraw-Hill.

Kositzke, J.A. (1990). A question of balance: Dehydration in the elderly. *Journal of Gerontological Nursing, 16*(5), 4-11.

Lamy, P. (1990). Adverse drug effects. *Clinics in Geriatric Medicine, 6*(2), 293-308.

Lamy, P. (1980b). *Prescribing for the elderly.* Littleton, MA: John Wright PSG.

Levine, M. (1986). New concepts in the biology and biochemistry of ascorbic acid. *New England Journal of Medicine, 314,* 892-902.

Lew, E., & Garfinkel, L. (1979). Variations in mortality by weight among 750,000 men and women. *Journal of Chronic Disease, 32,* 563.

Lindenbaum, J., et al. (1988). Neuropsychiatric disorders caused by cobalmin deficiencies in the absence of anemias or macrocytosis. *New England Journal of Nursing, 318,* 1728.

Lipkin, E.W. (1990). Enteral/parenteral alimentation. In W.R. Hazzard, et al. (Eds.), *Principles of geriatric medicine and gerontology* (2nd ed., pp. 269-303). New York: McGraw-Hill.

Lipschitz, D.A. (1994). Anemia in the elderly. In W.R. Hazzard, et al. (Eds.), *Principles of geriatric medicine and gerontology* (3rd ed.). New York: McGraw-Hill.

Logan, R.P., et al. (1991). One week eradication regimen for helicobacter. *Lancet, 338,* 1249.

Lowenstein, F.W. (1986). Nutritional requirements of the elderly. In E.A. Young (Ed.), *Nutrition, aging and health* (pp. 61-89). New York: Liss.

Miller, A.J., et al. (1987). *The national survey of oral health in the United States adults: 1985-1986* (U.S. Department of Health and Human Services, Public Health Service, National Institutes of Health, NIH Pub. No. 87-2868). Washington, DC: U.S. Government Printing Office.

National Research Council. (1989). *Recommended dietary allowances* (10th ed. rev.). Washington, DC: National Academy of Science.

Osato, E., et al. (1993). Clinical manifestations: Failure to thrive. *Journal of Gerontological Nursing, 19*(8), 29-34.

Osborn, C., & Marshall, M. (1993). Self-feeding: In nursing home residents. *Journal of Gerontological Nursing, 19*(3), 7-14.

Porth, C.M. (1990). *Pathophysiology: Concepts of altered health states* (3rd ed.). Philadelphia: J.B. Lippincott.

Reedy, D.F. (1988). How can you prevent dehydration? *Geriatric Nursing, 9*(2), 224-226.

Reif, T.R. (1987). Water and aging. *Clinics in Geriatric Medicine, 3*(2), 403-411.

Roe, D. (1987). *Geriatric nutrition* (2nd ed.). Englewood Cliffs, NJ: Prentice Hall.

Rosenberg, I. (1994). Nutrition and aging. In W.R. Hazzard, et al. (Eds.), *Principles of geriatric medicine and gerontology* (3rd ed.). New York: McGraw-Hill.

Rosenberg, I., & Miller, J. (1992). Nutritional factors in physical and cognitive function in the elderly. *American Journal of Clinical Nutrition, 55,* 1237S.

Shuster, M., & Mancino, M. (1994). Ensuring successful home tube feeding in the geriatric population. *Geriatric Nursing.*

Singer, H. (1991). *A study of the effect of touch during feeding on the food intake of dementia residents.* Unpublished master's study, Georgetown University, School of Nursing, Washington, DC.

Sodeman, W.A. (1989). Bowel habits. In W.A. Sodeman, T.A. Saladin, & W.P. Boyd (Eds.), *Geriatric gastroenterology* (pp. 85-108). Philadelphia: W.B. Saunders.

Sutnick, M.R. (1988). Dietary guidance for the elderly. *Clinics in Geriatric Medicine, 4*(1), 193-202.

Thompson, J.M., et al. (1989). *Mosby's manual of clinical nursing* (2nd ed.). St. Louis: Mosby.

Todd, B. (1989). Diuretics' dangers. *Geriatric Nursing, 10*(4), 212-214.

U.S. Department of Health and Human Services. (1992).

VanderJagt, D.J., Garry, P.J., & Bhagauan, H.N. (1987). Ascorbic acid intake and plasma levels in healthy elderly people. *American Journal of Clinical Nutrition, 46,* 290-294.

Viteri, F. (1988). Vitamin deficiencies. In Paige et al. (Eds.), *Clinical nutrition* (pp. 547-578). St. Louis: Mosby.

Weiffenbach, J., et al. (1990). Oral sensory changes in aging. *Journal of Gerontology, 48,* 45-121.

Williams, S.R. (1989). *Nutrition and diet therapy.* St. Louis: Times Mirror/Mosby.

Wu, W. (1994). Disorders of the esophagus. In W.R. Hazzard, et al. (Eds.), *Principles of geriatric medicine and gerontology* (3rd ed., pp. 683-692). New York: McGraw-Hill.

Yearick, E.S., Wang, M.S.L., & Pesias, S.J. (1980). Nutritional status of the elderly: Dietary and biochemical findings. *Journal of Gerontology, 35*(5), 663-671.

O sleep, O gentle sleep,
Nature's soft nurse, how have I frighted thee,
That thou no more wilt weigh my eyelids down
And steep my senses in forgetfulness?

WILLIAM SHAKESPEARE, *Henry IV, Part 2*

Sleep

■ Learning Objectives

On completion of this chapter, the reader will be able to do the following:

1. Identify the stages of normal sleep.
2. Understand how aging influences sleep patterns.
3. Describe sleep disorders that occur as people age.
4. Recognize what promotes or inhibits sleep in older adults.
5. Assess sleep patterns of older adults.
6. Develop a plan of care for an older adult experiencing a sleep pattern disturbance.
7. Identify appropriate nursing interventions for older adults with sleep pattern disturbances.
8. Promote healthy adaptation of older adults to changes in the sleep cycle caused by aging.

Sleep is a cyclic activity that is experienced by every human. At times this activity is a satisfying experience that one smiles about and rejoices in. At other times it is a distressing and frustrating experience that leaves one feeling at odds with the world. It is an experience to be longed for when one seeks rest and refreshment. At the same time, it can be a time-consuming and nonproductive experience. Nevertheless, sleep is a basic human need and is essential to the well-being of every person. Despite the recognition of the importance of "good sleep," few scientists are able to recite the elements that constitute good sleep, or provide a universal recipe for achieving a good sleep each time one decides to experience it. Many variables enter into each person's sleep experience, and each variable or set of variables can play a definitive role in each sleep experience.

Sleep is a fascinating and somewhat mysterious phenomenon in the daily experience of every human being. It occupies almost one third of a person's life and undergoes considerable variation in its patterns as a person grows and matures. In the early months of life, babies spend 17 of every 24 hours asleep. The total amount of sleep gradually decreases until adulthood, when the average person spends about 7 to 8 hours in sleep; in the later years of life, many individuals do not experience a period of unbroken sleep as they did in earlier adulthood.

425

The need for sleep must be met at regular intervals to preserve mental and physical well-being. However, there is much that is still unknown about sleep and its function. For instance, there is a wide variation in sleep duration and there is no universal standard for specifying the number of hours of sleep that each person requires. For older adults, sleep is a major health issue, and disturbed sleep or inadequate sleep is one of the most common complaints encountered by health professionals who care for older adults. Age is a significant variable in each person's experience of sleep; each person responds to the age factor and all of the related variables in different ways. It behooves each nurse who cares for older adults, as a responsible health care giver, to acquire as much knowledge as possible about sleep so that the person who is experiencing aging can learn to cope with the experience of sleep in a positive and constructive way.

■ Functions

Sleep is a period of relative unconsciousness, and although there is little research to support any particular functions of sleep, it seems to be a time when the body is repairing and restoring itself. The generally accepted functions of sleep are said to be recuperative and integrative (McCance & Heuther, 1990). The processes concerned with *recuperation,* such as repair, restoration, and growth, take place during deep sleep. The process of *integration* involves the brain's organizing and filing the day's activities and occurs during the more active stage of sleep, called "rapid eye movement" (REM) sleep. A number of physiologic processes are altered during sleep and have the potential to affect the health of the individual (Kryger et al., 1994; Thelan et al., 1994). Until quite recently, however, the physiologic basis for clinical treatment was derived almost exclusively from the wakeful state (Kryger et al., 1994). During sleep, there are changes in blood pressure, heart rate, respiration, and temperature. These vital signs may be increased or decreased, depending on the particular stage of sleep. Also, increases in the secretion of some hormones, such as the growth hormone, parathyroid hormone, thyroid-stimulating hormone, and adrenocorticotropic hormone (ACTH), have been noted, as have increases in cerebral blood flow and gastric secretion; renal volume, on the other hand, decreases (Kryger et al., 1994; McCance & Heuther, 1990).

■ Measurement

"Sleep is a state of consciousness distinct from waking during which we are generally unaware of our bodies and minds" (Shaver & Landis, 1994). The frequency and amplitude of brain waves distinguish sleep from waking and characterize specific stages of sleep; these waves can be recorded on a computer screen and paper (electroencephalogram [EEG]) and demonstrate what are generally classified as four stages of sleep. At the beginning of sleep, a short time is spent in stage 1—transitional sleep. Young and healthy people spend about 20% to 25% of sleep time in this stage. The person then enters a light sleep called stage 2, where 45% to 55% of sleep time is spent. About 13% to 23% of sleep time is then spent in stages 3 and 4—a deep sleep—and about 20% to 25% is spent in REM sleep (Box 16-1).

There are two major types of sleep: non-rapid eye movement (NREM) sleep and REM sleep. *NREM* sleep is a period of slow eye movement and normal muscle tension. There are four stages of NREM sleep: stage 1 is the lightest level of sleep, during which a person can be aroused easily; stage 2 is deeper than stage 1 but is still a light level of sleep; in stage 3, sleep becomes progressively deeper; and stage 4 is the deepest level. Stages 3 and 4 are often referred to as "slow-wave sleep" because of the characteristic brain waves, or as "deep sleep" because of the level of consciousness, which is markedly decreased. Stages 1 and 2 are called "light sleep" because of the light level of unconsciousness in, or the easy arousal from, these stages.

REM sleep is the dream state in which the person's eyes are constantly moving, although

> **BOX 16-1 TYPICAL NIGHT OF SLEEP**
>
> 20% to 25% in stage 1
> 45% to 55% in stage 2
> 13% to 23% in stages 3 and 4
> 20% to 25% in REM sleep

otherwise the person has almost no muscle tension. In fact, all but the eyes and the respiratory system show a form of paralysis in this state. This paralysis is nature's way of protecting the sleeping person from acting out the vivid dreams taking place. People who wake up immediately from a dream may experience a transient sleep paralysis, which only lasts a few moments and is a normal sensation. The REM period is characterized by a very active brain wave pattern, resembling the electroencephalogram of the wakeful state, described as an "alpha rhythm."

A night of sleep begins with an NREM period, which lasts for about 90 minutes before an REM period begins. Then the two types of sleep, REM and NREM, alternate with one another throughout the night, with the average cycle being about 90 to 100 minutes in the healthy adult. Four to six cycles occur during a usual night of sleep. As the night progresses, the periods of deep sleep shorten and the intervals of REM sleep lengthen. Overall, about 20% of total sleep is spent in REM periods. The pattern is approximately the same for both old and young adults.

■ Age-Related Changes

A number of physiologic dimensions are altered as a person ages, but contrary to popular belief, total sleep time does not change drastically. Total daily sleep duration values tend to be the same for healthy older and younger adults. Changes do

occur, however, in the quality and continuity of the sleep experience. Older adults experience less deep sleep, more frequent awakenings in the night, and an earlier awakening in the morning (Dowling, 1995). Modifications appear in the time spent in all of the various stages of the sleep cycle. As a person ages, less and less time is spent in the deep sleep stages 3 and 4. In fact, stage 4 may be completely absent in the older adult, and increasing time is spent in the light sleep stages 1 and 2. Not only is there a shift to more time in the lighter stages of sleep with older adults, but also, all stages appear to be lighter with advancing age, as indicated by easier arousal in stages 3 and 4 and a lower auditory arousal threshold during all stages.

Those processes that occur regularly over a 24-hour period are said to follow *circadian rhythms.* Although sleep is perhaps one of the most fundamental of the biologic processes characterized by such rhythms, its normal function is not completely understood (Kryger et al., 1994). Some questions have been raised regarding the effects of an aging circadian system on deterioration of sleep in older adults (Alward & Monk, 1995). It is still not clear how much of the obvious changes in the sleep cycles of older adults may be caused by the aging of the internal rhythm system and how much may be caused by other factors; further study is needed.

One of the most intriguing aspects of sleep research is that concerned with the pacemaker mechanism in the brain that influences the sleep-wake cycle (Figure 16-1). Much information has been gained in the past 20 years, but much more information is needed to understand the influence of circadian rhythm in our lives.

■ Influences on Sleep

A number of factors can enhance or disrupt the usual patterns of sleep for the older adult. These can be described as "direct" and "indirect" influences of aging on sleep. The *direct influences* are the normal physiologic changes that occur with the aging process, such as changes in the amount

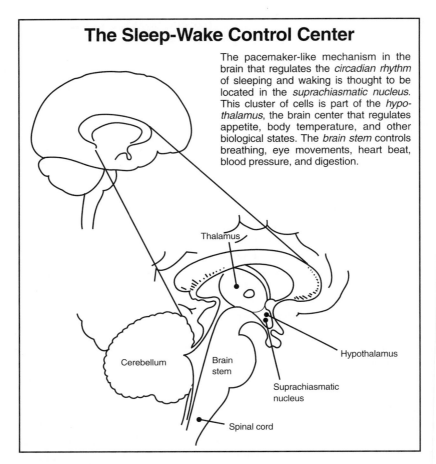

The Sleep-Wake Control Center

The pacemaker-like mechanism in the brain that regulates the *circadian rhythm* of sleeping and waking is thought to be located in the *suprachiasmatic nucleus*. This cluster of cells is part of the *hypothalamus*, the brain center that regulates appetite, body temperature, and other biological states. The *brain stem* controls breathing, eye movements, heart beat, blood pressure, and digestion.

Thalamus

Hypothalamus

Cerebellum

Brain stem

Suprachiasmatic nucleus

Spinal cord

FIGURE 16-1 The sleep-wake control center. Location of the brain mechanism that regulates circadian rhythms of sleep and waking. (From Harvard Health Letter. [1995, January]. *A special report: Sleep disturbance.* Boston: Harvard Medical School Health Publications Group.)

of time spent in the stages of NREM sleep and changes in the circadian rhythm. The *indirect influences* are further divided into the following:

1. *Internal events,* which are primarily physiologic or biologic in nature, such as diseases (e.g., heart disease and respiratory disorders) or reactions to medications
2. *External events,* which are social in nature, such as irregular schedule, physical environment, and family situations

The direct influences of age changes are not as well understood or as easily modified as are the indirect ones (Thelan et al., 1994).

It is difficult to interpret the impact of all the factors that influence the sleep patterns of older adults, but it is important to be aware of them. There are wide variations among individuals. Generalizations about the group should not be applied to an individual without first validating their applicability to that individual. Not all aging individuals change at the same rate, in the same way, or at the same time in their lives; in regard to sleep, some individuals hardly change at all. Bonnet and Arand (1989) raise the question of whether age changes in the sleep of older adults may cause chronic sleep deprivation or whether these changes may actually reflect decreased sleep need. Webb (1989) describes the changes in sleep that occur with aging as being pervasive, systematic, and usually irreversible.

Age-related changes clearly develop in most people. What remains unclear is whether these changes are an intrinsic or natural part of aging or whether they are the result of pathologic developments that have increased as the aging process has progressed. Sleep researchers identify this as a critical issue, because although some changes seem to be relatively innocuous, others, in the severe form (such as apnea), may be life threatening (Kryger et al., 1994).

■ Classification of Sleep Disorders

The Sleep Disorders Classification Committee, established in 1979 and composed of well-known sleep researchers, defined and classified an extensive list of sleep disorders in the journal *Sleep*. Their list is the generally recognized classification, and it comprises four main categories:

1. Disorders of initiating and maintaining sleep (DIMS)
2. Disorders of excessive somnolence (DOES)
3. Disorders of sleep-wake schedule
4. Dysfunctions associated with sleep, sleep stages, or partial arousals (parasomnias)

These classifications are based on symptomatic evaluations of patients and do not address the etiology of the disorder. There are also some disorders that have symptoms related to more than one category. A summary of these classifications with accompanying characteristics is provided by Buchholtz (1987).

DIMS, sometimes referred to as insomnias, are manifested by delayed sleep onset, frequent nighttime awakenings, and early morning awakening. Affected patients complain of fatigue and

general lack of energy but usually do not complain of excessive daytime sleepiness.

DOES, or *excessive waketime sleepiness (EWS),* cause patients to have difficulty staying awake during regular activities such as working and driving, manifesting themselves in histories of accidents and unsatisfactory work performance. Patients with these disorders may or may not have nocturnal sleep complaints, depending on the cause of the disorder, although frequent disruptions of nighttime sleep certainly can leave a person with excessive daytime sleepiness.

Disorders of the sleep-wake schedule (circadian rhythm disturbances) can be minor or severe. People with jet lag from changes in time zones, or people changing shifts or facing other disruptions in daily routine are able to adjust if given a few extra hours or days without serious responsibilities. Some patients in acute care units without day-night cues may have severe fragmentation of sleeping and waking, which can retard their recovery. These patients may complain of both DOES and insomnia because of the asynchrony between their sleep-wake schedule and the actual time of day.

Dysfunctions associated with sleep, sleep stages, or partial arousals (parasomnias) include a number of miscellaneous behaviors, such as *somnambulism* (sleepwalking), sleep-related headaches and seizures, *bruxism* (tooth grinding), nightmares, and cardiovascular symptoms. Usually, these behaviors only occur during sleep, and waking time is normal. Disturbances in sleep-wake schedule and sleep dysfunctions can also cause excessive sleepiness or disorders in initiating and maintaining sleep. There is some overlap in these categories.

■ Sleep Disorders in Older Adults

INSOMNIA

Insomnia is a frequent sleep complaint of older adults. It is usually described as the feeling that a person has not slept well or long enough. It is a symptom, not a definitive diagnosis, and may be expressed as difficulty in falling asleep (requiring more than 30 to 40 minutes), frequent awakenings during the night, or awakening too early in the morning and being unable to fall asleep again. Older adults are vulnerable to insomnia because of altered sleep patterns. The experience of insomnia may be that of *transient insomnia* that lasts only a few days, *short-term insomnia* that lasts a few weeks, or *long-term insomnia* that can last indefinitely.

The most frequently encountered form of sleeplessness is known as *learned insomnia,* in which the person learns to associate the bedroom with wakefulness. This can be precipitated by certain stressful events, mild depression, or some type of emotional problem.

Helping the older adult to cope with insomnia is a challenge and requires patient and persistent direction and support. Among the various techniques that may be used to help the insomniac are the following: lifestyle modification, sleep restriction to selected and scheduled hours, relaxation techniques, and drugs that are administered in a supervised and carefully monitored program.

Transient insomnia may be caused by a variety of temporary changes in a person's life, such as stress, minor physical conditions, travel, and new surroundings. By definition, transient insomnia is temporary, and it may correct itself or respond to reassurance and removal of the cause, when this is possible. As any adult is able to do, the older adult is often able to adapt to new circumstances or a new environment, or to cope with minor difficulties that are perceived as not long lasting. With the support of family, friends, or caregiver, the older adult is able to avoid becoming locked into this insomnia for any period of time.

Short-term insomnia can last as long as 3 weeks and may be precipitated by anxiety or by worries about social and personal losses that are prevalent in the lives of older adults. The death of a close relative or friend, social isolation, physical confinement, and excessive concern about health are some of the reasons for short-term insomnia. Professional help may be sought, or the person may use some individual strategies to try to alleviate the problem. Some people recognize that grief or worry is causing sleeplessness. They may seek out the companionship of close friends or other family members and also utilize home remedies, such as a glass of milk or a light snack at bedtime, a warm bath, soothing music, watching TV, prayer, or reading (e.g., the Bible or some type of meditative book). Some individuals, who have not been accustomed to living alone, develop a routine of calling some special person to say good night, or ask friends or family to call them at bedtime. On occasion, short-acting sleeping medications, particularly benzodiazepines (Bonnet & Arand, 1990), may be indicated to provide rest. These are neither the treatments of choice in general nor the first choices for treatment in older adults.

Long-term insomnia is the result of more permanent conditions, including such things as a noisy environment, chronic medical conditions, alcohol and other drug abuse, other sleep disorders, or psychiatric, emotional, or mental problems of long standing. In many cases, treatment of a known underlying cause will relieve the sleeplessness. However, the cause is not always known. Insomnia is a complex condition and requires careful assessment to help determine the best course for intervention. This is especially true when the insomnia has existed for an extended period and when there may be multiple factors influencing it. Good sleep usually means good health, and poor sleep may be the signal that there is some dysfunction or problem, such as a physical or psychologic disorder (Hauri & Linde, 1991).

A variety of medications are used periodically by people who experience sleeplessness. These should be taken with caution by anyone, especially by older adults, and not very frequently; these especially should not be taken routinely or frequently enough to become addictive. Each of the groups of sleeping pills has certain hazards associated with its use. One compound that continues to be recommended is tryptophan. This is an amino acid (a protein constituent) that is normally converted to the neurotransmitter serotonin. In 1989 the Food and Drug Administration (FDA) imposed a ban on the sale of isolated tryptophan after an impurity in one batch caused a rare blood disease that killed several people. Although the compound itself is probably harmless, it has no noticeable sedative properties (Harvard Mental Health Letter, 1994a; Tryptophan, 1990).

HYPERSOMNIA

Hypersomnia is classified as a member of the DOES grouping. People with this complaint are concerned that they sleep excessively. The person or a member of the family may report this, or it may be observed by a staff member. The condition may be caused by lack of sleep at night or by boredom, depression, physical confinement, or a number of other causes. If there is a continual feeling of tiredness, lack of energy, and irresistible sleepiness, the person could be suffering from narcolepsy, a chronic, little-known sleep disorder. *Narcolepsy* is a severe form of excessive sleepiness affecting 1 out of every 100 Americans. Over 50% of these cases remain undiagnosed. This condition may be called "sleep attacks," because the individual may find it impossible to remain awake and may fall asleep during almost any activity, even eating, walking, driving, or carrying on a conversation. Narcolepsy tends to be a condition of the early years, however.

Nonetheless, hypersomnia in general is not uncommon in older adults, although what appears to be hypersomnia may actually be a disturbance of the sleep-wake cycle brought on by some of the factors previously mentioned that have disturbed circadian rhythms. With older individuals, hospitalization or admission to a nursing home may cause this disturbance in sleep patterns. Most people will have some disruption in sleep, at least temporarily, if they are moved from their usual sleeping environment. For older individuals, this disruption tends to be more of a problem because of the decreased sleep efficiency, which may already be present, caused by age changes. *Sleep efficiency* is the proportion of time spent actually sleeping, in relation to the overall time spent in bed; this proportion is frequently reduced in older people.

NOCTURNAL MYOCLONUS

Nocturnal myoclonus, also called sleep-related myoclonus or periodic leg movement syndrome (PLMS), is characterized by repetitive leg contractions that occur in clusters during sleep; this is another dysfunction commonly associated with sleep in older adults. The clusters can last from 5 to 60 minutes, and the leg jerks occur at a rate of one every 30 seconds (Buchholtz, 1987). PLMS is sometimes called "restless legs syndrome" and may manifest itself as insomnia with sleep fragmentation.

Nocturnal myoclonus has multiple etiologies. Deficiency diseases such as calcium and potassium deficiencies and iron deficiency anemia can cause sleep-related myoclonus. Diabetes, uremia, withdrawal from some sedative or hypnotic medications, and abuse of caffeine or alcohol may also result in this condition. There are many cases in which there is no known cause, but there are also cases in which the condition occurs in patients with other sleep disorders. Polysomnography, a diagnostic test utilizing an EEG, an electromyogram (EMG), and an electrooculogram (EOG), is required for definitive diagnosis. There should be careful evaluation and search for any associated problems. Treatment involves correcting the underlying cause, if possible, followed by judicious use of medication to suppress the leg jerks. Most medications tend to suppress arousal rather than the contractions and should be used with caution because of the potential for increased drowsiness. Short-acting benzodiazepines are generally used when there is substantial nighttime sleep disruption (Bonnet & Arand, 1990; Snow et al., 1988). In some cases, light exercise before bedtime and quinine at bedtime might be helpful as well (Buchholtz, 1987).

SLEEP APNEA

Sleep apnea is a condition in which there are episodes of cessation of breathing during the night, sometimes as many as 300 times. Sleep apnea is a relatively recent discovery, which fits under the fourth classification of sleep disorder, as a dysfunction associated with sleep or sleep stages. It tends to affect mostly middle-aged, overweight men but may affect either sex at any age (Harvard Health Letter, 1995).

There are two types of sleep apnea: central and obstructive. In *central apnea,* the diaphragm contracts ineffectively or not at all, and thoracic breathing ceases. Respiration resumes as a result of arousal. In *obstructive apnea,* the oropharyngeal airway collapses or the pathway is obstructed by soft relaxed tissue, pressure builds up, and eventually the airway is cleared with a loud snorting sound (Figure 16-2). This condition is becoming more widely recognized in older adults (Ancoli-Israel, 1989; Bliwise et al., 1990; Harvard Health Letter, 1995), and it is potentially life threatening. Sleep apnea is characterized by daytime sleepiness because of interrupted sleep

FIGURE 16-2 Snorting occurs when dangling or loose tissue such as that of the *uvula, tonsils, adenoids,* or *tongue* vibrates during breathing. These tissues can also block the airway, causing obstructive sleep apnea. Poor muscle tone or excess weight around the neck can also lead to snorting and apnea by reducing the width of the trachea. (From Harvard Health Letter. [1995, January]. *A special report: Sleep disturbance.* Boston: Harvard Medical School Health Publications Group.)

at night. Ironically, the person with apnea may not be the one to identify his or her problem because the arousal periods are quite brief, though frequent. The sleep partner may be the one to recognize the sleep disturbance.

In addition to the loud snorting and excessive daytime sleepiness, signs and symptoms of sleep apnea are the following:

1. Broken sleep with frequent arousals
2. Unusual nighttime activity, such as sitting upright, sleepwalking, and falling out of bed
3. Nocturia
4. Morning headaches
5. Orthopnea
6. Cardiovascular signs (hypertension, irregular rhythm)
7. Mental and emotional signs (depression, memory changes, and anxiety)

The first clues to this disorder may be revealed when the patient's history is taken.

Several forms of treatment are available: surgery, drug treatment, position training, weight loss, and continuous positive airway pressure (CPAP) (Buchholtz, 1987; Harvard Health Letter, 1995; "Sleep apnea," 1989). CPAP, still a relatively new procedure, has become the treatment of choice. A mask is worn over the nose at night, through which a continuous flow of air, powered by a small compressor, is delivered by way of a length of large tubing. The device has been engineered so that the wearer can move and even sleep sideways while the airway is kept open by the continuous pressure. If the patient is cooperative and motivated, this treatment is quite successful. Use of CPAP is virtually free of complications and has been quite effective with older patients ("Sleep apnea," 1989; Thelan et al., 1994). See Figure 16-3 for an illustration of the use of CPAP.

SUNDOWN SYNDROME

A condition that occurs most often in people with cognitive dysfunction is "sundown syndrome," so called because it is more prominent

FIGURE 16-3 Continuous positive airway pressure, or CPAP. (From Sleep apnea: A new solution. [1989, July]. *Harvard Medical School Health Letter, 14*[9], 4.)

in the late evening. It is manifested by a state of increased confusion and disorientation, accompanied by wandering, talking, or inappropriate behaviors, at the usual bedtime. This may happen with an individual who, at other times of the day, is relatively alert and oriented. Although nurses in long-term care institutions have long been familiar with this phenomenon, it has not received a great deal of attention or study (Evans, 1987).

■ Effects of Acute and Chronic Illness on Sleep

Acute and chronic pathophysiologic conditions can disrupt sleep. Pain and discomfort from injuries and infections, to which older adults are prone, may result in problems of initiating and maintaining sleep, as well as dysfunction in the sleep-wake cycle. If the acute condition requires prolonged bed rest or enforced immobility, then sleep patterns can be seriously affected. Early ambulation and re-establishment of usual daily routines are especially important in averting sleep disturbances.

Chronic conditions are a part of the everyday life of many older adults. A number of older adults are afflicted with more than one chronic disorder. Heart conditions such as congestive heart failure (CHF), angina, and myocardial infarction (MI) may prevent restful sleep or may become exacerbated during sleep. Duodenal ulcers may be more active at night because of increased gastric secretions. Respiratory distress caused by chronic obstructive pulmonary disease (COPD) is often increased at night. Arthritic pain and stiffness intensify with the inactivity of sleep and may be the cause of frequent awakenings or difficulty in falling asleep. Urinary tract infections or diuretic therapy for cardiovascular conditions may cause nocturia, requiring frequent arousals for trips to the bathroom. Treatment of these disorders and other conditions that are secondary causes of sleep disruption often can effect dramatic improvement in the sleep pattern (Bliwise, 1989; Haponik, 1990).

Psychosocial problems and cognitive deficits also have an impact on sleep quality. Depression is a common problem in older adults and responds well to antidepressant therapy. However, investigators are unsure whether sleep changes that result from depression improve with therapy, because sleep response to antidepressant therapy has not been closely monitored (Hoch et al., 1992). Prolonged anxiety and life stresses are etiologic factors in sleep pattern disturbances, which, if recognized, may be successfully treated with supportive approaches.

Sleep is usually impaired in people with dementia, especially those with Alzheimer's disease (AD). The sleep impairment is probably caused by brain degeneration, which is a prominent feature of all dementias. "Disturbances of sleep and sleep-wake rhythms are a common clinical observation in AD; nighttime insomnia and wandering often become factors in the family's decision to institutionalize their demented relative" (Vitiello & Prinz, 1989, p. 290).

In the early stages of Alzheimer's disease, sleep-wake pattern changes are significant. These changes are apparent even before there is a marked decrease in cognitive functioning. As the disease progresses, so also do the sleep-wake changes, with a breakdown in circadian sleep-wake rhythm and an increase in daytime napping. There may be some benefit derived from minimizing daytime napping to increase nighttime sleep (Vitiello & Prinz, 1989). Overall, however, the outlook for improvement in sleep disorders caused by dementia is not promising, and this area needs further study. It is one of the most difficult aspects with which to cope in the care of the patient with Alzheimer's disease.

■ Drugs and Sleep

Older adults respond differently and less predictably to drugs than do younger people. "The combination of altered sleep, sleep pathologies and pharmacology in aging results in higher risk of drug induced insomnia and excessive daytime sleepiness among older persons" (Roehrs & Roth, 1989, p. 395). Pharmacokinetic processes of absorption, distribution, biotransformation, and elimination are altered in the older patient. Drug absorption seems to be the least affected of these four processes, even though there is a reduction in gastric pH and diminished gastrointestinal motility and emptying.

Distribution of drugs is altered significantly because of a decrease in lean body mass and a change in body composition, with an increased percentage of body fat and a decreased percentage of body water. There is a decline in plasma protein concentration, so there is less protein binding of some drugs.

Metabolism or biotransformation of drugs is slowed as a result of diminished liver function, which causes higher amounts of active drug to remain in the bloodstream for a longer period.

Elimination of drugs from the body is also altered, as a result of the decreased function of the kidneys, thus adding to the problem of accumulation of drugs in the body. The overall effect of all these changes in pharmacokinetics in older adults is "excessive, prolonged, and most importantly, adverse responses to standard doses of drugs" (Roehrs & Roth, 1989, p. 396). The number of older adults with drug-related sleep disorders is much larger than that of younger people. The most common symptoms of drug-related disorders are daytime sleepiness and nocturnal insomnia. See Table 16-1 for general categories of drugs that have an effect on the sleep-wake patterns of older individuals.

Drug therapy for older adults should involve judicious use, close supervision and monitoring, frequent evaluation, and early discontinuance. Although these are good guidelines for any individual who is taking medications, they are even more important for older adults because of multiple diseases, extensive drug use, and increased risk of drug interactions (Vestal, 1990).

Some authorities take the position that sedative-hypnotic drugs (sleeping medications) should not be prescribed for the older population at all (Ancoli-Israel, 1989), and many others agree that nonpharmacologic approaches should be thoroughly explored before sleeping medications are ordered (Gillin, 1990; Haponik, 1990; Vestal, 1990). It is much easier not to start taking medications for sleep than it is to stop, because dependence occurs so quickly. Nonetheless, sleeping medications have been and continue to be taken by older adults with sleep complaints (Gillin, 1990). The following substances have been utilized quite often by older adults to relieve sleeplessness.

Alcohol, although not considered a medication per se, has been widely used for years as a sleep aid, often self-prescribed. It can be relaxing and sleep promoting, but only on a limited basis. After the initial sleepiness wears off, there may be early and frequent awakenings. Alcohol also has serious side effects of tolerance, abuse, and dependence, which are well known. In addition to alcohol, *over-the-counter sleeping pills* are probably the most frequently used substances. These drugs are usually antihistamines and are not consistently effective.

Benzodiazepines, prescription medications, are probably the least harmful of the hypnotics and have become the drugs of choice to promote sleep. These drugs have been noted to reduce sleep latency (the time it takes to fall asleep), to reduce intervening awakenings, to increase total sleep time, and generally to improve personal satisfaction with sleep. The benzodiazepines are classified by the duration of the half-life of the drug's activity in the body, as follows: *long,* 20 to 100 hours; *intermediate,* 10 to 19 hours; or *short,* 3 to 9 hours. There is general agreement that the long-acting drugs should not be prescribed for older adults because of the prolonged hangover effect and the severe inhibition of daytime functioning (Gillin, 1990).

Intermediate- and short-acting benzodiazepines are the preferred drugs for use with older patients. Although triazolam, a short-acting preparation, has enjoyed recent popularity as the ideal sleeping pill, some serious drawbacks have been associated with its use (Gillin, 1990). Because it is so short acting, people wake up in a few hours and tend to take additional doses. Amnesia (lasting several hours) and other undesirable effects (such as hyperexcitability and daytime anxiety) have been reported (Gillin, 1990). The Public Citizen Health Research Group has recommended an intermediate-action drug, oxazepam, as the safest of the benzodiazepines for older adults because it seems to be less addictive than the others, has fewer side effects, and has a relatively short (12-hour) period of activity in the body (Wolfe et al., 1988). See Table 16-2 for a list of the benzodiazepines.

Barbiturates were formerly the standard sleeping pills but are rarely used now. These drugs were always somewhat problematic when used by older adults because of idiosyncratic effects (unexpected agitation, confusion, and wakefulness). The barbiturates are more hazardous than the benzodiazepines, with lethal overdoses not uncommon. The barbiturates also interfere with the metabolism of other drugs and are particularly dangerous when combined with alcohol (Gillin, 1990; U.S. Pharmacopeia, 1990).

Chloral hydrate, a drug that has been used clinically over a relatively long period, appears to

TABLE 16-1 Drugs and their potential effects on sleep-wake cycle

Category and generic name	Trade name	Effects
DEPRESSANTS		
Barbiturates		
Secobarbital	Seconal	Decreased slow-wave sleep, suppressed REM, increased onset of sleep and total sleep, rapid tolerance
Pentobarbital	Nembutal	
Narcotics		
Meperidine	Demerol	Suppressed REM, drowsiness, unusual dreams, sometimes insomnia
Morphine	Morphine	
Codeine	Codeine	
Benzodiazepines		
Flurazepam	Dalmane	Increased total sleep and onset, decreased REM and slow-wave sleep, residual daytime sleepiness
Oxazepam	Serax	
Triazolam	Halcion	
Alcohol		Decreased REM, early and frequent awakenings, apnea
TRANQUILIZERS		
Meprobamate	Miltown, Equanil	Daytime drowsiness, short-term memory loss
Hydroxyzine	Atarax, Vistaril	
ANTIPSYCHOTICS		
Thioridazine	Mellaril	Daytime drowsiness, confusion, impaired attention, short-term memory loss
Haloperidol	Haldol	
Chlorpromazine	Thorazine	
ANTIDEPRESSANTS		
Tricyclics		
Imipramine	Tofranil	Increased periodic leg movements, increased tiredness, suppressed REM
Monoamine oxidase inhibitors		
Isocarboxazid	Marplan	Improved sleep in depressed people
Phenelzine	Nardil	
STIMULANTS		
Methylxanthines	Caffeine, Theophylline	Delayed sleep onset, increased wakefulness
Amphetamines	Dexedrine	Delayed sleep onset, reduced total sleep and slow-wave sleep, frequent awakenings
ANTIHISTAMINES		
Diphenhydramine	Benadryl, Benylin	Daytime drowsiness, confusion, delirium

TABLE 16-1 Drugs and their potential effects on sleep-wake cycle—cont'd

Category and generic name	Trade name	Effects
ANTIHYPERTENSIVES		
Diuretics		
Chlorothiazide	Diuril	Frequent awakenings to urinate if drug is given late in
Hydrochlorothiazide	Esidrix	day
Furosemide	Lasix	
Beta-blockers		
Propranolol	Inderal	Insomnia, nightmares, hallucinations
Timolol	Blocadren	
Methyldopa	Aldomet	Daytime sleepiness
Clonidine	Catapres	Insomnia, fragmented sleep, suppressed REM
CARDIOVASCULAR DRUGS		
Digoxin	Lanoxin, Digoxin	Drowsiness, nightmares, hallucinations
Disopyramide	Norpace	Confusion, impairment of short-term memory

From Gillin, J. C. (1990, May). Sleeping pills. *Harvard Medical School Health Letter, 15,* 5-8. Roehrs, T. A., & Roth, T. (1989). *Drugs, sleep disorders and aging. Clinics in Geriatric Medicine, 5*(2), 395-404. United States Pharmacopeia (1990). *United States Pharmacopeia: Drug information for the consumer.* Rockville, MD: U.S. Pharmacopeial Convention. Wolfe, S. et al. (1988). *Worst pills, best pills: The older adult's guide to avoiding drug induced death or illness.* Washington, DC: Public Citizen Health Research Group.

TABLE 16-2 Benzodiazepines: sedative-hypnotic drugs

	Generic name and brand name	Half-life (hr)
Long acting	Diazepam (Valium)	100
	Flurazepam (Dalmane)	50-100
Intermediate	Lorazepam (Ativan)	12
	Temazepam (Restoril)	10-17
	Oxazepam (Serax)	3-21
Short acting	Triazolam (Halcion)	3

Adapted from U.S. Pharmacopeia. (1990). *United States Pharmacopeia: Drug information for the consumer.* Rockville, MD: U.S. Pharmacopeial Convention. Morgan. (1987).

be a safe drug for use in older adults. There are few side effects in the usual sleeping doses, and a number of physicians feel it is the least harmful of the sleeping medications for older people (Gillin, 1990). At this point there is no reported research in older adults to support or disprove these claims (U.S. Pharmacopeia, 1990).

As mentioned previously, use of sleeping medications for older people should involve judicious consideration, close supervision and monitoring, frequent evaluation, and early discontinuance (Haponik, 1990; Roehrs & Roth, 1989).

■ Nursing Process

ASSESSMENT

The assessment of the older adult with a sleep disturbance focuses on two main groups of data:

1. *Subjective data,* including a sleep history and if possible a sleep diary (Harvard Health Letter, 1995)
2. *Objective data,* including physical examination (with special attention to characteristics indicating that the person may have a sleep disorder), health record

BOX 16-2 SUGGESTED QUESTIONS FOR A SLEEP HISTORY

- What bothers you most about your sleep habits?
- How long have you had trouble sleeping, and what do you think started the problem? Did it come on suddenly?
- How would you describe your usual night's sleep? What time do you go to bed? When do you wake up?
- What is your bedroom like?
- What do you do in the few hours before bedtime?
- Do you follow the same sleep pattern during the week and on weekends? If not, how are weekends different?
- How well do you sleep on the first few nights when you're away from home? At home, do you sleep better in your bedroom or in another room in the house?
- Do you fall asleep at inappropriate times or in inappropriate places?
- What medications or drugs (such as alcohol or nicotine) do you use? Have you ever taken sleep medications? If so, which ones?
- Do you have physical aches and pains that interfere with sleep?
- Do allergies or nasal congestion bother you at night?
- Do you often have indigestion at night?
- Do you ever feel discomfort or a "fidgety" sensation in your legs and feet when you lie down? Do you have to get up and walk around to relieve the feeling?
- Do you ever have trouble breathing when you lie down, or do you awaken because it is hard to breathe?
- Does your bed partner or roommate mention that you snore loudly or gasp for air in the night?
- Do you ever awaken with a choking sensation or a sour taste in your mouth?
- Do you wake up with a headache or cramps in your legs?
- How have you been feeling emotionally? Does your life seem to be going as well as you would like?

Reprinted with permission from "Help for Geriatric Sleep Problems" by Dinner, et al., *Patient Care,* (June 15, 1992) pp. 166-192.

when available, systematic observations of sleep patterns on a 24-hour basis (when feasible and indicated), and use of specialized tests (such as polysomnograms and the Multiple Sleep Latency Test [MSLT]) when appropriate (Harvard Health Letter, 1995)

History

The *sleep history* may be the single most important piece of information in the assessment. It should be thorough and cover the patient's perception of the sleep experience, past and present sleep patterns, personal and family history of any

sleep disorders, and general health. Specific details regarding the sleep complaint are elicited: onset, duration, and what makes it better or worse. The effect of this disorder on the person's lifestyle is determined. Questions to ask are presented in Box 16-2. Eight broad areas (described in Box 16-3) need to be reviewed in any sleep pattern assessment, each of which contains both subjective and objective features. Data concerning these areas can be obtained from a variety of sources, including the patient, the family or close friends, the health history (if available), observations, physical examination, and diagnostic tests.

One of the first goals of the assessment is a specific determination of the duration of the complaint and its probable cause. Transient disturbances of less than 3 weeks' duration are probably caused by situational factors. More persistent problems (lasting longer than a month) require deeper assessment, looking at a combination of possible causes.

A sleep diary should be kept for 7 to 14 days to assist in determining the distribution of sleep, as well as its quantity and quality, over an average 24-hour period. Entries might include physical and mental activities, such as exercises, TV, reading, meals, intake of substances such as caffeine and alcohol, and daytime naps, as well as presleep state of mind, number of nocturnal awakenings, and time of morning awakening. (For a sample sleep diary, see Box 16-4.)

If a diary is used with an older adult, attention should be given to its practicality and ease of use. Requiring very frequent or extremely detailed entries could be a burden on an older adult and might defeat the purpose for which data are being collected. A way to enhance cooperation with this assessment tool is to enlist the older individual's aid in constructing it. This might also help to determine at the outset whether such a procedure is going to be successful.

Objective data The *physical examination* of the patient should include examination of several objective characteristics that are typically affected in the older adult with a sleep complaint, such as the person's behavior and appearance: Does the person appear tired or listless? Does there appear to be a reduction in the person's ability to perform daily tasks? Other signs might include irritability, agitation, and/or restlessness (Kartman & McFarlane, 1993). Some signs typically associated with sleeplessness when observed in younger adults would not be appropriate to consider in the examination of the older adult related to sleep problems. Drooping shoulders, dark circles under the eyes, and hand tremors are not uncommon findings in examining an older adult and may be unrelated to sleep patterns.

Systematic observations of individuals' sleep behaviors have been carried out in the long-term care setting as part of one reported research protocol (Bliwise et al., 1990). These observations appear to be an accurate method of validating sleep complaints and are less intrusive and expensive than polysomnographic studies would be for older patients. In such a protocol, characteristics such as mental status, functional capacity, and apnea or other physiologic symptoms, as well as intake of psychotropic medications, are observed at specified intervals and are recorded. This method of identifying potential predictors of sleep-wake dysfunction holds promise.

BOX 16-4 DATA FOR REVIEW AND DISCUSSION IN ASSESSING A PERSON'S SLEEP-WAKE EXPERIENCE: A SLEEP DIARY

A detailed sleep record can be a first step toward improving how you feel. Answer questions in part 1 at the end of a day, questions in part 2 the next morning, and questions in part 3 in the evening of the following day.

PART 1. ACTIVITIES DURING THE DAY

1. What exercise did you do? When and for how long?
2. What caffeine-containing foods and drinks did you consume? At what times?
3. How many alcoholic beverages did you drink? When?
4. How many cigarettes did you smoke? When?
5. How many sleep medications did you take? What dose and when?
6. What other medications did you take? What dose and when?
7. What did you eat for dinner, and when?
8. What after-dinner snacks did you eat, and when?
9. What were your evening activities?
10. What were your evening interactions with other people (in person and on the telephone)?

PART 2. MY NIGHT'S SLEEP

1. Before turning in, did you fall asleep somewhere other than in your bed?
2. What bedtime routine did you follow? (e.g., snack, brushing teeth, winding down by listening to the radio)
3. What time did you get in bed?
4. What time did you turn out the light and try to fall asleep?
5. About how long did it take you to fall asleep?
6. If you had difficulty falling asleep, what kept you awake? (e.g., couldn't stop thinking, pain, noise)
7. How many times did you wake up in the night? When? What woke you up?
8. About how long did you stay awake each time?
9. What did you do or think about during the time you were awake? (e.g., read, felt pain in knees, sat in living room, worried about paying bills)
10. What time did you wake up in the morning? Did you use an alarm clock?
11. What time did you get out of bed in the morning?
12. Altogether, how much sleep did you get during the night?
13. How would you rate the quality of your sleep? (e.g., sound, fitful, better or worse than usual)
14. How did you feel when you woke up? (e.g., refreshed, headachy, groggy, better or worse than when you went to bed)

PART 3. HOW I FELT THE NEXT DAY

1. In general, how was your mood? (e.g., great, irritable, depressed)
2. In general, how did you feel physically? (e.g., draggy, peppy, couldn't keep eyes open)
3. In general, how was your alertness and performance during the day? (e.g., worked hard, couldn't concentrate, felt interested in everything)
4. Did you take any naps? When and for how long?
5. Other comments or observations:

From Harvard Health Letter. (1995, January). *A special report: Sleep disburbance.* Boston: Harvard Medical School Health Publications Group.

Specialized tests *Diagnostic studies* may include sleep laboratory evaluation using polysomnography. This may be of benefit for some older individuals who have suspected sleep apnea or PLMS. When insomnia is persistent and does not respond to routine treatment, this type of assessment should be considered (Reynolds et al., 1986). As a general rule, however, it would not be an appropriate means of assessing an older adult's sleep problem because it is too intrusive and too expensive. In addition, it requires the use of a laboratory setting, which could be upsetting to an older individual. A polysomnogram involves multiple measurements recorded by electrodes placed in strategic areas to obtain data regarding brain waves (EEG), eye movements (EOG), and muscle tension (EMG) during sleep. The procedure is done in a sleep laboratory setting, and it generally takes at least 2 nights for the person to become accustomed to the apparatus.

A diagnostic tool sometimes used to assess daytime sleepiness is an objective measure called the Multiple Sleep Latency Test, MSLT (Carskadon et al., 1986; Richardson, 1990). It also utilizes electrophysiologic recordings, but it does so during a daytime period rather than at night. There are some indications that link increased tendencies to nap with sleep loss at night, and this test might be useful in validating that link.

Environmental assessment

The larger setting in which sleep takes place should also be considered in the sleep assessment. If older adults are living alone, do they feel safe? Is the home warm enough in winter and cool enough in summer? If people live with family members, is there adequate privacy? Is the sleeping area free from noxious stimuli, such as noise and light? Although older adults are often hard of hearing, they also have a lower auditory arousal threshold.

In acute care settings, multiple stimuli can affect the older adult's sleeping efficiency. In addition to higher levels of sensory stimuli, technical procedures and routines can disrupt an individual's usual pattern. Older adults do not do well for extended periods in acute care settings, and early discharge should be considered.

Nursing homes or long-term care institutions may contribute to some sleep disturbances, with high noise levels, incompatible roommates, unfamiliar routines, and poorly trained staff affecting the availability of a restful environment. On the other hand, institutions may provide the security that is lacking in a hostile or inadequate private or family home setting.

NURSING DIAGNOSES

The general nursing diagnosis accepted by the North American Nursing Diagnosis Association for describing sleep problems is *sleep pattern disturbance,* which describes the state in which disruption of sleep time causes discomfort or interferes with an individual's lifestyle (Kartman, 1993; Kartman & McFarlane, 1993).

Three nursing diagnoses concerning sleep disturbance result from the assessment of an older patient:

1. Sleep pattern disturbance related to pain and response to the critical care setting
2. Sleep pattern disturbance related to nocturia and frequent awakenings
3. Sleep pattern disturbance related to knowledge deficit

Further development of these diagnoses identifies specific related factors and defining characteristics.

Sleep pattern disturbance related to pain and response to the critical care setting may be evidenced by the following:

- Complaints of difficulty falling asleep, not feeling well rested, frequent interruptions in sleep
- Restlessness
- Disorientation, especially regarding time of day and actual day of the week and date

- Yawning, dozing during the day but being easily startled awake
- Complaints of awakening with pain, or pain with position changes

Sleep pattern disturbance related to nocturia and frequent awakenings may be evidenced by the following:

- Multiple nighttime trips to the bathroom
- Increased daytime sleepiness
- Fatigue and listlessness
- Verbal complaints of not feeling well rested
- Verbal complaints of interrupted sleep because of the need to go to the bathroom frequently
- Difficulty in going back to sleep after arousal

Sleep pattern disturbance related to knowledge deficit may be evidenced by the following:

- Increased use of nighttime medication for sleep, sometimes combined with alcohol, resulting in early morning hangover
- Verbal complaints of not feeling well rested and not getting a good night's sleep
- Thick, slurred speech, with mispronunciation and incorrect use of words, especially in early morning
- Lethargy, especially in the morning
- Daytime sleepiness, with frequent naps

PLANNING AND GOAL IDENTIFICATION

With the assistance of the patient, the members of the health care team, led by the nurse, review the assessment data that suggest that the patient has an alteration in sleep patterns. It is possible that the experience of pain is interfering with the experience of a satisfying sleep. The planned outcome defined by the team in this case will be that the pain will be controlled so that sleep can be experienced in a healthy way.

The experience of nocturia will interfere with healthy and satisfying sleep, unless controlled in a reasonable way. Achieving this goal or outcome will require controlling the amount, type, and time of liquid ingestion before bedtime. This usually means a change from the previous pattern of ingestion of fluids. Unless the patient is involved in examining this pattern and defining the outcomes that will be hoped for, it will be very difficult for the nurse and the health care team to achieve these outcomes alone—that is, without the cooperation of the patient.

Providing as much knowledge about sleep as possible, and about the patterns of life that alter or enhance the experience of sleep, will enable the patient to understand the outcomes that the health care team is defining and the goals the health care team is setting. This approach to the analysis of sleep patterns and the precise definition of behaviors to enhance and encourage sleep will enable the patient to develop living patterns, or patterns while awake, that will make the experience of sleep so much more comfortable and positive.

Planning involves the establishment of appropriate patient-centered goals that address the factors contributing to the sleep pattern disturbance. The patient, the family, and any other significant people providing care should be involved in the development of the plan of care. The long-term goal in all sleep pattern disturbances is to eliminate or to control as much as possible the disruption of sleep and its deleterious effects on the person's lifestyle (Kartman & McFarlane, 1993). Short-term goals for each of the three previously listed diagnoses focus on removing or modifying the related factors.

Short-term goals for sleep pattern disturbance related to pain and response to the critical care setting include the following:

1. Decrease in complaints of pain
2. Verbalization of satisfaction with sleep and rest
3. Increase in alertness and orientation, with accurate time awareness
4. Demonstration of a balance of sleep and waking periods at appropriate times
5. Discharge to regular patient unit

Short-term goals for sleep pattern disturbance related to nocturia and frequent awakenings include the following:

1. Description of the relationship of the
   diuretic medication to increased urination
2. Change in diuretic medication schedule
   to a decreased nocturnal action routine
3. Verbalization of increased satisfaction
   with sleep and rest
4. Appearance showing appropriate rest

Short-term goals for sleep pattern disturbance related to knowledge deficit include the
following:

1. Description of an understanding of internal and external factors that influence
   sleep
2. Demonstration of balance of sleep and
   activity
3. Verbalization of increase in satisfaction
   with sleep-wake patterns
4. Description of healthy sleep habits
5. Reduction or elimination of use of nighttime sedative and alcohol in the evening

IMPLEMENTATION

Reynolds and Kupfer (1994) suggest a broad
conceptual approach to the management of late-
life sleep disturbances, which captures the important principles underlying the care of older
patients. First, specific etiologic factors should be
identified, keeping in mind that, often, more
than one factor is producing a sleep-wake disruption. Second, patient and family education regarding age changes and sleep is vitally important. Third, because there seems to be a fragility
and brittleness to the circadian rhythm system in
older adults, these rhythms need to be reinforced
by enhancing time cues and stimulus control.
There has been some success in improving sleep
continuity by limiting the duration of sleep.

In addition, a short, regularly scheduled nap
may be permitted if necessary to overcome daytime sleepiness (Floyd, 1995). Fourth, the issue
of the timing of medications, both psychotropic
and nonpsychotropic, should be addressed to
determine the adverse effects of this timing on
the sleep-wake cycle. Finally, drug therapy for
sleep should only be used for specific conditions,
on a short-term basis, and with special attention
to adverse sleep effects.

Education of older adults, their families, and
their caregivers is one of the first interventions in
any plan of care and is an ongoing measure
throughout the course of treatment (Miller,
1990).

Most sleep disturbances respond to nursing
interventions. Nurses practice in varied settings
and often encounter patients who have some
problems with sleep. In general, older patients
and their families should be made aware that
some sleep pattern disturbance may not be preventable.

In intervention, the emphasis should be on
supporting the circadian rhythm of the sleep-
wake cycle and on avoiding tendencies to nap or
fragment sleep time during the usual waking
period. Although there are some indications that
daytime naps have little effect on the older
adult's nighttime sleep, in cases where there are
complaints of insomnia at night, frequent napping during the day should be discouraged
(Floyd, 1995). It is important to keep in mind
that prevention is the best intervention for sleep
disturbance.

Sleep disorders centers or *sleep clinics* are
specialized sleep facilities set up as part of a
hospital, a university, or some health care facility
to treat patients and to study sleep disorders.
These centers are a recent innovation for the
treatment of persistent and severe disorders. At
such facilities, a variety of specialists, such as
physicians, psychologists, psychiatrists, and sur-
geons, provide the appropriate treatment for the
particular disorder. Patients, typically seen as
outpatients, are given a thorough examination
and a battery of psychologic tests; then, after the

initial assessment, if deemed necessary, sleep patterns are recorded for 1 to 3 nights, to determine the etiology of the sleep disorder. The cost of this service varies considerably and can range from a few hundred to a few thousand dollars. In some cases, Medicare and/or an insurance company may assume the cost. This type of service is usually not required for older adults, but may occasionally be necessary for the older adult who has an intractable sleep disorder.

The National Institute on Aging (1990) has published some general recommendations for promoting or improving sleep in older adults. These can serve as a beginning in a patient-caregiver education program and offer sound advice for the population as a whole.

In the acute care setting

Older patients in the hospital, whether in critical care units or in intermediate care units, pose special problems in nursing care (Davis-Sharts, 1989). These patients are usually very ill and especially vulnerable to multiple system failures and complications. Because of the seriousness of their physical condition, plus the added dimension of a fast-paced acute care environment, older adults are predisposed to suffer the additional burden of a sleep disturbance. Several aspects of the hospital environment have the potential to alter the sleep of the older patient. Some of the more obvious are medications, the sensory overload of the critical care environment, and frequent interruptions of sleep.

Interventions in the hospital setting are concerned with providing the optimum treatment for the acute conditions of older patients while being aware of their increased vulnerability and susceptibility to sleep deprivation. Whenever possible, modify routines to decrease nighttime interruptions and to provide support for the older patient's usual bedtime schedule. Initiate and maintain control of unnecessary sensory stimulation, such as overhead lights, noise from equipment, and communication among personnel. Early discharge from critical care units to the quieter intermediate care units should be encouraged. In older adults, sleep can be influenced by the number and type of medications and the frequency of doses. Careful monitoring of sedatives and hypnotics for their effects on sleep is a responsibility of the nurse. Comfort measures such as back rubs, position changes, and modifications of environment can be utilized and relied upon at periodic intervals to help the patient experience the sleep that is needed.

The hospital setting is not an environment that encourages sleep. Sleep deprivation in acutely ill older adults can predispose them to greater risk of serious illness. Documenting the amount of uninterrupted sleep is an important part of keeping the older patient's record. Encouraging staff awareness regarding the essential need for extended periods of sleep for older patients could make a significant difference in the patient's well-being (Thelan et al., 1994).

In the nursing home

Residents of nursing homes are subject to many disruptions of sleep. In addition to the chronic health problems of the older resident, there are the added features of the institutional environment. In most cases this is not a homelike setting, and it requires creative approaches by the nurse to create a desirable sleep atmosphere. Careful gathering of assessment data from the resident and family will allow the nurse to individualize the sleep routine.

Research has documented increased sleep fragmentation in nursing home residents (Ancoli-Israel et al., 1989). Findings identified external environmental factors as being accountable for a substantial portion of sleep fragmentation, particularly such factors as being awakened at night by staff to administer medications or to change wet clothing and linens because of incontinence; noise from the other residents; and excessive amounts of time spent in bed during the day.

External factors can be controlled to promote a more sleep-conducive atmosphere. An education program for staff, resident, and family members regarding healthy sleep habits is a good beginning. Careful attention to the placement of disruptive patients and to structuring bedtime and medication schedules around a normal sleep-wake pattern is a nursing responsibility. Residents who are physically well and mentally alert need to be active during the day, thereby reducing their time spent in bed. For residents who are debilitated, activities such as games that are not physically demanding help provide enough daytime stimulation to promote nocturnal sleep.

Controlling temperature extremes, providing privacy and quiet, assisting with comfortable positioning in bed, and providing other comfort measures to relieve anxiety and pain are nursing interventions that encourage healthy sleep patterns. Use of reassurance and relaxation techniques at bedtime or use of late afternoon soothing baths may prove quite beneficial for some anxious residents. Providing soft music before bedtime from a tape recorder with an automatic shutoff is another measure to promote sleep (Miller, 1990). These and other interventions to promote satisfying sleep for nursing home residents will increase the residents' ability to function effectively and to find enjoyment in the daily activities of nursing home life.

In the private or family home

Interventions to promote sleep in the home need to be as individualized as the home settings. Teaching older adults, their families, and other caregivers about age changes and their effects on sleep is an important first step, as well as providing information on good sleep practices. Although the home is usually considered to be the ideal place for an older adult to reside, this environment still requires careful assessment concerning sleep pattern disturbances in older adults.

Older individuals may live alone or with relatives. They may or may not have control over the home environment. Some of the same concerns addressed in other settings, such as temperature control, may also be appropriate to consider in planning home interventions. Too much or too little sensory stimulation, inadequate provisions for privacy, or isolation could be factors in sleep pattern disturbance in the home setting. An important feature in the home setting is the involvement of the family or significant others in the assessment and management of sleep disruptions of their older family member.

Eating snacks containing the protein tryptophan (milk, cheese, turkey, etc.) has been suggested as a means of encouraging sleep in a natural way. The practice of taking large doses of tryptophan supplements is not recommended, however, because this practice has been implicated in adverse reactions, including myalgia, eosinophilia, and pneumonitis, in a number of people. Although tryptophan is an essential amino acid that has gained a reputation for having natural sedative properties, there is no body of research to support this claim. It is not natural to consume large quantities of a pure amino acid. The Food and Drug Administration halted the sale of tryptophan supplements in November 1989, after reports of toxic effects were made known (Tryptophan, 1990).

There is an additional concern for safety for older adults living alone. Although safety is a factor for older adults in all settings, it assumes greater importance for the person living alone and necessitates careful attention to the resources available for providing safety and security. Worry and anxiety concerning safety and welfare can be an ongoing obstacle to a good and restful sleep. A system of notification and monitoring to link the person living alone with the outside world is important to the person's sense of security. Outside noise may be a sleep-inhibiting factor, which can be dampened by heavy drapes or the use of earplugs. However, caution should be exercised when those living alone use earplugs because they might not hear the phone or the smoke alarm in an emergency.

Medications for sleep are often prescribed by physicians to manage sleep disturbances in older adults. The following important information

Health Promotion

- Maintain consistent daily schedule of awakening and going to bed.
- Limit daytime napping to 2 hours.
- Use the bed and bedroom only for sleeping.
- Eliminate consumption of caffeinated beverages in afternoon and evening hours.
- Maintain comfortable temperature in home and bedroom, and keep environmental stimuli to a minimum.
- Reduce stress and/or use relaxation techniques such as deep breathing to induce sleep.

concerning sleep-related medications should be emphasized with older adults, their families, and other caregivers:

1. Sleep-related medications are not for long-term use because their effectiveness is diminished after a few weeks; tolerance develops quickly, and withdrawal symptoms are quite unpleasant.
2. Many sleeping medications, including over-the-counter drugs, have adverse effects on the quality of sleep and on daytime functioning, causing drowsiness, lack of alertness, and sometimes dizziness, especially in older adults.
3. Alcohol is generally contraindicated and can have detrimental effects on sleep, even in moderate amounts. It should not be used in combination with other medications.
4. Combinations of other medications with sleeping medications can be dangerous (Buchholtz, 1987; U.S. Pharmacopeia, 1990).

For other sleep promotion tips, see the Health Promotion box.

EVALUATION

Evaluation of the patient's status, the nursing plan, and its implementation should be ongoing. The goals or expected outcomes should be achievable. One of the most important goals in sleep pattern disturbance is related to the diagnosis of knowledge deficit and subsequent patient control of circumstances related to the promotion of sleep. The patients' expressed perceptions of the effectiveness of the plan, of the interventions, and of personal satisfaction with the quality and quantity of the sleep experience are crucial elements in the evaluation.

REFERENCES

*Alward, R.R. (1995, April 3). Sleep hygiene tips. *Nursing Spectrum.*

Alward, R.R., & Monk, T.H. (1995). Sleep as a circadian rhythm: The impact of shift work. In *The American Nurse,* (Continuing Education Program: Vol. 27, No. 2, Pt. 3). Washington, DC: American Nurses' Association.

Ancoli-Israel, S. (1989). Epidemiology of sleep disorders. *Clinics in Geriatric Medicine, 5*(2), 347-362.

Ancoli-Israel, S. et al. (1989). Sleep fragmentation in patients from a nursing home. *Journal of Gerontology, 44*(1), M18-M21.

*Becker, P.M., & Jamieson, A.O. (1992). Common sleep disorders in the elderly: Diagnosis and treatment. *Geriatrics, 47,* 41-54.

Bliwise, D. (1989). Neuropsychological function and sleep. *Clinics in Geriatric Medicine, 5*(2), 381-387.

Bliwise, D., Carroll, J., & Dement, W. (1990). Predictors of observed sleep/wakefulness in residents in long term care. *Journal of Gerontology, 45*(4), M126-M130.

Bonnet, M.H., & Arand, D.L. (1989). Sleep loss in aging. *Clinics in Geriatric Medicine, 5*(2), 405-419.

Bonnet, M.H., & Arand, D.L. (1990). Use of triazolam in older patients with periodic leg movements, fragmented sleep and daytime sleepiness. *Journal of Gerontology, 45*(4), M139-M144.

---

*These references can be valuable for additional information.

Buchholtz, D. (1987). Sleep disorders. In T.M. Bayless, M.C. Brain, & R.M. Cherniak (Eds.), *Current therapy in internal medicine,* (pp. 1235-1239). Philadelphia: B.C. Decker.

Carskadon, M. et al. (1986). Guidelines for the multiple sleep latency test (MSLT): A standard measure of sleepiness. *Sleep, 9,* 519-524.

Colling, J. (1983). Sleep disturbances in aging: Theoretic and empiric analysis. *Advances in Nursing Science, 6* (1), 36-44.

Davis-Sharts, J. (1989). The elder and critical care: Sleep and mobility issues. *Nursing Clinics of North America, 24*(3), 755-767.

*Dinner, S.S., Erman, M.K., & Roth, T. (1992). Help for geriatric sleep problems. *Patient Care,* pp. 166-192.

Dowling, G. (1995). Sleep problems in older adults. In *The American Nurse,* (Continuing Education Program: Vol. 27, No. 3, Pt. 5). Washington, DC: American Nurses' Association.

Evans, L. (1987). Sundown syndrome in institutionalized elderly. *Journal of the American Geriatrics Society, 35*(2), 101-108.

Floyd, J.A. (1995, May-June). Another look at napping in older adults. *Geriatric Nursing, 16*(3), 136-138.

Gillin, J.C. (1990, May). Sleeping pills. *Harvard Medical School Health Letter, 15,* 5-8.

Haponik, E.F. (1990). Sleep problems. In W.R. Hazzard et al. (Eds.), *Principles of geriatric medicine and gerontology* (2nd ed., pp. 1213-1228). New York: McGraw-Hill.

Harvard Health Letter. (1995). *Sleep disturbance.* (Available from Harvard Medical School, Boston, MA 02117).

Harvard Mental Health Letter. (1994a, August). *Sleep disorders* (Vol. 11, No. 2, Pt. 1). (Available from Harvard Medical School, Boston, MA 02115).

Harvard Mental Health Letter. (1994b, September). *Sleep disorders* (Vol. 11, No. 3, Pt. 2). (Available from Harvard Medical School, Boston, MA 02115).

Hauri, P., & Linde, S. (1990). *No more sleepless nights.* New York: John Wiley and Sons.

Hoch, C.C. et al. (1992). Sleep disorders and aging. In J. Birren, R. Sloane, & G. Cohen (Eds.), *Handbook of mental health and aging* (2nd ed., pp. 557-581). San Diego: Academic Press.

Kartman, J. (1993). Sleep-rest. In J. Thompson et al. (Eds.), *Mosby's manual of clinical nursing* (3rd ed., pp. 1535-1537). St. Louis: Mosby.

Kartman, J., & McFarlane, E. (1993). Sleep pattern disturbance. In G. McFarland & E. McFarlane (Eds.), *Nursing diagnosis and intervention: Planning for patient care* (2nd ed., pp. 419-425). St. Louis: Mosby.

Kryger, M.Y., Roth, T., & Dement, W.C. (Eds.). (1994). *Principles and practices of sleep medicine* (2nd ed.). Philadelphia: W.B. Saunders.

McCance, K.L., & Heuther, S.E. (1990). *Pathophysiology: The biological basis for disease in adults and children.* St. Louis: Mosby.

McFarland, G.K., & McFarlane, E.A. (1993). *Nursing diagnosis and intervention: Planning for patient care* (2nd ed.). St. Louis: Mosby.

Miller, C.A. (1990). *Nursing care of older adults: Theory and practice.* Glenview, IL: Scott, Foresman.

Monk, T. (1989). Circadian rhythm. *Clinics in Geriatric Medicine, 5*(2), 331-346.

Monk, T.H. (Ed.). (1991). *Sleep, sleepiness and performance.* New York: John Wiley and Sons.

*Morgan, K. (1992). Sleep in normal and pathological aging. In J.X. Brodklehurst, R.C. Tollis, & H.M. Fillit (Eds.), *Textbook of geriatric medicine and gerontology* (4th ed., pp. 122-129). London: Churchill Livingstone.

National Institute on Aging. (1990). *Age page: A good night's sleep.* Bethesda, MD: U.S. Department of Health and Human Services, National Institutes of Health.

Reynolds, C., Hoch, C., & Monk, T. (1986). Sleep and chronobiologic disturbances in late life. In E.W. Busse & D.G. Blazer (Eds.), *Geriatric psychiatry* (pp. 475-488). Washington, DC: American Psychological Association.

*Reynolds III, C.F., & Kupfer, D.J. (1994). Sleep disorders. In J. Oldham & M.B. Riba (Eds.), *Review of Psychiatry* (Vol. 13). Washington, DC: American Psychiatric Press.

Richardson, G.S. (1990). Circadian rhythms and aging. In E.L. Schneider & J.W. Rowe (Eds.), *Handbook of the biology of aging* (3rd. ed., pp. 275-305). San Diego: Academic Press.

Roehrs, T.A., & Roth, T. (1989). Drugs, sleep disorders and aging. *Clinics in Geriatric Medicine, 5*(2), 395-404.

Shaver, J.L.F., & Landis, C.A. (1994). Understanding the behavior of sleep. In *The American Nurse* (Continuing Education Program: Vol. 26, No. 9, Pt. 1). Washington, DC: American Nurses' Association.

Sleep apnea: A new solution. (1989, July). *Harvard Medical School Health Letter, 14*(9), p. 4.

Sleep Disorders Classification Committee. (1979). Association of sleep disorders centers: Diagnostic classification of sleep and arousal disorders. *Sleep, 2,* 1-137.

Snow, T.L. et al. (1988). *Handbook of geriatric practice essentials.* Rockville, MD: Aspen Publishing.

Thelan, L.A. et al. (1990). *Textbook of critical care nursing: Diagnosis and management.* St. Louis: Mosby.

Thelan, L.A. et al. (1994). *Critical care nursing: Diagnosis and management* (2nd ed.). St. Louis: Mosby.

Tryptophan: Natural disaster. (1990, February). *Harvard Medical School Health Letter,* pp. 1-2.

U.S. Pharmacopeia. (1990). *United States Pharmacopeia: Drug information for the consumer.* Rockville, MD: U.S. Pharmacopeial Convention.

Vestal, R.E. (1990). Clinical pharmacology. In W. Hazzard, et al. (Eds.), *Principles of geriatric medicine and gerontology* (2nd ed., pp. 201-211). New York: McGraw-Hill.

Vitiello, M., & Prinz, P. (1989). Alzheimer's disease: Sleep and sleep/wake patterns. *Clinics in Geriatric Medicine, 5*(2), 289-299.

Webb, W. (1989). Age-related changes in sleep. *Clinics in Geriatric Medicine, 5*(2), 275-287.

Wolfe, S. et al. (1988). *Worst pills, best pills: The older adult's guide to avoiding drug induced death or illness.* Washington, DC: Public Citizen Health Research Group.

C H A P T E R   17

Where there is despair let me bring hope
Where there is darkness let me bring light
Where there is sadness let me bring joy

SAINT FRANCIS OF ASSISI

Cognition and Mood

■ Learning Objectives

On completion of this chapter, the reader will be able to do the following:

1. Discuss three mental disorders that are frequently experienced by older adults and the relationship between increasing age and the prevalence of these disorders.
2. Differentiate between two cognitive disorders, dementia and delirium, and specify their distinguishing features.
3. Differentiate between cognitive disorders and depression, a mood disorder.
4. Describe the effects of cognitive disorders and depression on the older individual.
5. Discuss the role of the caregiver of the cognitively impaired and/or depressed older person.
6. Discuss the assessment process as it applies to cognitive impairment and the use of instruments to assist in diagnosing the nursing needs of the cognitively impaired or depressed person.
7. Implement nursing interventions that meet the special needs of cognitively impaired older adults.

Just as the anatomic and physiologic changes of the aging process lead to increasing incidence of physical disorders such as arthritis and diabetes, and to sensory impairment from declining visual acuity and hearing loss, so, too, are the brain and other structures of the central nervous system subject to the normal degenerative changes of aging and to pathologic processes. The recognition of cognitive disorders in older adults, the institution of treatment where possible, and the provision of appropriate care and support for the individual, the family, and other caregivers is a major area of concern for all nursing professionals.

A person's state of health, genetic code, past experiences, educational background, cultural influences and beliefs, and current living conditions all influence the level of cognitive ability. Physical changes in the brain caused by the normal process of aging and selected pathologic conditions may affect the cognitive abilities of some older individuals. When cognitive abilities fall to a level that precludes people's ability to care for themselves, health problems are apt to occur.

Cognitive abilities vary among people and across the life span, with a wide range of differences. Language, attention, memory, orientation, visuospatial ability, conceptualization, and general intelligence are all manifestations of cognitive abilities (Albert, 1994).

The nursing care of an older person who has experienced a loss of cognitive ability is a significant challenge. The full knowledge, skills, and interpersonal strengths of the nurse are called upon when the nurse is caring for cognitively impaired people and their families. Society is not tolerant of those older adults who have lost vital cognitive abilities, nor is there a significant role for them within the larger society or even within family units. The fear of cognitive impairment is a recurrent theme in the conversations of the well older adult. Actually, many people of all ages are frightened by those who have suffered cognitive loss, and contact with them is avoided. Nonetheless, each cognitively impaired older person is a unique individual who has the same rights and privileges as any other person.

This chapter presents an overview of the normal structure and function of the neurologic system; age-related changes in the brain; the cognitive disorders of dementia and delirium; and the mood disorder of depression, which may be a symptom associated with cognitive loss or a separate and treatable condition. It also discusses the role of caregivers of cognitively impaired and depressed older adults followed by a description of the nursing process as it applies to the care of these older adults. It is hoped that this presentation may assist the reader in recognizing the complexity of providing nursing care to cognitively impaired or depressed older people.

■ Normal Structure and Function

The neurologic system is divided into two distinct systems, the central nervous system and the peripheral nervous system. The brain and the spinal cord make up the *central nervous system.* The *peripheral nervous system* is composed of the 12 cranial nerves, 31 paired spinal nerves,

and the autonomic nervous system, which is subdivided into the sympathetic and parasympathetic divisions. The complex functions of the nervous system encompass analysis of sensory information, response to the internal and external environment, control and coordination of motor function, emotional and intellectual functions, and regulation and communication among body systems.

BRAIN

The cerebrum, the cerebellum, and the brainstem are the three regions that make up the brain. The *cerebrum* consists of four lobes: frontal, parietal, temporal, and occipital; it is the largest part of the brain and controls the higher levels of intellectual functioning. The *cerebellum* functions as the control center for balance and coordination. The *brainstem* and the *spinal cord* form a continuous entity, with the 12 paired cranial nerves emerging from the brainstem. The brainstem comprises the pons, medulla oblongata, midbrain, and diencephalon. The brainstem functions as a connector of the different sections of the brain and as the transmitter of impulses between the spinal cord and the brain. The spinal cord is an important center for the 31 spinal nerves and for reflex action, and serves as the conduction pathway to the brain for sensory and motor impulses.

NEURONS AND NEUROTRANSMITTERS

Neurons are the specialized cells of the nervous system that receive and/or send neural data throughout the human system. *Neurotransmitters* function as a means of communication between neurons. The process of the transmission of information between two neurons involves the synthesis, storage, and release of one or more neurotransmitters (Poirer & Finch, 1994). Catecholamine neurotransmitters, such as dopamine, norepinephrine, and epinephrine, are thought to be involved in the control and modulation of emotion and attention. These neurotransmitters are involved in the control and modulation of visceral function and the cognitive function of attention. The neurotransmitter acetylcholine is thought to play a significant role in mental functions such as learning and memory (Nakamura, 1990). Serotonin, another neurotransmitter, is known to play a role in sleep and memory (Poirer & Finch, 1994). There are at least 30 known neurotransmitters. Science has not yet provided a complete understanding of the mechanism or the dynamics of neurotransmitters.

■ Age-Related Changes

CHANGES IN THE NEUROLOGIC SYSTEM

The neurologic system undergoes changes that are related to the aging process, but scientists disagree about what universal changes occur in the human brain and how these changes relate to cognitive function. The plasticity of the aging brain is without doubt a remarkable feature of the compensatory mechanism related to human aging. The brain undergoes an early period of growth, reaches a plateau of development and stability by adulthood, and then slowly enters a period of decline during senescence (Poirer & Finch, 1994). It has generally been thought that the brain atrophies as a result of the aging process. The most recent studies have challenged that general statement and have proposed that selected and restricted areas of the brain experience atrophy, rather than the entire brain (Poirer & Finch, 1994).

The extent of age-related neuron loss and the effect on function is not clear. Cotman (1990) states, "Neuron loss is not an inevitable consequence of aging, although it occurs." It appears that the age-related change most affecting neurons is shrinkage of large neurons (Terry et al., 1987). The result is a loss of large neurons, with an increase in smaller neurons. The loss is often restricted to specific areas of the brain and is often associated with the compensatory mechanism of dendrite formation (Poirer & Finch, 1994). There is scientific controversy regarding

the extent, location, and significance of neuron loss in the aging brain.

There is agreement that the following changes do occur in association with aging: some loss in brain volume and brain weight, enlargement of the ventricles, decrease in enzymes, loss of protein, loss of lipids, and alterations in the amount of and the receptors for some neurotransmitters. The importance of these age-related changes is unknown, as is the extent of their effect on each aging person's cognitive abilities.

Clinical changes exhibited by the older person that are revealed during the examination of the neurologic system and are attributed to the aging process include the following: (1) decreased sensation of vibrations, particularly in the legs, (2) less brisk deep tendon reflexes, with the ankle reflex often absent entirely; and (3) a decreased ability for upward gaze.

There is no doubt that aging brings change. Two examples of functional loss exhibited by most older people and attributed to neurologic age-related change are the slowing of response to tasks and the increase in time needed to recover from physical exertion (Cristofalo, 1990). Nonetheless, the ability of the human body to adjust to age-related alterations and the ability of the human spirit to be resilient in the face of physical loss must not be overlooked or devalued. Clinicians are concerned with the functional everyday abilities of the older adult. The nurse helps older people to adapt to change and to function in a manner that protects their health, promotes their well-being, and ensures their dignity.

CHANGES IN COGNITIVE AND AFFECTIVE FUNCTIONING

Cognitive functioning is the means by which individuals perceive and react to the world around them, based on the knowledge and skills they have learned and developed since birth, and that most people continue to acquire throughout their lives.

Even though it is normal for individuals to continue to learn from new and changing

Aging Alert
Nursing's challenge— care of the cognitively impaired older person
- Advocate thorough medical evaluation
- Protect existing level of health
- Promote well-being
- Preserve the dignity of the person

experiences, some changes in cognitive functioning do occur over time, as part of the aging process. These changes or declines do not develop uniformly, either across all areas of cognitive functioning, or at the same rate in all individuals. Some cognitive abilities are stable for many decades and decline late in life, whereas other abilities show change in middle age and then remain stable or show less decline with advancing age.

Memory is the first area of cognition to be affected, as the capacity of the brain to process, store, and retrieve information becomes less efficient. Cross-sectional studies have shown that by the age of 50 years, there is a significant decline in ability to recall relatively large amounts of information over long periods. By late in the sixth decade, proficiency declines at tasks that involve series completion. Scores on naming tests and intelligence tests begin to decline by age 70. Perceptual ability, such as the ability to copy complex three-dimensional designs, declines by the mid-60s, as do scores on tests requiring the individual to divide attention among different stimuli (Albert, 1994).

It should be emphasized that although these changes in cognitive functioning are a normal manifestation of aging, there is wide variation among individuals. Some individuals show little decline in cognition, even into their 80s, whereas others show some impairment by age 60.

In regard to affective functioning or change of mood, it is not a normal part of the aging process to develop symptoms of depression. Although older people tend to adhere more to routine, and their lives may become more restricted by physical limitations, most older people continue to have interests and to derive pleasure from life, even within a more limited sphere of activities and social contacts.

■ Common Health Deviations: Mental Disorders

The three most prevalent mental disorders of older adults are the following:

1. Dementia
2. Delirium
3. Depression

These three disorders may exhibit similar signs and symptoms, and the three may coexist within the same patient. The behaviors associated with them are often accepted as a normal part of the aging process, particularly in the older adult. Sometimes the symptoms result from, or are exacerbated by, treatments prescribed for medical conditions. Even though it might be possible to identify some underlying process, which could be treated to ameliorate the condition, this is often left undone. Mental disorders in older adults therefore present a major challenge in terms of accurate diagnosis and management.

Disorders that are the direct result of neurochemical, circulatory, and anatomic changes occurring in the brain are categorized as *organic* disorders and are the predominant form of cognitive illness affecting older adults. In this category are the various *dementias,* with symptoms progressing along a continuum from forgetfulness to a total lack of capacity for self-care, incontinence, and failure to recognize even close family members. These symptoms demonstrate a decline in *cognitive functioning,* or a diminished capacity to discern the common reality. Although symptoms of dementia may occur as the result of some underlying treatable condition, most dementias are progressive and largely unresponsive to treatment.

Delirium is an acute organic disorder, with impairment in cognitive functioning and change in level of consciousness. It is closely related to the dementias and results from either the physiologic effects of other conditions or the treatment administered for these conditions.

The major category of mental disorders, other than those directly attributable to organic processes, is the category described as *functional* disorders. These are diagnosed by identifying the behavioral and emotional symptoms exhibited by the patient, not because the symptoms occur independently of processes taking place in the brain, but because the etiology is unknown (American Psychiatric Association, 1994). The most common functional disorders in older adults are types of *depression,* characterized by loss of interest or pleasure in usual activities or pastimes. Depression can occur at any age, and older people may have a lifetime history of depressive episodes. Older adults are often subject to intense emotional stress from physical pain, disability, loss of independence, bereavement, and other life events associated with advancing age. Furthermore, there is evidence that direct changes in the biochemistry of the brain and the decline in hormone levels that occurs with aging may make older adults less able to cope with stress. Thus emotional stress, combined with the physiologic changes of aging, may put older individuals at risk for developing clinical depression for the first time in their lives.

In contrast with the dementias, depression may, in many cases, be successfully treated. Unfortunately, depression in older adults often manifests itself through signs and symptoms similar to those of dementia, such as memory impairment and self-neglect. In some individuals, both dementia and depression coexist and may be interrelated, with depression developing as a reaction to the stress of progressive loss of cognition caused by dementia.

Both cognitive and affective disorders in older adults can be devastating to the individual, causing loss of dignity, total dependence on others, and changes in behavior that are distressing and unacceptable to family, friends, and caregivers. These disorders are a major cause of institutionalization. They involve implications for the legal status of the individual and major concerns regarding access to and financing of long-term care, whether in nursing homes or in private or family homes. Therefore it is essential that people affected by these disorders receive an accurate diagnosis, so that appropriate treatment may be initiated, and care and support can be provided for the individuals and their families.

DEMENTIA

Dementia is a condition of deteriorating mentality, resulting in a loss of cognitive functioning. Cognitive impairment leading to a diagnosis of dementia should be differentiated from impairment resulting from other causes. *Dementia* is defined as being characterized by the following:

- A *deterioration* from a preexisting level of functioning. By comparison, mental retardation is a lifelong condition.
- A *global* deterioration of functioning, not just impairment of memory or speech, which may be caused by other neurologic conditions affecting specific areas of the brain.
- A state of *full consciousness* (i.e., the person is not comatose and is fully conscious when awake).

Generally, dementia is *not reversible,* although in some less common types of dementia, improvement may result when a precipitating cause, such as malnutrition, is identified and treated.

Prevalence

How common is dementia among older adults? The *prevalence rate,* or the number of cases of a disease found in a defined population at any point in time, is the product of two measures:

1. *Incidence rate*—the number of new cases occurring each year, per unit of the population

2. *Duration*—the length of time that individuals live with the disease

The incidence rate is usually estimated from the number of new cases diagnosed in a particular population. For every case in which a diagnosis of dementia is made, however, there may be an equal or greater number of comparably impaired people living in the community.

Longitudinal studies, in which the same individuals are assessed over a period of years, have established that the incidence of dementia increases with age. The prevalence rate more than doubles between the sixth and eighth decades of life. Projection rates anticipate significant increases, especially in the developed countries. By the year 2000 France is projecting a 9% increase in dementia victims, the United States a 42% increase, and Japan a 76% increase (Rocca et al., 1986). Similarly, studies of prevalence rates at a specific time, in different, older populations, consistently show higher rates of dementia in each successive decade of life. Table 17-1 summarizes the results of surveys carried out in three different settings.

The rates for those living at home and in the retirement community were derived from screening surveys for symptoms of cognitive impairment, carried out within the specific communities (Evans et al., 1989; Pfeffer et al., 1987). The rates determined in the National Nursing Home Survey of nursing homes throughout the United States use a physician's diagnosis of dementia (National Center for Health Statistics [NCHS], 1989). In other studies of the residents of specific nursing homes, up to 65% of residents of nursing homes meet the mental status criteria for dementia (Katzman, 1986).

Recent studies indicate that the prevalence of dementia has been increasing. This has occurred for two reasons:

1. Mortality rates in the older population have declined consistently over the past 30 years, leading to a major increase in the number of individuals age 75 and over, particularly those age 85 and older.
2. Those who develop the disease are likely to live longer because care is available to treat infections and other life-threatening conditions to which older adults are susceptible.

Study results have shown no consistent differences in rates of dementia between men and women or among races. There are, however, significantly more women than men with dementia because a higher proportion of women live to advanced old age. Dementia increases with age and is a major reason for loss of independence and for institutionalization. Risk factors that have consistently emerged from studies are the following: (1) family history of dementia, particularly in a sibling, (2) Down's syndrome, and (3) thyroid disease (Mayeux & Schofield, 1994). In a study of

TABLE 17-1 Reported incidence of dementia in different settings, by age

Type of residence	65 to 74 years	75 to 84 years	85 and over
Home*	3/100	19/100	47/100
Retirement community†	5/100	24/100	57/100
Nursing Homes‡	34/100	45/100	53/100

*Evans et al. (1989). Prevalence of Alzheimer's disease in a community population of older persons: Higher than previously reported. *Journal of the American Medical Association, 262*(18), 2551-2556.
†Pfeffer, R.I., Afifi, A.A., & Chance, J.M. (1987). Prevalence of Alzheimer's disease in a retirement community. *American Journal of Epidemiology, 125,* 420-436.
‡National Center for Health Statistics (1989). *The National Nursing Home Survey.* Washington, DC: U.S. Government Printing Office.

5055 subjects, higher education was found to be a buffering factor in respect to the development of dementia (Zhang et al., 1990). It is postulated that the attainment of higher education acts as a positive factor in delaying the clinical manifestations of the disease.

Symptoms and behaviors

Mental status decline, leading to a diagnosis of dementia, progresses along a continuum of deterioration in cognition, with associated changes in social, physical, and affective behaviors. Dementia is diagnosed when there are multiple cognitive deficits severe enough to cause impairment in occupational or social functioning and when the deficits represent a decline from a previously higher level of functioning. Also, according to recently published criteria, any cognitive deficits must be distinguished from the normal decline in cognitive functioning that occurs with aging in order to establish a diagnosis of dementia (American Psychiatric Association, 1994).

Progression of the disease and the dimensions of any one symptom vary from person to person, but the characteristic symptoms of dementia include the following:

1. Short- and long-term memory impairment (an individual is unable to learn new information, or to remember things that were well known in the past, such as birthdates or addresses)
2. Aphasia, or difficulty with the use of language (this may involve forgetting simple words or substituting one word for another with a similar sound)
3. Apraxia, or difficulty in performing motor activities, despite intact physical capacity for functioning
4. Agnosia, or failure to recognize or identify objects, despite intact sensory function
5. Disturbance in "executive functioning," that is, the ability to plan, organize, or think in abstract terms (this may be manifested as difficulty in defining words or in detecting similarities, as in comparing a dog and a lion)

Symptoms, behaviors, and progress of the disease vary from person to person, but *memory impairment* is the dominant symptom, particularly in the early stages of dementia. As the disease progresses, new information is rapidly forgotten, particularly when attention is distracted, and even long-term memory is retained only selectively. In advanced stages, memory impairment is so severe that individuals may forget the names of close relatives, their own home address, and their date of birth or age.

Aphasia, deficits in spoken and written language skills, frequently occurs. Language may become vague and imprecise, with use of long, rambling sentences to cover loss of words or inability to maintain attention on the topic. Repetitive questions or phrases may come to dominate speech. In the final stages, language and the ability to speak may be entirely lost.

Apraxia, difficulty with motor skills necessary to carry out everyday activities such as bathing, dressing, or eating, is a common symptom as the disease progresses. The person's appearance may become increasingly dirty and unkempt, a distressing symptom when a person was previously meticulous in grooming and behavior.

Agnosia, failure to recognize or identify objects even when sight, hearing, and other sensory systems are intact, means that the individual has increasing difficulty coping with the unfamiliar. Later, there is difficulty with formerly familiar activities, surroundings, and people. The individual may wander, become lost, and finally fail to recognize home and family members.

Disturbance in executive functioning or *impairment in abstract thinking* means that the individual cannot plan or undertake new tasks, and financial and other business affairs may fall into disarray. Judgment often fails as memory loss progresses, and the individual may be at increased risk for accidents. Water may be left running, pots may be left to burn on the stove, and traffic accidents are likely to occur if the individual continues to drive. The mortality rate from motor vehicle accidents for the population age 75 years and over is second only to the rate for those age 24 years and under, even though the number of miles driven by older adults is very low. The very highest mortality rates for motor vehicle accidents are for men age 85 years and over and men age 24 years and under (NCHS, 1990).

It is often reported that personality change occurs, with accentuation of earlier traits, the individual becoming more obsessive, impulsive, or paranoid. Alternatively, an active, energetic person may become apathetic and withdrawn. Along with personality change, social behavior and impulse control may also be affected, as exemplified by such things as inappropriate sexual advances and aggressive behavior.

Depression, anxiety, and other emotional disturbances often accompany the onset of dementia. As individuals become aware of cognitive decline, they may react with fear and withdrawal from social contacts and activities, especially as they recognize the potential for loss of control and as they lose self-esteem. Depressive symptoms associated with dementia further compound cognitive decline because memory impairment is a frequent symptom of depressive disorders in older adults.

In the final stages of a dementing disease, there is usually a total lack of capacity for self-care, with diminished psychomotor activity, visible generalized slowing of movement, incontinence of urine and feces, and almost total lack of communication and interaction with others.

Placement in a nursing home or other institution usually occurs when the person can no longer maintain hygiene or nutrition alone, or a spouse or other family member can no longer cope with the behavioral or personal care demands of the cognitively impaired person. If an accident, such as hip fracture, or other crisis occurs and the person is admitted to the acute care hospital, further physical and cognitive deterioration is likely to result. This may precipitate permanent institutional placement.

Etiology

Dementia is a complex of symptoms for which as many as 60 different causes have been identified (Katzman, 1986). The multiplicity of causes leads to the consideration of dementia as a number of different disease entities. It develops as the result of two different types of processes, giving rise to the use of the categories of primary and secondary dementias.

1. *Primary dementias*—These are the result of primary pathologic changes taking place within the cerebral cortex or the subcortical structures of the brain. Examples of dementing diseases resulting from these processes are Alzheimer's disease, multi-infarct dementia, and Parkinson's dementia. Less commonly, primary dementias may result from tumors of the central nervous system or from circulatory failure suffered during resuscitation from cardiac arrest.
2. *Secondary dementias*—These result from factors external to the brain, such as prescribed medications acting singly or in combination, metabolic disorders such as thyroid disease, or nutritional disorders that may be identified independently or in association with other conditions such as alcoholism.

A subcategory of the secondary dementias is delirium. *Delirium* is characterized by sudden onset of cognitive impairment, with change in level of consciousness, associated with the same etiologic factors as those associated with the secondary dementias.

Primary dementias

Alzheimer's disease Alzheimer's disease is the most common cause of dementia and is the most frequent postmortem diagnosis for hospitalized dementia patients (Mayeux & Schofield, 1994).

In 1907, a German physician (Alzheimer) published the autopsy findings from the brain of a woman suffering from progressive dementia who died at the age of 55. Her brain demonstrated degenerative changes, with tangled bundles of fibrils (*neurofibrillary tangles*) and clusters of degenerating nerve endings (*senile plaques*) in the cerebral cortex. Because of the age of the woman at death, Alzheimer's disease was, for many years, the diagnosis assigned to *presenile dementia* occurring in a few unfortunate individuals at relatively young ages.

There is evidence that from the beginning some pathologists were not convinced that Alzheimer's disease represented a process that was unique to those with dementia of early onset. However, it was not until some 60 years later, after there had been advances in examination of the anatomy of the brain using electron microscopy, that it was determined that the characteristic changes of Alzheimer's disease were found, at autopsy, in the brains of most individuals in whom dementia had been diagnosed. In the mid-1970s it was therefore proposed that the distinction between early- and late-onset dementia be dropped and that dementing disease for which no cause could be identified be renamed senile dementia—Alzheimer's type being referred to in the medical literature as SDAT, (senile dementia—Alzheimer's type). The preferred diagnosis for a progressive loss of cognitive functioning leading to dementia in those of more advanced age (i.e., senile dementia), as well as in younger people, has now become simply Alzheimer's disease.

There are relatively few signs and symptoms of Alzheimer's disease, and a diagnosis is usually made after other possible causes have been excluded. The following features tend to be characteristic of Alzheimer's disease:

- Slow, insidious onset
- Loss of *olfaction* (sense of smell) as an early symptom
- Lack of specific, focal neurologic signs until the later stages, when rigidity, slowing of movement, and abnormal gait may occur

- Deterioration in all areas of cognitive functioning, with associated changes in personality, mood, and behaviors

The types of anatomic postmortem findings originally identified by Alzheimer and others, including cerebral atrophy, have been found in the brains of both cognitively impaired and cognitively intact older people (Blessed et al., 1968). In 1977, however, the *neurotransmitter theory* of dementia was advanced by a team of British researchers who demonstrated that in those with dementia there are associated neurochemical changes in the brain, with decreases in the biochemical substances that transmit impulses within the central nervous system (Perry et al., 1978). Experimental studies in the area of neurotransmitters (including acetylcholine and somatostatin) and their associated enzymes are now directed toward pharmacologic replacement as a means of reversing or retarding the progress of dementia (Katzman, 1986).

Multi-infarct dementia The second largest diagnostic category of dementia is that caused by the effects of repeated small strokes or infarctions, which disrupt the blood supply to areas of the brain, and which cause deterioration and loss of cortical function in the affected areas. The severity of the symptoms is related to the amount and location of brain tissue of the cerebral hemisphere that has been destroyed.

In contrast with Alzheimer's disease, in which there are few identifiable physical findings, multi-infarct dementia is identified by the following characteristics (Hachinski et al., 1975):

- A history of high blood pressure
- Recurrent strokes or emboli, which may have affected other organs
- Rapid, as opposed to slow and insidious, onset
- A fluctuating course, with stepwise deterioration (a period of decline in cognitive functioning may be followed by some degree of improvement as compensatory brain function occurs)

- Relative preservation of personality
- Nocturnal confusion, compared with relative lucidity during the day
- Distinctive neurologic signs, such as weakness of the arms or legs, defects in the visual fields, or diminished reflexes (these vary from case to case, depending on the areas of the brain that have been affected)

Parkinson's dementia Parkinson's disease, a common neurologic disorder associated with dementia, is also known as *paralysis agitans.* It is a degenerative disease of the basal ganglia of the brain (also known as the extrapyramidal motor system) that leads to depletion of the neurotransmitter dopamine and produces diffuse neuromuscular symptoms, including tremor, rigidity, stooping posture, and *bradykinesia* (slowing of voluntary muscular movement). Parkinson's disease can be of two basic types:

1. Primary type—idiopathic disease, of unknown cause, which is the most common type of Parkinson's disease
2. Secondary type—classified according to metabolic, infectious, toxic, and vascular etiologies, such as viral encephalitis or exposure to substances, including manganese and some classes of drugs (in particular, the long-term administration of phenothiazine drugs [such as Thorazine] to control the symptoms of major mental disorders [such as schizophrenia] has been shown to induce Parkinson's disease)

Approximately 50% of those given a diagnosis of Parkinson's disease develop dementia. It is not known whether Parkinson's dementia derives directly from the pathologic changes of the disease itself, or whether the patients are already more susceptible to the development of Alzheimer's disease, because changes in the brain at autopsy are similar in both Parkinson's dementia and Alzheimer's disease (McDowell, 1994).

Whatever the cause, Parkinson's dementia is a frequent development in an already distressing and progressively disabling physical disorder. Unfortunately, some of the drugs developed to ameliorate the physical effects of Parkinson's disease may themselves have adverse effects on cognitive functioning.

Primary dementias caused by other central nervous system disorders A number of other disorders of the central nervous system are associated with progressive loss of cognitive functioning. These diseases tend to have low incidence and to be untreatable, but they have characteristic signs and symptoms that distinguish them from each other and from other causes of dementia. Included in this group are Creutzfeldt-Jakob disease (caused by a rare virus), Huntington's disease, and Pick's disease (both of which are hereditary disorders) (Gandy, 1994).

Secondary dementias

Progressive loss of cognitive functioning may result from physiologic changes brought about by diseases affecting organs of the body unrelated to the central nervous system; by nutritional deficiencies, sometimes associated with alcohol abuse; and by toxicity or interaction effects from prescribed or self-administered medications. In cases in which extrinsic factors are diagnosed and treated or removed, the patient will recover to the extent that irreversible changes in the brain have not occurred. It has been estimated that up to 20% of patients evaluated for dementia have potentially reversible disease (Cohen, 1985). Included among the risk factors for the secondary dementias are the following:

- Myxedema or hypothyroidism
- Alcoholism
- Metabolic and nutritional disorders
- Prescription and self-administered medications

Myxedema (hypothyroidism), brought about by deficient functioning of the thyroid gland, may lead to progressive cognitive impairment. Unfortunately, the cognitive loss may not be totally reversible, even after treatment with thyroid hormone.

Alcoholism is estimated to affect at least 10% of older adults and may be associated with a higher incidence of dementia in this population for a number of reasons (Bienenfeld, 1987).

Alcohol has a greater physiologic effect on older adults. A decrease in the proportion of body fluid in the aging body may result in a higher blood alcohol level in older people as compared with that of younger people who have ingested a similar volume of alcohol.

Alcohol interacts adversely with many prescribed medications. Alcohol abuse is commonly associated with poor eating habits, particularly with vitamin B_1 deficiency. This puts the individual at risk for the development of Wernicke-Korsakoff syndrome.

Metabolic and nutritional disorders, which create a lack of essential vitamins and other dietary nutrients, can cause degenerative changes in the brain, spinal cord, and peripheral nervous system. Older adults who live alone are at particular risk for malnutrition when physical and/or mental impairment leads to difficulty with grocery shopping or food cooking.

Several of the B vitamins are of particular importance for the integrity of the central and peripheral nervous systems. These are vitamin B_1 (thiamin), vitamin B_6 (pyridoxine), and vitamin B_{12}. Deficiency of pyridoxine can lead to confusion and progressive dementia. Lack of vitamin B_{12} is associated with degenerative changes in the spinal cord and associated neurologic symptoms, including confusion. *Wernicke's disease,* an encephalopathy causing global mental impairment resulting from thiamin deficiency, is a major emergency, which can lead to permanent loss of brain tissue and even death. It is associated with poor nutrition in chronic alcoholism and with

Korsakoff's syndrome, a profound loss of recent memory.

Prescribed and self-administered medications, acting alone or in combination, may lead to impairment in cognitive functioning. Older adults not only consume a higher volume and number of different medications than the rest of the population, but they are also at higher risk for the development of adverse reactions. Reasons for this include the following:

1. Differences in the ratios of body fat and water may cause prescribed medications given in the normal therapeutic dose to be retained longer and to have greater effects in older adults than in younger people.
2. Slowing of motility in the gastrointestinal tract may increase the absorption of some medications and may decrease that of others.
3. Drugs may be metabolized more slowly in the liver and eliminated less effectively by the kidneys.
4. Older adults may have difficulty following medication routines because of cognitive or physical impairment. Spoken directions may be forgotten, and written labels difficult to read.

Many classes of drugs that are prescribed for conditions such as glaucoma, hypertension, cardiac arrhythmias, and depression have been shown to produce neuropsychiatric side effects, including anxiety, hallucinations, or permanent cognitive impairment.

Medications designed to modify the control of the autonomic nervous system can alter the functioning of the central nervous system. Acetylcholine and norepinephrine are two primary neurotransmitters of the parasympathetic and sympathetic nervous system and are also active in the central nervous system. Anticholinergic and antiadrenergic medications, designed to inhibit the effects of acetylcholine and norepinephrine, therefore have the potential for causing impairment in brain function in susceptible subjects (Burks, 1979; Hollister, 1979).

The following are examples of drugs with known neuropsychiatric effects:

- Antihistamines, such as diphenhydramine (Benadryl)
- Antispasmodics with belladonna alkaloids, such as atropine and scopolamine
- Antidepressant drugs, including the tricyclic group, such as amitriptyline (Elavil) and imipramine (Tofranil)
- Antiparkinsonism drugs, such as benztropine (Cogentin) and trihexyphenidyl (Artane)

This short list of drugs with anticholinergic effects could be extended to include a range of widely prescribed medications of the same or different class, all with the potential for causing short- or long-term cognitive impairment. One study showed that during the course of a year these medications were prescribed for 60% of nursing home patients and 23% of older adults in private or family homes, with many patients receiving up to three of the medications at a time (Blazer et al., 1983). Data regarding drug use in institutionalized older adults showed a daily utilization of three to eight drugs and a higher use of psychotropics as compared with outpatient use (Schwartz, 1994).

The administration of several medications with potentially adverse effects on the central nervous system may precipitate the permanent cognitive impairment of dementia or may generate symptoms of delirium, which are reversed if the medication is withdrawn. Older adults are at particular risk for acute adverse reactions from medications superimposed upon progressive cognitive loss from underlying organic disease.

Diagnosis and management

Unfortunately, when dementia is diagnosed, in most cases there is no effective treatment to reverse or retard the progression of the disease. It is, however, important to try to determine the etiology in the hope that the cognitive loss is caused by some condition that may be amenable to surgical or medical intervention, such as pressure from a benign brain tumor, thyroid disease, or medication use.

To establish a diagnosis of dementia, to distinguish one type from another, and to determine potentially reversible causes of cognitive loss, it is necessary to consider a number of factors.

The first step is to document that an older adult is indeed cognitively impaired. Changes in lifestyle, unusual behavior, mild memory loss, and slowness in speech or in the performance of tasks need not indicate severe impairment in cognitive functioning. Neither does mild, transient disorientation following hospital admission for an acute illness or injury indicate a serious pathology. On the other hand, admission to the hospital for an unrelated illness is often the precipitating factor in the investigation of the mental status of the older adult when responses and behaviors are unusual or inconsistent.

A number of neuropsychiatric tests are designed to differentiate normal from abnormal cognition. Tests have been developed to cover all aspects of cognition, such as short- and long-term memory, abstract thinking, language and attention, response time, and others. In addition to more sophisticated testing, a number of screening tests have also been developed. These are of two types:

1. Patient questionnaires, which include tests of orientation to place and time, memory, and attention
2. Questionnaires for relatives or caregivers, requesting information about the patient's ability to perform normal activities of daily living, as well as information identifying emotional and personality changes

Both types of questionnaires are helpful in assessing mental status, as a basis both for deciding on further investigation and for planning care. Examples of these questionnaires are shown in the appendix to this chapter.

If cognitive functioning appears to be truly impaired, the process of arriving at a diagnosis of

Alzheimer's disease, versus other causes of dementia, is largely one of exclusion. Investigations are likely to include the following:

1. A careful history is taken from the patient or relative, to determine whether the onset of symptoms was insidious or sudden, and whether these symptoms are more obvious to the patient or to others. It is also necessary to document other physical or cognitive disorders. For instance, a history of high blood pressure or strokes would indicate that multi-infarct dementia should be considered.
2. The possibility of brain tumors or other space-occupying lesions in the brain is excluded, using radiologic and electroencephalography examinations.
3. Neurologic investigation is used to reveal whether the impairment is secondary to other central nervous system disorders, such as Parkinson's disease.
4. A laboratory workup is undertaken, checking renal, hepatic, and other body systems, to determine the overall health and nutritional status of the patient, and to consider whether dementia is secondary to other diseases, to vitamin deficiencies, to alcoholism, or to adverse reactions to medications.

The fact that an individual's loss of cognitive functioning is determined to have been caused by Alzheimer's disease does not preclude further impairment from other causes such as multi-infarct disease or adverse drug reactions. It has been shown that mixed Alzheimer's and multi-infarct dementia occurs in up to 20% of cases. The possibility of further impairment from nutritional or pharmacologic effects should not be overlooked, because the potential effects of cognitive loss from medications, malnutrition, or other causes will be greater where underlying impairment already exists.

A further issue in establishing a diagnosis is the determination of whether the impairment is delirium or dementia, or whether the two disorders coexist in the patient. It is only possible to determine this retrospectively, after any medications or conditions that might be responsible for inducing delirium have been eliminated or treated.

Management of patients with dementia, once reversible causes have been excluded, consists largely of symptomatic treatment and social support for the patient and family.

1. Since the neurotransmitter theory of dementia was advanced in the 1970s, a vast amount of neuropharmacologic research has been undertaken by academic researchers and the pharmaceutical industry with a view to developing drugs to retard or reverse the dementing process. In 1994 (Cognex), tacrine based on the cholinesterase inhibitor tetrahydroaminoacridine (THA), became the first drug treatment available for Alzheimer's disease. A clinical trial indicated that the drug had an effect, although very small, in reducing the rate of cognitive decline (Davis et al., 1992). However, many patients receive no benefit from the drug and there are significant adverse effects, particularly with regard to liver dysfunction.
2. Other medications may be useful in the symptomatic treatment of sleep disorders, agitation, and aggressive behaviors in more advanced stages of the disease. Antidepressants are also sometimes prescribed, particularly for depression associated with multi-infarct dementia. All drug use must be carefully regulated and the patient monitored for adverse effects.
3. Support for patients and families through individual counseling, group therapy, and self-help support groups may assist in maintaining the patient in the private or family home for as long as possible.

Thus far no truly effective drugs for reversing cognitive loss have been developed. However, if the ongoing research is successful, there will be radical changes in the clinical management of patients with dementia, and in particular those with Alzheimer's disease.

DELIRIUM

Delirium has been variously described as *acute brain syndrome, acute brain failure,* and *acute confusional states.* It is characterized by diffuse cognitive dysfunction, with changes in level of consciousness; it is caused by one or more organic etiologic factors; and it is frequently associated with hallucinations and delusions.

Delirium is an organic brain syndrome characterized by global cognitive impairment of abrupt onset, with disturbances of attention, reduced level of consciousness, increased or reduced psychomotor activity, and a disorganized sleep-wake cycle. Duration can be of a matter of a few hours or days, and seldom exceeds 1 month (Lipowski, 1994). Delirium differs from dementia, which is also a state of global cognitive impairment, in the following ways:

1. The onset of delirium is acute or subacute, whereas in dementia, the onset is insidious and the symptoms develop over months or years.
2. In delirium there is alteration in *level of consciousness,* usually shown by difficulty in staying awake, although hypervigilance can also occur. In contrast, dementia is characterized by a state of normal consciousness.
3. There are frequently changes and fluctuations in the symptoms of delirium, with lucid intervals, in which cognition and behavior appear normal, alternating with episodes of confusion, often during a 24-hour period. In dementia, there are no such major alterations in the level of cognitive functioning.
4. If the etiologic factors responsible for the onset of delirium can be identified and treated or withdrawn, improvement occurs in the general physical status of the patient and the state of delirium clears. In dementia, the changes are permanent and progressive.

The etiologic factors that have been implicated in the onset of delirium encompass virtually all diseases or therapeutic interventions with systemic effects, including cancer, chronic lung disease, and diabetes. Surgical interventions, particularly open heart surgery and surgery for hip fracture, are strongly associated with the development of delirium. Many classes of drugs, acting singly or in combination, and particularly exposure to alcohol and other mind-altering substances, are etiologic factors in the occurrence of delirium in certain older adults. Pre-existence of dementia or other organic brain disease has also been found to predispose patients to the development of delirium, and delirium and dementia may well coexist in an older patient. This makes accurate diagnosis difficult, and the relationship between loss of cognition caused by delirium and that caused by dementia can only be determined retrospectively (Foreman, 1986; Lipowski, 1987).

Delirium may occur after surgery or the initiation of treatment, or it may herald the onset of an acute medical emergency. Onset of delirium may be acute or *subacute* (with a slow increase in the number and severity of symptoms). Although it can and does occur at any age, the incidence is higher in older adults, as are mortality rates for those who develop delirium. The symptoms and behaviors associated with delirium can present major problems in the management of patients, who are at high risk for causing injury to themselves and others (Lipowski, 1994).

Prevalence

Although incidence rates for delirium vary, most reports indicate that its occurrence increases with advancing age. It is estimated that between 30% and 50% of older patients experience an episode of delirium during hospitalization. Delirium has been identified in 15% of older patients admitted to general medical wards (Francis & Kapoor, 1990), and up to 10% of nondelirious older patients go on to develop delirium during their hospitalization (Francis et al., 1990). Twenty-five percent of delirious patients have been found to be suffering from dementia, demonstrating that hospitalizations exacerbate the symptoms of mild dementia (Lipowski, 1994).

Symptoms and behaviors

Certain criteria guide the identification of delirium. The delirious patient may have the following:

- A reduced ability to maintain attention on external stimuli; distractibility, with the need to have questions repeated
- Disorganized thinking, as indicated by rambling, irrelevant, or incoherent speech
- A reduced level of consciousness, with difficulty in arousal or staying awake
- Illusions, hallucinations, or other perceptual disturbances
- Disorientation to person, place, or time
- Memory impairment
- Disturbance of the sleep-wake cycle, with insomnia at night or daytime sleepiness
- Increased or decreased psychomotor activity, with either agitation and restlessness or generalized slowing of movement and speech

Symptoms of delirium may be mild, moderate, or severe, with fluctuations in their severity. The essential features, however, are disorganized thinking and difficulty in sustaining or shifting attention. With attentional difficulties, the person is easily distracted by irrelevant stimuli so that it may be impossible to engage the person in conversation or to obtain answers to questions, even when the questions are repeated. Disorganized thinking is demonstrated by the inability to maintain a coherent stream of thought, with fragmented and disjointed speech, defective reasoning, and inability to perform or complete tasks.

There may be total disorientation to person, place, and time, accompanied by severe memory impairment. Because of shifting attention and incoherent speech, it may be difficult to accurately assess the disturbances of cognition.

There is almost always a disturbance of the sleep-wake cycle, usually involving some reduction in the level of consciousness, ranging from simple drowsiness to stupor or semicoma. In some instances, however, the individual becomes hypervigilant and remains awake for prolonged periods.

Illusions or hallucinations are symptoms of delirium that suggest perceptual disturbances. Equipment in the room may be misperceived, nonexistent people may be seen, and normal sounds may be misinterpreted. Frequently the illusions and hallucinations appear threatening to the patient.

Emotional disturbances seen with delirium include anxiety, fear, depression, irritability, anger, euphoria, and apathy, and in some instances, there are constant and apparently unprompted (or inappropriately prompted) changes of the patient's emotional state. Other characteristics of delirium include neurologic symptoms such as tremor and lack of coordination, as well as incontinence and other abnormal physical signs and symptoms, such as fever and electrolyte imbalance.

Fear, combined with psychomotor agitation and confusion, puts the patient at risk for self-injury or for aggressive behavior toward others. Behaviors such as pulling out intravenous lines, sutures, and catheters, or climbing or falling out of bed are not uncommon in patients with severe delirium.

In contrast with dementia, in which the level of cognitive functioning remains relatively constant, there is often marked fluctuation in level of consciousness and cognition, with lucid periods in which the patient may be attentive and coherent during the day, alternating with restlessness, hallucinations, and general mental deterioration at night.

It should be noted, however, that not all patients with delirium exhibit the more extreme symptoms just described. Prescribed medications may lead to the onset of mild, subacute delirium; without careful investigation, this is difficult to distinguish from early stages of dementia and may therefore go undetected. This is a particular risk for older adults living outside of institutional settings and should be considered when there is an observable decline in cognitive functioning of relatively sudden onset.

Etiology

Delirium is difficult to diagnose and therefore is also difficult to assign a single causal effect. However, the etiology can be delineated by distinguishing risk factors that predispose a person to developing delirium.

The most significant risk factor is age over 65 years, followed by chronic brain failure, either recognized or subclinical. Stress, both physical and emotional, manifested as hospitalizations, sleep loss, sensory deprivation, and any type of overload, is a precipitating event. Toxic systemic situations induced by drugs (especially anticholinergic drugs, alcohol, and sedative-hypnotic drugs) are frequent antecedents of delirium (Lipowski, 1994). In addition to the administration of these drugs, their withdrawal may also induce delirium in susceptible individuals. This phenomenon is clearly demonstrated with the use of alcohol. Acute intoxication with alcohol, or drunkenness, is delirium. However, withdrawal of alcohol from a physiologically dependent alcoholic patient leads to the onset of the syndrome known as delirium tremens. Similar effects may be found after the withdrawal of prescription drugs that have been taken for a prolonged period.

It has been observed that the potential causes of delirium encompass practically every condition and treatment that has general systemic effects. In acute care settings the onset of delirium often indicates a major underlying biochemical imbalance, which could prove fatal if untreated. Most physiologic changes can precipitate delirium; frequent causes include the following:

1. Organic brain disorders, including dementia, cerebral hemorrhage, or thrombosis
2. Cardiopulmonary disease resulting in low cardiac output, low blood oxygen levels (hypoxemia), or high carbon dioxide levels (hypercarbia)
3. Metabolic disorders associated with malnutrition, diabetes, or renal, hepatic, and other diseases leading to dehydration, electrolyte imbalance, or hypoglycemia

4. Postoperative states resulting from anesthesia, blood loss, pain, and other physiologic stresses
5. Congestive heart failure, pneumonia, urinary tract infection, and dehydration (Schor et al., 1992)

Delirium is therefore a complex, multifactorial syndrome. Not everyone with specific illnesses, biochemical imbalance, or exposure to multiple medications develops delirium, but the more predisposing etiologic factors affecting the individual, the greater the risk of onset.

Diagnosis and management

Delirium is an indicator of serious, life-threatening physiologic processes that can occur in patients at any age. Recent studies indicate that delirium tends to occur in older patients who are at increased risk for increased length of hospital stay, institutionalization, and mortality (Levkoff et al., 1992). All indications are that high mortality is associated with delirium. The sudden onset of severe delirium may be manifested either by symptoms of declining consciousness progressing to coma, or by agitation and hallucinations. These symptoms are not difficult to recognize, and they require immediate intervention to prevent fatal consequences. Close monitoring of the newly hospitalized older adult is important to detect less obvious symptoms of delirium.

Apparent difficulty in maintaining attention, distractibility, and drowsiness could be symptoms of delirium in older adults. Sudden changes in behavior in a demented patient, or apparent deterioration in mental status, may indicate adverse reaction to medication, the onset of acute infection, or some other physiologic reaction, with delirium superimposed on the dementia.

Use of mental status screening questionnaires can help in detecting symptoms of cognitive impairment (see the appendix to this chapter). However, the degree to which the loss of cognition is caused by delirium rather than dementia can only be determined after the delirium has cleared. There are no data to show whether delirium has long-term adverse effects, or whether cognitive functioning in older adults returns to predelirium baseline levels.

Treatment for delirium includes the following:

1. Physiologic support, including the maintenance of adequate hydration and nutrition, correction of electrolyte imbalance, adequate oxygenation, and ventilatory assistance, as clinically indicated
2. Full review of medication regimens to detect drugs that may be causing adverse effects on mental status (discontinue all suspect drugs, or reduce their dosage; it may be necessary to sedate the patient to relieve severe agitation and hallucinations)
3. Environmental support, which should include placing the patient in a bright, naturally lit room to allow the patient to distinguish day from night (constant reorientation to time, place, and person may prove helpful)
4. Constant monitoring of physiologic and mental status, being alert to the onset of further complications
5. Protection of the patient from self-injury

DEPRESSION

There is a traditional view, evident in writings from ancient Greece, and persisting until the present day, that depression is a normal and inevitable consequence of the aging process. The development of significant or persistent depressive symptoms, however, is not the normal emotional progression of the majority of older people, although older adults may have to adjust to changes in physical functioning and in family and social support systems. In spite of the stress caused by multiple changes and losses associated with aging, most older adults adjust to such life events, and they continue to maintain an interest in and derive pleasure from the world around them. It is therefore important that the signs and behaviors associated with depression be recognized and the illness treated, because the initiation of treatment will often be successful in relieving the symptoms of this debilitating and potentially fatal disorder.

Depression is a disorder of mood (affect). *Mood* is a pervasive and sustained emotion, which may dominate an individual's perception of the world. *Affect* is the observable behavior that expresses that emotion. Depressed mood is also termed *dysphoria* and is defined as a loss of interest or pleasure in usual activities and pastimes. The opposite mood is *euphoria,* one of elation or excitement. Everyone experiences changes of mood in reaction to life's events, but the essential feature of mood disorders and associated symptoms is that the mood is abnormally prolonged and affects the physical, psychologic, and social functioning of the individual.

Depression is classified as a *functional* disorder and can occur at any age. Depressive symptoms may be emotional, cognitive, social, and physical, and they include sadness, pessimism, self-criticism, slowed thinking, difficulty in concentrating, and disturbances of appetite and sleep. Depression frequently occurs for the first time in late life, although some individuals have a lifetime history of recurrent or chronic depressive illness. Unlike dementia, in which the symptoms are permanent and progressive, symptoms of depression vary in severity and duration within and among individuals over time. An individual who is depressed following the onset of an illness may adjust spontaneously and function normally some months later.

Prevalence

Reported rates of depression in older adults, like those of dementia, vary according to the population and the criteria used for defining the presence of the disorder. However, the prevalence of major depression is lower in late life than in midlife (Blazer, 1994). Studies to determine the prevalence of depression in the older population may be designed to include all individuals reporting relatively mild symptoms, or they may be limited to those individuals with manifestations of a major, disabling, depressive disorder.

For older adults living in the community in private or family homes, studies have shown a wide range of prevalence rates, from 3% to up to 27% (Blazer, 1994). Higher prevalence rates are found among older adults in institutions. The rate of mood disturbance among nursing home residents was found to be 42%, with rates of clinically diagnosed depression of 18% among those age 65 to 74 years, declining to 10% of those age 85 years and over (NCHS, 1989).

Symptoms and behaviors

In people of all ages, the manifestations of depression cover a variety of physical, emotional, and cognitive symptoms and behaviors, which range in severity from mild to severe. Furthermore, depressive symptoms in older adults will often be exhibited in ways that differ from those seen in younger people.

The criteria for arriving at a diagnosis of a major depressive episode are as follows (American Psychiatric Association, 1994):

1. Depressed mood most of the time, as indicated by looking and feeling sad, hopeless, or discouraged
2. Markedly diminished interest or pleasure in all or most activities—apathy, withdrawal, not caring
3. Significant weight loss or weight gain when not dieting
4. Insomnia or hypersomnia—difficulty sleeping or sleeping too much
5. Psychomotor agitation or retardation—excessive activity, usually nonproductive and repetitive, or slowing of physical reactions, movements, and speech
6. Fatigue or loss of energy
7. Feelings of worthlessness, low self-esteem, or inappropriate guilt
8. Diminished ability to think or to concentrate, or difficulty making decisions
9. Recurrent thoughts of death, thoughts of suicide, or suicide attempt

Many symptoms and behaviors may lead a clinician to suspect depression. Emotional symptoms associated with a depressed mood include the impulse to cry, irritability, fear and anxiety, a sense of failure, and feelings of emptiness, loneliness, or uselessness, as well as a loss of satisfaction with life. The emotional symptoms are converted into behaviors such as social withdrawal, crying or complaining, hostility, outbursts of aggression, suspiciousness, and uncooperativeness.

The appearance of the person is often indicative of depression. A stooped posture and unkempt appearance, as well as the more obvious sign of sad expression, may characterize depression. In severe depression there may be psychomotor retardation, demonstrated by slowing of speech and movement and a shuffling gait. Alternatively, psychomotor agitation may be observed, with restlessness, pacing, wringing of hands, or picking at skin.

Alteration in cognitive functioning, with symptoms ranging from difficulty concentrating to memory loss and confusion, may be the major manifestation of depression in an older adult. Unfortunately, although the individual may complain of memory loss and perform poorly in cognitive function testing, a misdiagnosis of dementia may be made because the patient is older. The cognitive loss experienced by depressed older adults is known as *pseudodementia*. If the underlying depression is recognized and treated, there will be recovery of cognitive functioning (Blazer, 1982).

The problem of distinguishing between depression and dementia is compounded by the fact that depression is frequently a symptom associated both with the various types of dementia and with delirium (American Psychiatric Association, 1994).

There is also a relationship between depression and symptoms of physical disorders. In some cases the individual may not admit to feelings of depression but may manifest the emotional distress through complaints of physical symptoms for which there is no underlying organic cause. Reported symptoms may be as diverse as headaches, musculoskeletal pain, or gastrointestinal disorders. This phenomenon, termed *somatiza-*

tion, occurs in depressed people of all ages, but is thought to be particularly common in older adults (Blazer, 1982).

However, depression is frequently associated with, and may be an early symptom of, a number of serious organic diseases, including diabetes, cancer of the pancreas, and thyroid disorders (Cohen, 1985). Therefore mental status assessments of those with somatic complaints and physical assessment of those with depressive complaints are essential.

Depression is not always recognized by the afflicted person, family members, or health care providers. Many individuals are depressed, but without admitting their feelings to themselves or to others, they are unable to understand the changes that affect their lives. Personality or behavioral changes often affect the quality of relationships with others. The depressed person either withdraws from, or is rejected by, those who would recognize and initiate help for the problem.

The denial of symptoms or withdrawal from social contact may be among the reasons why older adults are at higher risk for suicide than are members of all other age groups (21.6 per 100,000 for those age 65 and over, as compared with 12.8 per 100,000 for the total population). Among older adults, white men have far higher suicide rates than do members of all other groups, reaching 60.9 per 100,000 for those age 75 to 84 years, and 71.9 per 100,000 for those age 85 and over, as compared with 7.5 and 4.8 for women of comparable age (NCHS, 1990).

Suicide rates are strongly correlated with age, as exemplified by the high rates of suicide in white men over the age of 60. The highly susceptible person may be the widowed white man who is emotional, is alienated from family members, and has outlived friends. Suicide attempts are more likely to be successful in older adults than in younger people, and although the number of suicides among older people has increased consistently in recent years, the actual rate may be significantly higher than that officially recorded. This is because of underreporting by family and physicians and because older adults often resort to covert methods, such as giving up eating or taking an overdose of prescribed medications (Blazer, 1994).

Etiology

Depression does not have a single causal agent; rather, the etiology is best understood as a web of causality that includes biologic, psychologic, and psychosocial factors. Each individual experiences a unique intermixing of these complex elements, and some then experience a depressive disorder (Blazer, 1994).

Although there is evidence of genetic or familial predisposition to mood disorders, this has not been found to be a significant contributor to the onset of depression in late life (Blazer, 1982).

Biologic factors Pathophysiologic changes such as structural brain changes, disregulation of chemical messengers, hormonal feedback mechanisms, and changes in circadian rhythms are implicated in the development of depression. Abnormalities in norepinephrine and serotonin neurotransmitters are thought to contribute to mood disorders. At one time these neurotransmitters were reported to decline with aging; however, this theory has not found support in recent studies (Blazer, 1994).

Endocrine factors There is evidence that the endocrine system plays a role in the etiology of depression at all ages. High levels of cortisone, changes in estrogen and prolactin levels in women, and abnormal thyroid functioning and other endocrine disorders are all associated with behavioral changes and depressive symptoms.

Factors related to physical illness and medication Depression also occurs frequently in association with other cognitive and physical disorders. Physical disorders associated with depression include acute infections, Parkinson's disease, stroke, rheumatic disorders, and various types of cancer. Medications such as antibiotics, analgesics, antihypertensives, barbiturates, and benzodiazepines have all been implicated in the etiology of depression. Nutritional deficiencies and the use of alcohol are associated with depressive symptoms and with dementia and delirium. Alcohol is a depressant, and when individuals drink because they feel depressed, the problem is further compounded (Bienenfeld, 1987).

Psychologic factors Many theories of personality and of patterns of adjustment throughout the life cycle have also been developed to account for the etiology of depression. These include psychoanalytic, cognitive, and learning theories. *Psychoanalytic theories* of the relationship of depression to the aging process consider such possible causes for depression as thwarting of basic drives, loss of self-esteem, and regression to a more dependent state. *Cognitive theories* based on self-concepts postulate that the development of late-life depression is influenced by the individual's early life environment and by stressful events that lead to the formation of negative self-attitudes. *Learning theories* are based on the experiences of the individual and the individual's interaction with biologic and social factors. In particular, the model of "learned helplessness" hypothesizes that some older people, in a situation of chronic illness or institutionalization, become increasingly apathetic and withdrawn because of feelings of inability to influence the situation (Blazer, 1982).

Psychosocial factors Finally, there is the strong hypothesis that increased social stress and decreased social support contribute to the etiology of depression. One theory has divided stressors into (1) *predisposing factors* based on early experiences, which make an individual less able to cope with adversity, and (2) *precipitating factors,* associated with the onset of a depressive episode. In older adults, precipitating factors may include retirement, loss of a driver's license, death of a spouse, onset of illness, disability, and institutionalization (Blazer, 1982).

Conclusions Testing of the various theories of depression has led to inconsistent findings. This supports the notion that the etiology of depression is multidimensional, and that causes vary from person to person. Changes in physiologic processes associated with aging, social stress, and personality traits are all elements in the development of depressive symptoms.

Diagnosis and management

Older adults may not admit feelings of depression either to themselves or to others, and it may only be by careful observation of appearance and behaviors that depression becomes apparent. One problem is the difficulty of distinguishing symptoms of real physical disorders from symptoms of depression manifested as somatic complaints. The association of depressive symptoms with cognitive impairment necessitates a determination of whether the primary underlying disorder is depression, dementia, or delirium. Family members and caregivers frequently fail to accept depressive symptoms in older adults as abnormal and as indicative of a treatable disorder.

To detect depression in an older adult, the nurse should observe the older adult for any sudden or progressive change in appearance, speech, movement, or behaviors. Self-neglect, poor hygiene, weight loss, prolonged grieving, and unwillingness to socialize with family and friends may all indicate depression. When depression is suspected, the nurse should assess the mood of the person by using one of the depression screening questionnaires that have been developed for this purpose (see the appendix to this chapter).

Second, the nurse assesses changes in cognitive functioning, or complaints of memory loss or difficulty concentrating; all should be investigated. It is important to distinguish underlying dementia from depression appearing as dementia, because treatment of the depression will result in improvement of cognitive functioning. Screening for cognitive functioning may be helpful in distinguishing dementia from pseudodementia (see the appendix to this chapter). However, it may only be possible to arrive at a diagnosis of depression versus dementia retrospectively, by observing the response to a treatment regimen for depression.

Third, the nurse must recognize that physical disorders, such as infection, thyroid disease, and cancer, or medications may induce depressive symptoms. Therefore physical status, drug regimens, nutritional status, and use of substances such as alcohol should be investigated.

Fourth, the nurse must make the distinction between somatic complaints that are emotional in origin and those complaints that have a treatable underlying pathology. The patient's complaints, whatever the etiology, are always respected and treated with a concern for the well-being of the person. One study that investigated gastrointestinal complaints such as constipation and heartburn, a frequent focus of attention in older adults, found that, although there was no physical cause to account for more than half of such complaints, 46% did have some underlying treatable pathology (Cohen, 1985).

Individuals who manifest depression through somatic complaints, such as aches and pains and sleeping problems, are said to have little insight into their feelings and will therefore have difficulty accepting a diagnosis of depression (Blazer, 1982).

Treatment of depression in older adults, as in younger people, consists of four approaches, all of which may be conducted in conjunction with the others:

1. Medication regimens
2. Psychotherapy
3. Adjunct therapies (family)
4. Electroconvulsive therapy

Medications Three main classes of antidepressant drugs have been developed: tricyclic antidepressants, monoamine oxidase inhibitors, and selective serotonin reuptake inhibitors. They have been designed to effect biochemical changes in the brain, which increase the levels of those neurotransmitters thought to be linked to the etiology of depression.

The tricyclic antidepressants, so named because of their chemical structure, are the ones that have been most commonly used in older adults. Nortriptyline, desipramine, and doxepin are the most popular drug treatments for depressed older adults because of their effectiveness (Blazer, 1994). Unfortunately, although effective in the treatment of depression, many tricyclic drugs have a number of potential adverse interactions with other medications and potential side effects, including confusional states and postural hypotension, which can result in syncope and falls (Blazer, 1982; Hollister, 1979). To avoid these effects, the patient must be carefully monitored, and the dose slowly increased to reach therapeutic levels (Blazer, 1982).

Monoamine oxidase inhibitors (MAOIs), as a class of antidepressant medications, are seldom used in treating older adults. They may result in overstimulation of older people, inducing anxiety and agitation, as well as having the potential for life-threatening side effects, both alone and in interaction with other medications.

Selective serotonin reuptake inhibitors (SSRIs) specifically increase the amount of serotonin available at the neuronal synapses by selectively inhibiting the usual reuptake of the neurotransmitter in the synapses between brain cells. The resultant increase in serotonin at the neuronal junctions facilitates the antidepressant effect. Drugs of this class are being more frequently used in older adults, as in other age groups. The most well known is fluoxetine (Prozac), but others include paroxetine (Paxil, Seroxat) and sertraline (Zoloft). These drugs tend to have fewer adverse effects than do other antidepressants, but the effects may include agitation, insomnia, and gastrointestinal disturbances. Prozac tends to have a stimulant effect, whereas Zoloft is more sedative. Fluoxetine has a very long half-life, and side effects may persist for days following discontinuation of the drug (Blazer, 1994). The drug of choice therefore depends on the judgment of the physician as to the appropriate effect to be achieved in individual patients.

Other antidepressants that are not in the previously mentioned classes include trazodone (Desyrel), which is highly sedative, and bupropion (Wellbutrin), which can cause restlessness, anxiety, and agitation early in the treatment (Billig, 1995).

Three other types of medications may be used in the management of depression in older adults:

1. Low doses of stimulants, such as methylphenidate (Ritalin), may be used for the very apathetic person.
2. Tranquilizers such as the benzodiazepines, including lorazepam (Ativan) and diazepam (Valium), may be used for the mildly agitated. Major tranquilizers such as haloperidol (Haldol) are prescribed for those depressed people with severe agitation and psychotic symptoms.
3. Lithium is sometimes used to control repetitive depressive episodes, as well as bipolar or manic-depressive disorder (Blazer, 1982). Careful monitoring of older adults is required with use of this drug because of the risk of toxic confusional states (Hollister, 1979).

Psychotherapy Most people discuss with family and friends their feelings regarding illness, personal relationships, and conflicts, and they find these discussions therapeutic in helping to resolve a problem or to decide on a course of action. For the same reason, psychotherapy, or talking to express emotions, is advocated as an important modality in the management of depression. It may take the form of individual or group sessions, and it may either follow specific techniques suggested by trained psychotherapists or be conducted in a less structured way.

Cognitive and behavioral therapy can be helpful in the treatment of depressed older adults. One specific technique of cognitive therapy for the depressed older adult has been developed; it is time limited and has a problem-solving orientation that emphasizes present-day problems and coping skills (Blazer, 1994). Reminiscence therapy has also been advocated for older depressed people, with "life review" as a therapeutic tool.

More frequently, however, psychotherapy for older adults takes the form of less structured counseling or discussion of the problems or concerns of the depressed individual, with geropsychiatric clinical nurse specialists, social workers, physicians, and other caregivers. It is directed toward providing support, decreasing anxiety, orienting to reality, offering guidance and reassurance, and increasing socialization.

Adjunct therapies Other therapies that have been advocated and developed to assist in the recovery and maintenance of depressed older adults by improving physiologic function, motivation, socialization, and self-interest include the following (Blazer, 1982): (1) exercise and physical activity programs, which recognize the relationship between physical and mental health and may be designed to stimulate activity and endurance or to promote relaxation, and (2) occupational, art, and music therapy, which have been found to be therapeutic in the care and maintenance of depressed older adults.

Electroconvulsive therapy The use of electroconvulsive therapy for the treatment of depression was introduced more than 50 years ago, after it was observed that patients with both depression and epilepsy experienced remission of symptoms after epileptic seizures. Although the preferred course for management of depression is with medications and psychotherapy, electroconvulsive therapy is used as an adjunctive treatment in the management of major depressive episodes that do not respond to medication treatment, particularly where there are suicidal impulses.

This therapy may cause transient memory loss, with eventual return to normal memory functioning. A depressed older adult usually finds this amnestic period during treatment disturbing, because the fear of cognitive loss is profound in many depressed older adults (Blazer, 1994).

Healthy People 2000 Objectives

Increase to at least 45% the proportion of people with major depressive disorders who obtain treatment. (Baseline: 31% in 1982.)

From U.S. Department of Health and Human Services. (1990). *Healthy People 2000: National health promotion and disease prevention objectives* (DHHS Pub. No. [PHS] 91-50212). Washington, DC: U.S. Government Printing Office.

■ Family Systems as Caregiving Systems

Increased longevity has changed the composition of families, with most families having members in four generations and some having members in five or six generations. Every societal change brings unexpected benefits and unanticipated problems; perhaps modern societies will be judged on how they respond to the increased numbers of dependent members, both young and old. The following discussion is about families that are managing the care of an older family member and discusses the role of the nurse in assisting these families.

CAREGIVERS

Caregiving is crucial to the human experience. Infants will not thrive if they are deprived of human nurturing. *Marasmus,* a disease of infants in which there is a wasting away of human life, occurs at this tender age if no one provides physical and emotional care to the infant. Caregiving from the parent to the infant is anticipated by the parent and experienced by the infant. Other significant relationships, such as wife and husband, brother and sister, are also usually anticipated, and these carry the expectation of an intrinsic caring relationship that is mutually beneficial and reciprocal in terms of affection and exchange of services.

Caregiving for a cognitively impaired older adult does not have the characteristics of an adult relationship because of the impaired person's inability to reciprocate with appropriate affection and a meaningful exchange of services. Also, most people are unprepared for this change in a relationship with someone about whom they care deeply—someone with whom they may have shared a lifetime. Thus the nurse can understand the resistance shown by many people to the acknowledgment of cognitive impairment in an older family member.

At this time there is no known cure for the cognitive impairment associated with diseases that are classified as dementias. Until science provides either a cure for the condition or a mechanism to alleviate symptoms, such as insulin for diabetes, family caregivers will continue to provide the bulk of care for cognitively impaired older adults.

Cognitive impairment usually does not occur rapidly; it is usually an insidious process that slowly debilitates the individual. It has been shown through numerous studies that American families do not abandon their older relatives or impaired family members, and that most families continue over a significant period to care for their relatives at home (Brody, 1985; Shanas, 1979). Care given by families and friends represents the bulk of long-term care received by the nation's older adults. Many older adults are an integral part of informal networks of family and neighborhood. Whereas in the past they may have been providers in an intergenerational, reciprocal system of services spanning decades, now many are the worthy recipients of these services. The shift of services from one generation to the next is typically precipitated by the reluctant recognition of cognitive impairment in the older family member.

DESCRIPTIONS OF CAREGIVERS AND CAREGIVING

Informal family caregivers constitute an unacknowledged or at best underacknowledged part of the health care system by providing up to 80% of the home care for older adults. Caregiving activities cover a wide range of services that progress from helping with transportation and grocery shopping to 24-hour nursing care. Four common types of caregiving behaviors are provision of emotional support, of direct service, of linkage with a formal system of care, and of financial assistance (Horowitz, 1985). The amount and type of care given depends on the need of the older adult, and it usually increases over time (Stone et al., 1987). Families of impaired older adults turn to formal caregiving services only after requirements for care become more than they can handle alone (Soldo & Manton, 1985). Caregiver depression and caregiver exhaustion are often the predictors of older dementia patients being institutionalized, rather than overall change in the patients (Baumgarten et al., 1994; Gold et al., 1995).

Who are the caregivers and the potential caregivers? What happens to them while they provide care for their older relatives and friends? These are questions that researchers have been trying to answer for a decade.

Stone and Kemper (1990) report that 13.3 million Americans, one out of every six people 45 to 64 years of age, have a disabled parent or spouse. This large number of people are now or will be caregivers. Data from the 1982 National Long Term Care Survey provide estimates of family members, friends, and others who provide unpaid assistance to noninstitutionalized older people. The survey reports that 2.2 million unpaid caregivers are assisting 1.6 million older adults who are disabled and living outside of institutions. Twenty percent of older adult care recipients are 85 years old or older, and the average age is 78 years. Sixty percent are female; 40% live with a spouse only, 36% live with their spouse and/or children, and 11% live alone.

Forty-two percent report difficulty with up to five activities of daily living, and 69% report their own health status as poor or fair (Stone et al., 1987).

Data provide a complex picture of informal caregivers. Seventy-two percent of the caregivers are women; 23% are the spouse, 29% are daughters, and 20% are others, including daughters-in-law, grandchildren, other relatives, and nonrelatives. Husbands provide 13% of the informal care and are among the oldest caregivers, with an average age of 73 years, whereas the average age of all caregivers is 57.3 years. One third of the caregivers rate their health status as fair or poor, and one in three have incomes falling within the poor or near-poor range.

What services do the caregivers provide? This question has some interesting answers. Eighty percent of the caregivers provide services 7 days a week and spend an average of 4 hours a day in caregiving activities. The most frequently cited task is help with shopping and transportation; next is household tasks, with four out of five caregivers reporting this activity. Fifty percent administer medications, and over two thirds provide assistance with personal hygiene (Stone et al., 1987).

STRESS IN CAREGIVING

Notable is society's lack of awareness of the strains on the people providing the services within this informal caregiving system. It has been published and investigations have supported that there is serious stress inherent in caregiving (Biegel et al., 1991; Pearlin et al., 1990). Caregivers have repeatedly been found to have lower levels of social participation and of mental health than do their peers (Dura et al., 1991; George & Gwyther, 1986). *Caregiver burden* is a term that Zarit et al. (1986) have used to describe the extent to which caregivers view their emotional, physical, social, and financial health as suffering because of their caregiving responsibilities.

Factors shown to influence the perception of stress of the caregiver are history of the relationship with the care receiver, perceived support

Caregiving transcends many generations. *Courtesy Loy Ledbetter, St. Louis.*

from other family members, feelings of filial obligation, rigidity in caregiver and care receiver role performances, changes in lifestyle, and concerns for personal well-being (Baldwin & Stevens, 1990). The social isolation of the caregiver has been demonstrated to have a significant impact on the perceived burden that the caregiver experiences. Surprisingly, one study reported that family caregivers identified their greatest source of interpersonal stress as being other siblings (Suiter & Pillemer, 1993).

Many families, however, have extensive resources and are able to manage the care of an older impaired person without the perception of burden and with a feeling of accomplishment and satisfaction in the opportunity to care for one who has cared for them. Resources available to family caregivers include the following: respite care programs; in-home services; and support groups, counseling, and psychotherapy (Intrieri & Rapp, 1994). Not all caregiving experiences are negative, even for those who experi-

ence a great deal of stress during the time of the heaviest care demands.

The stress that caregivers are exposed to as they cope with the realities of caring for a cognitively impaired older relative is complex and at times difficult for the nurse to fully understand. Six areas of influence on the stress experienced by the caregiver are (1) the background and context of personal and family history; (2) the caregiving situation, including the behavior and status of the patient; (3) the stress inherent in the change in the caregiver's lifestyle; (4) the caregiver's emotional response to the caregiver role; (5) the available social support for the caregiver; and (6) the coping skills of the caregiver (Pallet, 1990; Pearlin et al., 1990). These areas of concern are important for the nurse to consider when assessing the strengths of the family caregiver and the ability of the caregiver to provide care and/or support.

Ensuring the ability of caregivers to provide safe physical, psychologic, and environmental care without jeopardizing their own health is the goal of nursing interventions (Phillips, 1989). Families vary in their abilities to cope with the stress of caregiving (Collins, et al., 1994; Piest, 1995). Studies have shown that the nature of the long-term relationship with the older adult is the primary indicator of institutionalization, rather than the overall progress of the cognitive loss. Some families are unable to manage the memory loss of the older person, whereas other families can accommodate more extremes of behavior, such as nighttime wandering. This difference in caring abilities must be recognized and incorporated into creative and caring nursing actions. People do the best they can at a particular time and with the resources they have available.

Five categories of family caregiving have been defined: four caregiving categories (anticipatory, preventive, supervisory, and instrumental) respond to the increasing degree of disability of the older adult; but the fifth category (protective) is a response to an emotional need and extends over the entire period of caregiving (Brower, 1987). The caregiver attempts to protect the older adult from the increasing awareness of the cognitive decline. Many caregivers are willing to risk physical harm rather than injure the older person's self-esteem. A frequent example of this type of choice is the adult child caregiver's decision not to intervene when the older parent is no longer cognitively able to drive an automobile. The caregiver is torn between sustaining the ego integrity of the parent and the physical risk that hazardous driving entails. This is a difficult situation in which the nurse and the physician have a responsibility to counsel patients and their families concerning the hazards involved if the cognitively impaired person continues to drive (Burke, 1994).

The nurse is a resource to individuals and their families as they cope with this difficult change in their lives (Phillips, 1989). The burden of adult caregiving is a significant social and health concern that results from demographic trends such as increased longevity, decreased fertility rates, and increased participation of women in the labor force (Baldwin, 1990). The increasingly common role of an adult child in a long-term caregiving relationship with an older parent is a new and complex role, which has brought with it the normative stress of caregiving (Brody, 1985).

■ Nursing Process

ASSESSMENT

The cognitive abilities of the older adult are assessed throughout the history taking and during the physical examination. The general appearance and behavior of the person provide the astute nurse with beginning clues to a change in cognitive abilities. The assessment of the neurologic system is an integral part of assessing the cognitive abilities of the older adult. The neurologic examination deals with the cranial nerves, motor and sensory function, deep tendon reflexes, and the mental and emotional status. The examination of the neurologic system is the same for older adults as it is for all adults, with the exception of the examiner's need to accept the older person's longer response time, both in physical and mental dimensions. The ankle reflex and the sensation of vibrations, especially in the lower extremities, may be absent, but these findings are considered within normal limits for the older adult. Mental status is assessed with screening tools, presented in the appendix to this chapter.

Factors that influence accurate assessment

If health care providers fear aging and especially if they fear cognitive loss or the loss of physical attractiveness, they may mislabel older patients. American culture values youth, physical attractiveness, and high levels of intellectual ability. This cultural value system makes it difficult to appreciate a physically unattractive, cognitively impaired older adult. It is essential to go beyond the limitations of a cultural view and to assess systematically all factors that affect an older person's cognitive abilities. It is equally important never to devalue a person because of limited cognitive abilities.

Another frequent type of lapse in diagnostic accuracy occurs in the opposite direction from that of overdiagnosing cognitive loss. Many gerontologic nurses err on the side of refusing to admit that, in fact, the patient is losing or has lost cognitive abilities (Palmateer & McCartney, 1985). For many nurses this problem originates in their value system; they center assessment on the strengths of the person without recognizing or accepting the reality of the losses. Recognizing cognitive loss does not negate the ability to see the strengths of an impaired person, nor does it serve the older adult to distort a cognitive assessment by providing extra clues and making excuses for incorrect answers to questions on mental status examinations. Accurate and knowledgeable assessment of all aspects of a person's cognitive functioning is a professional responsibility of the nurse. Nurses, along with all other health care providers, need to examine their attitudes, their values, and their assessment techniques, in order to accurately obtain and interpret clinical data.

Environmentally imposed time constraints concern all health care providers. Institutions that provide care for the nation's older adults are often driven by a view that "time is money." Therefore doing everything briskly is a sign of efficiency, and this swiftness is highly valued and rewarded. However, care of older people takes longer than does care provided to younger adults. Older patients need more time to respond to questions and to complete physical and mental tasks. It is the responsibility of nurses to ensure that sufficient time is provided for older adults to complete tasks in a manner that reflects their cognitive potential and allows for an accurate assessment of abilities.

Because of the wide variations in level of cognitive abilities, the nurse must attempt to ascertain the older person's prior level of func-

tion. Screening of the older person's mental status and cognitive abilities is accomplished through the use of observation skills and standardized screening tools. Consultation and referral for advanced testing is required for any older adult found to have new deficits in cognitive abilities.

History

Changes in behavior and function are significant clues in the assessment of cognitive abilities. Cognitive abilities vary widely throughout the population, and individual differences must be identified before establishing cognitive loss; change is the crucial determinant of loss. The recognition of cognitive loss may be reported by either the patient or the caregiver.

For most older adults the small amount of memory loss associated with aging does not affect daily living. For those older adults who have a disease process, such as a dementia, the process of cognitive loss is progressive, but for many, the slow nature of the process in the early stages of the disease allows an acceptable level of adaptation to occur.

Because of the multiple etiologies of cognitive loss, every aspect of the person's history is important to the diagnostic process. Physical ailments, malnutritional status, sleep deprivation, medication toxicity, sensory loss, grief, social isolation, and changes in physical and social environment may all contribute to changes in cognitive function. To accomplish a wholistic assessment, the nurse must obtain information about the physical, psychologic, social, and environmental domains that pertain to cognition.

Physical history and examination Any history of prior illnesses may be significant, and the patient's current physical status should be investigated, to search for any undetected relationship to the level of cognition.

A review of prescription and over-the-counter drugs is pursued to determine any possible relationship to the patient's cognition level. Mobility and abilities to perform activities such as personal grooming, dressing, toileting, and feeding are assessed, along with the patient's level of cognition.

Psychologic status Many conditions that affect cognition also influence the person's affect. Often it is behavior indicative of depression that brings the patient into contact with the health care system. Sometimes a sad and apathetic behavior pattern is viewed as a negative but normal and unavoidable result of growing older. Nothing could be further from the truth; depression is treatable even if it coexists with a mild dementia.

Just as there are varying degrees of cognitive loss, there are multiple patterns of response that people exhibit as they attempt to cope with this loss. The reaction of afflicted older adults to cognitive loss is influenced by their level of cognitive attainment, their level of social behavior, their personality, their relationships with close family members, and their living and work environments. Box 17-1 lists behaviors that older adults who are experiencing cognitive loss may exhibit.

Social interaction status Changes in cognition will affect the older person's ability to maintain usual social contacts. Playing bridge, counting change from a grocery clerk, keeping an appointment, answering a telephone, balancing a checkbook, traveling, and understanding nuances in speech such as might be required by a joke or a bit of gossip become increasingly beyond the capabilities of cognitively impaired older adults. These changes in ability cause an incremental shrinking of the social world available to the cognitively impaired older person. For many afflicted older adults, family members respond when the cognitive impairment is recognized and accepted as a legitimate condition.

The history of the patient's relationship with family members has an important influence on their abilities to accept cognitive loss as a legitimate condition. This may be especially true of family members who are not living with the

BOX 17-1 BEHAVIORS ASSOCIATED WITH COGNITIVE IMPAIRMENT

Mild to moderate behavioral changes
    Memory loss
    Hazardous behavior
        Driving
        Household dangers
        Financial problems
    Getting lost
    Nervousness and restlessness
    Suspiciousness
Severe behavioral changes
    Impaired communication or affective functioning
    Nocturnal confusion or sleep disturbances
    Personal self-care difficulties
    Wandering
    Catastrophic reactions

From Harvis, K. (1990). Care plan approach to dementia. *Geriatric Nursing, 11*(2), 76-79.

older patient. Daily contact with the older adult allows a more extensive and realistic assessment of the older adult's cognitive capabilities. Often, a mildly to moderately cognitively impaired older adult with adequate social skills can manage a superficial conversation quite well and can give an impression that all is well. For a visiting son or daughter, it is difficult to understand why the brother or sister living with or near the impaired older adult is upset and thinks that there is something very wrong with the older parent. It is important for the nurse to recognize the conflict family members may have as they take on the care and responsibility of an older parent, relative, or friend. The quality of relationships, rather than the quantity, is the relevant factor to be assessed.

Environmental status The home environment has personal meaning for each individual. A personal and social ordering of space has significance for the person and is recognized by society (Altman et al., 1984). For most people, sleeping occurs in the bedroom and cooking is done in the kitchen. Families may congregate around the kitchen table to share tales of the day's events, or they may sit on a front porch and watch the world go by. However, whatever the ordering and structuring of space, and whatever the significance and meaning attached, space is important to the cognitively impaired older adult. Wherever older adults live, whether in a private home or in a single room in an institution, their space has meaning for them, and it must be respected. Bernier and Small (1988) found that the behavior that nursing home residents considered most disruptive was the taking away of privacy and control over space in their rooms.

The attaching of significance to environmental objects is an individualized process and changes over time. A special table, a porcelain figurine, a special coffee cup, or a picture may have subjective meaning that is part of how the older adult defines a sense of self. There may be background or history related to an object that communicates the richness of the older person's journey through life. Often, questions or expressions of appreciation by nurses about objects in older adults' living areas may begin the process of sharing that can lead to greater understanding of the meaning attached to the object. Nurses should be open to opportunities to listen and to learn from older adults' expressions of the significance of the space and of the objects that make up their living environment.

The understanding of meaning attached to the environment and its relationship to the well-being of the cognitively impaired older adult is an essential and challenging facet of a wholistic assessment. Observation of behavior, listening to speech despite incoherence, and talking to relatives about the past relationship of the patient to the home environment may assist in understanding the personal significance that the environment has for the cognitively impaired patient.

NURSING DIAGNOSES

Nursing diagnoses are a result of the clinical judgment of the nurse, based on a deliberate process of data collection and analysis. Therefore the diagnosis guides nursing interventions, and the etiologies included in the diagnostic statement, along with the documentation of clinical data that substantiate the diagnosis.

Most of the time, the clinical data to support a diagnosis are observable and measurable. An example is the reporting of a physical change, such as "2-cm reddened area on left great toe." This type of physical data can be observed by another nurse in another environment at another location. Physical data are well understood and respected across the different health professions. Data regarding the patient's mental and emotional status are more difficult to define and are more difficult to communicate to others.

The communication of nursing diagnoses concerning the cognitive function of older patients is made difficult by (1) the diversity of the population, (2) the complexity of both the patient needs and the existing pathologies, and (3) the lack of specificity and conceptual clarity in these kinds of nursing diagnoses. Nonetheless, nurses must diagnose cognitive impairments in order to provide appropriate nursing care for the cognitively impaired older patients and their caregivers.

The following primary nursing diagnoses are applicable to many patients who are afflicted with cognitive impairment:

1. Confusion—acute confusional state or chronic confusional state
2. Altered thought processes
3. Alterations in sensory perception (visual, auditory, kinesthetic, gustatory, tactile, olfactory)

Diagnoses in the previous list are from the approved North American Nursing Diagnosis Association (NANDA) nursing diagnoses list, as are the following significant secondary nursing diagnoses:

1. Altered family processes
2. Ineffective denial
3. Caregiver role strain
4. Risk for caregiver role strain
5. Ineffective family coping
6. Dysfunctional grieving
7. Decisional conflict
8. Personal identity disturbance

These diagnoses are applicable in situations of early recognition of cognitive loss and throughout the period when the nurse is involved in the management of the nursing care for older cognitively impaired patients and their caregivers. Because of the increasing disability many of the cognitively impaired older persons experience, it is impossible to list all the secondary diagnoses that can result from the altered state of cognitive impairment. The alert nurse continually assesses and reassesses the physical, psychosocial, and environmental needs of the adult and the caregivers.

PLANNING AND GOAL IDENTIFICATION
Acute confusional state

Long-term goals include the following:

1. Patient will be free of any signs of confusion.
2. Patient will be aware of etiology of acute episode of confusion and will take appropriate measures to prevent further episodes.

Short-term goals include the following:

1. Patient will not harm self or others.
2. Patient will receive immediate and thorough interdisciplinary assessment to ascertain etiology of confusion.

Chronic confusional state

Long-term goals include the following:

1. Patient will receive environmental stimulation to maximize remaining cognitive abilities.
2. Patient will enjoy daily life.
3. Patient will be treated with dignity and compassion by all staff members.

Short-term goals include the following:

1. Patient will not harm self or others.
2. Patient will be treated with dignity and compassion by all staff members.
3. Patient will attend enjoyable activities.
4. Existing cognitive skills will be reinforced.

Altered thought processes

Long-term goals include having the patient be free of any signs of altered thought processes. Short-term goals include the following:

1. Patient will not harm self or others.
2. Patient will receive immediate and thorough interdisciplinary assessment to ascertain etiology of altered thought processes.
3. Patient will be treated with dignity and compassion by all staff members.

Alteration in visual sensory perception

Long-term goals include having the patient be free of any signs of altered visual perception. Short-term goals include the following:

1. Patient will not harm self or others.
2. Patient will receive immediate and thorough interdisciplinary assessment to ascertain etiology of altered visual perception.
3. Patient will be treated with dignity and compassion by all staff members.

IMPLEMENTATION
In the acute care setting

Acute confusional states are a common occurrence in hospitalized older patients. The patient experiencing an acute confusional state will probably have a medical diagnosis of delirium. Anticipatory mechanisms to identify patients at risk for developing acute confusional states are incorporated into admission assessments. These include identification of the patient's current mental status, prior reactions to hospitalization, and prior postoperative recovery patterns, as well as a detailed history of the use of alcohol and other mind-altering drugs by the older adult.

Early recognition of the fact that the patient is experiencing acute confusion is the next aspect of care. The older patient experiencing an acute confusional state may drift from periods of appropriate cognitive functioning to a state of perceptual disturbance and then to a full state of acute confusion. There is no standard, predictable pattern of behavior (Foreman, 1986).

After diagnosing an acute confusional state, the nurse initiates immediate consultation with the physician for the purpose of ascertaining whether there is a preventable cause of the confusion. It is necessary to review drugs, as well as to review the patient's physical status and physical parameters, such as blood gases, hydration levels, and signs of infection. Sleep-wake disturbances, levels of anxiety, nutritional status, levels of sensory stimulation, and many other factors may contribute to and may exacerbate the confusion.

Constant monitoring of the acutely confused patient ensures the safety of the patient. The environment should be structured so as to alleviate fears and to increase the patient's ability to recognize reality. Often the bedside environment of a modern acute care setting includes a frightening array of highly technologic beeping, flashing monitors, with little personal contact between the patient and the caring health professionals. Actually, because the business of caring for older patients in intensive care units is so demanding, hospitals limit the visitors who care most about the older patient to entering at prescribed and limited times.

Because there may be virtue in a continued orientation of older people during serious illness and subsequent hospitalization, it seems imprudent to exclude capable and mature family members from involvement in the care of their relative. Nurses can advocate use of creative methods of providing care to confused hospitalized older adults, which can involve concerned family members.

Protecting patients from pulling out their intravenous lines and ventilation tubes is important, but it is equally important to find an intervention that is less threatening and less injurious than restraining the already confused patient. The first thought should be, Is this line or tube necessary now? Is it part of current medical or nursing care? Consultation between nurses and physicians facilitates collaborative care of the confused patient. It may be appropriate for a family member to be in the room, to sit and hold the patient's hand, and to talk in a soothing and familiar voice. This constant orientation may be beneficial, and hearing a familiar voice may alleviate some of the patient's fear and anxiety. Restraints, if used, must be the last resort to protect the patient from harm. Many patients injure themselves trying to get out of bed when they are restrained, so constant monitoring is the only way to ensure the safety of the restrained older patient. The question to ask before applying restraints is, Would constant monitoring alleviate the need to restrain this patient?

The older patient who is experiencing an acute confusional state is usually hospitalized for an equally acute physical problem—perhaps for a surgical intervention such as a hip replacement. Problems are inherent in care provided by multiple specialists who may each have limited understanding of the comprehensive needs of the older patient. The growing potential for this type of problem increases the need for the one discipline (nursing) that understands the complexity of providing care to the unique and growing population of hospitalized older adults.

In the nursing home

Many of the residents of the nation's nursing homes are afflicted with chronic confusion. There are important areas of challenge for nurses who provide care to cognitively impaired nursing home residents. The ultimate challenge for the nurse is to improve the quality of life for residents who are chronically confused.

Detecting acute physical problems Changes in the pattern of behavior of a nursing home resident who is suffering from dementia may go unnoticed and unrecognized as the sign of an acute problem. Physical causes such as infections, pneumonia, heart attacks, and abdominal pain may be the etiology for an increase in the resident's confused state or a change in behavior. These types of problems, although very amenable to treatment, go unrecognized because of a lack of sensitivity on the part of the nursing staff to considering changes in behavior as a significant sign of a possible physical problem. Communication is difficult for older residents who have lost their cognitive abilities. They are unable to understand pain or discomfort and cannot communicate effectively with staff to call attention to their plight. The nurse must be alert and sensitive to the relationship between pathologic conditions and behavioral changes in cognitively impaired residents. Physical problems must always be considered and investigated when a significant behavior change occurs.

Management of behavior patterns Loss of independence, loss of contact with reality, loss of ability to care for oneself, and loss of a sense of self are the internal stresses that the confused nursing home resident faces on a daily basis. Externally, they face the stresses of an institutional environment: they usually must share their bedroom with another person; all the common living space, no matter how confining, is shared with others; and they confront changing members of nursing, housekeeping, and dietary staff who act as caregivers—some happily and lovingly, and others impersonally at best.

Behavior patterns exhibited by nursing home residents with chronic confusion can be divided into three categories: acting out behaviors, aberrant behaviors, and excess disabilities (Burgio et al., 1988). Specific situations that call for special management therapies include impaired abilities in communication, wandering, and catastrophic reactions (Harvis, 1990).

Impaired abilities in communication Confused residents vary in their abilities to communicate, and the pattern of communication usually contains aberrations. Difficulty in finding the correct word, saying the wrong word, not

being able to respond to a question, and being unable to express an emotion are all frequent experiences of the confused resident. This makes it difficult for meaningful communication to occur between the confused resident and the staff members. The nurse uses therapeutic techniques in communicating with the confused resident and acts as a role model for other staff. Valuing the personhood of the older nursing home resident who is confused is essential to the nurse's ability to teach others to communicate effectively.

Listening for the confused resident's meaning more than the words may help to clarify the true intent of the communication. Often, confused residents will call out a certain person's name or call for a long-lost parent. The nurse should avoid making an immediate response to the words of the resident, and should assess the mood and the intent of the communication. Is the resident seeking attention? Is there an unmet physical need (hunger, thirst, or an urge to use the bathroom)? Is the resident frightened by something unusual in the environment (the unexpected presence of a worker, a change in housekeeping staff, or newly assigned students in the unit)? If the answer to these assessments is negative, then the verbal communication (such as calling for a parent) may be the confused person's expression of profound loss. It is inappropriate to immediately reorient the confused person to the fact that they are in a nursing home and their parent is long since dead. This serves no purpose. The goal of nursing is to promote health, not to cause misery.

The calling out may be loud, annoying to others, and accompanied by pacing or other types of physical behavior. Walking with the resident and then slowing the pace may be the first step in the approach to understanding what the resident is trying to communicate. The ability to enter into the world of the confused person may be facilitated by taking on movements similar to those of the resident, such as walking or swaying with the person. This is a reflection of the rhythm that exists in normal communications; it is an unnoticed part of personal interactions, but significant to effective communication.

When it is ascertained that the confused person's calling out for a parent is not an indication of a more immediate concern, such as calling attention to pain, then the nurse can gently ask the resident questions, such as, "What was it like when you were a child? What color was your mother's hair?" Slowly move through the life cycle with questions and comments that are pertinent for the particular resident. If the resident is able to answer questions and is communicating in a meaningful way and still seems unable to relax, the nurse may ask further questions, such as, "Where were you when your mother died?" The resident might not be able to respond, but the nurse is at least trying to address a perceived need for solace related to unresolved grief over the loss of a parent. It is critical to go beyond mere words to reach the suffering that is under the veil of confused speech patterns. To understand the expression of emotion of a confused resident, the nurse tries to put meaning to movement and words and then validates the understanding with the resident. Box 17-2 illustrates a number of techniques that can be used in communicating with the confused nursing home resident.

Wandering Wandering behavior of confused nursing home residents may be an expression of intent, such as, "I'm leaving this place. I don't belong here," or an expression of longing for a valued adult role, such as, "The children will be waiting for me," or the resident simply may be lost. Residents who wander will also exhibit short attention span and constant motion (such as picking at clothes, or dressing and undressing); some also may be aggressive toward staff members.

Some residents move about aimlessly and quietly but stay within the institutional confines of the nursing home. Often, the quiet wanderer roams into other residents' rooms and takes

> ### BOX 17-2 TECHNIQUES FOR COMMUNICATING WITH CONFUSED NURSING HOME RESIDENTS
>
> 1. Listen closely to the words being spoken.
> 2. Observe the resident's movements.
> 3. Assess areas of emotional distress or physical need.
> 4. Gain the resident's attention before speaking.
> 5. Be aware of your facial expression, your body movements, and your mood.
> 6. Smile when you first establish eye contact.
> 7. Calmly call the resident by name.
> 8. Speak softly but distinctly to the resident.
> 9. Use simple, short sentences.
> 10. Be constantly aware of your spatial distance from the resident.
> 11. Use touch with caution, slowly at first, staying aware of the resident's response to touch.

belongings or explores bureau drawers, as if searching for a particular lost item. This behavior is a problematic one, especially for the resident whose room has been explored.

Other residents who exhibit wandering behavior may leave the area of the nursing home that is considered safe. This type of behavior is the most difficult for staff members to manage. It is important to remember that the resident is a confused person, not a disobedient child. One staff member should walk with the resident, listen, and respond to what the resident is saying. Walk at the resident's pace at first, by falling into step with the resident, and then try to slow the pace. Call the resident by name, touch her or his hand, and then move to stroking the arm if possible; next, gently redirect the walk back to the nursing home (Rader et al., 1985). The resident should never feel threatened; fear increases agitation and makes return more difficult.

Protecting the wandering person from injury is a significant area of concern. The nurse needs to know the resident and the pattern of behavior. The wandering behavior pattern may be severe during the first month of admission but change over time. Some wandering residents may establish a routine that they follow during their stay at the nursing home, and still others follow no predictable pattern except that they wander. Many nursing homes have special locked units that limit access and exit.

Nursing actions appropriate for residents who wander include physical identification of the resident, understanding of the resident's history, observing the wandering behavior, structuring the environment to meet the needs of this situation, alerting staff members and appropriate others regarding the resident's propensity to wander, taking a current picture of the resident for identification purposes, assigning staff members to walk with the resident on a regular basis, establishing valued activities for the resident (such as folding napkins), and, if possible, having the resident attend exercise classes.

Physical and chemical restraints are not appropriate therapies for the resident who wanders. Wandering is an expression of an unmet need that the staff members have not identified. The goals are to clarify the need of the resident and to protect the wandering resident from injury.

Catastrophic reactions The everyday life of a severely confused resident is a struggle. Dressing, bathing, toileting, and eating tax the resident's ability to coordinate thinking and doing. Often these everyday activities lead to the three categories of behavior cited by Burgio et al. (1988): (1) acting out behaviors, (2) aberrant behaviors, and (3) excess disabilities. It is essential for the nurse to reduce complex tasks to simple steps that the confused resident can understand and has the physical ability to perform.

Self-care disabilities and the frustration of the resident in attempting to accomplish such tasks as undressing can lead to agitated behavior. Overstimulation caused by repeated instructions, multiple questions, and multiple people can cause a reaction in the confused resident that is expressed by screaming, crying, refusing to cooperate, or striking out at staff members. Often the reaction occurs because of the difference in objectives of the resident and the staff. If the staff members have a fixed view of tasks in relation to time and are not able to allow deviations, the resident may be unable to accommodate, especially if the task or the timing of the task is unfamiliar. The nurse's role is to protect the resident from injury and from unnecessary distress.

In response to a resident's reaction, the nurse should attempt to quiet the resident by speaking softly and approaching quietly and in full view of the resident. It is helpful to reduce the number of people in the environment and to respond to the resident with a reassuring presence. The use of special techniques for communicating with confused residents is encouraged. After the resident has been comforted and has returned to a less agitated state, the care includes determining the factors that precipitated the event and establishing a plan that will avoid a recurrence (Mentes & Ferrario, 1989).

The quality of the confused resident's life in the nursing home can be enhanced by maintaining an ethical, humane, knowledgeable, and considerate delivery of nursing care. When the dignity of the confused resident is respected, the positive quality of life is assured.

Use of psychotropic drugs The effective management of older adults who are suffering from dementia is multifaceted and multidisciplinary. Nurses must be responsible and collaborative members of the health care team, who accept responsibility for the full process of care. Nurses are involved in varying degrees in the selection, administration, and evaluation of all drugs that are received by the cognitively impaired nursing home resident. Drugs are one aspect of a therapeutic plan of care, given for the treatment of behavior, not to cure the disease process.

Intensive and extensive pharmacotherapy occurs in nursing homes because of the large numbers of nursing home residents, their vulnerability, and the chronicity of their conditions. The Omnibus Reconciliation Act (OBRA) of 1987 was passed to protect nursing home residents and improve their care, with special provisions regarding the use of antipsychotic drugs. Studies in Baltimore and in Minnesota conducted after the 1990 implementation of OBRA reported a 33% decline in antipsychotic drug use (Garrad et al., 1995; Rovner, et al., 1992). Another important study demonstrated that an educational program, given to physicians, nurses, and other staff, that taught behavioral techniques and gradual reduction of antipsychotic drugs resulted in a significant decrease in the use of antipsychotic drugs and a significant reduction in the use of restraints (Ray et al., 1993).

On the other hand, the *undertreatment* of depressed residents is another well-documented, drug-related problem in the nation's nursing homes, and nurses need to become active advocates for treatment for those residents who are depressed (Avorn & Gurwitz, 1995).

Three major types of drugs frequently prescribed for nursing home residents are *antianxiety agents, antipsychotics,* and *antidepressants.* The benzodiazepines are most often prescribed for the older, anxious person and are considered the antianxiety drugs of choice. The half-life of these drugs is a significant factor in determining which drug is most efficacious for the older adult. Flurazepam (Dalmane) has a half-life that can extend over a 100-hour period. An older person will benefit from a drug with a short half-life, which minimizes drug accumulation. Side effects of benzodiazepines are drowsiness, lightheadedness, and dry mouth. Short-term use of the antianxiety drugs is preferred. If the resident has been taking the antianxiety drug for a long time (a year or more), the drug should not be discontinued abruptly, because there have been reports of seizures. It is possible to evaluate continued need for the drug. With physician consultation, it may be possible to slowly taper the resident off of the drug while evaluating the behavior for which the drug was originally prescribed (Maletta, 1988).

Antidepressants were described earlier in this chapter in relation to treatment of depression. Antipsychotic drugs are the third most frequent class of drugs used in the treatment of nursing home residents, and are used to treat those who have dementia and who experience acute catastrophic behavioral reactions, such as severe agitation (Phillipson et al., 1990). These drugs do not correct the intellectual deficits of the impaired older person, nor are the abilities of the person to perform daily life tasks improved by these drugs. Nonetheless, these drugs may provide symptomatic relief from delusions and hallucinations and the anxiety that accompanies these conditions (Maletta, 1988). Studies reviewing the efficacy of the antipsychotic drugs demonstrate mixed results. If any improvement occurs, it is moderate at best, with some studies finding no improvement over use of placebos (Barnes et al., 1982) and others finding the results of use of these drugs to be opposite those intended (Petrie, et al., 1982).

Because no single antipsychotic drug has been found to be more effective than another, the choice of drug is usually based on minimizing side effects and controlling dosages. The starting dose of any antipsychotic drug for an older person should be one fifth to one quarter of the normal dose. Haloperidol (Haldol) and thiothixene (Navane) are considered to be in the high-potency, low-sedation, high–anticholinergic effect, and low–extrapyramidal side effect group. Chlorpromazine (Thorazine) and thioridazine (Mellaril) are considered to be in the low-potency, high-sedation, high–anticholinergic effect, and low-extrapyramidal side effect group. (See Box 17-3 for specific side effects of antipsychotic drugs.)

Drugs are widely used in the treatment of people with dementia. Often it is the nurse's request to the physician that initiates the treatment of nursing home residents with antipsychotic drugs. All possible nonpharmacologic treatment modalities should be tried before resorting to drugs to control behavior. If a drug is used, it must be periodically reevaluated in light of the resident's condition. If it is noneffective, it should be discontinued. If the behavior for which the drug was given has disappeared, then the dosage of the drug can be tapered down to protect the resident from potential damaging side effects. The nurse is the health care provider most able to make the clinical judgments necessary in monitoring the nursing home resident who is receiving antipsychotic drugs. Treatment should not harm a person; a drug should not be used to act as a chemical restraint. The nurse is an advocate for the patient's welfare and initiates and supports appropriate treatment of nursing home residents who are afflicted with behavior problems secondary to confusion.

In the private or family home

One function of the nurse in the care of the noninstitutionalized confused older adult is to serve as a consultant to the caregiver. Often the home care nurse will be attending the older adult for a condition other than confusion; however, the person's confused state is a major determinant of the overall health and well-being of the caregiver. The nurse assesses, assists, and cares for the dyad of the older patient and the caregiver (Phillips, 1989).

CARE OF THE OLDER DEPRESSED PATIENT

Depression may be a masked condition that the caregiver and health professionals miss. Twenty-seven percent of an older community population reported depressive symptoms (Blazer et al., 1983), although the incidence of major depression in the noninstitutionalized older adult population may be as low as 3% (Blazer, 1994). Physical illness may be the precipitating factor in the occurrence of depression in the older patient. The high suicide rate in this population must be recognized as a potential risk factor when care is being provided to the older adult.

Behavior problems such as refusal to eat, constipation, somatic complaints, and being critical and envious of others may be signs of depression in an older adult, rather than the classic signs of sadness and a depressed mood (Dreyfus, 1988). Depression may be a secondary effect of a number of physical conditions (Box 17-4), and it may also be a side effect of a number of drugs (Box 17-5). Assessment consists of a review of all possible physical conditions and a complete review of both prescription and over-the-counter drugs that the older person may be taking. Specific tools for assessing depression, such as the Geriatric Depression Scale, are helpful in assessing the condition and in tracking the patient's response to treatment (see the appendix to this chapter).

The older adult may be vulnerable to the development of depression because of failing

BOX 17-4 CONDITIONS THAT MAY MANIFEST THEMSELVES WITH DEPRESSIVE SYMPTOMS

Collagen-vascular conditions
   Giant cell arthritis
   Gout
   Periarteritis nodosum
   Rheumatoid arthritis
   Systemic lupus erythematosus
Endocrine conditions
   Acromegaly
   Diabetes mellitus
   Hyperadrenalism
   Hyperparathyroidism
   Hyperthyroidism
   Hypoadrenalism
   Hypoglycemia
   Hypoparathyroidism
   Hypopituitarism
   Hypothyroidism
Gastrointestinal conditions
   Cirrhosis
   Inflammatory bowel disease
   Pancreatitis
   Whipple's disease

Hypovitaminosis
   Ascorbic acid
   Folate
   Iron
   Niacin
   Pernicious anemia
   Pyridoxine
   Thiamin
Infectious conditions
   Brucellosis
   Encephalitis
   Hepatitis
   Influenza
   Malaria
   Pneumonia
   Syphilis
   Tuberculosis
Metabolic conditions
   Decreased bicarbonate
   Hyperkalemia
   Hypocalcemia

Hypokalemia
Hypomagnesemia
Hyponatremia
Increased bicarbonate
Uremia
Neoplastic conditions
   Intracranial
   Leukemia
   Lymphoma
   Oat cell carcinoma
   Pancreatic
Neurologic conditions
   Chronic subdural hematoma
   Huntington's disease
   Multiple sclerosis
   Organic brain syndrome
Miscellaneous
   Amyloidosis
   Psoriasis
   Sarcoidosis
   Wilson's disease

---

physical health, loss of loved ones through death, loss of social support, and the awareness of time constraints. Erikson's eighth stage—"ego integrity versus despair"—points to the importance of the concept of time. Older adults who are able to integrate and accept aging are viewed as coming to an acceptance of their life's course. On the other hand, older adults who are unable to accept their life course are faced with the reality of a limited amount of time to significantly alter their life. Such a person, in Erikson's view, experiences despair. Whatever the causes of depression, it is paramount that the nurse be able to assess affected older patients and refer them for treatment. Depression is a treatable condition, not an inherent result of old age.

Often the treatment for noninstitutionalized, older, depressed patients consists of antidepressant medications. The most common cardiovascular side effect of the tricyclic antidepressants is orthostatic hypotension. Of all the tricyclic antidepressants, nortriptyline (Pamelor, Aventyl) causes the least hypotension (Chutka, 1990). Other side effects of medications used in the treatment of late-life depression are shown in Table 17-2.

Drugs with anticholinergic effects may have a detrimental effect on the already vulnerable cognitive abilities of the older adult. These drugs can cause delirium in highly sensitive patients. Other anticholinergic side effects that occur over a longer period and therefore are not easily

BOX 17-5 DRUGS THAT MAY CAUSE DEPRESSION AS A SIDE EFFECT

Analgesics and anti-inflammatory
agents
  Ibuprofen
  Indomethacin
  Baclofen
  Opiates
  Pentazocine
  Phenacetin
  Phenylbutazone
Anticonvulsants
Antihistamines
Antihypertensive agents
  Clonidine
  Guanethidine
  Hydralazine
  Methyldopa*
  Propranolol
  Reserpine*

Antimicrobials
  Ampicillin
  Cycloserine
  Dapsone
  Griseofulvin
  Isoniazine
  Methronidazole
  Nalidixic acid
  Nitrofurantoin
  Procaine penicillin
  Streptomycin
  Sulfonamides
  Tetracycline
Antiparkinsonian agents
Cytotoxic agents
Hormones
  Adrenocorticotropic
    hormone (ACTH)*
  Corticosteroids*
  Estrogen

Immunosuppressive agents
Tranquilizers
  Barbiturates*
  Major tranquilizers
  Minor tranquilizers*
Miscellaneous
  Alcohol*
  Amphetamine withdrawal*
  Caffeine
  Cimetidine
  Digitalis
  Disulfiram
  Fenfluramine
  Halothane
  Inderal*
  Methysergide
  Methrizamide
  Phenylephrine

*High incidence.

TABLE 17-2 Drugs used to treat late-life depression

		Side effects	
Drug	Dose (mg)	Sedative	Anticholinergic
1. Doxepin (Sinequan, Adapin)	50-75	+ + +	+ + +
2. Nortriptyline (Pamelor, Aventyl)	25-50	+ +	+ +
3. Desipramine (Norpramin)	25-50	+	+
4. Trazodone (Desyrel)	100-150	+ + +	0
5. Fluoxetine (Prozac)	20	0	+ +

Adapted from Blazer (1990). Depression. In *Gerontology*. New York: McGraw-Hill.

identified as adverse effects of the drug are dysarthria, decreased gut motility, decreased bladder emptying, decreased visual accommodation, and increased cardiac rate (Maletta, 1988).

Other aspects of treatment for the depressed older adult may be derived from cognitive-behavioral treatment techniques that help the older adult to deal with the here-and-now issues of life. Daily activities and daily diaries engage the older adult in life and begin to reestablish social skills lost through disuse. Assisting older adults in regaining the ability to solve problems through their own actions may help them to feel a sense of self-worth.

Life review therapy is another treatment modality that may help certain older people to master the task of enjoying a mentally healthy old age. *Life review* therapy is considered to be a psychoanalytical intervention and should be instituted by a qualified specialist in mental health. This therapy may include reminiscence as a portion of the process of life review (Butler, 1963).

The single modality of reminiscence is considered a psychosocial intervention and may be used with both alert and cognitively impaired older adults (Burnside, 1988). The focus may be on a variety of subjects that the patient may find beneficial. Subjects can range from the meaning of life to a discussion of trips, or the focus can be directed by a leader of a reminiscence group to topics such as current events or art objects. Demonstrating the ability to listen and to respect the older person's reminiscence is the first step in the nurse's intervention that leads to a significant one-to-one relationship. The goals of reminiscence are to increase self-regard, to improve problem-solving abilities, and to enhance self-understanding. These goals are congruent with needs of most depressed older adults, and therefore, if the patient is a willing participant, reminiscence is an appropriate nursing intervention that is within the scope of nursing practice.

NEEDS OF THE CAREGIVER

The stresses involved in the caregiver role are complex and not easily understood. The nurse should assess five major factors relating to caregiver stress: (1) personal history within the family context of the caregiver-patient relationship, (2) the caregiver's subjective appraisal of stress, (3) change in the caregiver's lifestyle, (4) mastery of the caregiver role, and (5) available social support. These areas of concern are important for the nurse to consider when assessing the strengths of the family caregiver and his or her abilities to provide care and/or support. Several

assessment tools are available for assessing caregiver stress. Three assessment tools are included in the appendix to this chapter to allow the reader to review what has been used in the recent past to assess the caregiver role (Kosberg & Cairl, 1986; Lawton et al., 1989; Zarit et al., 1980). These three scales were developed with a practice orientation for the purpose of assessing the hidden stress experienced by caregivers of older adults. The nurse must be aware of the importance of a systematic assessment of caregivers and the need to be available to the caregiver as an educator and supportive helper.

Legal concerns may present problems for many caregivers. The nurse can suggest that the caregiver discuss with the older adult the option of securing a durable power of attorney for health issues. This allows the caregiver to say how the older adult would have requested to be treated if the person were able to speak for himself or herself. The caregiver should be advised to seek legal advice for interpretations of the laws of a particular state and for legal alternatives that can be used for the benefit of the older adult and the caregiver (Weiler & Buckwalter, 1988).

The twofold goal of nursing interventions involving caregivers of a cognitively impaired older adult is, first, to ensure safe physical, psychologic, and environmental care for the older adult, and second, to safeguard the ability of caregivers to maintain their own health and happiness.

EVALUATION

Evaluation is governed by the stated goals developed during the planning phase. If correctly stated, the goals are observable, measurable, and patient centered. The nursing process is continuous and is centered on the goals of nursing, to provide comfort and to promote, maintain, and restore health. The confused older adult is in need of nursing care on a continuing basis, and the profession of nursing has an obligation to ensure the quality of that care, no matter what the patient's residential setting.

REFERENCES

Albert, M.S. (1994). Cognition and aging. In W.R. Hazzard, R. Andres, E.L. Bierman, J.P. Blass, W. Ettinger, & J. Halter (Eds.), *Principles of geriatric medicine and gerontology* (3rd ed., pp. 1013-1020). New York: McGraw-Hill.

Altman, Lawton, & Wohlwill. (1984). *Elderly people and the environment.* New York: Plenum Press.

American Psychiatric Association. (1994). *Diagnostic and statistical manual of mental disorders DSM-IV* (4th ed.). Washington, DC: Author.

Avorn, J., & Gurwitz, J.M. (1995). Drug use in the nursing home. *Annals of Internal Medicine, 123*(3), 195-205.

Baldwin, B. (1990, July). Family caregiving: Trends and forecasts. *Geriatric Nursing,* 172-174.

Baldwin, B., & Stevens, G. (1990). Family caregiving: Education and support. In C. Eliopoulos (Ed.), *Caring for the elderly in diverse care settings.* Philadelphia: J.B. Lippincott.

Barnes, R., et al. (1982). Efficacy of antipsychotic medications in behaviorally disturbed and dementia patients. *Psychiatry, 139,* 1170-1174.

Baumgarten, M., Hanley, J., Infante-Rivard, C., Battista, R., Becker, R., & Gautier, S. (1994). Health of family members caring for elderly persons with dementia: A longitudinal study. *Annals of Internal Medicine, 120*(2), 126-132.

Bernier, S., & Small, N. (1988). Disruptive behaviors. *Journal of Gerontological Nursing, 14*(2), 8-13.

Biegel, D., Sales, E., & Schulz, R. (1991). *Family caregivers in chronic illness.* Newbury Park, CA: Sage Publications.

Bienenfeld, D. (1987). Alcoholism in the elderly. *American Family Physician, 6*(2), 163-169.

Billig, N. (1995). *Growing older and wiser: Coping with expectations, challenges and change in the later years.* New York: Lexington Books.

Blazer, D.G. (1982). *Depression in late life.* Toronto: Mosby.

Blazer, D.G. (1994). Depression. In W.R. Hazzard, R. Andres, E.L. Bierman, J.P. Blass, W. Ettinger, & J. Halter (Eds.), *Principles of geriatric medicine and gerontology* (3rd ed., pp. 1063-1070). New York: McGraw-Hill.

Blazer, D.G., Federspiel, C.F., Ray, W.A., et al. (1983). The risk of anticholinergic toxicity in the elderly: A study of prescribed practices in two populations. *Journal of Gerontology, 38*(1), 31-35.

Blessed, G., Tomlinson, B.E., & Roth, M. (1968). The association between quantitative measures of dementia and of senile change in the cerebral grey matter of elderly subjects. *British Journal of Psychiatry, 114,* 797-811.

Brody, E. (1985). Parent care as a normative family stress. *Gerontologist, 25*(1), 19-29.

Brower, B. (1987). Intergenerational caregiving: Adult caregivers and their aging parents. *Advances in Nursing Science, 9,* 20-31.

Burgio, L., Jones, L., Butler, F., & Engel, B. (1988). Behavior problems in an urban nursing home. *Journal of Gerontological Nursing, 14,* 31-34.

Burke, M. (1994). Nurse Practitioner: *Journal of Primary Health Care, 19*(2), 9-16.

Burks, T.F. (1979). Autonomic agents: Neuropsychiatric side effects of drugs in the elderly. *Aging, 9,* 69-78.

Burnside, I. (1988). *Nursing and the aged: A self-care approach* (3rd ed.). St. Louis: Mosby.

Butler, R. (1963). The life review, an interpretation of reminiscence in the aging. *Psychiatry, 26,* 25-28.

Chutka, D. (1990). Cardiovascular effects of the antidepressants: Recognition and control. *Geriatrics, 45*(1), 55-67.

Cohen, G.D. (1985). Toward an interface of mental and physical health phenomena in geriatrics: Clinical findings and questions. In C.M. Gaitz & Samorajski (Eds.), *Aging 2000: Our health care destiny: Vol. 1. Biomedical issues.* New York: Springer-Verlag.

Collins, P., Stemmel, Wang, & Givern. (1994). Caregiving transitions: Changes in depression among family caregivers of relatives with dementia. *Nursing Research, 43*(4), 220-225.

Cotman, C. (1990). The brain: New plasticity/new possibility. In R. Butler, M. Oberlink, & M. Schechter (Eds.), *The promise of productive aging: From biology to social policy* (pp. 70-85). New York: Springer.

Cristofalo, V. (1990). Biological mechanisms of aging: An overview. In W. Hazzard, R. Andres, E. Bierman, & J. Blass (Eds.), *Principles of geriatric medicine and gerontology.* New York: McGraw-Hill.

Davis, K.L., Thal, L.J., Gamzu, E.R., et al. (1992). A double-blind, placebo-controlled multicenter study of tacrine for Alzheimer's disease. *New England Journal of Medicine, 327*(18), 1253-1259.

Dreyfus, J. (1988). Depression: Assessment and interventions in the medically ill frail elderly. *Journal of Gerontological Nursing, 14*(9), 27-36.

Dura, J.R., et al. (1991). Anxiety and depressive disorders in adult children caring for demented parents. *Psychology Aging, 6,* 467.

Evans, D.A., Funkenstein, H.H., Albert, M.S., et al. (1989). Prevalence of Alzheimer's disease in a community population of older persons: Higher than previously reported. *Journal of the American Medical Association, 262*(18), 2551-2556.

Folstein, M.F., Folstein, S.E., & McHugh, P.R. (1975). "Mini–mental state": A practical method for grading the cognitive state of patients for the clinician. *Journal of Psychiatric Research, 12,* 189-198.

Foreman, M.D. (1986). Acute confusional states in hospitalized elderly: A research dilemma. *Nursing Research, 35*(1), 34-38.

Francis, J., & Kapoor, W. (1990). Delirium in hospitalized elderly. *Journal of General Internal Medicine, 5,* 65.

Francis, J., et al. (1990). A prospective study of delirium in hospitalized elderly. *Journal of the American Medical Association, 263,* 1097.

Gandy, S. (1994). The degenerative disorders of the nervous system. In W.R. Hazzard, R. Andres, E.L. Bierman, J.P. Blass, W. Ettinger, & J. Halter (Eds.), *Principles of geriatric medicine and gerontology* (3rd ed., pp. 1063-1070). New York: McGraw-Hill.

Garrad, J., Chin, V., & Dowd, B. (1995). The impact of the 1987 federal regulation on the use of psychotropic drugs in Minnesota nursing homes. *American Journal of Public Health, 85*(6), 771-776.

George, L., & Gwyther, L. (1986). Caregiver well-being: A multidimensional examination of family caregivers of demented adults. *Gerontologist, 6,* 253-259.

Gold, D., Reis, M., Markiswiez, D., & Andres, D. (1995). When home caregiving ends: A longitudinal study of outcomes for caregivers of relatives with dementia. *Journal of the American Geriatrics Society, 43,* 1.

Hachinski, V.C., Iliff, L.D., Zilkha, E., et al. (1975). Cerebral blood flow in dementia. *Archives of Neurology, 32,* 632-637.

Hamilton, M. (1967). Development of a rating scale for primary depressive illness. *British Journal of Social and Clinical Psychology,* 278-296.

Harvis, K. (1990). Care plan approach to dementia. *Geriatric Nursing, 11*(2), 76-79.

Hollister, L.E. (1979). Psychotherapeutic drugs: Neuropsychiatric side effects of drugs in the elderly. *Aging, 9,* 79-88.

Horowitz, A. (1985). Family caregiving in the frail elderly. In C. Eisdorfer (Ed.), *An annual review of gerontology and geriatrics* (Vol. 5). New York: Springer.

Intrieri, R.C., & Rapp, S.R. (1994). Self-control skillfulness and caregiver burden among help-seeking elders. *Journal of Gerontology, 49*(1), 19-23.

Jacobs, J.W., Bernhard, B.A., Delgado, A., & Strain, J.J. (1977). Screening for organic mental syndromes in the medically ill. *Annals of Internal Medicine, 86,* 40-46.

Katzman, R. (1986). Alzheimer's disease. *New England Journal of Medicine, 314*(15), 964-973.

Kosberg, J., & Cairl, R. (1986). The cost-of-care index: A case management tool for screening informal care providers. *Gerontologist, 26*(3), 273-278.

Lawton, P., Klebian, M., Moss, M., Rovine, M., & Glicksman, A. (1989). Measuring caregiving appraisal. *Journal of Gerontology, 44*(3), 61-71.

Levkoff, S.E., et al. (1992). Delirium: The occurrence and persistence of symptoms among elderly hospitalized patients. *Archives of Internal Medicine, 152,* 334.

Lipowski, Z.J. (1987). Delirium (acute confusional states). *Journal of the American Medical Association, 258*(13), 1789-1792.

Lipowski, Z.J. (1994). Delirium. In W. Hazzard, A. Andres, E. Bierman, J. Blass, W. Ettinger, & J. Halter (Eds.), *Principles of geriatric medicine and gerontology* (3rd ed., pp. 1021-1026). New York: McGraw-Hill.

Maletta, G. (1988). Management of behavior problems in elderly patients with Alzheimer's disease and other dementias. *Clinics in Geriatric Medicine, 4*(4), 719-747.

Mayeux, R., & Schofield, P. (1994). Alzheimer's disease. In W. Hazzard, A. Andres, E. Bierman, J. Blass, W. Ettinger, & J. Halter (Eds.), *Principles of geriatric medicine and gerontology* (3rd ed., pp. 1035-1050). New York: McGraw-Hill.

McDowell, F.H. (1994). Parkinson's disease and related disorders. In W. Hazzard, A. Andres, E. Bierman, J. Blass, W. Ettinger, & J. Halter (Eds.), *Principles of geriatric medicine and gerontology* (3rd ed., pp. 1051-1062). New York: McGraw-Hill.

Mentes, J., & Ferrario, J. (1989). Calming aggressive reactions: A preventive program. *Journal of Gerontological Nursing, 15*(2), 22-27.

Moore, J.T., Bobula, J.A., Short, T.B., et al. (1983). A functional dementia scale. *Journal of Family Practice, 16,* 499-503.

Nakamura, S. (1990). The brain: Neurochemical aspects. In R. Butler, M. Oberlink, & M. Schechter (Eds.), *The promise of productive aging: From biology to social policy* (pp. 85-101). New York: Springer.

National Center for Health Statistics. (1990). *Health, United States, 1989.* Hyattsville, MD: U.S. Public Health Service.

National Center for Health Statistics. (1989). In Hing, E., Sekscenski, E., & Strahan, G. (Eds.), *The National Nursing Home Survey, 1985: Summary for the United States. Vital and health statistics* (Series 13, No. 97, DHHS Pub. No. [PHS] 89-1758). Washington, DC: U.S. Government Printing Office.

Pallet, P. (1990). A conceptual framework for studying family caregiver burden in Alzheimer's-type dementia. *Image, 22*(1), 51-58.

Palmateer, L., & McCartney, J. (1985). Do nurses know when patients have cognitive deficits? *Journal of Gerontological Nursing, 11*(2), 10-12.

Pearlin, L., Mullan, J., Semple, S., & Skaff, M. (1990). Caregiving and the stress process: An overview of concepts and their measures. *Gerontologist, 30*(5), 583-591.

Perry, E.K., Tomlinson, B.E., & Blessed, G. (1978). Correlation of cholinergic abnormalities with senile plaques and mental test scores. *British Medical Journal, 2,* 1457-1459.

Petrie, et al. (1982). Loxapine in psychogeriatrics. A placebo and standard controlled clinical investigation. *Journal of Clinical Psychopharmacology, 2,* 122-126.

Pfeffer, R.I., Afifi, A.A., & Chance, J.M. (1987). Prevalence of Alzheimer's disease in a retirement community. *American Journal of Epidemiology, 125,* 420-436.

Pfeiffer, E. (1975). A short portable mental status questionnaire for the assessment of organic brain deficit in elderly patients. *Journal of the American Geriatrics Society, 23,* 433-441.

Phillips, L. (1989). Elder-family caregiving relationships: Determining appropriate nursing interventions. *Nursing Clinics of North America, 24*(3), 795-807.

Phillipson, M., Morganville, J., Jeste, D., & Harris, M. (1990). Antipsychotics. *Clinics in Geriatric Medicine, 6*(2), 411-422.

Piest, S. (1995). Rewards, costs and coping of African American caregivers. *Nursing Research, 44*(3), 147-152.

Poirer, J., & Finch, C. (1994). Neurochemistry of the aging brain. In W. Hazzard, A. Andres, E. Bierman, J. Blass, W. Ettinger, & J. Halter (Eds.), *Principles of geriatric medicine and gerontology* (3rd ed., pp. 1005-1012). New York: McGraw-Hill.

Rader, J., Doan, J., & Schwab, M. (1985). How to decrease wandering: A form of agenda behavior. *Geriatric Nursing, 6*(4), 196-199.

Ray, Taylor, Meador, Lichtenstein, Griffin, Fought, Adams, & Blazer. (1993). Reducing antipsychotic drug use in nursing homes: A controlled trial of provider education. *Archives of Internal Medicine, 153*(6), 713-721.

Reisberg, B., Schneck, M.K., Ferris, S.H., et al. (1983). The brief cognitive rating scale: Findings in primary degenerative dementia. *Psychopharmacology Bulletin, 19,* 47-50.

Rocca, W., et al. (1986). Epidemiology of clinically diagnosed Alzheimer's disease. *Annals of Neurology, 19,* 415.

Rovner, S.W., Edelman, B.A., Cox, M.P., & Shmuely, Y. (1992). The impact of antipsychotic drug regulations on prescribing practices in nursing homes. *American Journal of Psychiatry, 149*(10), 1390-1392.

Schor, J.D., et al. (1992). Risk factors for delirium in hospitalized elderly. *Journal of the American Medical Association, 267,* 827.

Shanas, E. (1979). Social myth as hypothesis: The case of the family relations of old people. *Gerontologist, 19,* 3-9.

Soldo, B., & Manton, K. (1985). Health status and service needs of the oldest old: Current patterns and future trends. *Milbank Memorial/Fund Quarterly/Health and Society, 63,* 286-319.

Stone, R., Cafferata, G., & Sangl, J. (1987). Caregivers of the frail elderly: A national profile. *Gerontologist, 27*(5), 616-626.

Stone, R., & Kemper, P. (1990). Spouses and children of disabled elders: How large a constituency for long-term reform? *The Milbank Memorial/Fund Quarterly/Health and Society, 67*(34), 485-506.

Suiter, J., & Pillemer, K. (1993). Support and interpersonal stress in the social network of married daughters caring for parents with dementia. *Journal of Gerontology, 18*(1), 81-89.

Terry, R., DeTeresa, R., & Hansen, L. (1987). Neocortical cell counts in normal human adult aging. *Annals Neurology, 21,* 530-539.

Weiler, K., & Buckwalter, K. (1988). Care of the demented client. *Journal of Gerontological Nursing, 14*(7), 26-31.

Williams, J.M. (1987). *Cognitive behavior rating scales.* FL: Psychological Assessment Resources.

Yesavage, J.A., Brink, T.L., Rose, T.L., et al. (1983). Development and validation of a geriatric depression screening scale: A preliminary report. *Journal of Psychiatric Research, 17,* 37-49.

Zarit, S., Reever, K., & Back-Peterson, J. (1980). Relatives of the impaired elderly: Correlates of feelings of burden. *Gerontologist, 20,* 649-655.

Zarit, S., Todd, P., & Zarit, J. (1986). Subjective burden of husbands and wives as caregivers: A longitudinal study. *Gerontologist, 26*(3), 273-278.

Zhang, M., et al. (1990). The prevalence of dementia and Alzheimer's disease in Shanghai: Impact of age, gender, and education. *Annals of Neurology, 27,* 428.

Zung, W.W.K. (1965). A self-rating depression scale. *Archives of General Psychiatry, 12,* 63-70.

BIBLIOGRAPHY

Abraham, I., & Neundorfer, M. (1990). Alzheimer's: A decade of progress, a future of nursing challenges. *Geriatric Nursing, 11*(3), 116-119.

Colman, P.D., & Flood, D.G. (1987). Neuron numbers and dendrite extent in normal aging and Alzheimer's disease. *Neurobiological Aging, 8 ,* 521.

Folstein, M., Anthony, J.C., Parhad, I., et al. (1985). The meaning of cognitive impairment in the elderly. *Journal of the American Geriatrics Society, 33,* 228-235.

Ford, C.V., & Folks, D.G. (1985). Psychiatric disorders in geriatric medical/surgical patients: Part II. *Southern Medical Journal, 78*(4), 397-402.

Fox, P. (1989). From senility to Alzheimer's disease: The rise of the Alzheimer's disease movement. *Milbank Quarterly, 67*(1), 58-102.

Gallagher, D., Rose, J., Rivera, P., Lovett, S., & Thompson, L. (1989). Prevalence of depression in family caregivers. *Gerontologist, 4,* 438-448.

Hirst, S., & Metcalf, B. (1989). Whys and whats of wandering. *Geriatric Nursing, 10*(5), 237-238.

Kolcaba, K., & Miller, C. (1989). Geropharmacology treatment: Behavioral problems extend nursing responsibility. *Journal of Gerontological Nursing, 15*(5), 29-35.

Nagley, S., & Dever, A. (1989). What we know about treating confusion. *Applied Nursing Research, 1,* 80.

Smith, L.W., & Dimsdale, J.E. (1989). Postcardiotomy delirium: Conclusions after 25 years? *American Journal of Psychiatry, 146,* 452-458.

Wolanin, M., & Phillips, L. (1981). *Confusion: Prevention and care.* St. Louis: Mosby.

■ Appendix: Screenings

SCREENING FOR DEMENTIA AND DELIRIUM

Over the years, numerous tools have been devised to test individuals of all ages in the various dimensions of cognitive functioning, including memory, conceptualization, verbal fluency, and motor performance. The administration of many of these tests requires specialized neuropsychologic training and equipment. In recent years, however, several questionnaires have been developed specifically for preliminary assessment of cognitive functioning in older adults. They were designed to test for signs of the existence of organic brain disease, resulting in either dementia or delirium.

Among the most commonly used test questionnaires are the following:

1. The Short Portable Mental Status Questionnaire (SPMSQ) (Pfeiffer, 1975) (shown in this appendix)
2. The Mini–Mental State Examination (MMSE) (Folstein et al., 1975)
3. The Cognitive Capacity Screening Examination (CCSE) (Jacobs et al., 1977)

All of these questionnaires are easily administered at the bedside and can provide nurses and other health care professionals with some information on the patient's level of cognitive functioning. It should be stressed, however, that low scores on these test instruments provide only an indicator of the existence of organic brain syndromes. Lack of education, language difficulties, and poor hearing also may lead to low scores in individuals without significant impairment. Similarly, there is evidence of lack of sensitivity in these instruments for detecting impairment in individuals with higher levels of education, even though behaviors would indicate that impairment exists.

Follow-up neurologic or psychiatric assessment is therefore always required when individuals obtain low scores, to establish that there is real impairment. Similarly, when there are symptoms and behaviors associated with dementia or delirium, without obvious loss of cognitive functioning as evidenced by preliminary screening, further investigation should be undertaken.

The SPMSQ is shown herein. It has an advantage over the MMSE in that it does not require the patient to write and can therefore be more easily administered to patients with physical impairments or restricted mobility. It also has an advantage over the CCSE, in that it is shorter and less demanding on the patient.

It should be noted that the SPMSQ does have adjustment scores for level of education, as well as for race.

Caregiver-relative questionnaires

Loss of cognitive functioning resulting from dementia is important to the extent that it affects the physical and social functioning of the individual and the person's relationships with other people. Observations by family members and other caregivers are therefore important in determining the level of functional impairment shown by an older adult, particularly where the individual is resistant to testing, or where loss of cognition is suspected but not detected by preliminary screening tests.

Several instruments have been developed for assessment of the severity of symptoms of dementia by family members or other caregivers. These include the following:

1. The Functional Dementia Scale (Moore et al., 1983)
2. The Cognitive Behavior Rating Scale (Williams, 1987)
3. The Brief Cognitive Rating Scale (Reisberg et al., 1983)

The Brief Cognitive Rating Scale assesses impairment in concentration, recent and remote memory, orientation, social functioning, and self-care. It is, however, administered by a trained observer during a structured clinical interview. An alternative is the Cognitive Behavior Rating Scale, which asks a family member to rate the severity of symptoms, covering orientation, memory, aggression, need for routine, and other symptoms and behaviors. The length of this instrument, which has more than 100 items, may be unacceptable to many caretakers.

The Functional Dementia Scale (shown in this appendix) has advantages over the other two. It has only 20 items to be rated by the caregiver, covering activities of daily living, orientation, and emotional factors. It is therefore easily completed and can provide useful supplementary information in determining the level of impairment in the person being assessed.

SCREENING FOR DEPRESSION

Older adults seldom complain of feeling depressed. They often go to primary care physicians with somatic complaints of insomnia, constipation, or lack of energy. Some may be seen by social workers when they seek assistance for perceived financial or other problems that are precipitated by depression. The depressed patient in the hospital or nursing home may appear to the nursing staff as apathetic and uncooperative. Depression screening instruments or tests are therefore valuable in detecting symptoms of depression in older adults.

There are two types of depression scales—those that are self-rated and those that are rated by an interviewer or observer. Among the screening tests that have been devised are the following:

1. The Geriatric Depression Scale (Yesavage et al., 1983)
2. The Zung Self-Rating Depression Scale (Zung, 1965)
3. The Hamilton Rating Scale for Depression (Hamilton, 1967)

The Hamilton scale has the disadvantage that it must be administered by a trained observer, and the Zung self-rating scale may be somewhat confusing to many older people because each symptom must be ranked on a 4-point scale. Furthermore, neither was specifically designed for detection of depression in older adults.

In contrast, the Geriatric Depression Scale was designed to include items that are characteristic of depressive symptoms and behaviors in older people and was tested for reliability against the Hamilton and Zung scales. It requires only simple yes-or-no answers and can be self-administered. If an older adult has poor vision or reading skills, another person, without specialized training, may ask the questions.

Of the 30 questions on the Geriatric Depression Scale, 20 indicate depression when answered yes, and 10 indicate depression when answered no. A depression score of 0 to 10 is considered to be in the normal range. A score of 11 or more is indicative of clinical depression and merits further evaluation of the patient to determine whether a clinical depression does exist and treatment should be initiated.

SCREENING FOR CAREGIVER STRESS

Three assessment tools are included herein to assist the nurse in providing an opportunity for caregivers to express their needs and concerns. The degree of stress or burden can only be inferred through these tools. The tools may be helpful in providing the caregiver with a sense that others are experiencing similar stresses and that their negative feelings, if any, are not abnormal.

The tools are as follows:

1. The Burden Interview (Zarit et al., 1980)
2. The Cost-of-Care Index (Kosberg & Cairl, 1986)
3. The Caregiver Appraisal Scale (Lawton et al., 1989)

SHORT PORTABLE MENTAL STATUS QUESTIONNAIRE (SPMSQ)
ERIC PFEIFFER, M.D.

Instructions: Ask questions 1-10 in this list and record all answers. Ask question 4A only if patient does not have a telephone. Record total number of errors based on ten questions.

+	−

1. What is the date today? _____
                         Month   Day   Year

2. What day of the week is it? _____

3. What is the name of this place? _____

4. What is your telephone number? _____

4A. What is your street address? _____
   (Ask only if patient does not have a telephone)

5. How old are you? _____

6. When were you born? _____

7. Who is the president of the United States now? _____

8. Who was president just before him? _____

9. What was your mother's maiden name? _____

10. Subtract 3 from 20 and keep subtracting 3 from each new number, all the way down.

_____ Total Number of Errors

To Be Completed by Interviewer

Patient's Name: _____ Date: _____

Sex: 1. Male   Race: 1. White
        2. Female   2. Black
                           3. Other

Years of Education: _____ 1. Grade School
                                   2. High School
                                   3. Beyond High School

Interviewer's Name: _____

From Pfeiffer, E. (1975). SPMSQ for the assessment of organic brain deficit in elderly patients. *Journal of the American Geriatrics Society, 23,* 433-441.

INSTRUCTIONS FOR COMPLETION OF THE SHORT PORTABLE MENTAL STATUS QUESTIONNAIRE (SPMSQ)

Ask the subject questions 1 through 10 in this list and record all answers. All responses to be scored correct must be given by subject without reference to calendar, newspaper, birth certificate, or other aid to memory.

Question 1 is to be scored correctly only when the exact month, exact date, and the exact year are given correctly.

Question 2 is self-explanatory.

Question 3 should be scored correctly if any correct description of the location is given. "My home," correct name of the town or city of residence, or the name of hospital or institution if subject is institutionalized, are all acceptable.

Question 4 should be scored correctly when the correct telephone number can be verified, or when the subject can repeat the same number at another point in the questioning.

Question 5 is scored correct when stated age corresponds to date of birth.

Question 6 is to be scored correct only when the month, exact date, and year are all given.

Question 7 requires only the last name of the president.

Question 8 requires only the last name of the previous president.

Question 9 does not need to be verified. It is scored correct if a female first name plus a last name other than subject's last name is given.

Question 10 requires that the entire series must be performed correctly in order to be scored as correct. Any error in the series or unwillingness to attempt the series is scored as incorrect.

From Pfeiffer, E. (1975). SPMSQ for the assessment of organic brain deficit in elderly patients. *Journal of the American Geriatrics Society, 23,* 433-441.

SCORING OF THE SHORT PORTABLE STATUS QUESTIONNAIRE (SPMSQ)

The data suggest that both education and race influence performance on the mental status questionnaire and they must accordingly be taken into account in evaluating the score attained by an individual.

For purposes of scoring, three educational levels have been established: (1) persons who have had only a grade school education; (2) persons who have had any high school education or who have completed high school; (3) persons who have had any education beyond the high school level, including college, graduate school, or business school.

For white subjects with at least some high school education, but not more than high school education, the following criteria have been established:

0-2 ERRORS	INTACT INTELLECTUAL FUNCTIONING
3-4 ERRORS	MILD INTELLECTUAL IMPAIRMENT
5-7 ERRORS	MODERATE INTELLECTUAL IMPAIRMENT
8-10 ERRORS	SEVERE INTELLECTUAL IMPAIRMENT

Allow one more error if subject has had only a grade school education.
Allow one less error if subject has had education beyond high school.
Allow one more error for black subjects, using identical education criteria.

From Pfeiffer, E. (1975). SPMSQ for the assessment of organic brain deficit in elderly patients. *Journal of the American Geriatrics Society, 23,* 433-441.

FUNCTIONAL DEMENTIA SCALE

Patient _____

Circle one rating for each item:

Observer _____

1 None or little of the time
2 Some of the time
3 Good part of the time
4 Most or all of the time

Position or relation to patient _____

Facility _____ Date _____

1 2 3 4 [01] Has difficulty in completing simple tasks on own, e.g., dressing, bathing, doing arithmetic
1 2 3 4 [02] Spends time either sitting or in apparently purposeless activity
1 2 3 4 [03] Wanders at night or needs to be restrained to prevent wandering
1 2 3 4 [04] Hears things that are not there
1 2 3 4 [05] Requires supervision or assistance in eating
1 2 3 4 [06] Loses things
1 2 3 4 [07] Appearance is disorderly if left to own devices
1 2 3 4 [08] Moans
1 2 3 4 [09] Cannot control bowel function
1 2 3 4 [10] Threatens to harm others
1 2 3 4 [11] Cannot control bladder function
1 2 3 4 [12] Needs to be watched so doesn't injure self, e.g., by careless smoking, leaving the stove on, falling
1 2 3 4 [13] Destructive of materials around him, e.g., breaks furniture, throws food trays, tears up magazines
1 2 3 4 [14] Shouts or yells
1 2 3 4 [15] Accuses others of doing him bodily harm or stealing his possessions when you are sure the accusations are not true
1 2 3 4 [16] Is unaware of limitations imposed by illness
1 2 3 4 [17] Becomes confused and does not know where he/she is
1 2 3 4 [18] Has trouble remembering
1 2 3 4 [19] Has sudden changes of mood, e.g., gets upset, angered, or cries easily
1 2 3 4 [20] If left alone, wanders aimlessly during the day or needs to be restrained to prevent wandering

From Moore, Bobula, Short, et al. (1983). A functional dementia scale. *Journal of Family Practice, 16,* 499-503.

GERIATRIC DEPRESSION SCALE

Choose the best answer for how you felt over the past week

1. Are you basically satisfied with your life?   yes/no
2. Have you dropped many of your activities and interests?   yes/no
3. Do you feel that your life is empty?   yes/no
4. Do you often get bored?   yes/no
5. Are you hopeful about the future?   yes/no
6. Are you bothered by thoughts you can't get out of your head?   yes/no
7. Are you in good spirits most of the time?   yes/no
8. Are you afraid that something bad is going to happen to you?   yes/no
9. Do you feel happy most of the time?   yes/no
10. Do you often feel helpless?   yes/no
11. Do you often get restless and fidgety?   yes/no
12. Do you prefer to stay at home, rather than going out and doing new things?   yes/no
13. Do you frequently worry about the future?   yes/no
14. Do you feel you have more problems with memory than most?   yes/no
15. Do you think it is wonderful to be alive now?   yes/no
16. Do you often feel downhearted and blue?   yes/no
17. Do you feel pretty worthless the way you are now?   yes/no
18. Do you worry a lot about the past?   yes/no
19. Do you find life very exciting?   yes/no
20. Is it hard for you to get started on new projects?   yes/no
21. Do you feel full of energy?   yes/no
22. Do you feel that your situation is hopeless?   yes/no
23. Do you think that most people are better off than you are?   yes/no
24. Do you frequently get upset over little things?   yes/no
25. Do you frequently feel like crying?   yes/no
26. Do you have trouble concentrating?   yes/no
27. Do you enjoy getting up in the morning?   yes/no
28. Do you prefer to avoid social gatherings?   yes/no
29. Is it easy for you to make decisions?   yes/no
30. Is your mind as clear as it used to be?   yes/no

From Yesavage, Brink, Rose, et al., (1983). Development and validation of a geriatric depression screening scale: A preliminary report. *Journal of Psychiatric Research, 17,* 37-49.

THE BURDEN INTERVIEW

1. I feel resentful of other relatives who could but who do not do things for my spouse.
2. I feel that my spouse makes requests that I perceive to be over and above what s/he needs.
3. Because of my involvement with my spouse, I don't have enough time for myself.
4. I feel stressed between trying to give to my spouse as well as to other family responsibilities, job, etc.
5. I feel embarrassed over my spouse's behavior.
6. I feel guilty about my interactions with my spouse.
7. I feel that I don't do as much for my spouse as I could or should.
8. I feel angry about my interactions with my spouse.
9. I feel that in the past, I haven't done as much for my spouse as I could have or should have.
10. I feel nervous or depressed about my interactions with my spouse.
11. I feel that my spouse currently affects my relationships with other family members and friends in a negative way.
12. I feel resentful about my interactions with my spouse.
13. I am afraid of what the future holds for my spouse.
14. I feel pleased about my interactions with my spouse.
15. It's painful to watch my spouse age.
16. I feel useful in my interactions with my spouse.
17. I feel my spouse is dependent.
18. I feel strained in my interactions with my spouse.
19. I feel that my health has suffered because of my involvement with my spouse.
20. I feel that I am contributing to the well-being of my spouse.
21. I feel that the present situation with my spouse doesn't allow me as much privacy as I'd like.
22. I feel that my social life has suffered because of my involvement with my spouse.
23. I wish that my spouse and I had a better relationship.
24. I feel that my spouse doesn't appreciate what I do for him/her as much as I would like.
25. I feel uncomfortable when I have friends over.
26. I feel that my spouse tries to manipulate me.
27. I feel that my spouse seems to expect me to take care of him/her as if I were the only one she/he could depend on.
28. I feel that I don't have enough money to support my spouse in addition to the rest of our expenses.
29. I feel that I would like to be able to provide more money to support my spouse than I am able to now.

From Zarit, S., Reever, K., & Back-Peterson, J. (1980). Relatives of the impaired elderly: Correlates of feelings of burden. *Gerontologist, 20,* 649-655.

COST-OF-CARE INDEX

	Strongly disagree	Disagree	Agree	Strongly agree
1. I feel that meeting the psychologic needs of my elderly relative for feeling wanted and important is not (will not be) worth the effort.	1	2	3	4
2. I feel that my elderly relative is (will be) an overly demanding person to care for.	1	2	3	4
3. I feel that caring for my elderly relative has negatively affected (will negatively affect) my family's or my physical health.	1	2	3	4
4. I feel that as a result of caring for my elderly relative I do not (will not) have enough time for myself.	1	2	3	4
5. I feel that caring for my elderly relative is causing me (will cause me) to dip into savings meant for other things.	1	2	3	4
6. I feel that meeting the health needs of my elderly relative is not (will not be) worth the effort.	1	2	3	4
7. I feel that my elderly relative tries (will try) to manipulate me.	1	2	3	4
8. I feel that caring for my elderly relative has negatively affected (will negatively affect) my appetite.	1	2	3	4
9. I feel that caring for my elderly relative puts (will put) a strain on family relationships.	1	2	3	4
10. I feel that my family and I must give up (will have to give up) necessities because of the expense to care for my elderly relative.	1	2	3	4
11. I feel that caring for my elderly relative disrupts (will disrupt) my routine in my home.	1	2	3	4
12. I feel that caring for my elderly relative has caused (will cause) my family and me much aggravation.	1	2	3	4
13. I feel that meeting the daily needs of my elderly relative is not (will not be) worth the effort.	1	2	3	4
14. I feel that caring for my elderly relative has caused me (will cause me) to be physically fatigued.	1	2	3	4
15. I feel that my family and I cannot (will not be able to) afford those little extras because of the expense to care for my elderly relative.	1	2	3	4
16. I feel that my elderly relative makes (will make) unnecessary requests of me for care.	1	2	3	4
17. I feel that meeting the social needs of my elderly relative for companionship is not (will not be) worth the effort.	1	2	3	4
18. I feel that caring for my elderly relative has caused me (will cause me) to become anxious.	1	2	3	4
19. I feel that caring for my elderly relative interferes (will interfere) with my friends or friends of my family coming to my home.	1	2	3	4
20. I feel that caring for my elderly relative is (will be) too expensive.	1	2	3	4

From Kosberg, J., & Cairl, R. (1986). The cost-of-care index: A case management tool for screening informal care providers. *Gerontologist, 26*(3), 273-278.

MEASURING CAREGIVER APPRAISAL

Subjective caregiving burden

Your health has suffered because of the care you must give [IP]?*

Isolated and alone as a result of care for [IP]?

You will be unable to care for [IP] much longer?

You have lost control of your life since [IP's] illness?

Very tired as a result of caring for [IP]?

Nervous or depressed when with [IP]?

Taking care of [IP] gives me a trapped feeling.

Embarrassed over [IP's] behavior?

Angry when you are around [IP]?

[IP] seems to expect you to take care of [her] as if you were the only one [she] could depend on?

You don't have enough money to care for [IP] in addition to the rest of your expenses?

Resentful of other relatives who could but who do not do things for [IP]?

You wish you could just leave the care of [IP] to someone else?

Impact of caregiving

Your social life has suffered because you are caring for [IP]?

Because of the time you spend with [IP], you don't have enough time for yourself?

It's hard to plan things ahead when [IP's] needs are so unpredictable.

It's mostly [IP's] needs that determine how my days are spent.

[IP] asks for more help than [she] needs?

[IP] currently affects your relationships with other family members in a negative way?

Caring for [IP] doesn't allow you as much privacy as you would like?

Uncomfortable about having friends over because of [IP]?

Caring for [IP] has interfered with your use of space in your home?

Caregiving mastery

I can fit in most of the things I need to do in spite of the time taken by caring for [IP].

Uncertain about what to do about [IP]?

Reassured knowing that as long as you are helping [IP], [she] is getting proper care?

You should be doing more for [IP]?

You could do a better job in caring for [IP]?

In general, I feel able to handle most problems in the care of [IP].

I am pretty good at figuring out what [IP] needs.

Nothing I can do seems to please [IP].

Taking responsibility for [IP] gives your self-esteem a boost?

[IP] is beyond being helped by most things I do for [her].

The things I do for [IP] keep [her] from getting worse.

I can take care of [IP] with no help, or I could—if I had to.

MEASURING CAREGIVER APPRAISAL—cont'd

Caregiving satisfaction
  You really enjoy being with [IP]?
  [IP] shows real appreciation of what you do for [her]?
  [IP's] pleasure over some little thing gives you pleasure?
  Helping [IP] has made you feel closer to [her]?
  It makes you happy to know that [IP] is being cared for by [her] family?
  You take care of [IP] more because you want to than out of a sense of duty?
  [IP's] old self is showing through in spite of [her] current condition?
  The knowledge you are doing your best gets you through the rough times with [IP]?
  I do pretty much what I have to do, not what I want to do, in relation to [IP].
Cognitive reappraisal (traditional caregiving ideology)
  A strong reason for taking care of [IP] is to be true to family traditions?
  Taking care of [IP] is a way for you to live up to religious principles?
  A strong reason to care for [IP] is to provide a good model for your own children to follow?
  You think of the help you give [IP] as an opportunity to repay [her]?

From Lawton, P., Klebian, M., Moss, M., Rovine, M., & Glicksman, A. (1989). Measuring caregiving appraisal. *Journal of Gerontology, 44*(3), 61-71.
*Identified patient.

More humane, we assert, than to take care of the hurt,
Is the plan of removing the danger.

AUTHOR UNKNOWN, *Parable of the dangerous cliff*

Safety

■ Learning Objectives

On completion of this chapter, the reader will be able to do the following:

1. Discuss the concept of safety as it applies to the older adult.
2. Discuss the incidence of injury in the older population.
3. Recognize the older adult who is at risk for falling.
4. Discuss interventions to diminish the risk of falling for older adults.
5. Identify the susceptibility of the older adult to sustaining an injury as a result of a traffic accident and/or burns.
6. Recognize signs and symptoms of elder abuse.
7. Discuss the use of restraints with older patients.

Safety generally connotes protection from hazards to health and well-being. More specifically it can mean protection from unintentional injury or harm to one's physical or psychologic well-being. Safety, despite various definitions, is a recognized universal human need. Maslow (1954) listed safety, as a human need, right after the most basic physiologic needs such as food, air, and water. In this context, higher social needs of love and belonging can be realized only after physiologic and safety needs have been met. Safety provides a sense of stability and manageability to one's world—in other words, security.

The risk of actual injury or harm is variable at any given time for any given individual. In turn, a person's susceptibility to harm or injury will be affected by that individual's own personal characteristics, as well as the offending agent and the environment of the agent and susceptible person (host). Epidemiologically derived models that consider the interrelationship of hazardous agent, host (person), and environment are helpful in providing a wholistic framework for examining hazards to safety. Box 18-1 provides an example of an epidemiologic model of factors involved in safety. Activities to promote safety will employ methods to control the hazardous

BOX 18-1 FACTORS INVOLVED IN SAFETY

AGENT

Kinetic force
Thermal energy
Electrical energy
Gravitational energy
Radiation
Chemicals
Microbes

PERSON

Consciousness
Cognitive and emotional status
Developmental stage
Knowledge
Physiologic status
Health status
Nutritional status
Biologic defense mechanisms
Attitude

ENVIRONMENT

Space
Ventilation
Cleanliness
Sanitation
Lighting
Temperature
Weather
Shelter
Furnishings
Pets
Other people

agent, decrease the susceptibility of the host, and/or modify environmental factors.

Because numerous factors pose hazards or threats to one's health and well-being, this chapter will focus on those that have particular relevance to older people: unintentional injuries, particularly falls; automobile accidents; and abuse. The use of physical restraints as they relate to safety in older adults also will be discussed.

■ Ethical Considerations

As people age, they experience age-related changes that alter what constitutes a threat or risk to their safety. The family home environment can be dangerous for an older adult, not because the aspects of the home have changed, but because of the change in the physical abilities of the older adult. Older adults with intact cognitive abilities may choose to take the risk of staying in their familiar home environments, with full knowledge of increased risk. The dilemma for others, especially family members and health care providers, is the definition of what constitutes the acceptable level of risk for older adults.

Balancing the rights of individuals and the need to provide for their safety is not an easy task and may pose ethical dilemmas for older adults, their families, and health care providers. An ethical dilemma exists when one must choose between two equally desirable or undesirable alternatives. Resolving such a dilemma requires consideration of a number of ethical principles. Autonomy, beneficence, and nonmaleficence are ethical principles that are considered in making decisions about the older adult's safety.

Autonomy refers to an individual's right to determine his or her own course of existence, as long as that right does not infringe on the autonomy of another (Beauchamp & Childress, 1994). Most Western ethicists view autonomy as the supreme and overriding principle in ethical decision making. Exercise of the right of autonomy requires rational decision making. For some older adults the capacity for rational decision making may be compromised or diminished. In these cases the decision making may have to be assumed by another.

In the older adult with diminished decision-making capability, not all areas of self-determination are necessarily compromised to the same degree. Those assuming decision making for the older adult must use care to ensure that the individual maintains the right to self-determination whenever and wherever possible. Overriding an individual's right to self-determination and exercise of autonomy is rarely, if ever, justified.

Beneficence and its corollary principle of nonmaleficence require one to do good for others and to do no harm (Beauchamp & Childress, 1994). In the case of those with diminished decision-making capabilities, those assuming the decision making must weigh the risk of doing harm against the benefits of any given action. Most ethicists concede that the duty to prevent harm is stronger than the duty to do good (Hogstel & Gaul, 1991).

This chapter is written within the framework of acceptance of the older adult's individual right to make choices. When there is a question of the extent of risk inherent in the decision or in the older adult's behavior, family members and care providers must employ ethical principles to guide their actions. The right to be treated with dignity is a basic human right, and it must rarely be breached in the name of safety and beneficence by violating principles of autonomy or nonmaleficence.

Chapter 22 provides a more detailed discussion of ethical principles related to the care of older adults.

■ Injury

Accidents are usually viewed as random events in which individuals have little or no control either to prevent them or to influence their outcome. On the other hand, injury can be thought of as having three phases of development: preevent, event, and postevent. Injury prevention is possible in the preevent phase and may decrease the number of serious injuries. Whether the term *unintentional injury* or *accident* is the label

Health Promotion

Increase vigilance for potential injury when these psychosocial factors are present
- Cognitive impairment
- Depression
- Grief
- Anniversary date of significant loss
- Psychologic stress
- Anger
- Loss of social roles, or social isolation
- Loss of independence
- Hazardous behavior

used to describe these random events, the prevention of their occurrence is a significant challenge for nursing and is the main focus of this chapter.

Unintentional injuries (accidents) are the seventh leading cause of death in people over 65 years of age, and their incidence increases dramatically with advancing age. The rate for those age 65 and older is twice that of middle-aged people (U.S. Census Bureau, 1994). In the over-85 age group, it is the fifth leading cause of death. Close to two thirds of all injury-related deaths and more than 80% of hospitalizations resulting from injury involve unintentional injuries (U.S. Department of Health and Human Services [USDHHS], 1991). Motor vehicle accidents account for half of the deaths resulting from unintentional injuries, and falls are the second most frequent cause of injury-related death. Unintentional injuries cost the United States close to $400 billion each year, with one third attributable to falls and 28% to motor vehicle accidents (U.S. Census Bureau, 1994).

FALLS

Falls and fall-related injuries account for a considerable amount of morbidity and death in older adults. Longer recovery periods and greater severity of injuries related to falls in older people pose particularly serious threats to the older person's health and functional abilities. Although most falls do not result in serious physical injury or death (Nevitt et al., 1991), they very often lead to decreased physical and social activity and loss of confidence in functional independence.

Falls in older adults are a major risk factor for hip fracture. Four physical factors have been found to be related to increased risk of fracture: inability to rise from a chair without using arms, a faster resting pulse, poor depth perception, and poor low-frequency contrast sensitivity (Cummings et al., 1995). The number of hip fractures (200,000) yearly in the United States is substantial, costly, and serious. Hip fractures lead to death in 12% to 20% of cases, and the mortality rate increases with age. Those over 80 years of age have a mortality rate from falls 8 times greater than those 60 years of age or under (Urton, 1991). Only about a fourth of older adults who sustain a hip fracture will fully recover (Ross, 1991). Box 18-2 lists some of the more serious physiologic, psychosocial, and functional consequences of falls.

Most falls occur in the home. Stairs account for a large proportion of falls, and most serious falls on stairs occur during descent. Many falls occur because the older individual misses the last step. The risk of falling is generally recognized to be significantly greater for hospitalized older adults than for other hospitalized age groups. In the nursing home population, more than one half of the ambulatory nursing home residents fall during a 1-year period (Tinetti, 1990).

A myriad of environmental and personal factors contribute to fall susceptibility. Poorly or inappropriately soled footwear; unstable furniture; elevated bed positions; side rails; highly polished floors; loose floor coverings (e.g., scatter rugs and broken tiles); dimly lighted bathrooms, halls, and stairways; clutter, ice, water, or grease in walking areas; use of ambulatory assistive devices; and even pets are environmental factors that have been generally cited as contributing

BOX 18-2 CONSEQUENCES OF FALLS

PHYSIOLOGIC

Fractures, especially of the hip, wrist, vertebrae, and ribs
Soft-tissue injury: hematomas, lacerations
Concussion, subdural or epidural hematoma
Exacerbation of arthritis or cardiovascular or pulmonary problems
Death

PSYCHOSOCIAL

Loss of confidence
Depression
Fear of falling
Social withdrawal
Dependency
Compromised autonomy
Institutionalization

FUNCTIONAL

Immobility, which may lead to the following:
   Thrombosis
   Dehydration
   Contracture
   Pressure ulcers
   Urinary and bowel incontinence or retention
   Infection
Deconditioning
Decreased righting reflex

Adapted from Hough, J.C. (1992). Falls and falling. In R.J. Ham & P.D. Sloane (Eds.), *Primary care geriatrics: A case based approach* (2nd ed., pp. 362-379). St. Louis: Mosby.

Aging Alert
Factors to address when older adults have complaints of instability and/or falls

Assessment and treatment of physical injury
Treatment of underlying conditions
Provision of physical therapy and education
    Gait retraining
    Muscle strengthening
    Aids to ambulation
    Properly fitted shoes
    Adaptive behaviors
Alteration of the environment
    Safe and proper-sized furniture
    Elimination of obstacles
    Proper lighting
    Rails (stairs, bathroom) (Figure 18-1)
Provision of increased assistance and monitoring

to falls (Brady et al., 1993; Keene-Payne, 1994; Ross, 1991). Being 75 years of age or older, having a history of falls, and having gait problems are personal factors that have been identified repeatedly in the literature as increasing the risk of falls (Brady et al., 1993). Sensory impairments, diminished position and postural control, decreased muscle strength and coordination, increased bone fragility, and alterations in gait are age-related physiologic factors that may increase fall susceptibility. Many medications have also been identified as increasing the risk of falling. Examples include diuretics, antihypertensives, hypoglycemics, sedatives, and psychotropic drugs. The older person's risk of falling may be compounded further by cognitive deficits; urinary or bladder dysfunction; cancer; or cardiovascular, cerebrovascular, or neurologic diseases.

TRAFFIC INJURIES AND BURNS

The same physiologic changes that increase older people's risk of falls, such as decreased response time, sensory impairments, and alterations in the musculoskeletal, nervous, and cardiovascular systems, increase their risk of traffic accidents and burns. Approximately 25% of accidental deaths in those over the age of 65 are attributed to motor vehicle accidents, whereas burns account for about 8%. Injuries incurred from motor vehicle accidents and burns affect multiple organ systems and can quickly overwhelm the older person's physiologic reserves. Increased metabolic, cardiopulmonary, renal, and immunologic requirements of injury have more severe consequences and result in higher case mortality rates for older people, as compared to younger people with similar injuries.

The older person's driving an automobile is often a vital link in maintaining independence and a necessity for socializing and obtaining goods and services (Carr, 1993). However, deficits in visual-spatial skills, psychomotor coordination, cognition, and attention increase the risk of traffic accidents. Intersections are particularly hazardous to older adults, whether as pedestrian or as vehicle passenger or driver (Figure 18-2). Curb height, increased complexity of visual and auditory stimuli at intersections, and increased time needed for crossing on foot are factors that increase the risks to older adults. There are some indications that older drivers tend to ignore red lights and more often disregard the right-before-left priority at intersections than do younger drivers (Schlag, 1993). Identifying conditions that increase the likelihood of vehicle accidents and modifying driving practices or seeking alternative transportation should be included in any attempt to ensure the safety of older people.

Burns are another category of injury that poses a significant safety threat to older adults. Decreased sensory perception (hearing, vision, touch, and smell), decreased reaction time, and decreased mobility and agility make older adults

FIGURE 18-1 Handrails and non-skid surfaces in hallways help the older adult to avoid accidents. *Courtesy Loy Ledbetter, St Louis.*

particularly prone to burn injuries (Potter, 1993). The most common burn injuries are scalds (from hot baths, showers, fluids on the stove) and flame burns (from ignition of clothing, flammable liquids, house fires) (Reynolds, 1994). Smoking, cooking, heating, and use of electrical equipment account for a large percentage of older adult burn casualties. Because of the poor prognosis associated with burns in older adults, a greater effort needs to be directed toward prevention (Reynolds, 1994).

■ Abuse and Neglect

Two million older Americans are abused or neglected each year (Gilman, 1993), and the number of reports has been increasing annually. Furthermore, it is estimated that only between 1 in 8 and 1 in 14 cases are reported (Tatara, 1995). A significant problem in identification of abuse has been the lack of a clear definition. Elder abuse is defined by state laws, yet definitions vary considerably from state to state.

Most broadly, the terms *elder abuse* and *elder neglect* refer to any action that brings harm to people over the age of 65. Elder abuse is further categorized into three broad areas: (1) domestic elder abuse, (2) institutional elder abuse, and (3) self-neglect or self-abuse. Domestic elder abuse occurs in the older person's own home or the home of a caregiver and usually consists of any of five types of maltreatment (Box 18-3) of an older person by someone with a special relationship to the person (e.g., a spouse, a sibling, a child, a friend, or a caregiver) (Tatara, 1995). *Institutional abuse* generally refers to any of the five types of maltreatment when they occur in residential facilities (nursing homes, foster homes, group homes, and assisted living facilities) for older people. The perpetrators of institutional abuse are usually paid caregivers or others with a legal or contractual obligation to provide care and protection to the older person. *Self-neglect* or *self-abuse,* on the other hand, refers to older people's conduct that threatens

FIGURE 18-2 Crossing a busy intersection can be hazardous to the older adult. *Courtesy Loy Ledbetter, St. Louis.*

Health Promotion
Measures to prevent fire and burns

- Do not smoke in bed or when sleepy.
- When cooking, do not wear loose-fitting clothing (robes, nightgowns, pajamas).
- Set hot water thermostat at 120° Fahrenheit.
- Install a portable hand fire extinguisher in the kitchen.
- Keep access to outside doors unobstructed.
- Identify emergency exits in public buildings.
- If considering moving to a boarding home or foster home, check to see that it has smoke detectors, a sprinkler system, and fire extinguishers.
- Wear clothing that is nonflammable or treated with a flame-retardant finish. Wear less flammable materials of animal hair, wool, or silk.
- Avoid the use of electrical extension cords and do not overload electrical outlets.
- Install and maintain smoke detectors.
- Do not store flammable materials in the home.
- Call in an alarm before attempting to extinguish a fire, regardless of its size.

their own health or safety and is often the result of physical or mental impairment. Examples include the refusal to eat or to seek and receive appropriate medical and personal care.

The majority of confirmed cases of elder abuse are self-abuse, whereas approximately 16% are physical abuse (Tatara, 1995). Elder abuse or neglect occurs in all racial, religious, and socioeconomic groups. Those at highest risk appear to be female, living with the caregiver, and dependent on the caregiver for personal care, health care, and financial decision making. More than two thirds of elder abusers are family members, and over one third are the adult children of the abused older person. The median age of the victims was 76.4 years and those over the age of 80 accounted for more than one third of the victims in 1994 (Tatara, 1995).

A complex variety of factors contributes to the occurrence of elder abuse, and no single theory best explains its occurrence. However, abuse is generally attributed to a combination of personal, psychosocial, and economic factors that affect interpersonal and intrafamilial relationships. Caregiver stress, in combination with other factors such as unresolved conflicts with the older person, inadequate coping skills, emo-

tional problems, financial burden or concerns, and lack of family and community support, may lead to frustration and abuse or neglect. Stress and frustration may be heightened by the increasing mental and/or physical disabilities of the older person and thus lead to abuse. Other theories propose that the abuse is part of a learned behavior of violence toward others and is the expression of a normative behavior pattern in some families. Among abusers, a high incidence of mental and emotional problems that have led to their dependence on the older person for finances and housing has been observed

---

BOX 18-3 TYPES OF DOMESTIC ELDER ABUSE

1. Physical abuse: nonaccidental use of physical force causing bodily injury, pain, or impairment.
2. Sexual abuse: nonconsensual sexual contact of any type with an older adult.
3. Psychologic or emotional abuse: willful infliction of mental or emotional anguish by threat, humiliation, intimidation, or nonverbal abusive conduct.
4. Neglect: intentional or nonintentional failure by the caregiver to fulfill caregiver duties or obligations, such as providing adequate food, companionship, assistance with activities of daily living (ADLs), clothing, medication, or recreational opportunities.
5. Financial or material exploitation: intentional manipulation of the older adult to obtain funds, property, or other material resources or the unauthorized use of them.

Adapted from Tatara, T. (1995). *Elder abuse: Questions and answers* (5th ed.). Washington, DC: National Center on Elder Abuse.

(All, 1994). In these cases it may be that the abuse is an inappropriate response of the adult children to their own inadequacies. The abuse may be the result of the abuser's poor self-control or ineffective coping mechanisms. Regardless of the etiology, abuse and neglect can pose significant risks to the safety of the older adult and should be considered in any effort to meet the safety needs of the older adult.

Elder abuse laws exist in all 50 states, and more than 85% of the states include provisions for mandatory reporting of abuse or suspected abuse. Health care personnel are designated as mandated reporters of suspected elder abuse in most states with a mandatory reporting law. Most statutes require confidentiality for people who report suspected abuse and protect reporters from civil or criminal liability (Tatara, 1995).

■ Restraints

Physical devices, euphemistically labeled *protective devices,* have been used for years to restrain and protect people. Vests, belts, wrist ties, mitts, straitjackets, side rails, nets, and locked geriatric chairs are just some of the devices used to control wandering, prevent falls, facilitate treatment, and control disruptive and agitated behavior. Yet the use of such devices may, more often than not, be a form of physical and psychologic abuse that violates the dignity and autonomy of the restrained person (Strumpf & Evans, 1991). Rather than promoting safety, in many instances such devices cause depersonalization, unintentional injury, diminished quality of life, and even death (Brower, 1991; Miles & Irvine, 1992; Strumpf & Evans, 1992; Weick, 1992). Between 100 and 200 deaths a year are associated with the use of physical restraints (Weick, 1992). In fact, "restraints are an under recognized, under reported, avoidable, and proximate cause of death in at least 1 in 1,000 nursing home deaths" (Miles & Irvine, 1992, p. 762).

Growing research findings indicate that the hazards of restraint use outweigh perceived benefits. Those who exhibit confusion, poor judgment, or behavioral problems and have concurrent physical impairments are those most likely to be restrained (Mion & Strumpf, 1994; Tinetti et al., 1992). Those who exhibit behavioral problems of verbal and physical aggression are not only the most likely to be restrained, but also the least likely to be released from restraints or appropriately monitored and attended to while restrained—in other words, neglected by staff (Schnelle et al., 1992). Furthermore, restraint use has been linked to impeded mobility; loss of muscle strength, balance, and gait; new-onset bowel and bladder incontinence; pressure ulcers;

nerve injuries; contractures; and nosocomial infections (Janelli et al., 1994; Mion & Strumpf, 1994; Tinetti, 1990; Tinetti et al., 1992). Restraints do not appear to decrease injuries from falls or wandering and actually increase the seriousness of injuries in those who do fall (Mion & Strumpf, 1994; Tinetti et al., 1992). Significant psychologic distress, confusion, depression, anger, fear, loss of self-esteem, and increased agitation may also be related to restraint use. Despite an increased awareness of the physical, psychologic, and ethical problems of restraint use, the practice continues, and conflicts between the decision to restrain and the preservation of patient dignity and autonomy persist (Scherer et al., 1991).

Use of restraints must be accompanied by more rigid and explicit criteria for their use, proper application by trained personnel, and more staff monitoring of the restrained person. Otherwise, their use may be abusive, unnecessary, and punitive and actually constitute a greater risk to safety than any problem they are meant to control. The Omnibus Budget Reconciliation Act (OBRA) of 1987, the Health Care Financing Administration (HCFA), the Commission on Accreditation of Rehabilitation Facilities (CARF), and, more recently, the Joint Commission on Accreditation of Healthcare Organizations (JCAHO) and the Food and Drug Administration (FDA) have set forth standards and guidelines regarding restraint use (Stolley, 1995; Weick, 1992). In addition to recommendations for thorough evaluation of the need for restraints, appropriate application, and documentation related to their use, these standards and guidelines require development and implementation of suitable alternatives to the use of restraints (CARF, 1992; HCFA, 1992; U.S. FDA, 1992). See Box 18-4 for a practice protocol developed to address these standards and guidelines.

The movement of many health care facilities to becoming virtually "restraint-free environments" is increasing. Since passage of the Nursing Home Reform Law of OBRA in 1987, the preva-

lence of restraint use in nursing homes has declined 47% to 54% ("Nursing Homes Report," 1992; Strumpf & Evans, 1992). That still means that nearly a quarter million U.S. older adults are being restrained to their beds or chairs. Nurses can continue the movement to safer, more humane protection of older people only with diligent assessment of older people's behavior and awareness and implementation of alternative interventions.

Companionship, supervision, the elimination of bothersome treatments, environmental manipulation, psychosocial interventions, diversion, and physical activities must be considered and tried before physical restraint. See Box 18-5 for more specific examples of restraint alternatives.

Consistent with Maslow's ideas, safety and security are needs for all humans, but they are important to older people in a unique way. Activities that are often taken for granted by younger people can become major challenges as people age. All age groups are concerned about controlling hazardous agents, decreasing the susceptibility of the host, and/or modifying the environment. Approaches to each and all of these factors take on a different degree of emphasis for the older adult.

Injuries, accidents, falls, burns, and abuse are threats to the comfort and well-being of older adults. It behooves the health care provider to be aware of the hazards that precipitate any one or more of these events. Preventing these incidents enables greater comfort for the older person, as well as fewer challenges in the provision of health care.

There is increased awareness of the problems that can and do result in the use of restraints in the care of older adults. The creative health care provider is willing to accept the challenge of coping with the health care of the older adult through means other than the use of restraints.

Care of the person who may be prone to any or several of these threats to safety and security requires a systematic, orderly pursuit of care,

BOX 18-4 NURSING STANDARD OF PRACTICE PROTOCOL: USE OF MECHANICAL RESTRAINTS WITH OLDER ADULTS

I. Background

   A. Physical restraint is the use of any manual method or physical or mechanical device that the older person cannot remove, that restricts the older person's physical activity or normal access to his or her body, and that

      1. Is not a usual or customary part of medical, diagnostic, or treatment procedure indicated by the older person's medical condition or symptoms

      2. Does not serve to promote the older person's independent functioning

   B. The standard of care for institutionalized older people is nonuse of mechanical restraints, except under exceptional circumstances, after all reasonable alternatives have been tried.

   C. Risk factors involved in use of mechanical restraints in the institutional setting include the following:

      1. Fall risk

      2. Tubes or intravenous (IV) lines that need stability

      3. Severe cognitive or physical impairments

      4. Diagnosis or presence of a psychiatric condition

      5. Surgery

      6. Lack of staff education regarding restraint use

   D. Morbidity and mortality risks associated with mechanical restraint use include the following:

      1. Nerve injury

      2. New-onset pressure ulcers

      3. Pneumonia

      4. Incontinence

      5. Increased confusion

      6. Inappropriate drug use

      7. Strangulation or asphyxiation

   E. Appropriate alternatives exist to the use of mechanical restraints.

II. Assessment parameters

   A. Request information about the use of mechanical restraints from preinstitutional settings.

   B. On admission, identify as "at risk for restraint use" any older person who is agitated, at risk for falling, or disrupting therapy.

   C. Use one-to-one observation or behavior monitoring logs to identify and document specific risks. For example, for fall risk, assess impaired cognition, poor balance, impaired gait, orthostatic hypotension, impaired vision and hearing, and the use of sedative and hypnotic agents.

III. Care strategies

   A. Prevention

      1. Develop a nursing plan tailored to the older person's presenting problem or problems and specific risk factors.

      2. Consider and implement several alternative interventions.

      3. Refer to occupational and physical therapy for self-care deficits or mobility impairments; use adaptive equipment as appropriate.

      4. Document use and effect of alternatives to restraints.

Continued

BOX 18-4 NURSING STANDARD OF PRACTICE PROTOCOL: USE OF MECHANICAL RESTRAINTS WITH OLDER ADULTS—cont'd

B. Treatment
1. Use restraints only after exhausting all reasonable alternatives.
2. Obtain informed consent from the older person or the person's guardian before using restraints.
3. Use restraints only under the supervision of a licensed health care provider and only for a strictly defined period.
4. When using restraints do the following:
   a. Choose the least restrictive devices.
   b. Use the correct size and follow manufacturer's directions.
   c. Reassess the older person's response at least every hour.
   d. Remove restraints at least every 2 hours.
   e. Renew orders every 24 hours.
5. Modify the care plan to compensate for restrictions imposed by restraint use:
   a. Change person's position frequently and provide skin care.
   b. Provide adequate range of motion.
   c. Assist with ADLs, such as eating and use of toilet.
6. Continue to address underlying condition or conditions that prompted restraint use (e.g., gait impairment). Refer to gerontologic nurse specialist, occupational or physical therapist, etc., as appropriate.

IV. Evaluation of expected outcomes
A. Older person: Mechanical restraints will be used only under well-documented, exceptional circumstances, after all reasonable alternatives have been tried.
B. Health care provider: Providers will use a range of interventions other than restraints in the care of older people.
C. Institution
1. Incidence and prevalence of physical restraint use will decrease.
2. Use of chemical restraints will not increase.
3. The number of serious injuries related to falls, agitated behavior, and other problems indicating use of restraints will not increase.
4. Referrals to occupational and physical therapy will increase, as will availability of adaptive equipment.
5. Staff will receive ongoing education on the prevention of restraint use.

V. Follow-up to monitor condition
A. Document incidence of restraint use on an ongoing basis.
B. Educate caregivers to continue assessment and prevention.
C. Identify older people's characteristics and care problems that continue to be refractory, and involve consultants (e.g., gerontologic nurse specialist, recreational therapist) in devising an expanded range of alternative approaches.

Adapted from: Mion & Strumpf, L.C.N. (1994), Use of physical restraints in the hospital setting: Implications for the nurse. *Geriatric Nursing, 15*(3), 127-131.

BOX 18-5 ALTERNATIVES TO RESTRAINT USE

Provide companionship and supervision.

- Have staff, family, friends, or volunteers stay with the patient.
- Assess times that the older person needs more individual attention (typically early evening and at night) and intervene accordingly.
- Answer call bells promptly.

Change or eliminate bothersome treatments.

- Initiate oral (as opposed to IV or nasogastric [NG]) feedings.
- Remove catheters and drains as soon as possible.
- Provide more frequent nasal, oral, and skin care to reduce irrigation.

Modify the environment.

- Modify the amount of light in the room to reduce glare, accommodate visual deficits, and avoid interruption of sleep.
- Position the bedside tables, personal articles, and commode for easy patient access.
- Move the patient nearer the nurses' station, unless the situation triggers agitation or worsens confusion.
- Keep the bed at its lowest height or place the mattress on the floor so that the older person can move about freely in bed without falling.
- Leave the bed rails down if the older person tends to climb over them, or use half rails to prevent the patient's rolling out of bed.
- Reduce environmental stimulation, such as unnecessary noise or use of the wall intercom (many older people have difficulty understanding what is said over an intercom).
- Keep the call button accessible and review its use frequently.
- Use special furniture (low bed, special chairs).

Use reality orientation and psychosocial interventions.

- Involve the patient in conversation and therapeutic communication to elicit feelings, fears, and perceptions.
- Explain procedures to reduce fear and misperceptions.
- Provide reality links when appropriate (TV, radio, calendar, clock, newspaper).
- Use relaxation techniques (therapeutic touch, massage, warm baths).

Offer diversionary and physical activities.

- Use TV, radio, or music appropriate to the older person's preferences and cognitive status.
- Enlist the aid of a recreational therapist.
- Schedule appropriate exercise and ambulation into the daily routine.
- Institute training in ADLs.
- Use physical and occupational therapy to increase strength and endurance and promote a sense of accomplishment.

Continued

BOX 18-5 ALTERNATIVES TO RESTRAINT USE—cont'd

Design creative alternatives.

- Use rocking chairs to provide diversion and expend energy.
- Use music, audiobooks, or videotapes chosen specifically for the patient to reduce agitation or to provide diversion.
- Use a pressure-sensitive bed or chair pads with alarms for alerting staff to an unsteady patient who is standing without help.
- Develop, implement, and periodically evaluate toileting routines to eliminate sense of urgency and reduce falls related to elimination.
- Consult with other disciplines for other suggestions.

Adapted from Evans, L., et al. (1993). Limiting use of physical restraints: A prerequisite for independent functioning. In E. Calkins, et al. (Eds.), *Practice of geriatrics* (2nd ed.). Philadelphia: W.B. Saunders. Stolley, J.M. (1995). Freeing your patients from restraints. *American Journal of Nursing, 95*(2), 27-31. Strumpf, N., et al. (1992). Physical restraint of the elderly. In C. Chenitz, et al. (Eds.), *Clinical gerontological nursing* (pp. 329-344). Philadelphia: W.B. Saunders. Strumpf, N., et al. (1992). *Reducing restraints: Individualized approaches to behavior.* Huntington Valley, PA: Whitman Group.

---

whether in the acute care setting, the long-term care facility, or the person's own home. This care is best achieved by following the nursing process: assessing, diagnosing, identifying goals or outcomes, implementing, and evaluating.

■ Nursing Process

ASSESSMENT

Data for the identification of threats to safety are obtained from individual and environmental assessments. A comprehensive health history is necessary and should include both a medical and social history with information on existing medical conditions and their past and current treatment; over-the-counter and prescription drug use; previous falls (Box 18-6); and any episodes of vertigo or dizziness. The physical assessment should encompass the cardiovascular, neurologic, and musculoskeletal systems. Postural blood pressures, performance-based assessment of posture, and sensory-motor testing are essential (Kane et al., 1994) (Box 18-7).

Environmental assessment (Box 18-8) should identify any item or factor that puts the older person at risk, such as scatter rugs, inadequate lighting, clutter, or wet floors. Environmental assessments are most easily accomplished in institutional settings. For those living at home, some information on the environment may be obtained from the older adult, caregiver, or family member. In some cases an in-home assessment may need to be arranged through a home care agency such as a visiting nurses association.

There is no easy formula for the assessment of abuse and neglect of an older person. One reason is that both the older victim and the abuser tend to deny the mistreatment. Older women who are cognitively impaired and exhibit difficult behaviors such as wandering, belligerence, and insomnia should be considered at greatest risk for abuse or neglect. Unexplained bruises or burns, poor skin care, severe dehydration, malnutrition, poor hygiene, and the patient's fearful response to the caregiver should alert the health care provider to the possibility of abuse or neglect. Other cues are listed in Box 18-9. Caregiver characteristics should also alert the health care provider to the increased risk of abuse or neglect (Box 18-10).

BOX 18-6 KEY POINTS IN HISTORY FOR OLDER ADULTS WITH PREVIOUS FALLS

General medical history
Medications (especially antihypertensives, diuretics, sedatives and hypnotics, and psychotropic agents)
Patient's thoughts on the cause of the fall
    Was patient aware of impending fall?
    Was it totally unexpected?
    Did patient trip or slip?
Circumstances surrounding the fall
    Location and time of day
    Witnesses
    Relationship to changes in posture, turning of head, cough, urination
Premonitory or associated symptoms
    Lightheadedness, dizziness, vertigo
    Palpitations, chest pain, shortness of breath
    Sudden focal neurologic symptoms (weakness, sensory disturbance, dysarthria, ataxia, confusion, aphasia)
    Aura
    Incontinence of urine or stool
Loss of consciousness
    What is remembered immediately after the fall?
    Could the patient get up, and if so, how long did it take?
    Can loss of consciousness be verified by a witness?

BOX 18-7 EVALUATING THE OLDER ADULT FOR RISK OF INJURY: KEY ASPECTS OF THE PHYSICAL EXAMINATION

Vital signs
    Fever, hypothermia
    Respiratory rate and quality
    Pulse and blood pressure (lying, sitting, standing)
Skin
    Turgor
    Pallor
    Trauma
Eyes and Ears
    Visual acuity
    Hearing acuity
Cardiovascular
    Arrhythmias
    Carotid bruits
    Signs of aortic stenosis
    Carotid sinus sensitivity
Musculoskeletal
    Muscles (weakness, rigidity, spasticity)
    Posture
    Degenerative joint disease
    Strength and range of motion
    Deformities
Fractures
Podiatric problems (calluses; bunions; ulcerations; poorly fitted, inappropriate, or worn-out shoes)
Neurologic
    Mental status
    Focal signs
    Peripheral innervation (especially position sense)
    Cerebellar (especially heel-to-shin testing and coordination)
    Resting tremor, bradykinesia, other involuntary movements
    Gait
Stability when standing, reaching, bending, rising from a chair, or being hugged (performance-based posture)

When abuse is suspected, it is imperative to interview the older person in a private setting apart from the caregiver. Many victims fear reprisal from the abuser, abandonment, or nursing home placement. It is important to ask direct questions such as "Has anyone harmed you?" or "Have you been confined against your will?" (O'Brien, 1992).

In some instances an abuse assessment tool may be helpful in screening for possible abuse or neglect. Box 18-11 presents an elder abuse

BOX 18-8
ENVIRONMENTAL ASSESSMENT

1. Poorly lighted stairwells, halls, or bathrooms
2. Stairs with weak or absent banisters
3. Absence of grab bars near bathtub
4. Glare in hallways
5. Absence of a working smoke alarm
6. Wet floors and/or waxed floors
7. Poorly placed extension cords
8. Throw rugs
9. Clutter
10. Inappropriate footwear and long clothing
11. High beds
12. Improper use of walking aids
13. Restraints and protective devices

BOX 18-10 CAREGIVER CHARACTERISTICS ASSOCIATED WITH ABUSE OR NEGLECT OF OLDER PEOPLE

- Has history of abusive or violent behavior
- Is substance abuser or alcoholic
- Has mental or physical impairment
- Has unrealistic expectations of self and/or older person
- Is socially isolated
- Is sole caregiver
- Is experiencing prolonged or extensive burden of care
- Lacks family or community support
- Is dependent on older person for money, housing
- Was a child abuse victim

BOX 18-9 CUES INDICATING ABUSE OR NEGLECT

- Unexplained trauma
- Delay or neglect in treating medical problems
- Noncompliance with medications or treatment plans
- Conflicting histories from caregiver and older person
- Inappropriate or bizarre explanation of an injury
- Long delay in treatment of an injury
- History of being accident prone or multiple visits to emergency room or ambulatory care clinics

screening tool developed by an elder abuse assessment team at Beth Israel Hospital in Boston for emergency room use (Fulmer et al., 1984). This screening tool allows the nurse to perform a comprehensive, systematic assessment. A problem with the tool is the lack of definitive parameters in differentiating among the points on the scale from very good to very poor. Also, there is no effort made to distinguish between abuse and neglect; rather, the goal is to detect those older adults who are receiving inadequate care in their caregiving situation.

NURSING DIAGNOSES

Data obtained from the assessment are logically clustered, and diagnoses that can be validated by the data are formulated. High risk for injury and altered protection are diagnoses that might be appropriately used to label the clustered data (Carroll-Johnson, 1991). At times it will be more useful to specify the type of injury within the diagnostic statement—for example, high risk for injury from a fall or high risk for injury related to inappropriate caregiving.

Define characteristics or those subjective and objective data that indicate the presence of a condition that corresponds to a given diagnosis (McFarlane, 1993). For the older person with a

BOX 18-11 SCREENING TOOL FOR ABUSE

Date: _____ Person completing form:_____

Payment status (please check one):

____ Blue Cross/Blue Shield _____ Medicaid _____ Medicare _____ Private payment _____ Other

Residence (please check one):

____ Home _____ Name of nursing home ____ Other (e.g., son/daughter's home)

Accompanied by: ____ Family ____ Friend ____ Alone ____ Nursing home personnel

Reason for visit: ____ Cardiac ____ Changed mental status ____ Fall ____ GI

Orthopedic ____ Other (please state)

Current mental status: ____ Oriented ____ Confused ____ Unresponsive

---

1. *General assessment*

	Very good	Good	Undecided	Poor	Very poor	No basis for judgment
a. Clothing						
b. Hygiene						
c. Nutrition						
d. Skin integrity						

Additional comments: _____

_____

_____

_____

_____

_____

_____

_____

Continued

BOX 18-11 SCREENING TOOL FOR ABUSE—cont'd

	Definite evidence	Probable evidence	Uncertain	Probably no evidence	No evidence	No basis for judgment
2. *Physical assessment*						
a. Bruising						
b. Contractures						
c. Decubiti						
d. Dehydration						
e. Diarrhea						
f. Impaction						
g. Lacerations						
h. Malnutrition						
i. Urine burns/excoriations						

Additional comments: _____

_____

_____

_____

_____

_____

	Totally independent	Mostly independent	Uncertain	Mostly dependent	Totally dependent	No basis for judgment
3. *Usual lifestyle*						
a. Administration of medications						
b. Ambulation						
c. Continence						
d. Feedings						
e. Maintenance of hygiene						
f. Management of finances						
g. Family involvement						

BOX 18-11 SCREENING TOOL FOR ABUSE—cont'd

Additional comments: _____

_____

_____

_____

_____

4. *Social assessment*
   - Narrative statement regarding older person–identified social problems: _____

   _____

   - Family or nursing home perception of problem: _____

   _____

	Very good quality	Good quality	Uncertain	Poor quality	Very poor quality	No basis for judgment
a. Financial situation						
b. Interaction with family						
c. Interaction with friends						
d. Interaction with nursing home personnel						
e. Living arrangement						
f. Observed relationship with care provider						
g. Participation in daily social activities						
h. Support systems						
i. Ability to express needs						

Additional comments (recent changes in life situation): _____

_____

_____

_____

_____

Continued

BOX 18-11 SCREENING TOOL FOR ABUSE—cont'd

5. *Medical assessment*

	Definite evidence	Evidence	Possibility	Probably no evidence	No evidence	No basis/not applicable
a. Duplication of similar medications (e.g., multiple laxatives, sedatives)						
b. Unusual doses of medication						
c. Alcohol or other substance abuse						
d. Greater than 15% dehydration						
e. Bruises and/or fractures beyond what is compatible with alleged trauma						
f. Failure to respond to warning of obvious disease						
g. Repetitive admissions because of probable failure of health care surveillance						

NOTE: ATTACH DESCRIPTION OF ANY ADDITIONAL PHYSICAL FINDINGS.

Additional comments (if either 5a or 5b has been answered in the affirmative, please elaborate and be *as specific as possible*): _____

_____

_____

_____

_____

_____

_____

_____

_____

_____

BOX 18-11 SCREENING TOOL FOR ABUSE—cont'd

	Definite evidence	Evidence	Possibility	Probably no evidence	No evidence	No basis/not applicable
6. *Summary assessments*						
a. Evidence of financial and/or possession abuse						
b. Evidence of physical abuse						
c. Evidence of psychologic abuse						
d. History of recent life crisis						

Additional comments: _____

_____

_____

_____

_____

	Yes	No
7. *Disposition*		
a. Referral to elder assessment team		
b. Referral to clinical advisor		

8. General comments (nursing home contact person and date): _____

_____

_____

_____

_____

_____

_____

From Fulmer, T., Street, S., & Carr, K. (1984). Abuse of the elderly: Screening and detection. *Journal of Emergency Nursing,* *10*(3), 131-140.

high risk for injury, defining characteristics may include any of the following:

- Sensory impairment: visual, auditory, tactile, olfactory
- Cognitive impairment
- Physical impairment: reduced muscle mass, muscle weakness, musculoskeletal system abnormalities or limitations; peripheral neuropathies, irregular heart rhythms; dehydration, electrolyte disorders; malnutrition; anemia, fever
- History of falls, family violence, affective disorder, drug abuse
- Unexplained or repeated trauma
- Recent environmental change
- Declining functional ability
- Lack of safety education
- Family stress: interpersonal, material, financial
- High fall-risk appraisal profile
- Fatalistic attitude

PLANNING AND GOAL IDENTIFICATION

The planning phase of the nursing process involves specifying expected patient goals or outcomes. The goals or outcomes will guide the nurse in selecting appropriate interventions to achieve the desired goals or outcomes.

Identification of goals or outcomes for older people at high risk for injury will facilitate the nurse's ability to develop and evaluate nursing interventions. Individualized goals and outcomes may also be thought of as subcategories of national health goals for older adults, because the health of the nation ultimately depends on the health of individuals. Prevention of injury is one of the major strategies identified for improving the health of the nation (USDHHS, 1991). Objective 9.4a of *Healthy People 2000* is to reduce the number of fall-related deaths and injuries to no more than 14.4 per 100,000 people age 65 to 84 (1987 baseline 18). This would require a 20% decrease from the 1987 figures. A related and equally relevant objective is 9.21: to increase to at least 50% the proportion of primary care providers who routinely provide age-appropriate counseling on safety precautions to prevent unintentional injury. Counseling is particularly urged for individuals at increased risk for motor vehicle injury, alcohol and other drug users, and patients whose medical conditions diminish motor vehicle safety. Objective 7.12 focuses on increasing the use of protocols for identifying, treating, and referring victims of violent and abusive behavior, including older adults. These broad, long-range objectives should be kept in mind as more specific, individualized goals and outcomes are formulated. Examples of more specific goals and outcomes include but are not limited to the following:

- The older adult will remain injury free.
- The older adult or caregiver will be able to identify factors or people that increase the potential for injury (e.g., falls, motor vehicle accidents, neglect, or abuse).
- The older adult or caregiver will eliminate physical risks from the environment (e.g., loose carpeting, poorly lighted areas, or unnecessary restraints).
- The older adult or caregiver will install and maintain safety devices (e.g., railings, grab bars, elevated toilet seats, or smoke detectors).
- The older adult will engage in appropriate exercises to promote and maintain flexibility and mobility.
- The older adult will demonstrate appropriate use of devices to enhance mobility.
- The older adult will discontinue behaviors that place him or her at risk for injury (e.g., driving at night, on major highways, or during peak traffic hours; climbing on chairs; or wearing inappropriate footwear).
- The older adult will obtain regular periodic evaluation of hearing, vision, and functional ability.
- The older adult or caregiver will utilize appropriate community services or agencies (e.g., Adult Protective Services, Meals on Wheels, transportation services, or home health aides).

IMPLEMENTATION

The four broad areas of the OMAHA system nursing intervention scheme can provide the nurse with guidance for organizing and implementing interventions for the older adult at risk for injury (Martin & Scheet, 1992). Although originally developed for use in community health settings, these categories can be very helpful to nurses in other settings. The four categories of interventions are as follows: (1) health teaching, guidance, and counseling; (2) treatments and procedures; (3) case management; and (4) surveillance.

In the acute care setting

Older patients are at significant risk for sustaining an injury as a result of a fall during the time they are hospitalized. Any decline in the physical condition or mental status of an older patient should be identified as a risk factor. Precipitating factors, especially the interaction of physical and environmental hazards such as a sense of urgency to urinate at night when unfamiliar side rails are in place, can increase the occurrence of falls. Studies have found a relationship between falls and a sense of urgency in older, hospitalized patients (Janken et al., 1986). Most nurses' ability to assess and identify those who might fall are relatively well developed; the difficulty is in developing realistic interventions that will decrease the number of falls.

Labeling the patient's chart to alert staff to the fact that the patient is classified as being at high risk for falling, with subsequent close monitoring, is a standard intervention. Scheduling accompanied trips to the bathroom is another frequently used intervention. Educating patients to be aware of the risk of falling and to take precautions, such as always dangling legs before getting out of bed, is an important intervention that often may be overlooked. The use of restraints has been demonstrated to be counterproductive in preventing falls. Furthermore, the use of side rails contributes to falls rather than being an instrument of protection. The ordinary hospital, with its high-tech and high-speed orientation, may be viewed as a hazardous environment for many older patients. Falls by older patients in acute care settings are difficult problems that require continued education of staff, patients, and families, as well as constant surveillance. Clinical nursing research should investigate interventions that both decrease the number of falls and maintain the dignity and autonomy of the older patient.

In the nursing home

All of the interventions used in the acute care setting can be utilized in the nursing home. The major difference is the transitional nature of the hospital experience. The hospital is an acute, time-limited experience. In contrast, the nursing home may well be the older person's residence for an extended period; it is *home,* which should be a safe haven, not a dangerous harbor.

The second category of the OMAHA interventions—treatments and procedures—would include nursing activities aimed at identifying risk factors for injury and preventing, decreasing, and/or alleviating signs and symptoms of injury. Examples of interventions in this category might include such actions as implementing alternatives to physical restraints; instituting a fall protection protocol; or modifying or making recommendations for the modification of the environment. Surveillance, another OMAHA intervention classification, will also be effective and necessary in a long-term care facility setting.

The resident who is independent is clearly more at risk for falling than the resident who is confined to bed or to a wheelchair. Meeting the safety needs of nursing home residents is a difficult problem for all health care professionals because of the conflicting goals of seeking to protect the resident from sustaining an injury as a result of a fall and seeking to meet the resident's need for a sense of independence. The nursing staff must make the adjustments in the environment that are necessary to diminish the likelihood of falling, while fostering the independence and preserving the dignity of the older resident.

In the private or family home

Case management, the third category of the OMAHA system nursing intervention scheme, includes nursing activities involving advocacy, coordination, and referral. Many times, the case manager will be a nurse making a home visit.

Prevention of falls may not be the primary reason for the home care visit, but the nurse should always be alert to the older person's increased risk of falling. Intervention in the pre-injury phase is an appropriate independent nursing action. Observation of the patient's physical abilities and detection of significant changes are key functions of the home care nurse's visit.

The house in which the family and the patient have been living may be assessed by the nurse as having many hazards. It is good for the nurse to stress that there is a need to reassess the home environment because of the changes in the patient's abilities. This approach may be less threatening to family members who may regard an assessment of their home as an unwarranted intrusion and as a judgment that they have not provided a safe environment for their family member. Working within the family structure and with the community of the homebound older person is crucial to the nurse's effectiveness.

Many older people live alone in an apartment or in a house. The nurse must remember the importance of preserving the patient's dignity and self-esteem, along with assisting the patient to maintain a safe environment. In regard to home hazards, with some support, teaching, follow-up, and appropriate referral, the nurse can make a significant impact in the area of prevention of falls.

Patients need to have information concerning the effects of drugs that they are taking, and they need to consider their risk of orthostatic hypotension. Instruction concerning how to decrease the effects of orthostatic hypotension, such as dangling feet before getting out of bed and rising slowly from a sitting or a reclining position, is important in the prevention of falls.

Nurses are among the few professionals who are welcomed into older adults' homes. Nurses have the opportunity to make a significant difference in older people's efforts to remain in an independent living arrangement. The prevention of injury from falls should always be a segment of every nurse's visit when home care is provided for an older person.

EVALUATION

The last step of the nursing process is evaluation. Goals or outcomes and nursing interventions are planned to reduce the risk of injury. The evaluation of the extent to which these goals or outcomes have been achieved indicates the effectiveness of the interventions. Evaluation of outcome achievement is ongoing and should be used to direct further assessment, outcome revision, and/or changes in interventions. Data for the evaluation of outcomes may come from reassessment of the patient and environment, subjective reports from the older adult and caregiver, chart reviews, and incident reports.

REFERENCES

All, A.C. (1994). A literature review: Assessment and intervention in elder abuse. *Journal of Gerontological Nursing, 20*(7), 25-31.

Beauchamp, T., & Childress, J.E. (1994). *Principles of biomedical ethics* (4th ed.). New York: Oxford University Press.

Brady, R., Chester, F.R., Pierce, L.L., Salter, J.P., Schreck, S., & Radziewicz, R. (1993). Geriatric falls: Prevention strategies for the staff. *Journal of Gerontological Nursing, 19*(9), 26-32.

Brower, H.T. (1991). The alternatives of restraints. *Journal of Gerontological Nursing, 17*(2), 18-22.

Carr, D.B. (1993). Assessing older drivers for physical and cognitive impairment. *Geriatrics, 48*(5), 46-51.

Carroll-Johnson, R.M. (Ed.). (1991). *Classification of nursing diagnoses: Proceedings of the Ninth Conference.* Philadelphia: J.B. Lippincott.

Commission on Accreditation of Rehabilitation Facilities. (1992). *Standards manual for organizations serving people with disabilities.* Tucson: Author.

Cummings, S.R., Nevitt, M.C., Browner, W.S., Stone, K., Fox, K.M., Ensiud, K.E., Cauley, J., Black, D., & Vogt, T.M. (1995). Risk factors for hip fracture in white women. *New England Journal of Medicine, 332*(12), 767-773.

Fulmer, T., Street, S., & Carr, K. (1984). Abuse of the elderly: Screening and detection. *Journal of Emergency Nursing, 10*(3), 131-140.

Gilman, L. (1993). Elder abuse. *American Health, 1*(7), 84.

Health Care Financing Administration. (1992). *State operations manual.* Baltimore: U.S. Department of Health and Human Services.

Hogstel, M.O., & Gaul, A.L. (1991). Safety of autonomy: An ethical issue for clinical gerontological nurses. *Journal of Gerontological Nursing, 17*(3), 6-11.

Janelli, L.M., Kanski, W.G., & Neary, M.A. (1994). Physical restraints: Has OBRA made a difference? *Journal of Gerontological Nursing, 20*(6), 17-21.

Janken, J., Reynolds, B., & Sweich, K. (1986). Patient falls in the acute care setting: Identifying risk factors. *Nursing Research, 35,* 215-219.

Kane, R.L., Ouslander, J.G., & Abrass, I.B. (1994). *Essentials of clinical geriatrics* (3rd ed.). New York: McGraw-Hill.

Keene-Payne, R. (1994). Hospitalized older adults. In M.O. Hogstel (Ed.), *Nursing care of the older adult* (3rd ed., pp. 250-264). Albany, NY: Delmar.

Martin, K., & Scheet, N. (1992). *The OMAHA system: A pocket guide for community health nursing.* Philadelphia: W.B. Saunders.

Maslow, A. (1954). *Motivation and personality.* New York: Harper.

McFarlane, E.A. (1993). Nursing diagnosis: The critical link in the nursing process. In G.K. McFarland & E.A. McFarlane (Eds.), *Nursing diagnosis and intervention* (2nd ed., pp. 10-20). St. Louis: Mosby.

Miles, S.H., & Irvine, P. (1992). Deaths caused by physical restraints. *Gerontologist, 32,* 762-766.

Mion, L.C., & Strumpf, N. (1994). Use of physical restraints in the hospital setting: Implications for the nurse. *Geriatric Nursing, 15*(3), 127-132.

Nevitt, M.C., Cummings, S.R., & Hudes, E.S. (1991). Risk factors for injurious falls: A retrospective study. *Journals of Gerontology, 46,* M164-M1701.

Nursing homes report decreased restraint use. (1992). *American Geriatrics Society Newsletter, 21*(2), 1.

O'Brien, J.G. (1992). Elder abuse. In R.J. Ham & P.D. Sloane (Eds.), *Primary care geriatrics: A case based approach* (2nd ed.). St. Louis: Mosby.

Potter, P., & Perry, A. (1993). *Fundamentals of nursing* (3rd ed.). St. Louis: Mosby.

Reynolds, C.A. (1994). Emergency care. In M.O. Hogstel (Ed.), *Nursing care of the older adult* (3rd ed., pp. 265-287). Albany, NY: Delmar.

Ross, J.E. (1991). Iatrogenesis in the elderly: Contributors to falls. *Journal of Gerontological Nursing, 17*(9), 19-23.

Scherer, Y.K., Janelli, L.M., Kanski, G.W., Neary, M.A., & Morth, N.E. (1991). The nursing dilemma of restraints. *Journal of Gerontological Nursing, 17*(2), 14-17.

Schlag, B. (1993). Elderly drivers in Germany: Fitness and driving behavior. *Accident Analysis and Prevention, 25*(1), 47-55.

Schnelle, J.F., Simmons, S.F., & Ory, M.G. (1992). Risk factors that predict staff failure to release nursing home resident from restraints. *Gerontologist, 32,* 767-770.

Stolley, J.M. (1995). Freeing your patients from restraints. *American Journal of Nursing, 95*(2), 27-31.

Strumpf, N.E., & Evans, L.K. (1991). The ethical problems of prolonged physical restraint. *Journal of Gerontological Nursing, 17*(2), 27-30.

Strumpf, N.E., & Evans, L.K. (1992). Alternatives to physical restraints. *Journal of Gerontological Nursing, 18*(2), 4, 27-30.

Tatara, T. (1995). *Elder abuse: Questions and answers* (5th ed.). Washington, DC: National Center on Elder Abuse.

Tinetti, M.C. (1990). Falls. In W. Hazzard, R. Andres, E. Bierman, & J. Blass (Eds.), *Principles of geriatric medicine and gerontology* (2nd ed., pp. 1192-1199). New York: McGraw-Hill.

Tinetti, M.C., Liu, V., Marottolil, R.A., & Ginter, S.F. (1992). Mechanical restraint use among residents of skilled nursing facilities: Prevalence, patterns, and predictors. *Journal of the American Medical Association, 265,* 468-471.

Urton, M.M. (1991). A community home inspection approach to preventing falls among the elderly. *Public Health Rep, 106*(2), 192.

U.S. Department of Health and Human Services, Public Health Service. (1991). *Healthy people 2000: National health promotion and disease prevention objectives— Full report, with commentary* (DHHS Pub. No. [PHS] 91-50212). Washington, DC: U.S. Government Printing Office.

U.S. Food and Drug Administration. (1992). *FDA safety alert: Potential hazards with restraint devices.* Rockville, MD: U.S. Department of Health and Human Services.

Weick, M.D. (1992). Physical restraints: An FDA update. *American Journal of Nursing, 92*(11), 74-80.

The soul has no rainbow
If the eyes have no tears.
NATIVE AMERICAN SAYING

Cancer in the Older Adult

■ Learning Objectives

On completion of this chapter, the reader will be able to do the following:

1. Understand the problem of cancer, its myths, and its biases as they relate to the older adult.
2. Discuss biologic aspects of aging as they relate to cancer incidence, morbidity, and mortality.
3. Recognize major issues (e.g., age, gender, extent of disease, and comorbidity) that may influence decisions concerning eligibility for screening, extent of diagnostic workup, treatment, and treatment aggression for the older adult experiencing cancer.
4. Address (1) the major therapeutic modalities employed in cancer treatment; (2) the major cancers affecting the older adult; and (3) the nurse's role in caring for the older adult experiencing cancer.
5. Identify patterns of care for the older adult, family, and community experiencing cancer.
6. Project future goals for approaches to cancer prevention, control, treatment, and research in the older adult.

The burden of cancer is disproportionately carried by the older adult. It is a leading cause of morbidity and death in individuals over 65 years of age. Age is the most important determinant of cancer risk. The overall cancer incidence rate for individuals 65 years of age or older is 2085.3 per 100,000, compared to a rate of 193.9 per 100,000 for individuals younger than 65 years of age (Miller et al., 1994). With projections that one in five individuals will be over 65 by the year 2020, cancer presents a major health problem. Nursing is well positioned to play a role in all aspects of

cancer care, from prevention, through active treatment, to providing care at the end of life. The purposes of this chapter are to frame the problem of cancer within the context of aging, to identify the major issues related to providing care to this population, and to discuss strategies that may be helpful to nurses caring for older adults, families, and communities experiencing cancer.

Older adults faced with a diagnosis of cancer pose a challenge to those responsible for their care. The individual over age 65 generally has one or more coexisting conditions, physical disabilities, and/or psychologic alterations that may complicate management of care (Monfardini & Yancik, 1993). In addition, access to health care may be compromised because of lack of or insufficient financial and insurance resources, lack of social support, and lack of knowledge about specifics of care requirements. Myths and biases related to treating older adults with cancer pose significant barriers to early detection and appropriate treatment and management. Ageism is a major bias that interferes with appropriate care of the older adult. Ageism is defined as negative attitudes toward or beliefs about aging and the older adult (Berkman et al., 1994). Ageism in oncology can lead to unwarranted discrimination in screening practices, treatment decisions, and health care practices. Myths and biases held by practitioners, patients, families, and communities can perpetuate this discrimination. Additional myths and biases are presented in Box 19-1.

It is important that those caring for the older adult understand how the biologic processes of aging may affect cancer incidence, morbidity, and mortality. It has long been appreciated that cancer is a disease of aging; however, research initiatives have focused primarily on determining the specific mechanisms of carcinogenesis rather than on the process of aging. Further, it is important to recognize that cancer and aging differ, in that cancer originates from alterations in a single clone, whereas aging is a phenomenon that affects the entire organism (Cutler & Semsei, 1989). Miller (1994) makes several important observations about normal aging and disease. First, he distinguishes between "normal" aging and actual disease. Second, he suggests that although the effects of aging may not become obvious until the last decades of life, the process of aging is occurring throughout the life of an adult. Third, he concludes that the changes that occur throughout life reflect this aging process and not necessarily disease (Miller, 1994). These assertions are of particular importance in deter-

mining the presence or absence of cancers in the early stages and will be addressed in greater detail later in the chapter.

■ Theories of Aging and Cancer Incidence

That host defense mechanisms change with aging has been recognized for more than 50 years. The relationship of these changes to the occurrence of certain diseases, such as cancer, is less well understood (Schwab et al., 1989). Numerous theories of cancer and aging have been suggested. Among the age-related etiologic factors involved in these theories are the following: (1) decreased immune surveillance; (2) longer duration of carcinogenic exposure; (3) increased susceptibility of cells to carcinogens; (4) decreased DNA repair; (5) oncogene activation or amplification; and (6) defects in tumor suppressor genes (Cohen, 1994). Figure 19-1 depicts the multistage process of carcinogenesis and aging.

DECREASED IMMUNE SURVEILLANCE

Alterations in the functions of the immune system occur with aging. Specifically, there is significant evidence for a loss of tumor-specific immunity with advancing age in animal models (Cohen, 1994). However, the data that link this occurrence to humans remain circumstantial. It is most likely that many factors contribute to the decreased homeostasis seen in aging and contribute to the incidence of cancer as an individual ages. Such factors include, for example, DNA damage, decreased DNA repair, altered cell proliferation, decreased DNA methylation, altered immunosurveillance, alteration in protein synthetic capacity, alterations in genomic regulation, and decreased metabolic proficiency (Cohen, 1994).

Active debate continues as to whether low immune responses of the older adult contribute to vulnerability to cancer (Miller, 1991). The role of immune function in cancer causation remains controversial, possibly more as it relates to the incidence of lymphoid malignancies than to that of solid tumors (Cohen, 1994).

BOX 19-1 MAJOR MYTHS AND BIASES

	Myths and biases	Facts and examples
Causation myths	Cancer is contagious	Cancer is not contagious in the same sense as an infectious disease; some cancers can be transmitted genetically; selected viruses are associated with higher incidence of cancer.
	Cancer is incurable; is synonymous with death and pain	Cancer diagnosed at early stages is highly curable. Pain is a late symptom of cancer and is controllable in the majority of patients.
	Cancer is caused by personal vulnerabilities (e.g., stress and unhealthy behavior)	Stress, in and of itself, most likely does not cause cancer; however, its influence on the immune system may contribute to one's susceptibility. Cancer is not caused by physical injuries (e.g., cuts, bruises, or bumps to a body part). Smoking, high-fat diets, and lack of exercise are a few factors associated with increased incidence of cancer.
Treatment myths	Treatment is painful and should be avoided	Pain and discomfort from treatment are usually of short duration, and treatment should not be avoided because of fear of pain.
	Older adults have less pain and tolerate it better	No evidence exists that pain sensitivity decreases with age or that older adults tolerate pain better.
	Pain medication causes addiction	Narcotics to control pain from cancer do not cause addiction. Tolerance may develop, requiring increased doses. Adequate management of pain frees patients to perform activities of daily living.
	Surgery causes metastasis	Occasionally, "seeding" may occur, but it is rare.
	Radiation therapy is dangerous, painful, and a treatment of last resort	Side effects from radiation therapy in older adults have been successfully managed; radiation is an effective therapy for symptom control in more advanced disease.
	Chemotherapy is very dangerous	Chemotherapy can be safely administered to older adults in doses similar to those for younger adults when consideration is given to alterations in physiologic status and presence of comorbidity.
Biases	Ageism, associated with inadequate treatment	Example: Studies suggest that older adults are screened less often and receive less aggressive therapy than younger adults.
	Belief that rehabilitation is not necessary in older adults	Activity, involvement in therapy, and choice are associated with decreased morbidity and depression.
	Cultural biases, associated with increased incidence, morbidity, and mortality	Example: Latinos attribute cancer to such factors as sugar substitutes, bruises, microwave ovens, eating spicy foods, breastfeeding, and antibiotics. Breast self-exam is contrary to moral beliefs in conservative Hispanic communities.

From Berkman, B., Rohan, B., & Sampson, S. (1994). Myths and biases related to cancer in the elderly. *Cancer, 74* (Suppl. 7, 2004-2008. Reprinted by permission of Wiley-Liss, a division of John Wiley and Sons, Inc.

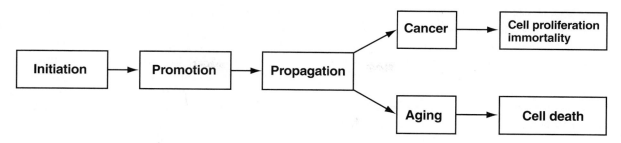

FIGURE 19-1 Multistage carcinogenesis process and aging.

LONGER DURATION OF CARCINOGENIC EXPOSURE

It has been suggested that the elapse of time caused by aging allows for the cellular alterations responsible for the development of a neoplasm. However, time as a sole factor is not sufficient to explain the phenomenon. The time necessary for a mutated cell to evolve into a clinically detectable tumor is estimated at 10% to 30% of the maximum life span for a given animal species (Cohen, 1994). Given this observation, it seems unlikely that longer duration of carcinogenic exposure alone is sufficient to cause cancer in the older adult.

INCREASED SUSCEPTIBILITY OF CELLS TO CARCINOGENS

Aging cells vary in their susceptibility to differing amounts of carcinogens. Data from experiments in laboratory animals are contradictory. Results from some experiments suggest that the occurrence of cancer is dose related, whereas others suggest a relationship of cancer occurrence to age of the animal (Cohen, 1994). Data from studies in humans are also inconclusive.

DECREASED DNA REPAIR

Laboratory experiments suggest that fibroblasts engage in sufficient activity to maintain cellular integrity; however, DNA synthesis and replication are absent. It has been suggested that this laboratory observation provides a reasonable model that may explain cellular aging of the individual.

ONCOGENE ACTIVATION OR AMPLIFICATION AND TUMOR SUPPRESSOR GENE LOSS

The data in this area are limited. There is some evidence that oncogene activation or amplification may be increased, resulting in increased initiation or promotion. Inactivation of cancer suppressor genes as a result of DNA damage may also contribute to the development of neoplasia (Cohen, 1994).

CONCLUSION

It seems clear that what is known remains inconclusive. It is also apparent that some combination of the preceding factors, possibly with the addition of others, will be found to account for the development of neoplasia in the older adult. Recent literature suggests that future research should be specifically directed at studying the process of aging and that findings from this research might provide more insight into tumor biology, therapeutic management, and improved outcomes (Holmes et al., 1991; Miller, 1991). Miller (1994) stated that if one were able to modify the rate of aging in humans, such as can be achieved in some animals, greater benefit might be realized to the health of humans than if diseases such as cancer, cardiovascular diseases, and diabetes were totally eliminated.

■ Screening and Treatment

Issues that face older adults with a potential risk for a diagnosis of cancer include age, gender, extent of disease, and presence of comorbidities. These issues affect decisions concerning cancer control, adequate and appropriate treatment, and rehabilitation. Further, these issues have the potential to complicate care for this group of individuals from biologic, psychologic, and sociodemographic perspectives. Alterations in body systems, changes in psychologic and social support, diminished resources, and altered mobility all affect the capacity of the older adult to cope with a diagnosis of cancer.

Although the primary purpose of this chapter is to address the nursing care of individuals over age 65 faced with a diagnosis of cancer or a potential diagnosis, two factors should not be overlooked. First, older adults are a heterogeneous group. Their care needs are complex and multifaceted and require the coordination of many disciplines. Second, although chronologic age is the one most important factor in increasing an individual's risk for cancer, in and of itself, it is probably the least important factor in developing therapeutic approaches to care for people experiencing cancer. This is due, in part, to the fact that biologic aging is a process that occurs at a variable pace. Although the patterns of these biologic changes are easily recognized, when they occur and to what extent are highly variable among individuals. Therefore the many factors that may influence this pace (e.g., biologic, psychologic, and social) must be considered when planning therapeutic approaches for this group. Figure 19-2, the *Comprehensive Gerontologic Model,* depicts the relationship of these factors (Cohen, 1994).

The *Comprehensive Gerontologic Model* provides a framework or guide for analyzing the factors that may influence decisions for the older adult at risk for the development of cancer. The model depicts the relationship of the individual to cancer from biologic, psychologic, and social perspectives and demonstrates how therapy, while targeting the cancer, also affects the entire person. This interactive model clearly demonstrates the narrowness of relying on chronologic age as the sole criterion for making management decisions and points to the need to consider a multitude of factors. Decisions concerning management of the older adult at risk for cancer are made across the entire wellness-illness trajectory. Decisions also center around whether or not to screen for cancer, whether to pursue a diagnostic workup, and whether to treat at all, and if so, how aggressively to treat (Cohen, 1994). Nurses, physicians, and other health care professionals must weigh each of these factors when making management decisions across the entire spectrum of cancer care for the older adult.

■ Management of the Older Adult at Risk for Cancer

DECISION TO SCREEN THE OLDER ADULT FOR CANCER

The American Cancer Society (ACS) has provided guidelines for cancer screening since 1980. These guidelines provide recommendations for the type of examination to be performed, who should be targeted (i.e., gender and age), and the frequency of the examination. Controversy exists concerning effectiveness of mass screening. Opponents to mass screening suggest that there is a lack of clear evidence as to the benefit to the individual from screening (Brawley, 1995). Proponents, on the other hand, suggest that cancer screening has many public health benefits in addition to the potential for early detection of cancer (Padberg, 1995).

Even in the context of the controversy, the ACS recommendations have been accepted by a wide variety of health care practitioners, professional organizations, federal agencies, and the general public. It is generally accepted that the ACS guidelines have had a positive impact on the early detection and diagnosis of cancer. Therefore nurses must be knowledgeable about such contro-

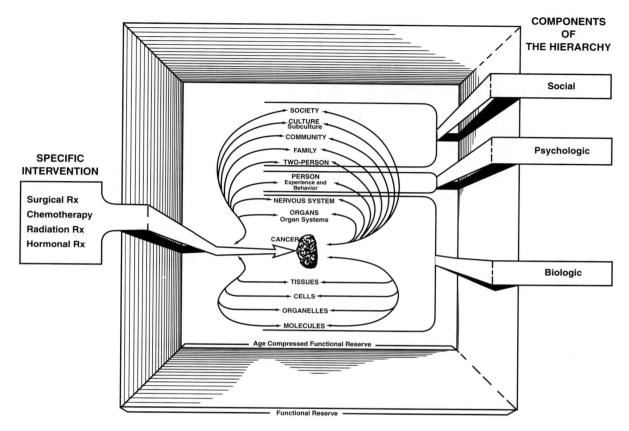

FIGURE 19-2 Comprehensive Geriatric Model. (From Cohen, H.J. [1994b]. Oncology and aging: General principles of cancer in the elderly. In W.R. Hazzard, et al. [Eds.], *Principles of geriatric medicine and gerontology* [3rd ed., p. 85]. New York: McGraw-Hill.)

versies, pay particular attention to changes in the recommendations, and be prepared to educate patients and their families about the current guidelines.

As can be seen in Table 19-1, recommendations for cancer screening frequently begin after age 50 (Fink, 1991). Only recently have upper age limit restrictions been lifted from screening guidelines. It must be recognized that screening for cancer is not an exact science and decisions concerning whether or not to screen rely on a comprehensive evaluation of each individual.

Factors that should be considered when deciding whether or not to screen include the cost of the test, the specificity and sensitivity of the test, the ability to treat the cancer if a diagnosis is made, and the discomfort and potential risk to the individual from the test. Evaluation of these factors contributes to the screening decisions made for all individuals, not just the older adult. In addition to the preceding factors, other factors that influence a screening decision for an older individual include the presence or absence of comorbidity, ability to perform activities of daily

TABLE 19-1 American Cancer Society recommendations

| Examination | Target population | | Interval |
	Gender	Age	
Sigmoidoscopy (preferably flexible)	M and F	50 and older	Every 3 to 5 years (per physician's recommendations)
Fecal occult blood test	M and F	50 and older	Every year
Digital rectal examination	M and F	40 and older	Every year
Pap test	F	18 and older; currently or having been sexually active	Every year (may be performed less frequently, at discretion of provider, after three or more consecutive negative examinations)
Pelvic examination	F	18 to 40	Every 1 to 3 years with Pap test
		40 and older	Every year
Endometrial tissue sample	F	At menopause (high-risk women*)	At menopause
Breast self-examination	F	20 and older	Every month
Clinical breast examination	F	20 to 40	Every 3 years
		40 and older	Every year
Mammography†	F	40 to 49	Every 1 to 2 years
		50 and older	Every year
Health counseling and cancer checkup‡	M and F	20 and older	Every 3 years
	M and F	40 and older	Every year

Adapted from *Guidelines for the cancer related checkup* (ACS, 1992).
*History of infertility, obesity, failure to ovulate, abnormal uterine bleeding, or estrogen therapy.
†Begin screening mammography at age 40.
‡Includes examination for thyroid, testicular, prostate, ovarian, head and neck, skin and lymph node cancers.

living (ADLs), and life expectancy. Although determining life expectancy for a particular individual is ambiguous, some attempt should be made to correlate the life expectancy with the potential for development of a specific cancer in the future. The decision to treat is separate from deciding how aggressive that treatment should be. The prevention of morbidity and enhancement of quality of life as a result of early detection must be weighed carefully against the morbidity caused by screening. For example, there is no reason not to screen for breast cancer regardless of age in an otherwise healthy individual. It may make more practical sense to screen a healthy 75-year-old, who may have a life expectancy of 7 to 10 years, than to screen a 55-year-old who has severe debilitating cardiovascular disease, suffers from diabetes, and has a limited life expectancy. Breast cancer can be detected relatively inexpensively, with little discomfort or risk. The early detection of a small breast cancer in the older adult can result in effective treatment and minimal impact on quality of life. On the other hand, undetected breast cancer has the potential to cause significant morbidity, requiring more extensive therapy and costing more. Health care professionals must weigh the costs and benefits of screening for a particular individual, with a particular risk profile, within the context of that person's preferences. Recommendations exist for screening for many cancers, and these serve only as a starting place for the practitioner. "Differences in decisions may be entirely appropriate in certain situations but must be based on specific individualized patient information, not on categorical decisions made on the basis of chronological age" (Cohen, 1994b, p. 84).

To serve their purpose effectively, guidelines must be individualized. Three other factors influence decisions regarding screening for cancer. First, the older adult may choose not to participate in routine cancer screening. This decision may be related to lack of complete information about a particular screening test (e.g., a perception that, because of age, screening is not necessary), fears or other myths or biases about cancer or a cancer diagnosis (see Box 19-1), or inability to pay for screening tests. Second, physicians and other health care professionals may also lack correct information concerning eligibility for screening. Third, older individuals tend to be seen for episodic rather than preventive services. Therefore physician and patient alike tend to focus more on attending to presenting symptoms than on whether or not an individual has had a Pap test or mammogram. Educating physicians and the public about the value of early detection of cancer in the older adult is essential.

DECISION TO DIAGNOSE CANCER IN THE OLDER ADULT

Once the decision has been made to screen the older adult for a particular type of cancer, one must next decide which screening tests should be used for the purpose of diagnosis. Again, more than just the older adult's chronologic age should be considered when making this decision. The decision should consider the social, psychologic, and biologic factors portrayed by the comprehensive gerontologic model (see Figure 19-2). In addition, the following factors should be evaluated when making a decision concerning whether to pursue diagnosing a cancer: (1) the efficacy of the screening test, its cost, and its potential for causing morbidity; (2) how extensive the workup should be (or how many tests to include); and (3) the availability of appropriate treatment once a diagnosis is made. The preferences of the older adult individual, in consultation with the appropriate health care provider, are an integral part of this decision-making process.

Consider the following case scenario: A 75-year-old woman comes to the clinic complaining of a breast lump that she says she discovered while doing her monthly breast self-examination. She is in good health with no significant comorbidities, is married, and is fully active. The goal in this situation is to obtain clear-cut evidence as to whether or not a malignancy is present. The primary decision that faces the practitioner in this scenario is whether to order a diagnostic mammogram or to go directly to a biopsy. The practitioner must weigh the risks and benefits of choosing one or both of these diagnostic tests.

The previously discussed paradigm may provide some guidance in evaluating whether one or both of these diagnostic tests should be used. The mammogram has a high specificity and sensitivity, is of relatively low cost, and is generally risk-free. If a diagnosis of breast cancer is made, efficacious treatment is available. There are no significant factors described in this case that would preclude the use of a mammogram for this particular individual. The major factor that needs consideration is whether a mammogram is needed given the fact that a clinically palpable lump is present. If the additional clinical information that might be obtained from the mammogram would possibly alter approaches to therapy, then a decision to perform this diagnostic test seems appropriate. If, however, no additional treatment-relevant information is expected, then not to perform a mammogram may be an appropriate decision. Because the mass is clinically palpable, a biopsy is the only method available that will provide conclusive data as to whether or not it is malignant, what its cytologic characteristics are, and if prognostic parameters are present. Therefore, in this situation, it may be most appropriate to avoid the expense and possible discomfort of a mammogram.

If there is any question about whether the lump might be cystic, either a needle aspiration or a sonogram might be appropriate. However, the addition of the mammogram would only be important to detect occult disease in either the affected breast or the contralateral breast. These factors must be weighed within the context of the social, psychologic, and biologic parameters of the individual. The possible discovery of an occult cancer, which might not be clinically detectable for many years, may not be a sufficient reason to proceed with extensive diagnostic testing. This reasoning may be appropriate even in a healthy 75-year-old individual such as the one discussed in the scenario. Decisions such as this remain controversial.

Additional factors that might influence a decision to have additional diagnostic tests include when the individual had her most recent mammogram, and the existence of financial and insurance constraints. It is beyond the scope of this chapter to discuss all the possible scenarios that might influence decisions concerning what approach or approaches to take to make a diagnosis. It is essential, however, to discuss each possible approach with the patient, discuss the risks and benefits of each approach, and present expected outcomes from each approach. Providing accurate information is essential so that the older adult is equipped with sufficient data with which to make an informed decision.

DECISION TO TREAT THE OLDER ADULT WITH A DIAGNOSIS OF CANCER— AND HOW AGGRESSIVELY

Research suggests that a significant age bias exists in relation to treatment decisions for the older adult (Bergman et al., 1991; Greenfield et al., 1987; Guadagnoli et al., 1990; Mor et al., 1985; Samet et al., 1986; Yancik et al., 1989). This age bias is reflected in decisions physicians make concerning whether or not to treat the older adult with cancer, the type of therapy offered, and the aggressivity of this therapy. Findings from studies suggest that physicians tend to offer older women more conservative therapy and refer them to specialists less frequently than they do comparable younger women. Although older women may refuse chemotherapy and certain types of surgical procedures more frequently than do younger women, these decisions tend, in part, to be related to the type of recommendations made by the physician. Chronologic age should not be the sole factor used in deciding on cancer treatment in the older adult (Ganz, 1993).

Consider the following case scenario: The 75-year-old woman described in the previous scenario received a biopsy with a resultant diagnosis of infiltrating ductal carcinoma of the breast. The interaction of the biologic, social, and psychologic factors should guide decisions concerning appropriate treatment options. In addition, patient factors (e.g., personal preferences and physician recommendations) need to be carefully weighed. Other factors include expected outcomes from each therapy, impact of the chosen therapy on the patient's quality of life, and economic factors.

Assume that the following therapies are equivalent in this situation. The possible approaches to treatment include breast-conserving therapy alone (removal of the mass), breast-conserving therapy with radiation therapy, or modified radical mastectomy. Also, the addition of chemotherapy and/or tamoxifen may be considered. Just as the decisions to screen and to diagnose are made independently, so are treatment decisions. The first decision is to treat the local disease. A decision must be made as to which of the approaches will afford the individual the best local control of her breast cancer, with the least morbidity and maintaining the best quality of life. Second, the decision of whether or not to treat the woman with chemotherapy is dependent on the characteristics of the tumor and the presence or absence of tumor-positive axillary nodes. In most situations tamoxifen is prescribed for postmenopausal women with a diagnosis of breast cancer. Each of these decisions is made within the context of what is in the best interest of the individual woman. The decision concerning the extent of therapy, in particular, whether to treat the older adult with adjuvant radiation or chemotherapy, remains uncertain. Little data exist for the older person concerning the outcome from aggressive treatment for the various cancers. This lack of data is due, in part, to the lack of clinical trials that include a significant sample of older adults in the study (Ganz, 1993). Therefore studies that include a significant sample of older individuals are needed. Data from these studies would assist providers and patients in the difficult treatment decisions with which they are often faced.

The health care team must weigh the interaction of a composite of factors when determining the efficacy of screening, making decisions concerning which tests to use for diagnosis, and deciding whether to and how aggressively to treat the older adult. Throughout this process the preferences of the older adult must be included in the decision-making process.

■ Major Therapeutic Modalities

The major therapeutic modalities used in the treatment of cancer include surgery, radiation therapy, chemotherapy, hormonal therapy, and biologic therapy. The choice of therapy is dependent on such factors as the type of cancer, the extent of disease at diagnosis (i.e., presence or absence of metastasis), tumor aggressivity, and the presence of certain prognostic factors.

SURGERY

Surgery has been and remains one of the mainstays of cancer therapy. Its use can be traced to ancient times. For example, at the beginning of the Christian era, surgery for breast cancer was described by Leonides (De Moulin, cited in Lippman et al., 1989). Although surgery is frequently the first approach to therapy, an enhanced understanding of tumor biology, introduction of new therapeutic techniques, earlier stage of disease at diagnosis, and a greater reliance on interdisciplinary approaches to care have all contributed to changing the overall complexion of cancer therapy (Kalinowski, 1993). Surgery is used to establish a diagnosis of cancer, to determine the extent of disease (stage), to treat the primary cancer with curative intent, and to provide palliation in more advanced stages of disease. Although in some situations surgery is the only therapy, it must be remembered that it is a local therapy. Therefore surgery is frequently followed by additional therapies that are discussed in the following sections. The use of combination therapy in the older adult has not been well studied. Clinical trials that examine the effects of combination therapies on quality of life and morbidity and mortality in the older person are needed.

Two major factors may influence the choice of surgery as a therapeutic modality in the older adult. First, research has demonstrated that surgery in the older adult carries morbidity and mortality similar to those seen in the younger adult when controlled for comorbid conditions and other physiologic parameters (Cohen, 1994). Second, older adults may choose surgery over other modalities, such as radiation therapy. This choice is frequently related to a desire to treat the cancer in the most expeditious manner and "get on with one's life." This choice of surgical treatment over more time-consuming breast-conserving surgery with adjuvant radiation therapy was observed in older women with a diagnosis of breast cancer who described their experiences during participation in focus groups (C.B. Burnett, B. Kraling, & J.H. Rowland, personal communication, 1995).

RADIATION THERAPY

Radiation therapy is a local modality that can be used as primary therapy with curative intent, as

Aging Alert
Warning signs for potential surgical complications
- Existence of comorbid conditions
- Extensive surgery
- Psychologic distress or fear of surgery
- Potential risk of anesthesia
- Potential for infection

Aging Alert
Warning signs of complications from radiation therapy
- Skin: potential dryness, desquamation, infection
- Mucous membranes: sloughing, alterations in taste, decreased saliva
- Alterations in nutrition, weight loss
- Target organ injury (e.g., cardiac or pulmonary)
- Weakness and/or fatigue

adjuvant therapy with surgery and/or chemotherapy, or as palliative therapy. Radiation therapy, particularly in the older adult, may be the initial treatment of choice to help decrease tumor size and reduce the need for extensive surgery that may convey significantly more morbidity. In some situations (e.g., in prostate and breast cancers), radiation therapy and surgery have been shown to provide equivalent outcomes with regard to overall survival. Choices that have emerged in such therapies are particularly beneficial to the older adult for whom biologic, social, and psychologic factors may limit the feasibility of one particular modality. The side effects that accompany radiation therapy must be considered when suggesting this as a therapeutic modality. The effects of radiation therapy on normal tissue are said to be more pronounced in the older adult (Cohen, 1994). It should be remembered that side effects from radiation therapy are generally limited to the site at which the therapy is delivered. However, when radiation therapy is delivered to organs that are experiencing the normal decline that occurs with aging (e.g., salivary glands, mucous membranes, and skin), the effects potentially will be magnified. Fatigue is another type of side effect experienced by most people who receive radiation therapy. In the older adult,

fatigue may result in significant alterations in the quality of life and the ability to carry out ADLs.

CHEMOTHERAPY

Chemotherapy administration poses significant management problems for all individuals, not just older adults. A major reason for the problems relates to the issues of pharmacokinetics and pharmacodynamics. Pharmacokinetics refers to the action taken by the body on the drug, and pharmacodynamics refers to the action of the drug on the body (Egorin, 1993). The pharmacodynamic effects of chemotherapy are both therapeutic and potentially toxic. Drug therapy in general is designed to have a maximum therapeutic effect with little or no side effects. In cancer chemotherapy, this goal is modified somewhat. The aim is still to have a maximum therapeutic effect; however, there is an expectation that there will be side effects. The level or degree of side effects is closely monitored.

No studies have clearly demonstrated a difference in tumor response from chemotherapy in older versus younger adults (Cohen, 1994). However, in the older adult the dosing is complicated by (1) the effects of normal aging on body systems, (2) the presence of comorbid conditions, and (3) polypharmacy. The changes associated with normal aging may affect the processes of absorption, distribution, metabolism, and excretion. Specifically, the changes may include decreases in body tissue mass, decreases in renal and hepatic functioning, changes in gastric absorption and motility, and alteration in bone marrow reserve (Egorin, 1993). Measuring the effects of these changes is less than an exact science and requires the practitioner to carefully evaluate the physiologic age of the individual.

The effects of comorbidity and polypharmacy are frequently linked. For example, the older adult is more likely to have made long-term use of such agents as allopurinol, barbiturates, or acetaminophen that may minimize or exaggerate age-related hepatic changes (Egorin, 1993).

Clearly, providing for the correct dose that produces an appropriate therapeutic level within some acceptable range of toxicity is essential. To achieve this goal, approaches to therapy must be individualized. As stated earlier, chronologic age, in and of itself, is not a sufficient parameter to guide therapeutic management. Physiologic age, to the extent possible, needs to be determined by assessing body system functions. Table 19-2 provides an overview of body systems, alterations related to aging, assessment factors for chemotherapy, and some of the major chemotherapy drugs that affect those systems.

Health care professionals must be willing to accept the underlying principle inherent in cancer chemotherapy that there will be some toxicity. Underdosing as a means to prevent side effects may cause patients more harm in that they are receiving medication designed to kill cancer cells in less than therapeutic doses. Decisions to treat with chemotherapy must be made with the older adult, providing sufficient information so that informed decisions are possible. Nurses must be able to monitor the response to the drug, record and treat its side effects, and educate patient and family concerning their individual responsibilities.

Aging Alert

Warning signs of complications from chemotherapy

- Nausea and vomiting resulting in malnutrition
- Depletion in marrow reserve resulting in infection
- Alopecia resulting in alterations in body image
- Pain as a result of therapy
- Constipation as a result of altered elimination
- Mucositis

■ Future Goals in Cancer Prevention, Control, and Treatment

Projections on the number of older adults by the year 2030 indicate that there will be more than 55 million people 65 years of age or older. This number will account for approximately 20% of the population (Monfardini & Yancik, 1993). Also, an increased number of individuals will be at risk for the development of cancer. Improved treatments for cardiovascular diseases and those of infectious origin result in more individuals surviving and subsequently being at risk for cancer. The significant increase in older adults who will require cancer care clearly makes research on aging a national priority.

A variety of initiatives have evolved in response to these factors. The significance of these factors for nursing lies in the implications for clinical practice and research. Specifically, nurses in general, as well as advanced practice nurses, will need to educate themselves to the needs of the older adult as they relate to aging and the potential development of cancer, and to develop

TABLE 19-2 Chemotherapy and the older adult

System	Alterations related to aging	Assessment factors	Therapeutic measures
Cardiovascular	Decreased compliance and elasticity in both peripheral vessels and heart; decreased maximum heart rate; increased peripheral vascular resistance	Blood pressure; pulse; electrocardiogram volume	Doxorubicin
Pulmonary	Decreased elasticity; decreased ciliary activity; decreased respiratory muscular strength	Tidal volume; vital capacity in total oxygen consumption; sensitivity skin test	Bleomycin
Wound healing	Slower healing due to decreased cell proliferation and collagen production and to decreased skin thickness and loss of subcutaneous tissue; decreased muscle and bone weight and mass	Mobility	Surgery resulting in immobility
Endocrine	Changes most likely to occur during time of stress (increase in basal and stimulated plasma norepinephrine concentrations; impaired release of insulin resulting in impaired use of glucose)	Blood chemistry	Surgery and chemotherapy
Central nervous	Loss of neurons in cerebral cortex, cerebellum, and hippocampus; lipofuscin pigment accumulation; loss of brain weight and cerebral blood flow; confusion; postoperative delirium	Mental status; peripheral neuropathy	Cerebellar toxicity from cytosine, arabinoside; peripheral toxicity from vincristine
Special senses	Visual and hearing changes; changes in taste and smell; decreased pain sensation	Hearing and visual testing before, during, and at completion	Chemotherapy; radiation therapy to head and neck
Hematopoietic	Diminished hematopoiesis during increased demand	Complete blood counts	Chemotherapy; radiation therapy
Gastrointestinal	Decreased nausea	Nutritional status	Cyclophosphamide
Hepatorenal	Decreased drug metabolism	Liver function tests; creatinine clearance	Platinum methotrexate

From Cohen, 1994a.

BOX 19-2 RESEARCH REGARDING PATTERNS OF CARE FOR OLDER ADULT CANCER PATIENTS

National Institute of Medicine priority areas	Subjects of National Cancer Institute and National Institute on Aging funded projects
Basic biomedical research	Altered drug metabolism and enhanced toxicity
	Pharmacokinetics and metabolism of antineoplastic agents
Clinical research	Toxicity of chemotherapy
	Patterns of care and incidence of comorbidity
Behavioral and social research	Analysis of relationships between age, diagnosis, and treatment
	Symptom management
	Social support and relation to outcome
Research on the delivery of health services	Variations in patterns of medical care between older adults and the young
	Effects of age on stage of disease at diagnosis
Research in biomedical ethics	Decision making in older adults and responses to treatment
	Physicians' attitudes toward treatment of older adults and relation to treatment choice
General	Survey in patterns of care in radiation therapy

appropriate intervention strategies designed to meet these needs. Collaboration among nurses and other health care personnel is essential to this process.

In 1984 the National Institutes of Health's National Cancer Institute (NCI) and the National Institute on Aging supported 11 projects designed to identify patterns of care for older adult cancer patients. These projects focused on the natural history of cancer in the older adult; treatment patterns; the interaction of comorbidity, aging, and cancer; and the professional skills necessary to provide optimum cancer care for the older adult (NCI, 1987). Findings from these studies provided some of the first information concerning patterns of care for individuals age 65 years and older. Box 19-2 summarizes these initiatives.

In 1991 the Institute of Medicine of the National Academy of Sciences released a report that delineated 15 high-priority research areas designed to increase knowledge of the aging process and enhance understanding of factors that contribute to quality of life (QOL) in the older adult (Lonergan & Krevans, 1991). Of the 15 areas, the majority of them are relevant to the individual at risk for the development of cancer. These areas focus on biologic aspects of oncogenesis, prevention and control, clinical management, social and psychologic factors, ethical issues concerning allocation of resources and treatment decisions, and access to and costs of care. Box 19-3 summarizes these areas.

In 1991 the U.S. Department of Health and Human Services (USDHHS) published *Healthy*

BOX 19-3 A NATIONAL AGENDA FOR RESEARCH ON AGING: RELEVANCE TO CANCER

High-priority research areas	Specific research areas
Basic biomedical research	Cellular regulation and repair
Clinical research	Prevention, management, and rehabilitation
	Mismanagement of medications: lack of compliance; polypharmacy; underdosing and overdosing
	Interaction of age-dependent physiologic changes and cancer
	Health service delivery systems designed to reduce morbidity and mortality
	Targeted diseases such as cancer, infectious diseases, and diminished immunologic competence
Behavioral and social research	Relations among social, psychologic, and biologic factors in aging
	Effects of changes in the social structure on performance, productivity, health, and well-being
Research on the delivery of health services	Long-term care and continuity of care
	Cost and financing of care
	Availability of drug therapy and its costs
	Prevention of disability and disease and promotion of health
Research in biomedical ethics	Decisions on life-sustaining therapies
	Decision making concerning appropriateness and availability of therapies
	Equity of access to care, clinical trials, and research
General	Adequate resources for delivery of appropriate care
	Sufficient funds for centers of education and research
	Increased support for research infrastructure

Adapted from Lonergan, E.T., & Krevans, J.R. (1991). A national agenda for research on aging. *New England Journal of Medicine 324*(25), 1825-1828. Copyright 1991. Massachusetts Medical Society. All rights reserved.

People 2000: National Health Promotion and Disease Prevention Objectives. A major focus of this initiative was to provide health promotion and disease prevention guidelines for major diseases across the life span and among special populations. The most important aspect of health promotion among older people is to maintain health and functional independence (US-DHHS, 1991). Determining why cancer incidence and death rates differ with advancing age is the only high-priority research need that specifically focuses on older individuals. Five "key

Healthy People 2000 Objectives

General categories		Specific categories
General health status	17.1	Increase years of healthy life to at least 65 years. (Baseline: An estimated 62 years in 1980.)
Risk reduction	21.1f	Increase to at least 40% the proportion of adults aged 65 and older who have received . . . all of the screening . . . appropriate for their age and gender . . .
Key services: general	8.8	Increase to at least 90% the proportion of people aged 65 and older who had the opportunity to participate during the preceding year in at least one organized health promotion program through a senior center, lifecare facility, or other community-based setting that serves older adults.
Key services: breast cancer screening	16.11	Increase to at least . . . 60% those aged 50 and older who have received [a clinical breast examination] within the preceding 1 to 2 years. (Baseline: 25% of women aged 50 and older "within the preceding 2 years" in 1987.)
Key services: cervical cancer screening	16.12b	Increase to at least 95% the proportion of women aged 70 and older with uterine cervix who have ever received a Pap test, and to at least 70% those who received a Pap test within the preceding 1 to 3 years. (Baseline: 76% "ever" and 44% "within the preceding 3 years" in 1987.)
Key services: fecal occult blood testing	16.13	Increase to at least 50% the proportion of people aged 50 and older who have received fecal occult blood testing within the preceding 1 to 2 years, and to at least 40% those who have ever received proctosigmoidoscopy. (Baseline: 27% received fecal occult blood testing during the preceding 2 years in 1987; 25% had ever received proctosigmoidoscopy in 1987.)
Key services: primary care	16.14	Increase to at least 40% the proportion of people aged 50 and older visiting a primary care provider in the preceding year who have received oral, skin, and digital rectal examinations during one such visit. (Baseline: An estimated 27% received a digital rectal exam during a physician visit within the preceding year in 1987.)

From U.S. Department of Health and Human Services. (1990). *Healthy People 2000: National health promotion and disease prevention objectives* (DHHS Pub. No. [PHS] 91-50212). Washington, DC: U.S. Government Printing Office.

Health Promotion
Cancer prevention

- Avoid overexposure to the sun.
- Eliminate smoking.
- Cut down on excessive alcohol use.
- Eat a diet high in fruits, vegetables, and fibers.
- Exercise daily.
- Participate in regular screenings and self-examinations to detect cancers at an early stage. Early detection can lead to a better prognosis.

services and protection objectives" that specifically target older adults are presented in the *Healthy People 2000 Objectives* box.

The Oncology Nursing Society has long been a champion of care issues for special populations. In 1992 the organization published a fact sheet on cancer and the older adult. This fact sheet serves as a resource for nurses, other health care providers, and other disciplines interested in care of the older adult with cancer. The background material summarizes major issues of concern in providing care to this population. Some of these issues include insufficient financial resources that influence compliance with treatment regimens; problems related to more advanced stage of disease at time of diagnosis as a result of delay in seeking health care; lack of accurate and complete information about cancer, its risks, and the need for early detection and treatment; and limited access to care (*Fact Sheet,* 1992). Also in 1992, the society published the *Oncology Nursing Society Position Paper on Cancer and Aging* (Boyle, et al., 1992), which delineated ten position statements that serve to guide the nurse caring for individuals 65 years of age or older throughout their experiences with cancer. Box 19-4 presents these statements.

A number of research initiatives supported by the NCI and the American Cancer Society have subsequently focused on various aspects of older adult cancer care (NCI, 1987, 1993). Most recently the Agency for Health Care Policy and Research funded an initiative designed to examine the care and cost outcomes of older adult women with a diagnosis of early-stage breast cancer (PORT, 1994). The American Cancer Society has convened several conferences that focus on older adults at risk for cancer and on issues surrounding their diagnosis, treatment, and supportive care (Cancer, 1991 & 1994). Relevance of the guidelines and findings from these conferences has been discussed throughout the chapter.

National attention on issues facing the older adult with cancer, partly as a result of lobbying efforts by groups such as the American Association of Retired Persons (AARP), has contributed to changes in approaches to care and to dispelling myths and biases. Research initiatives have been supported by the federal government and professional organizations. Future research efforts must continue to focus on the special needs of the individual facing a diagnosis of cancer. In particular, efforts must be championed toward enhancing the early detection of cancer throughout the individual's life span. Nursing's role in this effort is clear. Primary care and political advocacy are but two areas in which nurses are well positioned to effect change.

■ Cancer Risk Assessment

Because the incidence of cancer increases with age, performing a cancer risk assessment in older adults is as important as it is in younger individuals. Basic elements of a cancer risk assessment include obtaining a detailed personal and family medical history (White & Spitz, 1993). In addition, the nurse should obtain information about the older adults' level of understanding of cancer and their potential risk, physical ability to perform routine screening procedures (e.g., breast self-examination), and desire to participate in cancer screening.

BOX 19-4 POSITION STATEMENTS ON CANCER AND AGING,
ONCOLOGY NURSING SOCIETY (1992)

1. It is imperative that oncology nurses recognize personal biases toward aging and older adults that may interfere with the delivery of quality nursing care.
2. It is imperative that oncology nurses advocate cancer prevention and early detection activities for older adults.
3. It is imperative that oncology nurses acknowledge the dynamic and complex interrelationships between cancer and aging that affect cancer nursing care.
4. It is imperative that oncology nurses intervene to prevent or minimize the unique age-specific sequelae of cancer and its management.
5. It is imperative that oncology nurses integrate comprehensive gerontologic assessment into the nursing care of older adults.
6. It is imperative that oncology nurses assess the availability and capability of the support networks of older patients and their significant others.
7. It is imperative that oncology nurses increase communication with colleagues about older adults with cancer to enhance problem solving in a variety of settings and at different points along the cancer continuum.
8. It is imperative that oncology nurses consider age-related factors that affect learning and performance of self-care activities related to the cancer experience.
9. It is imperative that oncology nurses maximize their advocacy role in ethical decision making relative to quality of life of older people with cancer.
10. It is imperative that oncology nurses recognize the effects of health care policy on the nursing care of older adults who have or who are at risk for cancer.

A goal of cancer risk assessment is to avoid the consequence of missed opportunities. Missed opportunities result if there is a failure to perform cancer risk assessment when an opportunity presents itself. These missed opportunities occur when an individual seeks episodic or chronic care from a provider, sees a provider who assumes that primary health care needs are being given by another provider, relies on misinformation concerning efficacy of screening for the older adult, and/or is fearful of and resistant to having screening examinations performed. Data suggest that compliance with screening guidelines can be increased if these examinations are incorporated into routine health care (Mandelblatt et al., 1993). This section focuses on elements of a cancer risk assessment and describes approaches designed

to incorporate this assessment for older adults into routine care so as to avoid these missed opportunities.

A variety of reminder systems have been reported that are designed to increase the frequency with which an older adult is screened for cancer. Some of these include chart reminder flow sheets, personal contact by telephone and/or mail, and other, more general approaches such as use of clinic posters, mass media, and community agencies. A recent study found that when nurse practitioners (NPs) personally approached underserved older women attending a primary care clinic about participating in breast and cervical cancer screening, the compliance rate was significantly higher for those approached by the NP than for those seeing physicians who were using a standard chart reminder card (Mandelblatt et al., 1993). Findings such as these have significant implications for nursing practice. These findings suggest that nurses are well positioned to perform a cancer risk assessment on patients who are attending a clinic for routine or episodic care; to determine the date of a previous mammogram, Pap test, digital rectal examination, prostate-specific antigen (PSA), stool blood test, and/or sigmoidoscopy; to recommend appropriate screening tests that are consistent with ACS guidelines; to schedule necessary screening tests; and to follow up to ensure that the appropriate tests have been obtained. Refer to Table 19-1 for recommended ACS screening guidelines.

■ Nursing Process

ASSESSMENT

Assessment of cancer risk status is appropriate whether a patient is being seen for the first time in a clinic, is being admitted to an acute care setting, or is a resident of a long-term care facility. It is essential to carefully differentiate between normal symptoms of aging and those that suggest early-stage cancer. Cancer checkups, as recommended by the ACS, should be completed every year for individuals over 40 years of age. This checkup includes collection of standard demographic information (e.g., age, gender, marital status, height, weight, alcohol and/or smoking history, and exposure to environmental risk factors); recording of personal and family history of cancer; a physical assessment for cancers of the breast, ovary, prostate, lymph nodes, oral cavity, skin, testicles, and thyroid according to recommended ACS guidelines (Mettlin & Dodd, 1992); recording of changes in body functions (e.g., weight loss, blood in stools, and changes in appetite); and assessment of general cancer knowledge, myths and biases, cultural factors, previous screening behavior patterns, and changes in cognition and physical ability that might influence ability to perform self-examination. See Table 19-3. For the purpose of

example, many of the responses used in the table are vague and might easily give the impression of merely reporting symptoms associated with normal aging.

NURSING DIAGNOSES

The potential for development of cancer exists for all older adults. A review of the findings from the assessment will enable the nurse to determine a cancer risk profile for the individual patient. The data may reveal a strong family history of cancer (i.e., first-degree relatives with a history of breast, ovarian, and colorectal cancers), significant environmental exposure to known carcinogens, long history of tobacco use, or severe sunburns as a young child or adult. Although many of the familial cancers would be expected to have occurred at an earlier age, a strong family history might be an indication that members of the family other than the patient are at increased risk. It would be important to gather specific information concerning age at onset, type of cancer, and outcome for each affected individual so that appropriate action might be taken.

To accurately determine a person's cancer risk, a variety of factors, including the individual's age, must be considered (Fink, 1991; Frank-Stromberg & Rohan, 1992):

HIGH RISK FOR THE DEVELOPMENT OF BREAST CANCER

- Age
- Family history of breast cancer or genetic predisposition
- Young age at menarche, first full-term pregnancy after 30 years of age, late menopause
- Nulliparity
- History of ovarian or colorectal cancer
- Alcohol use

RISK FOR THE DEVELOPMENT OF OVARIAN CANCER

- Age
- History of breast or colorectal cancer

TABLE 19-3 Cancer risk assessment for the older adult

Assessment factors	Sample questions	Possible responses	Action
Demographic factors date of birth, gender, height and weight (changes), marital status	Has your weight changed in the past 6 months?	Lost 10 lb	Assess changes in eating and bowel habits
Date of last exam Reason for current exam	What was the date of your most recent health exam? What brought you to the clinic today? What do you expect from today's visit?	May 1, 1995 Tired all the time, no appetite To find out what's wrong	Assess changes in emotional, sleep, and physical activity patterns
Smoking history: cigarettes, cigars, pipes, other	Do you currently use any tobacco products? Have you ever used any tobacco products? How many cigarettes do you smoke a day?	Yes	Assess presence or absence of cough, sputum, shortness of breath
Alcohol history: amount, type, frequency	Do you currently drink alcohol? What type? How many drinks per week?	15 to 20 Yes Wine 5 glasses a week	Is this your usual amount?
Nutrition history	How would you describe your eating habits? What types of food do you eat a lot of? What foods do you avoid?	Nibble frequently Chicken Meat No	Assess whether easily satiated, feelings of bloating, stool composition
History of cancer	Have you ever been diagnosed with cancer?		
Family history of cancer	Has anyone in your family been diagnosed with cancer? If yes, obtain details of age at diagnosis and primary site	Yes (father: colon; sister: ovarian)	Assess personal risk factors for these and other familial cancers
Cancer knowledge, cultural biases and myths	Can you describe what you think cancer is? What do you believe causes cancer? Do you think that you are at risk for cancer?	Refer to Box 19-1	Correct misinformation, myths, and biases
Cognitive and physical abilities	Have you noticed any changes in your ability to take care of yourself (either emotional or physical)?	Arthritis limits mobility and sensation	Plan for teaching self-examination methods according to limitations

545

- Family history of ovarian cancer
- Low parity

RISK FOR THE DEVELOPMENT OF CERVICAL CANCER

- Multiple sexual partners
- Intercourse before age 20
- HPV infection (human papilloma virus)
- Smoking

RISK FOR THE DEVELOPMENT OF COLORECTAL CANCER

- Personal or family history (first-degree relatives) of polyps
- History of polyposis syndromes
- High-fat diet
- Personal history of inflammatory bowel disease

RISK FOR THE DEVELOPMENT OF PROSTATE CANCER

- Age
- Being black North American man

RISK FOR THE DEVELOPMENT OF ORAL CANCER

- Poor dental hygiene
- Tobacco use
- Alcohol use

RISK FOR THE DEVELOPMENT OF LUNG CANCER

- Age
- Smoking
- Asbestos and other environmental or occupational exposures

RISK FOR THE DEVELOPMENT OF MELANOMA AND NONMELANOMA SKIN CANCERS

- Age
- Dysplastic nevi
- Family history
- Being white and fair-skinned
- Severe sunburns, particularly before age 18

The risk for development of cancer and the stage at which it is diagnosed may be influenced by frequency and adequacy of cancer screening. A woman who has not had a Pap test since the birth of her last child, or a man who avoids a digital rectal examination of his prostate, increases the chances that disease, when detected, will be at a more advanced stage. Therefore the nurse compiles the data gathered in the initial assessment and determines appropriate action for screening.

PLANNING AND GOAL IDENTIFICATION

Compliance with cancer screening guidelines is the primary desired outcome or goal. Increased knowledge on the part of the patient about cancer, its causes, and its risks is another desired outcome, which contributes to compliance with screening guidelines.

Providing the older adult with feedback is a key aspect of conducting a cancer risk assessment. This feedback provides older adults with an opportunity to ask questions concerning their understanding of the findings from the assessment and enables the nurse to validate the findings. A plan might include a review of the assessment at the time it is conducted or the scheduling of a future meeting. Studies that have looked at compliance with screening guidelines—in particular, guidelines for mammograms—show that tests that are performed at the time of an initial visit, rather than scheduled in the future, have a higher compliance rate (Mandelblatt et al., 1993). One might suggest from these findings that immediate discussion of the findings from the cancer risk assessment with the older adult would have a greater impact on compliance. Therefore it is suggested that at least a preliminary review of the assessment be conducted on the same day it is completed. If feasible, set aside time for discussion of the results of the cancer risk assessment at the conclusion of the examination, and inform the patient beforehand of this arrangement.

Discuss possible approaches to cancer screening and risk behavior modification with the patient after reviewing the findings from the assessment. Assist the patient in setting achievable goals that consider demographic, personal, social, and fiscal factors.

IMPLEMENTATION

Intervention strategies include education of the older adult about cancer, cancer screening tests, and self-examination. Provide the individual with appropriate educational materials (e.g., copies of ACS cancer screening guidelines or other NCI and ACS publications), resource telephone numbers (1-800-4-CANCER, National Institutes of Health, or local ACS and screening clinics), and information on availability of financial assistance.

Strategies have been developed for increasing compliance with guidelines among economically disadvantaged older adults. These include the elderly educator (EE) method, adaptation for aging changes (AAC) method, and combination method (Weinrich et al., 1992). The elderly educator method was designed to use older adults as educators in an ACS colorectal cancer program (Weinrich et al., 1992). The underlying tenet of this approach is that through the use of role models with whom individuals can identify, common myths and misinformation concerning colorectal screening can be dispelled. The adaptation for aging changes method uses approaches to education that account for changes occurring with aging (i.e., increased time needed for processing information, and changes in sensory abilities, such as visual acuity and tactile sensitivity). The combination method is the EE and AAC methods combined. The findings from the study clearly demonstrate that the combination method produces a higher level of participation in colorectal screening by socioeconomically disadvantaged older adults. Nurses can adapt these methods to develop and implement intervention strategies for the variety of cancers for which approaches to screening and early detection are available.

EVALUATION

Evaluation of intervention strategies provides information necessary both for improving the ef-

fectiveness of the educational approach and ultimately for improving older adults' adherence to cancer screening guidelines. Evaluation will uncover factors that influence compliance—for example, lack of comprehension of educational material, altered sensory or motor ability necessary to perform self-examination, cultural factors, lack of desire, or a combination of factors that contribute to misunderstanding the importance of carrying out these screening behaviors.

Knowledge of personal cancer risk and appropriate screening guidelines can be evaluated by a test designed to measure comprehension. Return demonstrations can be used to determine an individual's ability to perform self-examination procedures. Evaluation of compliance with cancer screening guidelines can be accomplished by checking with individual patients (verbal report) during routine primary or episodic care, checking patient records to see if the results of a screening test have been reported, or checking with the relevant department (e.g., x-ray or laboratory) for the test results.

In summary, the nursing process provides an organized approach to performing a cancer risk assessment. A cancer risk assessment should be carried out for any individual over 40 years of age; however, it increases in importance for those over 65. Patients need to be made aware that they are never too old to alter outcomes; for example, stopping smoking can always have beneficial effects. Practitioners need to be educated on the fact that patients are never too old to be screened for cancer. The combination of patient and practitioner education about cancer prevention and control is one approach that will work toward decreasing morbidity and mortality from those cancers for which screening is efficacious.

REFERENCES

Bergman, L., Dekker, G., van Kerkhoff, E.H.M., Peterse, H.L., van Dongen, J.A., & van Leeuwen, F.E. (1991). Influence of age and comorbidity on treatment choice and survival in elderly patients with breast cancer. *Breast Cancer Research and Treatment, 18*, 189-198.

Berkman, B., Rohan, B., & Sampson, S. (1994). Myths and biases related to cancer in the elderly. *Cancer, 74*(Suppl. 7), 2004-2008.

Boyle, D.M., Engelking, C., Blesch, K.S., Dodge, J., Sarna, L., & Weinrich, S. (1992). Oncology Nursing Society position paper on cancer and aging: The mandate for oncology nursing. *Oncology Nursing Forum, 19*(6), 913-933.

Brawley, O.W. (1995). Are mass cancer screenings effective? Con. *ONS News, 10*(1), 7.

Cohen, H.J. (1994a). Biology of aging as related to cancer. *Cancer, 74*(Suppl.), 2092-2100.

Cohen, H.J. (1994b). Oncology and aging: General principles of cancer in the elderly. In W.R. Hazzard, E.L. Bierman, J.P. Blass, W.H. Ettinger, J.B. Halter, & R. Andres (Eds.), *Principles of geriatric medicine and gerontology* (3rd ed., pp. 77-89). New York: McGraw-Hill.

Cutler, R.G. & Semsei, I. (1989). Development, cancer and aging: Possible common mechanism of action and regulation. *Journals of Gerontology, 44*(1), 25-34.

Egorin, M.J. (1993). Cancer pharmacology in the elderly. *Seminars in Oncology, 20*(1), 43-49.

Fact sheet: Cancer and the elderly. (1992, April). Oncology Nursing Society.

Fink, D.J. (1991). Guidelines for the cancer related checkup: Recommendations and rationale. Reprinted from *American Cancer Society textbook of clinical oncology.* (91-50M, No. 3347-PE). Atlanta: American Cancer Society.

Frank-Stromberg, M. & Rohan, K. (1992). Nursing's involvement in the primary and secondary prevention of cancer: Nationally and internationally. *Cancer Nursing, 15*(2), 79-108.

Ganz, P.A. (1993). Age and gender as factors in cancer therapy. *Clinics in Geriatric Medicine, 9*(1), 145-155.

Greenfield, S., Blanco, D.M., Elashoff, R.M., et al. (1987). Patterns of care related to age of breast cancer patients. *Journal of the American Medical Association, 257,* 2766-2770.

Guadagnoli, E., Weitberg, A., Mor, V., Silliman, R.A., Glicksman, A.S., & Cummings, F.J. (1990). The influence of patient age on the diagnosis and treatment of lung and colorectal cancer. *Archives of Internal Medicine, 150,* 1485-1490.

Holmes, F.F., Wilson, J., Blesch, K.S., Kaesberg, P.R., Miller, R., & Sprott, R. (1991). Biology of cancer and aging. *Cancer, 68*(Suppl.) 2525-2526.

Kalinowski, B.H. (1993). Surgical therapy. In S.L. Groenwald, M.H. Frogge, M. Goodman, & C.H. Yarbro (Eds.), *Cancer nursing: Principles and practice* (3rd ed., pp. 222-234). Boston: Jones and Bartlett.

Lippman, M.E., Lichter, A.S., & Danforth, D.N. (1989). *Diagnosis and management of breast cancer* (p. 96). Philadelphia: W.B. Saunders.

Lonergan, E.T., & Krevans, J.R. (1991). A national agenda for research on aging. *New England Journal of Medicine, 324*(25), 1825-1828.

Mandelblatt, J., Traxler, M., Lakin, P., Thomas, L., Chauhan, P., Matseoane, S., Kanetsky, P., & Harlem Study Team. (1993). A nurse practitioner intervention to increase breast and cervical cancer screening for poor, elderly black women. *Journal of General Internal Medicine, 8*(4), 173-178.

Mettlin, C. & Dodd, G.D. (1992). Guidelines for the cancer related checkup: An update. Reprinted from *Ca-A cancer journal for clinicians, 41,* 279-282. (92-10M, No. 3402).

Miller, R.A. (1991). Gerontology as oncology: Research on aging as the key to the understanding of cancer. *Cancer, 68*(Suppl.), 2496-2501.

Miller, R.A. (1994). The biology of aging and longevity. In W.R. Hazzard, E.L. Bierman, J.P. Blass, W.H. Ettinger, J.B. Halter, & R. Andres (Eds.), *Principles of geriatric medicine and gerontology* (3rd ed., pp. 3-18). New York: McGraw-Hill.

Monfardini, S., & Yancik, R. (1993). Cancer in the elderly: Meeting the challenge of an aging population. *Journal of the National Cancer Institute, 85*(7), 532-538.

Mor, V., Masterson-Allen, S., Goldberg, R.J., et al. (1985). Relationship between age at diagnosis and treatments received by cancer patients. *Journal of the American Geriatrics Society, 33,* 585-589.

Padberg, R.M. (1995). Are mass cancer screenings effective? Pro. *ONS News, 10*(1), 7.

PORT. (1994). *Care, costs, and outcomes of localized breast cancer in elderly women.* (Report 1 RO1 HSO8395-0115). Agency for Health Policy and Research.

Samet, J., Hunt, W.C., Key, C., et al. (1986). Choice of cancer therapy varies with age of patient. *Journal of the American Medical Association, 255,* 3385-3390.

Schwab, R., Walters, C.A., & Weksler, M.E. (1989). Host defense mechanisms and aging. *Seminars in Oncology, 16*(1), 20-27.

Weinrich, S.P., Weinrich, M.C., Boyd, M.D., Atwood, J., & Cervenka, B. (1992). Effective approaches for increasing compliance with American Cancer Society recommendations in socioeconomically disadvantaged populations. In *Proceedings of the Second National Conference on Cancer Nursing Research.* Atlanta: American Cancer Society. (92-50M, No. 3320.01-PE).

White, L.N., & Spitz, M.R. (1993). Cancer risk and early detection assessment. *Seminars in Oncology Nursing, 9*(3), 188-197.

Yancik, R., & Ries, L.G. (1994). Cancer in older persons. *Cancer, 74*(Suppl. 7), 1995-2003.

Yancik, R., Ries, L.G., & Yates, J.W. (1989). Breast cancer in aging women: A population-based study of contrasts in stage, surgery, and survival. *Cancer, 63,* 976-981.

BIBLIOGRAPHY

Annas, G.J. (1992). Breast cancer screening in older women: Law and patient rights. *Journals of Gerontology, 47*(Special issue), 121-125.

Baulch, Y.S., Larson, P.J., Dodd, M.J., & Deitrich, C. (1992). The relationship of visual acuity, tactile sensitivity, and mobility of the upper extremities to proficient breast self-examination in women 65 and older. *Oncology Nursing Forum, 19*(9), 1367-1372.

Blesch, K.S. (1991). Cancer treatment responses in older adults: Challenges in treatment and management. In *Proceedings of the Sixth National Conference on Cancer Nursing Research.* Atlanta: American Cancer Society. (92-50M, No. 4503.02-PE).

Cancer facts and figures. (1995). New York: American Cancer Society. (95-375M, No. 5008.95).

Cassel, C.K. (1992). Breast cancer screening in older women: Ethical issues. *Journals of Gerontology, 47*(Special issue), 126-130.

Derby, S.A. (1990). Cancer in the older person. In P. Ashwanden, A.E. Belcher, E.A. Hubbard Mattson, R. Moskowitz, & N.E. Riese (Eds.), *Oncology nursing: Advances, treatments into the twenty-first century* (pp. 141-162). Rockville, MD: Aspen.

National Institutes of Health, National Cancer Institute, Division of Cancer Prevention and Control. (1989). Breast cancer detection, management and sequelae in elderly women: Request for applications, centers and community oncology.

Rimer, B.K., Ross, E., Cristinzio, C.S., & King, E. Older women's participation in breast screening. *Journals of Gerontology, 47*(Special issue), 85-91.

Weinrich, S.P., & Weinrich, M.C. (1986). Cancer knowledge among elderly individuals. *Cancer Nursing, 9*(6), 301-307.

C H A P T E R 20

An aged man is but a paltry thing
A tattered coat upon a stick unless
Soul clap its hands and sing, and louder sing
For every tatter in its mortal dress

WILLIAM B. YEATS

Loss, Bereavement, and Care of the Dying Person

■ Learning Objectives

On completion of this chapter, the reader will be able to do the following:

1. Define the concepts of loss, bereavement, and grief.
2. Describe the relevance of these concepts (loss, bereavement, and grief) to the older population.
3. Describe the phases of bereavement, including the physical, psychologic, social, and spiritual manifestations of each.
4. Describe emotional responses to dying, using a dynamic model of coping responses.
5. Describe nursing roles related to care of the dying older person and the person's family in various care settings.
6. Describe the care of a person experiencing spiritual distress in relation to death.
7. Apply the nursing process to the care of the bereaved and the care of the dying person.

All nurses who work with the older population encounter the significant topics of loss, bereavement, and care of the dying person, either directly or indirectly, and with varying degrees of frequency in their professional practice. Therefore it is important for nurses who work with the older population to have a solid base of knowledge about these topics and an understanding of the practical application of them through the nursing process. Although the subjects of loss, bereavement, and care of the dying person are related, they are also separate and different. Because of this, this chapter is divided into two discrete parts: the first part includes background knowledge about loss, bereavement, and dying; the second part focuses on the care of the dying person or the family in various settings. Each part of the chapter provides theoretic and practical information relating to the specific topic being addressed.

■ Loss and Bereavement

To live is to experience loss. Loss and the accompanying state of bereavement and the resulting grief responses are universal, yet painful, facts of life. Rituals for mourning have been established in every culture. Although the concept of loss pertains to a variety of situations and causalities, the focus of this chapter is on loss of a person, or of a relationship with a person, as a result of death.

As a group, older people are especially likely to be affected by loss and bereavement. Indeed, to age is to experience numerous physical, psychologic, and social changes that are defined as losses by most people. Multiple occurrences such as involuntary retirement, loss of social roles, financial insecurity, and changes in living arrangements, combined with the primary types of losses of death of a spouse, child, or close friend and the reality of declining health, do indeed challenge even the most healthy and successful aging person. For many older adults there will be times of grief and bereavement in response to loss. An acceptance of the understanding that grief and bereavement have physical as well as psychologic dimensions is becoming commonplace.

Older people are often faced with multiple losses within a short period. Such bereavement overload stresses the adaptation capacity of most people. One of the most frequent causes of bereavement in the older person is the death of a spouse. This problem primarily affects women because of their greater longevity, in addition to the fact that women are often younger than their husbands. Death of a spouse is generally accepted to be one of the most stressful life experiences.

Functional impairments and physical symptoms such as feeling lonely, sleep disturbances, medical illness, and searching for a deceased loved person have been reported in the extant literature (Grimby, 1993; Prigerson et al., 1995). In a study of older men and women who had experienced the death of a spouse, half of the subjects reported feeling the presence of the deceased loved one and over a third reported seeing, hearing, and talking to the deceased person. These types of experiences were very frequent and found to be helpful for the older grieving person (Grimby, 1993). It is most helpful for the nurse to be aware and accepting of different grief reactions that may at other times be considered abnormal behavior.

This portion of this chapter presents a model of bereavement and guidelines for providing care to the bereaved individual, based on the nursing process. Throughout, the emphasis is on nursing's unique perspective on bereavement and on bereavement care. The content in this portion of the chapter should be of value in planning bereavement care, not only for the older bereaved person, but also for people of any age who have lost someone.

INTEGRATIVE THEORY OF BEREAVEMENT

Numerous theories of bereavement have been developed over the years since Freud proposed his theory of grief in the 1917 work *Mourning and Melancholia*. A recent theory that seems to have much to offer nursing because of its clarity and comprehensiveness is the integrative theory of bereavement (Figure 20-1). This theory builds not only upon earlier theories, but also upon empiric research. Catherine M. Sanders, a clinical psychologist and researcher who has worked in the area of loss and bereavement since 1968, has proposed the integrative theory of bereavement (Sanders, 1989).

Characteristics of the integrative theory of bereavement include the following (Sanders, 1989):

- An awareness that each psychologic event that occurs during the process of grief also has a biologic counterpart that determines the physical well-being of the individual
- A viewpoint that sees bereavement as adaptive rather than debilitative
- An accounting for previously existing personality traits
- A consideration of internal and external moderator variables as having implications for the outcome of bereavement

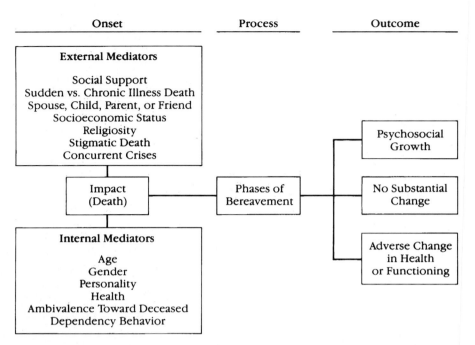

FIGURE 20-1 Integrative theory of bereavement. (Used with permission from Sanders, C.M. [1989]. *Grief: The mourning after—Dealing with adult bereavement.* New York: John Wiley and Sons. p. 39.)

- The notion of motivation (making the decision of whether to survive the loss)
- The identification of five phases of the bereavement process, each with characteristic symptoms
- The identification of emotional, biologic, and social levels of functioning during bereavement (Table 20-1)
- An acceptance of the fact that the length of time it takes to complete the bereavement process is variable, and often longer than expected

PHASES OF BEREAVEMENT

The integrative theory of bereavement specifies the five phases of bereavement shown in Table 20-1, and described as follows.

Phase 1: Shock

The initial response to a loss is shock. This is true whether the death is sudden and unexpected or is anticipated. A number of factors determine the length and intensity of the phase of shock. Such factors include the level of attachment to the deceased, the circumstances of the death, and the presence or absence of supportive people (Sanders, 1989).

General characteristics of the shock phase may include disbelief, confusion, restlessness, feelings of unreality, regression and helplessness, and a state of alarm. Specific manifestations of this phase may include dryness of the mouth and throat, need for sighing, loss of muscular power, weeping, uncontrolled trembling, startle response, sleep disturbance, loss of appetite, ego-

TABLE 20-1 Tripartite levels in the phases of bereavement

Phases	Levels		
	Emotional	Biologic	Social
1. Shock	Impact	Trauma	Egocentricity
2. Awareness of loss	Anxiety	Acute stress	Regression
3. Conservation and withdrawal	Despair	Chronic stress	Withdrawing
4. Healing	Gaining control	Healing	Identity restructuring
5. Renewal	New level of functioning	Recovery	Renewal

Used with permission from Sanders, C.M. (1989). *Grief: The mourning after—Dealing with adult bereavement.* New York: John Wiley and Sons. p. 40.

centricity, preoccupations with thoughts of the deceased, and psychologic distancing (Sanders, 1989).

Sanders (1989) states that "the shock phase is variable and may be as brief as a few minutes or extend for many days. Typically, it ends when the funeral rituals are over."

Phase 2: Awareness of loss

Once the shock phase has passed, the bereaved individual is left with the acute pain of loss. General characteristics of this phase may include the following: separation anxiety, conflicts, the acting out of emotional expectations, and prolonged stress. Specific manifestations of phase 2 may include yearning, crying, anger, guilt, frustration, shame, sleep disturbance, fear of death, oversensitivity, dreaming, disbelief and denial, and searching for and sensing the presence of the person lost (Sanders, 1989). "Searching" refers to the tendency of people who are bereaved to search for the lost person in familiar places. "Sensing the presence" refers to experiences wherein the bereaved have a "sense" of the deceased being present or actually report seeing an image of the deceased. These experiences are generally comforting to the bereaved person (Sanders, 1989).

Because of the emotional intensity associated with phase 2, it is an extremely exhausting

Grief. *Courtesy of Loy Ledbetter, St. Louis.*

experience. The bereaved person experiences a need to withdraw and conserve energy—this pushes the griever into phase 3 (Sanders, 1989).

Phase 3: Conservation and withdrawal

Phase 3 is a time of withdrawing and can appear to be similar to clinical depression. It is an especially difficult time for many bereaved people. General characteristics of phase 3 may include withdrawal, despair, diminished social support, and helplessness. Specific manifestations of this phase may include weakness, fatigue, increased need for sleep, weakened immune system, hibernation, obsessional review, grief work, and the turning point (Sanders, 1989).

Sanders (1989) proposes that at the end of phase 3, the bereaved person makes a choice, either consciously or unconsciously, to move in one of three directions. The person decides either to move forward, to remain in the status quo, or to die. According to Sanders, many older people who have lost spouses elect the second option—that of remaining in the status quo and not making major changes, which would require more strength and energy than they feel they have available.

Phase 4: Healing

Phase 4 is analogous to the healing that occurs in a physical wound. General characteristics of phase 4 may include assuming control, identity restructuring, and relinquishing roles. Specific manifestations of this phase may include physical healing, increased energy, sleep restoration, immune system restoration, forgiving, forgetting, searching for meaning, closing the circle, and hope (Sanders, 1989).

"Closing the circle" refers symbolically to the fact that the open wound of bereavement is closing. Thus healing is occurring (Sanders, 1989).

Phase 5: Renewal

In phase 5 the bereaved person reaches a new, higher level of functioning. Sanders (1989) states,

Grief is akin to a death and resurrection experience. As part of the old dies with the old life, there is almost simultaneous preparation for a rebirth into a new one. And when it comes, so does a deeper compassion for others, as well as a new strength that pervades the entire lifestyle (p. 98).

General characteristics of phase 5 may include new self-awareness, accepting responsibility, and learning to live without. Specific manifestations of this phase may include revitalization, functional stability, caring for physical needs, living for oneself, anniversary reactions, loneliness, and reaching out (Sanders, 1989).

Sanders proposes that bereavement is influenced by a variety of internal and external mediators. Internal mediators include age, gender, personality, health, ambivalence toward the deceased, and dependency behavior. External mediators include social support; sudden death versus chronic illness; whether the deceased was a child, spouse, parent, or friend; socioeconomic status; religiosity; whether death was stigmatic; and whether there were concurrent crises (Sanders, 1989).

It is a professional nursing responsibility to provide nursing-based bereavement care for any person who has sustained a significant loss and with whom the nurse has established a professional caring relationship. As is true in any situation where the patient experiences a specific need, the nurse proceeds to assess the patient situation, diagnose the problems, determine a plan of care, implement the plan, and evaluate its effectiveness.

■ Nursing Process in the Care of the Bereaved Person

ASSESSMENT

Assessment of the bereaved person requires knowledge of the bereavement process, skill in communication techniques, compassion, and adequate time. Being alert to nonverbal cues, as well as to what is said, is especially important.

The assessment form presented in Figure 20-2 can be used as a guide for collecting and organizing pertinent patient data. Additional data relevant to internal and external mediators, as suggested by the integrative theory of bereavement, may also be included. For example, the nurse may assess the circumstances surrounding the death or the degree of ambivalence that the survivor holds toward the deceased. Also, on the basis of the assessment made, it will probably be possible to identify the person's phase of bereavement. When the complete patient data are collected and analyzed, the nurse defines the appropriate nursing diagnoses.

NAME OF BEREAVED _____ DATE OF BIRTH _____

ADDRESS _____ PHONE _____

NAME OF DECEASED _____ DATE OF BIRTH _____

RELATIONSHIP TO DECEASED _____ DATE OF BIRTH _____

LENGTH OF RELATIONSHIP _____ ANNIVERSARY _____

PRIMARY NURSE _____

LIVING ARRANGEMENTS

OWN HOME _____ APARTMENT _____ OTHER _____

LIVING WITH _____ RELATIONSHIP _____

_____

_____

PHYSICAL STATUS

1. Sleeping pattern _____

2. Appetite _____ Weight-gain _____ loss _____

3. Substances used — alcohol _____ change in intake _____

cigarettes _____ change in intake _____

drugs _____ change in intake _____

4. Appearance — neat _____ unkempt _____

5. Health _____

ACTIVITY LEVEL

Increased _____ Decreased _____ Employed _____

Hobbies _____

PSYCHOLOGICAL EMOTIONAL STATUS

1. Affect: Appropriate _____ Flat _____ Labile _____

2. Expression of grief: Discussion of loss _____

guilt _____

anger _____

suicide _____

SUPPORT SYSTEMS

1. Family _____

2. Clergy _____

3. Quantity of contacts _____

4. Perceived quality of contact _____

ADDITIONAL CONCERNS

1. Other losses _____

2. Financial _____

3. Living arrangements _____

4. Major problems _____

OVERALL IMPRESSION

_____

_____

PLAN/INTERVENTION STRATEGY

_____

_____

_____

_____

SIGNATURE _____

DATE _____

FIGURE 20-2 Bereavement—initial assessment form. (From Amenta. [1986]. *Nursing care of the terminally ill.* [pp. 247-262]. Philadelphia: Lippincott-Raven Publishers.)

NURSING DIAGNOSES

Numerous nursing diagnoses may be associated with bereavement in older adults. Among the possible nursing diagnoses are the following:

- Dysfunctional grieving
- Anxiety
- Denial, ineffective
- Fear
- Health maintenance, altered
- Role performance, altered
- Social interaction, impaired
- Spiritual distress (distress of the human spirit)

For each diagnosis, the nurse records the appropriate cause or related factors according to the patient data gathered during the assessment. The nursing diagnosis that is most directly related to bereavement following a loss is that of dysfunctional grieving. However, the focus of this chapter is on normal bereavement. By changing this from an actual nursing diagnosis to a potential nursing diagnosis (i.e., potential for dysfunctional grieving), it is possible to maintain the emphasis on normal bereavement.

PLANNING AND GOAL IDENTIFICATION

The plan of care depends on the nursing diagnoses identified as a result of the assessment. The nursing goals and strategies described here are meant to facilitate normal grieving and to prevent dysfunctional grieving.

Long-term goals for a diagnosis of potential for dysfunctional bereavement include the following:

1. The person will accommodate to the loss.
2. The person will reinvest in a new life.

Short-term goals include the following:

1. The person will verbalize feelings.
2. The person will cope adequately with the immediate physical and psychologic demands of bereavement.
3. The person will verbally acknowledge the loss.
4. The person will agree to use available social support.

IMPLEMENTATION

Nursing interventions for the bereaved span all settings. The major responsibilities of the nurse are encouragement and support, as this is an attempt to acknowledge loss. This may be accomplished by being physically and psychologically present and available to provide a sense of security. The nurse demonstrates an understanding of the loss and provides freedom to express the loss in an individual and unique way. If the person gives evidence of experiencing spiritual pain, the nurse can acknowledge presence of the pain and encourage the expectation that eventually it will subside.

There may be need for support and assistance in verbalizing feelings about the loss. To enable the verbalization, the nurse gives the person permission to identify, accept, and express all of the various emotions connected with grief. Opportunity can be provided for the person to cry or to talk if need be. It is not unusual to review and re-review the situation without interruption.

Nurses can provide the grieving person with factual information about bereavement. Realistic and practical help with immediate problems resulting from the loss can assist in moving through the grieving process. The person may experience frustration with self or others, and it is important to encourage patience.

Allow grievers to give themselves a respite from their grief, and encourage them to accept help and consolation from others. Maximum utilization of social support networks can often be key in the person's adaptation to loss. When appropriate, the nurse can provide information about bereavement support groups.

Accommodating to loss can be accomplished by helping the griever to develop a perspective on what it will mean to resolve the grief. This may include helping the person to develop a new identity and to learn new life skills. The nurse can help the person (1) to develop a new relationship with the deceased, based on the changed reality; (2) to find and utilize ways to replenish self; and (3) to identify secondary losses resulting from the death of a loved one.

Reinvesting in life is a difficult change, but the nurse is in an optimal position to effect change. The nurse can give the person permission to engage in new activities and new relationships. However, it is important not to rush or force the process of reinvestment.

EVALUATION

Evaluation of care is achieved by comparing the actual outcomes with the expected outcomes. However, there are several problematic areas in evaluating the effectiveness of nursing care to meet bereavement outcomes. One problem is that the process of bereavement requires time. Often, several years are required for healing after a significant loss. Another problem is that each person's bereavement pattern is unique. Utilizing knowledge of the phases of bereavement like a recipe is simply not appropriate; it is disrespectful of the person's particular responses. The somewhat subjective nature of the entire process of bereavement makes a broadly general, rather than a narrowly specific, evaluation more appropriate.

■ Care of the Dying Person

Bianchi (1985) writes of a young nurse who is dying in a hospital; she speaks to those who are caring for her:

I know you feel insecure, don't know what to say, don't know what to do. But please believe me, if you care, you can't go wrong . . . Don't run away . . . all I want to know is that there will be someone to hold my hand when I need it. I am afraid. Death may be routine to you, but it is new to me . . . If only we could be honest, both admit of our fears, touch one another. If you really care, would you lose so much of your valuable professionalism if you even cried with me? Just person to person? Then, it might not be so hard to die.

This genuine call for compassion in tangible forms of listening, touching, and being present for the dying person is the challenge calling all nurses to respond to the needs of the dying person.

Dying is a personal and lonely experience. Older people may have faced their own mortality before they are faced with the actual experience of impending death. But it is dangerous to assume that any individual is well prepared for and accepting of death in spite of the fact that many are. Several factors can be operative in older adults that may help them to face their own death: a philosophic attitude that tends to accept all of what life offers (including death); having had multiple opportunities to encounter and learn to cope with death, through personal losses of parents, friends, perhaps a spouse, and possibly even children; a developmentally appropriate timing of death for the individual; and support from religious beliefs, including the concept of life after death (Bohnet, 1986).

Several factors may hinder an older person's ability to face death: multiple losses that have occurred in close succession and have left the person emotionally depleted, lack of support because many significant others have preceded the person in death, and lack of attention to needs because of the incorrect assumption that all older people accept death easily.

This section of the chapter describes the range of emotional responses within the person who is facing death, the usual fears of the dying individual, and the various nursing roles with the dying person and family members that are appropriate in the settings of hospital, nursing home, and private or family home. This part of the chapter includes application of the nursing process to the care of the dying older person.

EMOTIONAL RESPONSES TO DYING
Models of response: Kübler-Ross and Kaye

Much remains to be discovered about the actual emotional needs of the dying person. Nevertheless, there is an increased public and professional awareness that such needs are, in fact, important. Kübler-Ross brought the subject to popular attention in 1969, when she described the five stages

BOX 20-1 DYNAMIC MODEL OF COPING RESPONSES

Emotion	Closed response	Open response
1. Fear	Denial	Facing fears
2. Anger	Guilt, blame	Fighting the illness
3. Sadness	Misery	Grieving, adjusting
4. Dependency	Helplessness	Participation
5. Search for meaning	Hopelessness	Seeking sense of purpose

Reproduced by permission from Kaye, Peter: *Notes on Symptom Control in Hospice and Palliative Care,* First Edition, 1989, Hospice Education Institute. Essex, Connecticut, p. 85.

of coping with the dying process: denial, anger, bargaining, depression, and acceptance.

Kaye (1989) presented a dynamic model of coping responses to dying (Box 20-1). Kaye purports that the dying person is often experiencing several emotions simultaneously, and also that the person's methods of coping can be flexible and vary in their degree of openness. The model does *not* propose various stages or phases through which the dying person proceeds.

Rather, the model specifies both a "closed response" and an "open response" for each of the commonly occurring emotions that may accompany the process of dying. In general, open responses tend to be more adaptive, but at times, a closed response may be more appropriate. Kaye (1989) states,

Each coping response is like a door—open, closed, or partly open. Very rarely can a person keep all doors open all the time, nor is this necessarily healthy. Closed coping responses are not necessarily harmful. (Any coping response that allows a person to function without harming others, and to adjust to illness, should be encouraged.) Most people keep some doors open, and others partly closed, to maintain equilibrium (p. 86).

It is appropriate for coping strategies to change as the situation changes.

Fears of the dying person

Anxiety is to be expected in most if not all people who are dying. Because anxiety is vague in nature and not related to a specific threat, the primary way in which to assist a dying person to deal with anxiety is to help the person isolate particular fears, which then can be addressed. Although it is a nearly universal experience for the dying person to have fears, the particular fears that are of most concern are specific to each person.

An awareness of the fears most often expressed by the dying person should promote more sensitive attention to the person's needs. Common fears include the following (Rando, 1984):

- Fear of the unknown
- Fear of loneliness
- Fear of loss of family and friends
- Fear of loss of self-control
- Fear of loss of body parts and disability
- Fear of suffering and pain
- Fear of sorrow
- Fear of regression
- Fears of mutilation, decomposition, and premature burial

Often, being able to verbalize a particular fear helps to relieve some of the terror that may be associated with it. Once a fear is shared with the nurse, then a plan can be developed to deal with that particular fear. For example, in dealing with the fear of the unknown, it is important to answer honestly all questions that can be answered. It is also important to help the dying person differentiate between those questions that are answerable and those that are not answerable in this lifetime. In another example, when helping people deal with the fear of loss of self-control, it is essential to encourage and allow them to retain control whenever and wherever possible. A final example is helping the person deal with the fear of sorrow. Rando (1984) states,

Sources of sorrow must be identified and worked through individually, rather than all at once, and it must be made clear that grief is acceptable and necessary. On the other hand, intervention should also focus on enabling the dying patient to experience the joys and pleasures that remain possible, especially since all losses do not occur simultaneously (p. 237).

■ Nursing Process with the Dying Older Adult

Providing wholistic, individualized nursing care for the dying older adult is an important factor that can contribute greatly to a "good" or "appropriate" death experience for the dying person, as well as for the family. Whether in a direct or an indirect caregiving role, the nurse is in a key position to provide and promote excellent, compassionate care for the dying person. This care includes attention to the physical, the psychosocial, and the spiritual needs of the person. Attention to the physical needs of the dying person will generally be based upon a *care* model rather than on a *cure* model. Concepts such as palliative care and symptom control are relevant to the physical care of the dying older person. Good basic nursing care, with attention to needs such as nutrition, elimination, sleep, mobility, skin and mouth care, and pain management, will provide significant comfort for dying people and will show respect for their physical

being. The nursing assessment and interventions related to these physical needs are fundamental to nursing practice and are not detailed here. The focus in this section is on the psychosocial and spiritual needs of the dying older person.

ASSESSMENT

Assessment of psychosocial and spiritual needs of any person requires both skill and perceptiveness; this is especially true of assessment of these needs in the dying older person. The nurse collects data about these needs by observing behavior, by listening to what is said spontaneously, and by sensitive questioning of the dying person and the family or other personally significant individuals. Rigidly following a narrowly defined assessment guide would be counterproductive in this situation. Box 20-2 suggests questions to ask in performing a psychosocial and spiritual assessment. At the completion of preliminary data collection and analysis, appropriate nursing diagnoses are identified. The proper statement of a nursing diagnosis would include both the general diagnostic category, such as fear, and the relevant etiologic or related factors.

The sensitivity of the nurse should undergird all assessment and intervention with the dying older adult. This sensitivity embraces the understanding that dying people have the right to their unique experiences of dying. Such an understanding respects, allows, and accepts differences in emotional responses to dying. This understanding also directs the nurse to develop goals in collaboration with each person's wishes, to the extent that this is possible.

NURSING DIAGNOSES

Selected nursing diagnoses that may be identified in the dying older person are as follows:

- Anxiety
- Denial
- Fear
- Impaired social interaction
- Spiritual distress

BOX 20-2 PSYCHOSOCIAL AND SPIRITUAL ASSESSMENT OF THE DYING OLDER ADULT

1. Does the person understand that he or she is dying?
2. How is the person behaving?
3. What coping strategies is the person using?
4. Are the coping strategies effective for the person?
5. What are the person's emotional reactions?
6. How is the person managing her or his emotions?
7. Does the person feel supported by family or significant others?
8. Is the person able to ask for and to receive assistance for meeting his or her needs?
9. Is the person able to grieve for impending losses?
10. Is the person able to begin to say good-bye to significant others?
11. Is the person able to settle business affairs (e.g., make a will)?
12. What does the person fear most about dying?
13. Is the person where she or he wishes to be (i.e., home, hospital, nursing home)? If not, why not?
14. How is the person's age influencing his or her responses to dying?
15. Does the person express concern about the meaning of her or his life, impending death, or belief system?
16. Does the person express concern about his or her relationship with a higher being, if any?
17. Does the person seek spiritual assistance?
18. Does the person express a sense of powerlessness, hopelessness, guilt, punishment, or abandonment?
19. Does the person express a desire for forgiveness?
20. Does the person express inner conflict about his or her beliefs?
21. Is the person able to participate in her or his usual religious practices, if any?

Adapted from Haber, J., Leach, A.M., Schudy, S.M., & Sideleau, B.F. (1982). *Comprehensive psychiatric nursing* (2nd ed.). New York: McGraw-Hill, Gordon. (1989). *Manual of nursing diagnosis 1988-1989.* St. Louis: Mosby.

PLANNING AND GOAL IDENTIFICATION

In response to each individual's nursing diagnoses, the appropriate care is planned. For each nursing diagnosis, both expected outcomes and nursing interventions are developed. For example, in this section the selected nursing diagnosis is spiritual distress. This particular nursing diagnosis was selected for several reasons: It is a nursing diagnosis that is less familiar to most nurses than are a number of the other nursing diagnoses, such as anxiety or fear; it tends to be more global and encompassing than many of the other nursing diagnoses; and it is a critically important issue in the nursing care of the dying older adult, yet its existence often goes unrecognized and therefore untreated. In this example, the nursing role in caring for a person with spiritual distress incorporates a unique wholistic perspective. The nurse can make a major contribution to assisting the dying person in that person's area of need and should never assume that simply calling in the clergy is the extent of the nurse's responsibility.

For a diagnosis of spiritual distress, the short- and long-term goals include the following:

1. Patients will express a positive meaning in their existence and present circumstances.
2. Patients will express decreased feelings of guilt and experience a sense of forgiveness and hope.
3. Patients will express comfort in their relationship with a higher being, if any, and in relationships with significant others.
4. Patients will accept self.
5. Patients will participate as fully as possible in whatever rituals, sacraments, or spiritual practices are of importance to them.
6. Patients will state feelings of being at peace.
7. Patients will experience a sense of integration and completion.

IMPLEMENTATION

The following general nursing interventions are appropriate for use:

Spend time with the person on a regular basis, to develop a relationship.

- Be totally present and available to the person.
- Use active listening and other attentional skills.
- Use effective communication skills.
- Be open and accepting.
- Be sensitive to the suffering of the person.
- Convey compassion and empathy.
- Provide care with an attitude of humility.
- Use touch, as appropriate.

The nurse can encourage introspection and reflection, listening patiently to personal searchings. The nurse should encourage the patients to identify and draw upon inner resources, helping them to find a way to express suffering, as well as the current meaning of their lives. Above all, the nurse should promote realistic and appropriate hope.

Patients should be encouraged to discuss their views of a higher being. The nurse communicates verbally and nonverbally an acceptance of the patient's views, feelings, and beliefs, and expresses utmost respect for the dying person.

Contact with significant others should be encouraged, to promote a sense of connected-ness between the person, significant others, and a higher being, if relevant. The nurse explores ways to help the person to say good-bye to significant others. Acceptance of self is important for the dying patient. Through the process of life review, the nurse listens as the person articulates anger, despair, fear, and loneliness and works toward self-forgiveness.

The nurse should respect the dying person's preference for and participation in rituals, sacraments, or spiritual practices. If requested and appropriate, the nurse prays with the person or reads scripture or other religious literature to the person. If the nurse is not comfortable with this level of involvement, the nurse may advocate on behalf of the patient's spiritual beliefs and may refer the person to the spiritual advisor of choice.

Special interventions such as relaxation techniques and music therapy may be appropriate, to help some patients achieve a peaceful state. The nurse may also be with the person quietly at times when verbal communication is not possible or desired.

The nurse supports dying patients' efforts to work toward both internal and external integration, helping people to identify with and accept, as well as to move beyond, their own suffering. Accept the tears and complaints found necessary by many people as they move toward integration.

It is difficult for the patient and the nurse to cope with the emotional, as well as the cognitive, dimensions of dying, especially if the patient and the nurse have not had an opportunity to discuss the complex emotions that can accompany dying. The extent to which these discussions can proceed will depend, to a great extent, upon the setting in which the nurse cares for the dying patient and upon the ability of the nurse to generate thoughts, feelings, and expressions from the patient during the caregiving activities.

In the acute care setting

In the hospital setting, the primary role of the nurse is usually that of direct caregiver for the dying older person. The nursing process is the framework within which the nurse provides wholistic care to address the physical, psychologic, and spiritual needs of the dying person.

To function with competency in the care of the dying patient, the nurse determines the policies of the institution, as well as the pertinent laws that govern the jurisdiction in which the patient is located. Attorneys and other members of bioethical committees are available to answer questions and to provide legal and ethical advice when necessary.

Assessment of the emotional and cognitive status of the patient is performed by the nurse to determine whether the patient is able to participate in choosing the care measures to be used as dying becomes more imminent. It is advisable to discuss the patient's specific wishes and preferences as soon as possible; in fact, the most desirable time for such discussion is before admission to the acute care setting, if possible.

If the patient is able to participate in discussions about care, the nurse provides a clear explanation and ensures the patient's understanding of options available. The many technologies present in today's acute care settings present a complex challenge to the nursing team as they cope with educating the patient about the choices available.

One of the options for the patient to consider is that of selecting a "code" or a "no code" status in relation to the life-saving or life-supporting measures preferred. The nurse must understand the implications of these options and determine with certainty that if the patient states a choice in this matter, the patient has emotional and cognitive awareness of this statement of choice. This is an area in which the nurse will want to involve the patient, the family, the physician, and other significant persons in arriving at a conclusion that is consistent with the wishes of the patient and that is communicated to all members of the care team.

The needs of the grieving family members are as important as the needs of the dying patient. The nurse is responsible for addressing these while rendering direct care to the dying patient. Assessing and diagnosing, as well as planning for and meeting, these multiple needs are the components of wholistic care of the dying person. In conjunction with the early phases of developing the plan of care for the seriously ill person and the family, there should be discussion about delineation of responsible people, agreement about advance directives, definition of a person to assume power of attorney for the dying, and attention to other pertinent legal, ethical, and business matters. Although these topics are emotionally laden, the family members should be supported by the nurse and encouraged to deliberate on these subjects and to make decisions about them while the patient is able to participate in the discussions, especially if these issues have not yet been discussed. Depending upon the nurse's assessment of the coping resources of the family, they may be referred to appropriate individuals or to agencies within the community for further support.

In any setting, control of pain becomes one goal of the health care team in the care of the dying patient. The goal of treatment is to prevent the experience of pain. The dying patient should not have to encounter the anxiety caused by pain and the frustration of the cycle of calling for the nurse, experiencing pain symptoms again, and waiting for relief. Analgesics delivered by constant infusion pumps have provided many dying patients with a sense of control and a level of comfort. When nurses ensure scrupulous adherence to round-the-clock dosing schedules, they provide a level of comfort and a sense of security that pain will be controlled. These two methods of delivering analgesics eliminate the cycle that allows the analgesic to wear off and the pain to return. The nurse serves as an advocate to ensure that the dying person will not experience undue physical pain that can be controlled by analgesics.

In the nursing home

When caring for a dying person in a nursing home, the nurse assumes many of the same responsibilities that are assumed in the acute care setting, except that the complex technology is not present in the nursing home. The dying older person has usually been part of the nursing home setting for a longer time than the dying older patient has been in the hospital, so the death of a person in a nursing home is different. Most of the time, the dying person has made the deliberate choice to die in the nursing home. With full recognition of this fact, the nursing home staff respect this choice of the resident. The resident's family, too, is usually involved in the choice that is made.

The terminally ill or dying person in the nursing home needs continued attention from the staff personnel. It is important that residents be treated and cared for as *living* persons for as long as they live, and that communications and interpersonal relationships be maintained in the same manner as before the terminal illness. If a staff member is uncomfortable with the care of a dying older adult and there is evidence of avoidance behavior, it is the responsibility of the nurse to recognize the staff member's discomfort and to initiate plans and strategies to help the staff member deal with and correct the discomfort. Dying people need to feel the presence of others, both family and caregivers. They need to be assured that people are available to comfort them and to care for them physically, psychologically, and spiritually.

To provide the best care for the dying person, the staff members have specific needs that must be met so that they can give the resident the care that is needed. Communication channels must be maintained efficiently. The true status of the resident should be communicated to the staff personnel so that they can deal with resident needs realistically. Some of the staff members may never have been present at the death of a person, so they may need instructions, support, and comfort in this situation. The instructions should include telling the staff members what might be expected in terms of the resident's status (whether changes can occur, whether improvement can be expected). Sup-

port and encouragement are necessary for the novice caregiver in such a situation. The more successfully the nurse can provide these dimensions of care, the more the novice caregiver, as well as the veteran caregiver, can feel a sense of fulfillment when the needs of the dying person are successfully met.

Several means of instruction are available for the nurse to use in teaching staff members in the nursing home to care for the dying. Clinical conferences are effective means to set forth the information needed by the staff; there can be opportunities for them to ask questions and to share with the clinical teacher their concerns and worries about performing in this difficult role. Following the classroom dialogue, the nurse can perform mock demonstrations for small groups of the staff. When a dying person is present in the nursing home, the nurse can role-model care at the bedside of the person, using all the skills of communication, touch, providing physical comfort measures and spiritual literature readings, and various other care activities appropriate to the specific needs of the person. Through classroom discussions, clinical demonstrations, and role modeling, the professional nurse uses unique skills to effectively prepare the nursing staff to meet the needs of the dying person in the nursing home.

When the dying person has been a member of the nursing home community for quite a while, there usually have been liaisons and linkages established with other residents of the nursing home.

When a person is terminally ill in the nursing home, other residents need to be informed appropriately. Older people are realistic about life and death, and they can often handle these experiences better than younger people give them credit for being able to do. If the occasion permits, some residents may wish to visit their friend who is terminally ill. As they grieve about the imminent loss of another friend, almost as if a family member is dying, the residents deserve sympathy and support in their experience; it is the professional nurse and the staff who will provide this.

In the private or family home

In each situation of caring for a dying patient, the nurse is dealing with unique beliefs and values, according to the life experiences of each older person. Also distinctly individual in such a situation is the influence of culture with each dying person. This becomes a highly influential aspect of care when the nurse cares for a dying patient in the person's own home. *Hospice care* signifies a care perspective that recognizes that death is inevitable and near and that cure is not within present human capacity. Inpatient hospice beds are few in the United States, but outpatient hospices provide coordinated services for those persons who are dying at home and have a caregiver present. Medicare and some commercial health insurances will reimburse for some of the formal hospice services.

The territory of the patient and the parameters of personal space are identified readily in the home, making the care of the dying older adult in the home quite different from that in the hospital or in the nursing home. Often there is a favorite chair, a specific furniture arrangement, a particular way to arrange and to place linen or clothing, or a pattern of activity that the patient prefers. Identification of and respect for these preferences are crucial to providing the best possible care for the dying older adult. One important aspect of the care of the dying patient at home is the control of pain. This crucial aspect of care of the dying person at home has been successfully managed by the use of transdermal system of administering fentanyl. The drug is available to the person over a 72-hour period and allows for continuous administration for a stable control of pain (Schmitz et al., 1994). The nurse must be an advocate to ensure that pain is recognized, deemed treatable, and controlled by appropriate and effective methods.

Direct care for the dying person is the responsibility of the family or other caregiver, as a rule.

The nurse may assist with the caregiving activities, but the most important role of the nurse is that of supporting the caregivers, helping them to develop plans of care, suggesting strategies of care that may be more acceptable to the patient, and monitoring and evaluating the results of the interventions. The nurse should express positive regard for the courage and the strengths of the caregiver, comment on the significance of that care to the patient, and help the caregiver to experience a renewed sense of accomplishment.

The patient should be encouraged to experience the warmth and love of relationships that have sustained life and to enjoy the simple pleasures that being at home allows. Acting as a resource person is a valuable role for the nurse. The family and the patient often need supplies and equipment to facilitate their caregiving activities; the nurse can obtain these. Also, the nurse can provide the family with suggestions for consultants in the community who can help address patient needs, such as dietary needs, personal care needs, spiritual needs, and so on. Other community resources can be identified and utilized as specific needs are noted.

The astute nurse will be attuned to the needs of caregivers, as well as to the patients' needs. If the terminal illness is prolonged, caregivers will appreciate a periodic respite from the daily activities. The nurse can recognize this need and initiate measures that will provide the caregivers respite while the continued needs of the patient are met. Often the caregivers are experiencing the physical demands of providing care for the dying person while dealing with their own grief and impending loss; the nurse is in a strategic position to help both patients and caregivers.

■ Conclusion

Whether the setting is the hospital, the nursing home, or the person's own home in the community, the experience of dying is difficult, complex, and challenging. It is an experience that is viewed quite differently by different age groups. Older adults have usually witnessed the death of friends and loved ones, and they realize, as they age, that they are approaching the time when crises can occur. To a greater or lesser extent, older people can become reconciled to this; in fact, they may develop a view of the terminal illness as a spiritual crisis rather than strictly a medical crisis. Younger people, including the middle aged, usually are less aware of the approach of terminal illnesses and death. Such an event is not imminent for them, they reason. Nonetheless, the young or middle-aged health care giver, though younger than the older patient, recognizes and acknowledges these differences in perspectives resulting from differences in age.

For the older patient, it is important to have an opportunity to discuss individual views and preferences. Providing an opportunity for the older person to assert personal beliefs and choices will facilitate a more comfortable experience and peace of mind as the end of life approaches. Family and caregivers, too, can experience comfort in knowing that they proceeded with the care of the patient as the highest priority.

EVALUATION

Consistent with the evaluation of other nursing activities related to care of older adults, the nursing activities performed for the dying patient should be periodically examined and reviewed to ensure achievement of goals. Because the experience of caring for the dying patient is often emotion laden, it is one of the more difficult experiences to evaluate. Nursing staff and families can benefit, however, when the nurse assumes a leadership role and identifies those activities that yield satisfying outcomes for the patient and family. These are the activities the nurses can rely upon in similar situations in the future, to assist in goal achievement.

The health care system in the United States is oriented toward achieving wellness and restoring health. When caring for the older person who is dying, reality orientation is necessary. If the family and staff can review the care of the dying person and be satisfied that quality care was provided and that the patient's perceptions, attitudes, and responses to dying were constantly considered, then the evaluation activities can confirm that the patient's rights were respected, the patient's needs were met, and the dying experience was as comfortable and peaceful as the nursing staff could provide.

REFERENCES

Bianchi, E. (1985). Death preparation as life enhancement. In *Affirmative aging*. Minneapolis: Winston Press.

Bohnet, N.L. (1986). The dying elderly. In M.O. Amenta & N.L. Bohnet (Eds.), *Nursing care of the terminally ill* (pp. 227-233). Boston: Little, Brown.

Grimby, A. (1993). Bereavement among elderly people: Grief reactions, post-bereavement hallucinations and quality of life. *Acta Psychiatric Scand, 87*(1), 72-80.

Kaye, P. (1989). *Notes on symptom control in hospice and palliative care*. Essex, CT: Hospice Education Institute.

Kübler-Ross, E. (1969). *On death and dying*. New York: Macmillan.

Prigerson, H.S. et al. (1995). Complicated grief and bereavement-related depression as distinct disorders: Preliminary empirical validation in elderly bereaved spouses. *American Journal of Psychiatry, 152*(1), 22-30.

Rando, T.A. (1984). *Grief, dying, and death: Clinical interventions for caregivers*. Champaign, IL: Research Press.

Sanders, C.M. (1989). *Grief: The mourning after— Dealing with adult bereavement*. New York: John Wiley and Sons.

Schmitz, P., Lynn, J., & Cobbs, E. (1994). The care of the dying patient. In W. Hazzard, E. Bierman, J. Blass, W. Ettinger, & J. Halter (Eds.), *Principles of geriatric medicine and gerontology* (3rd ed.). New York: McGraw-Hill.

Our society must make it right and possible for old people not to fear the young or be deserted by them, for the test of a civilization is the way that it cares for its helpless members.

PEARL S. BUCK

Legal Perspectives on Planning for Older Adults

■ Learning Objectives

On completion of this chapter, the reader will be able to do the following:

1. Discuss the legal aspects of planning that will help older adult patients manage their affairs, and plan for their potential inability to manage their own affairs.
2. Identify the public benefit programs that may assist the older adult.
3. Describe the main regulations governing nursing homes.

It is a sad reality that many older adults in the United States are not enjoying "the best that is yet to be," which Browning claimed for old age. Whereas many are at home, depending on themselves, their families, or the community for support, large numbers are residents of institutions established to provide the necessary support. Caregivers in these institutions have an opportunity to assist older adults by encouraging them to plan for some of the difficulties they will face as they age. Knowledge of the various planning devices available is not usually gained in practice but must be acquired through study. Outlining this information is the purpose of this chapter.

The chapter presents information helpful to caregivers attempting to assist older adults in planning for the various physical, mental, and financial challenges they will encounter as they age. Because the caregiver usually has a close, nurturing relationship with the older adult, there is an opportunity to offer advice and counseling that may be more welcomed and more carefully considered than the same advice offered through advertisements for various commercial planning services. This relationship between older adult and caregiver often makes the caregiver a source of information for the older adult's family, as well, and dictates that the caregiver have an awareness of such topics as legal competency and of the financial, health care, and housing issues that may arise and for which planning is possible. Encouraging planning, if successful, may result in the older adult's being able to maintain independence and a degree of financial security, which will be much more satisfactory than the restricted life that might have resulted from arrangements made on the older person's behalf by well-intentioned caregivers. (As an aside, it should be noted that many of the legal devices enabling planning for future contingencies are equally applicable to younger people.)

Incapacity may come upon anyone because of illness or accident; having made one's desires known in advance will lessen the burden on the caregivers and will improve the chances that decisions are made as the incapacitated person would have wanted. Although older adults are not the only ones concerned about the future. The main focus of this chapter, however, is to provide caregivers with information useful for encouraging older adults to be informed about the choices that can be made in advance of a loss of capacity to make choices. There are specific steps that the family of an already incompetent older adult can take to better manage the care of the older adult.

The premise that underlies the necessary planning is that the older adult is able to make the necessary decisions and understand the ramifications of the plans put in place. The person must have the legal capacity to make these decisions. If the older adult is not competent when the caregiver or family is attempting to plan for the future, an opportunity has been missed. Timely planning is a means of ensuring that older adults continue to have the benefit of their important right to make choices affecting their life. The peace of mind that comes to the person who has considered the eventualities and made choices about how they should be managed is a valuable asset that is relatively easy to obtain.

■ Mental Capacity

Because mental capacity is essential to making effective plans, it is appropriate to introduce the legal view of the concept on which so much is founded. Of all the concerns that aging brings, the most worrisome to older adults and their families is often the loss of those mental capabilities that mark one as capable or competent. The fear of loss and the actual loss are major factors in aging, but planning for them is possible. Before the various planning devices are addressed in the following sections, this section discusses capacity and the concept of a "surrogate."

Definitions of the vital human capability known as *capacity,* or *competency,* are varied:

- From a legal dictionary: "Ability to understand the nature and effects of one's acts" (*Black's Law Dictionary,* 1983).
- From a medical dictionary: "In psychiatry, the mental ability to distinguish right from wrong and to manage one's own affairs" (*Stedman's Medical Dictionary,* 1990).
- From a state statute: " 'Incapacitated person' means any adult who is impaired by reason of mental illness, mental retardation, physical illness, or disability, advanced age or other causes to the extent that the adult lacks sufficient understanding or capacity to make, communicate, or carry out responsible decisions concerning his or her well-being" (*Code of Virginia,* § 63.1-55.2).
- From a medical text: "The term *competency* has many meanings in the law. In the medical context, the term is used to describe a patient's capacity to give informed consent to medical treatment" (Mewhinney, 1994).

From the differences in these definitions it is clear that the concepts of "competency" or "capacity" are poor guides for the assessments caregivers must make about the capabilities of their loved ones or family members. Trying to determine at what point people have a lessened mental capability for participating in managing their affairs and their own treatment is extremely difficult for all concerned. In all cases, however, the caregivers must have a well-considered opinion as to whether the older adult is sufficiently aware of the nature of the issues in question. The older adult has the right to determine the issues and make the decisions. However, in cases where the caregiver concludes that the person is not sufficiently aware to make such determinations, decisions must be made by a surrogate, a person empowered to act on behalf of the older adult. If such a person has not been designated by prior planning, a surrogate will have to be sought from the courts.

As in making all effective decisions, capacity is required in persons who are attempting to surrender, in advance of incapacity, some of their decision-making powers to another. The person who is receiving these powers, and who will exercise them on behalf of the older adult, is often called a surrogate decision maker. Other terms are used with slightly different meanings depending on the nature of the powers granted or the instruments used to grant the powers. These terms, such as *trustee, attorney in fact, personal representative, guardian,* or *conservator,* will be explained as they arise in the discussion, but at this point a definition of the term *surrogate* may be helpful.

The term *surrogate* is commonly applied to the person who is assisting the older adult by making certain decisions on the older adult's behalf. The standard dictionary definition applies: "A person or thing that is substituted for another, a substitute" (Morris, 1979).

This is a deceptively simple definition. There are many aspects to consider with regard to surrogates. In the context of this heading there may be one or more surrogates making various decisions on behalf of the older adult. The surrogate must become fully informed, with the caregiver's assistance, and then provide the decision, based on informed consent, that the older adult is unable to give. Surrogates may act because they have been given some sort of power to do so. They may have been given the power by the patient, if there has been planning, or they may have been given the power by the laws or the courts, if the incapacity preceded the establishment of the surrogate. In general, powers of the surrogate to act may currently be in effect, that is, the surrogate may act at present for the patient; or they may become effective in the future, for example, when the power to act is effective only after the older adult becomes incapacitated. Surrogates are limited in their abilities to act for the older adult to the specific powers that have been granted. Guardians and conservators are granted powers by the courts, after the older adult's capacities have diminished to a specified level and a judicial proceeding has taken place.

Specific types of planning can be done by a competent person to mitigate some of the difficulties that aging (or an accident) may bring to the fore. The following are descriptions of the major tools available for managing personal decisions while older adults still have the capacity to participate in planning for their own affairs. Legal procedures to implement several planning objectives in areas such as health care, finances, or residency are discussed. The section also presents an overview of some of the programs available to assist older adults in meeting their financial obligations and a brief look at the nursing home regulatory environment. The second section, on guardians and conservators, assumes that no surrogate has been empowered to make the necessary decisions and presents an overview of when, why, and how guardians are appointed. Also presented are some of the considerations that are important in selecting a guardian as well as overview of some laws that have been passed to protect the incompetent person from abuse or to permit families to make certain decisions although no guardian has been appointed.

The following discussions attempt to present the common, national view of the topic discussed, but the thoughtful caregiver will recognize that details, often important ones, do vary by jurisdiction. Federal, state, and even local rules or regulations may sometimes make a course of action easier or more difficult to put in place, more or less effective, or even legal or illegal. From the information presented in this chapter, the caregiver should have a sufficient background to recognize when to have a more specialized expert assist with the desired action.

■ Planning Techniques

Families and caregivers often only begin to explore what legal steps can be taken to assist in making decisions for an older adult, or in managing their various affairs, when signs of poor decisions or an inability to make decisions become evident. This is regrettable, because proper planning best proceeds when time and resources are devoted to it early, and not under the pressure of having a failing loved one. Anticipating a decline, family members and health care providers can encourage the older adult to consider the problems that may arise through loss of capacity as the person ages. All concerned may be encouraged if it is the older adult who realizes the potentialities and instigates the planning process.

Employing the best planning techniques requires the knowing participation and agreement of the person granting some of his or her decision-making powers to another. It is possible that the older adult whose capacity is minimally impaired may concur in the appointment of a guardian or conservator, although such agreement is not required if the court makes the finding of incapacity. In all of the arrangements made, the older adult is a full participant in, and often the instigator of, the establishment of the surrogate and the one who determines which powers will be surrendered and to what degree.

Many legal instruments involve the term *power,* a term that needs to be understood. Although the guardianship powers may be awarded by the court to the surrogate with or without the consent and assistance of the older adult, the powers are established with the con-

sent and assistance of the competent older adult. The power of the surrogate may not become effective immediately and may not be needed while the older adult is competent, or it may become effective because the older adult has decided to employ the benefits of having a surrogate to make life easier. It is in the best interests of the older adult to retain as much autonomy in decision making as that person is capable of managing. But as this capability declines, or is anticipated to decline, the older adult can make various types of grants of decision-making power to surrogates. Such grants of power are made by legal instruments, observing applicable laws and procedures. Almost all types of decision-making powers may be granted, and the terms of the granting instrument, also usually called a "power," will provide both the scope and limitations of the powers granted. Caregivers need to remember at all times, however, that powers not specifically given by the older adult are retained and may not be assumed by health care providers without some type of due process. Older adults can empower a surrogate to make health care decisions on their behalf.

HEALTH CARE PLANNING

Health and health care are topics of great interest to older adults. Recognizing their changing physical condition and suffering various age-related diseases or injuries, older adults are concerned about their abilities to stay actively involved in the decisions concerning their medical treatment. They sense that well-meaning family, friends, or caregivers may begin to make decisions that they feel they can, and should, still make. Maintaining their autonomy is important to them, and helping them to do this is an important aspect of providing care. After a brief review of an important law concerning the patient's rights, this section addresses two legal devices that can be used to make known the older adult's desires for receiving health care.

The section concludes with a brief look at the issues surrounding death.

The caregiver will be called upon to assist many older individuals in various settings. Many will be able to manage all aspects of their care and the management of their affairs. The caregiver, in these cases, will help to maintain this state of affairs for as long as possible. In these cases the planning techniques discussed previously are appropriate. However, the caregiver will also encounter older adults who are alert and oriented but who are soon likely to experience a decline in their mental and physical functioning such that their legal capacity to formulate and communicate decisions about their care, treatment, and financial affairs will be diminished. For these older people, planning for incapacity is an important consideration and should be discussed openly as part of the care planning process. Although it is inappropriate for caregivers, for example, a nursing home, to require that residents execute living wills or other advance directives, residents should be fully aware of the options that are available to them. The caregiver can assist in providing this awareness, and in protecting the older adults' right to make their own choices.

In June of 1990 the United States Supreme Court issued its decision regarding the Nancy Cruzan "right to die" case. The Court affirmed the right of a competent person to refuse life-sustaining treatment (including hydration and nutrition), but held that states may determine the degree of proof required before a patient's wishes set forth in an advance directive are honored. In response to the court's decision, Congress enacted the Patient Self-Determination Act on October 26, 1990. The act empowers patients to receive necessary information concerning health care decisions; it does not provide for any new rights (Huntington & Fry-Revere, 1991). Box 21-1 gives a summary of the provisions.

At this time 41 states and the District of Columbia have living will or advance directive statutes that express the state's view of the proof required of the patient's wishes. Caregivers should be knowledgeable concerning the law in the state where they practice. The following are two common instruments of advance directives: living wills and durable powers of attorney.

Living wills

One way for incapacitated individuals to maintain control over what decisions are made about their health care and financial matters is to issue instructions in advance. In each state there may be several legally recognized and accepted mechanisms for doing so.

One type of advance directive is the living will. *Living will* is the popular name for declarations or directives created by state law, often referred to as "natural death acts," that permit individuals to direct their health care in the event of terminal illness or irreversible condition. Most living wills direct that in the event of a diagnosis of terminal illness, extraordinary medical care should not be initiated or should be withdrawn so that the process of dying will not be artificially prolonged. Many living wills make provision for the continuation of care necessary for comfort, dignity, and the relief of pain.

In states that have created natural death acts, state law will set forth the requirements that must be met to create a legally valid living will. Generally, the document must be signed in the presence of at least two disinterested witnesses. A few states require that if the person signing the living will lives in a nursing home, one of the witnesses must be the long-term care ombudsman. In some states the document must be notarized.

There are a number of limitations on the usefulness of a living will to direct and control health care decisions after the onset of incapacity. A major consideration is the fact that a living will applies only to individuals who are terminally ill. Many states have enacted additional specific restrictions on their application. In California and Oklahoma, a living will is valid only if it is signed after a diagnosis of terminal illness has

---

BOX 21-1 PATIENT SELF-DETERMINATION ACT OF 1990: RESPONSIBILITIES OF HEALTH CARE PROVIDERS

Hospitals, nursing facilities, providers of home health care or personal care services, health maintenance organizations (HMOs), and hospice programs certified by Medicare or Medicaid must do the following:

- Maintain written policies and procedures with respect to all adult individuals receiving medical care by or through the provider or organization
- Provide written information to each individual concerning the individual's rights under state law (whether statutory or as recognized by the courts of the state) to make decisions concerning medical care, *including the right to accept or refuse medical or surgical treatment and the right to formulate advance directives,* and the written policies respecting the implementation of such rights
- Document in the individual's medical record whether or not the person has executed an advance directive
- Not condition the provision of care or otherwise discriminate against an individual based on whether or not the individual has executed an advance directive
- Ensure compliance with the requirements of the state law respecting advance directives at facilities of the provider or organization
- Provide for education for staff and the community on issues concerning advance directives

The written information should be provided to an adult individual as follows:

- For hospitals, at the time of inpatient admission
- For nursing facilities, at the time of admission
- For home health care or personal care services, in advance of the individual's coming under the care of the provider
- For hospices, at the time of initial receipt of hospice care
- For HMOs, at the time of enrollment

Adapted from American Hospital Association Section for Aging and Long Term Care Services (1991).

---

been made. In several states a living will is not effective if the patient is pregnant. In other states, artificial hydration and nourishment are specifically excluded from the definition of extraordinary care and cannot be withheld or withdrawn under the general authority of an otherwise valid living will.

Durable powers of attorney

Another type of advance directive is the durable power of attorney. A traditional power of attorney is a voluntary delegation of authority to another person, usually called the "attorney in fact," to act on behalf of the person making the delegation, usually referred to as the "grantor." Under traditional legal principles, because the delegation of authority is voluntary and can always be revoked, a power of attorney is effective and valid only so long as the grantor remains competent to effectuate a revocation. Thus the traditional power of attorney is not an effective tool as an advance directive because it lapses upon the incapacity of the grantor.

In recent years, states have enacted legislation to create powers of attorney that endure past the time when the grantor becomes incapacitated—hence the term *durable power of attorney.* The advantage of a durable power of attorney is that it is more flexible than a living will. It can be drafted to encompass both health care decisions and financial transactions, it can be general or specific, and it allows the grantor to authorize a person (chosen by the grantor) to execute the grantor's instructions.

There are a number of variations among state laws regarding the requirements for creating a valid durable power of attorney. In a handful of states a special form must be used. In others the document must be notarized. In at least two states a durable power of attorney must be approved by a judge, whereas other states require that the document be filed in a specified government office.

Although durable powers of attorney are an extremely valuable tool for issuing advance directives, they may be of limited utility for nursing home residents. The majority of nursing home residents have no involved family or friends and therefore have no one whom they would feel comfortable appointing to act on their behalf. In such instances it may still be useful for the resident to commit to writing a statement of desires and intentions regarding health care and other matters. Should the resident become incapacitated at a later date and a surrogate be appointed by a court, the written statement of desires and intentions will be important evidence of the resident's concerns to guide the surrogate in exercising substituted judgment on behalf of the resident.

Consent and dying

In the 1990s the people of the United States have begun a serious discussion of several questions concerning the older adult's right to die, the family's right to insist upon treatments prolonging life, and the physician's role in opposing such treatments or in assisting the patient to die. The following is a discussion of these issues from the legal point of view, leaving the medical and ethical considerations aside for discussion elsewhere.

Informed consent The purpose of informed consent is to allow patients to exercise their decision-making skills in relation to their health care. For older people to be able to give consent, they must be competent and informed, yet not coerced. The health care provider has a responsibility to communicate pertinent information in a manner that the person is able to understand. The rationale for each treatment, medication, or diagnostic test needs to be explained, along with the risks and benefits. Many times older adults may find themselves choosing an option that is not favored by the health care team. To be free of coercion means having the freedom to disagree but still be assured of continued support and treatment from the health care team.

The problems with informed consent as a practical, everyday device are many. Older patients may not be willing to accept responsibility for this type of decision making, especially in light of the fact that their socialization process as young adults taught them not to question a physician's recommendations. Another serious problem that is a result of a similar socialization process is the negative attitude of many health care professionals toward the abilities of patients to make the "right decision." Time constraints experienced by all health care providers leave little time to explain options properly and answer questions. Many times patients sign informed consent forms without truly understanding what they have just signed.

Perhaps improvements regarding simplified language, longer time intervals before signing, and obligatory confirmation of understanding of content will make the process of true informed consent a reality.

Family consent laws In some states, family consent laws provide family members with clear legal authority to make health care decisions for relatives who are incapacitated. Where such laws exist, the need to proceed with a petition in court may be obviated.

Family consent laws are different in every state. In some states, family members may make all health care decisions, whereas in others, a family member's authority to make health care decisions for an incapacitated relative is limited to situations in which a physician has certified that the patient is terminally ill. There is also usually a requirement that before a family member is authorized to act, the resident or patient must be certified as lacking capacity to make a health care decision. State law specifies both who can make such a certification and how.

Although physicians labor with a respect for life, which is the impetus for saving many lives, on occasion it appears to the medical provider that further treatment would be useless. The term often used is *medical futility*. And the issue is being debated "in multiple arenas: in courtrooms, in legislative halls, and at the bedside" (Darr, 1995). It is an issue that will call for understanding on the part of caregivers, patients, and patients' families if the difficult circumstances surrounding death are not to be made more extreme by arguments, lay and legal, over the bed of the dying person.

Even more emotionally charged is the issue of physician assistance in dying. The courts and legislatures are already grappling with this issue, in part because of the activities of Jack Kevorkian, M.D., and such groups as the Hemlock Society. The issue is a continuing and complex one, and one that our society is having a difficult time resolving. But it is also one about which a caregiver may be questioned by patients or their families. It is also one in which a caregiver may become personally involved through circumstances. Therefore it would be prudent to have thought through the issues as they apply to the patient involved, and to have formed one's views and reached an opinion calmly, before being asked in a difficult situation for advice, opinion, or assistance.

It may be helpful in trying to form conclusions in this area for the caregiver to reflect on the patient and to attempt to see the patient's view. Although not always agreeing with the patient's conclusions, the caregiver can always seek to enhance patient autonomy and respect any advance directives put in place by the patient for ensuring a death with dignity.

FINANCIAL AND PROPERTY MANAGEMENT PLANNING

Often compounding the problems that challenge older adults with respect to failing health is the situation of failing financial abilities. The costs of necessities such as food, lodging, and medical care often take an ever-increasing share of the older adult's income as prices rise and inflation takes its toll. Preserving savings and minimizing costs are ever-present goals that take careful management. Many older adults recognize this situation and desire to make plans to manage their finances and property.

One of the most common signs that people are thinking of their own death is their interest in making a will. Wills are commonly understood as disposing of the person's estate after death, offering an opportunity for the deceased to influence the disposition of the property, and serving as a last communication of the person's wishes. Although wills may be prepared by individuals on their own behalf, such wills often encounter difficulties in probate because of their failure to meet some arcane requirement of state law. Will law is notorious for its unique development in each state and for its complexities of execution. Older adults should be advised to obtain legal assistance in the preparation of their wills. Preparing a will is an overt step that a person takes toward acknowledging his or her mortality, and it is usually the first step of a planning nature that people take in response to their recognition of the fact that there are things they can do to influence how their affairs will be managed when they are no longer capable of managing them themselves. The peace of mind that comes from having taken a concrete step toward the uncertain future is important and may serve to make the person more inclined to make other types of plans.

The older adult may also take any of the steps that all citizens are entitled to take to manage their affairs. A "trust," a type of surrogate, to manage property, including real estate properties, can be established. A trust is a "person" as seen by the law and so can act as a surrogate for another person. Of course, there is a real person who takes the actions on behalf of the older adult, the "trustee," and the trustee can exercise the trust powers either now or in the future. If a trust is established by a living person, the powers and the resources given the trustee are detailed in a document called an "inter vivos" (living) trust, which is effective when signed. If the trust is established in the will of a person who has died, the powers and the resources given the trustee are detailed in a document called a "testamentary" trust, which is effective upon the death of the person making the will and trust. Trusts are also classified as revocable and nonrevocable, depending on whether the grantor has retained the power to modify or revoke the trust. For example, an older adult can prepare a revocable living trust that allows him or her the flexibility of revoking the trust if not satisfied with the arrangement, but that becomes irrevocable upon the older person's loss of capacity. The different types of trusts can have similar effectiveness in managing the affairs of the older adult, but choosing the type of trust to use has income and estate tax consequences and therefore requires professional assistance.

There are often specific things that the older adult or the surrogate can do to better manage the available resources, or to prepare for the eventual need to qualify for the Medicaid program discussed in a later section. For example, the older adult, or the older adult's surrogate, may be advised to prepare, and perhaps pay for, funeral arrangements in advance. Such a step often has the benefit of allowing older adults to express their desires in an effective way, whereas wills, which may contain instructions, are often not located or read until after the burial. And prepayment eases the burden survivors face in making decisions as to arrangements while under the stresses related to the death of the older person. Prepayment of funeral arrangements also removes countable assets from the Medicaid calculations.

Two types of commercial offerings are widely available to assist the older adult with financial concerns. Long-term care insurance is offered by various health insurance companies in response to the perceived concern on the part of older adults and their families regarding meeting the large, and increasing, costs of long-term care. These are insurance-type contracts designed to provide funds for paying the expenses of care provided in nursing homes or at home. Long-term care contracts are complex contracts with both a potential impact on the older adult's Medicaid eligibility and tax implications. A qualified advisor should be consulted in the selection and purchase of such insurance.

Another type of contract, sometimes confused with the long-term care insurance, is the contract for continuing care. This is a contract for services, such as care and housing, and it is discussed in the section on living arrangements.

Reverse mortgages are, in effect, loans on the equity of the older adult's home. These mortgages are offered by banks and have many of the characteristics of a typical mortgage, such as interest payments and claim on the property by the lender. The unique feature is that the amount borrowed is not paid all at once to purchase the home and repaid with interest over time, but rather, the amount "borrowed" is paid monthly to the borrower in amounts dependent on the interest rate, value of the equity, and term of the loan. Upon the death of the borrower, or sale of the home if earlier, the lender recoups the loan and interest from the value of the home that is then sold. As with the long-term care insurance, these are complex contracts and obtaining professional assistance is advised before assuming such a loan.

Representative payees

Many older adults live on the income provided from the federal Social Security Administration. The amount of this income is based on the person's, or spouse's, earnings and contributions to Social Security. Anyone advising the older adult needs to have a basic familiarity with that person's Social Security entitlement and to ensure that the payments are properly received and used for the person's care. If the older adult needs assistance in receiving or managing these payments, another type of surrogate may be appropriate. This type of surrogate is granted power, not by the courts, but by the government. Also, this type of power is granted when the capacity of the older adult has declined, but when legal declaration of incapacity and a legal proceeding are not required. When individuals become unable to manage their money and are receiving some specific federal benefit payments, they, or someone acting on their behalf, make an administrative application to the agency making the payments, for example, the Social Security Administration. By this application it is arranged to have the benefits paid to a third party on behalf of the beneficiary. The person to whom the benefits are sent is called a "representative payee," and that person is responsible for using the benefits only for the personal interest and well-being of the beneficiary. A representative payee may be appointed only when there is clear evidence that a beneficiary is unable to manage benefits properly. However, there is no requirement that the beneficiary be declared or adjudicated incompetent. The Social Security Administration, the Veteran's Administration, and the Office of Personal Management all make provisions for the appointment of representative payees.

Benefits programs

Since the Great Depression, various federal administrations have proposed, adopted, or modified programs designed to aid those people in the United States who need assistance. These programs have varied in funding strategy from outright grants to imaginative savings programs to insurance-type programs. A majority of these programs have tried to address the needs of those who require medical care for which they do not have the money. These programs have come to be a main source of financial assistance for older adults today. One, the Medicare program, is used by most older adults, and another, the Medicaid program, is used by many.

The national desires for balanced budgets and health care reform were joined in the various reform proposals of the mid-1990s. The actions proposed in federal and state legislatures will result in many changes—some, perhaps, incompatible—being enacted and shaping the manner in which care will be rendered to older adults. Although it is still too early to tell what the results of current congressional drives for change will be, it is certain that future planning has been complicated. The following sections are the major provisions of existing programs that benefit older adults.

The Medicare program Medicare is the principal health care insurance for individuals who are 65 years old or older or who are disabled. Unlike Medicaid, it is not a needs-based program. Eligibility is not based on income. The program is funded through payroll deductions and by some premiums paid by beneficiaries. It is administered by the federal Health Care Financing Administration (HCFA), which contracts with private insurance companies known as "intermediaries" or "carriers" to carry out the day-to-day operations of the program.

Although many older adults believe that, once they reach age 65, Medicare will pay for most, if not all, nursing home care, in fact, Medicare payments for nursing home services are only about 4% nationally. This is because Medicare covers only the first 100 days of skilled nursing care.

The criteria for determining whether someone qualifies for skilled care services are specified in federal regulations. Basically, a person is not entitled to Medicare coverage unless that person occupies a bed in the nursing home that is certified as a skilled care bed under the provisions of the Medicare program. In addition, the skilled care services needed by the resident must be ordered by a physician, they must be needed on a daily basis, and they must be the type of services that can be safely and effectively performed only by, or under the supervision of, professional or technical personnel, such as a registered nurse, licensed practical nurse, speech therapist, or physical therapist. The overall condition of the resident must be considered. The restoration potential of the resident is not the deciding factor in determining whether skilled services are needed. Even if full recovery or medical improvement is not possible, a resident may still need skilled services to prevent further deterioration or to preserve current capabilities.

Federal regulations give many examples of skilled care. These include observation and assessment of a resident's changing condition, management and medical evaluation of a care plan, injections, gastrostomy feedings, insertion of catheters, treatment of some specific skin disorders, applications of sterile dressings involving prescription medications, and various physical therapies.

Determinations of noncoverage made under the Medicare program are appealable. The steps that a beneficiary must take to appeal a Medicare determination vary, depending on the type of coverage involved and the amount in controversy. Generally the first step is to request a reconsideration. This is a paper review, but beneficiaries usually have the opportunity to submit additional evidence at this point. Many denials are reversed at this stage. If the beneficiaries do not prevail at the reconsideration stage, they may be able to request a hearing before an administrative law judge. The next step is the appeals council, which is also a paper review. Finally, some cases may be appealed to the U.S. Federal District Court.

Sometimes Medicare coverage is denied informally because the nursing home has made its own determination that services provided to the resident do not meet the criteria for coverage under the Medicare program and fails to submit a claim. In such cases, residents have a right to challenge the nursing home's initial assessment that skilled care services are not required and demand that the nursing home submit a claim to Medicare for a formal eligibility determination. As a result of recent litigation, nursing homes that participate in Medicare must provide residents with a uniform skilled nursing facility denial notice whenever the nursing home has determined that a resident does not require services or levels of care covered by the Medicare program, and it must inform the resident of the right to appeal the initial determination directly to Medicare (*Sarrassat v. Sullivan,* 1989).

The Medicaid program   The nation's single largest payor of nursing home care is the Medicaid program. Medicaid, also called "medical assistance," is a joint federal-state program under Title XIX of the Social Security Act. It is operated and partially funded by each state to pay necessary medical care—including nursing home care—for the poor. Some requirements and broad limits are set by the federal government, but within those limits, state Medicaid rules and benefits vary tremendously.

To qualify for Medicaid in a nursing home, residents must be at least 65 years old, or blind or disabled (as defined under the Social Security Act). They must be in need of intermediate or skilled nursing home care, and they must meet the state's limitations on income and assets. The eligibility rules will generally be similar to the rules for eligibility under the federal Supplemental Security Income (SSI) program, except that state variations also exist.

If a resident is eligible for Medicaid, the program will help pay for an unlimited number of days of medically necessary skilled nursing care and intermediate care. The total monthly payment to the nursing home is established by the Medicaid program, and it differs from nursing home to nursing home. Except for a few deductions, a Medicaid resident must pay all monthly income to the nursing home. The state then pays the balance of the monthly Medicaid payment amount established for the particular nursing home.

Deductions from monthly income that the resident does not have to pay to the nursing home include the following:

- A "personal needs allowance" for non-medical needs such as clothing, sundries, and reading material (The federal personal needs allowance minimum, as of 1989, is $30, but states may set higher levels.)
- A monthly allowance to maintain the resident's home, if the resident is returning within a short period and does not have a spouse living there (This deduction can last only 6 months.)
- An allowance for the resident's spouse, if the spouse's own income is below a specified amount
- The monthly cost of medical insurance premiums (including Medicare premiums) and other medical services not covered by Medicaid (e.g., over-the-counter drugs, eyeglasses, dentures, and hearing aids)

A person who is eligible for the Medicaid program benefits may also qualify for benefits from the Social Security Administration under the Supplemental Security Income program. This is a program based on need, and an application must be filed to obtain benefits.

The Veterans Administration The Veterans Administration (VA) will pay for skilled or intermediate nursing home care in private nursing homes for (1) veterans in VA hospitals in need of direct discharge to a nursing home and (2) other veterans in need of admission to a nursing home for a "service-connected disability." The VA must make the determination that the disability is service connected, meaning that it involves an injury or disease incurred or aggravated in the line of duty during active service.

The usual limit for VA coverage is 6 months. However, the VA has discretion to extend this limit under some medical and economic circumstances. The VA also operates its own nursing units. Eligibility for admission to these units is more liberal, at least in theory, than for admission to private nursing homes.

Other programs Many states provide assistance to older adults for their needs and financial obligations through various programs of fuel assistance, property tax relief, home care, meals on wheels, or rent assistance. These programs, as well as Medicaid, are potential sources of help that older adults may be hesitant to use because of a perceived stigma of being "on the dole." An advisor would be doing a service to older adults by reminding them of the many years they have worked and paid the taxes that support these programs, and by encouraging them to make any appropriate applications. Of course, any surrogate appointed to act for the older adult should also be familiar with these entitlements. There is wide variation in eligibility requirements and in benefits available, but some state office, often called an office of aging, will be able to provide the detailed information required.

LIVING ARRANGEMENTS

The final discussion of planning techniques concerns the older adult's choice of residence. Today older adults live in various settings, many in their own homes, some with relatives, some in hospitals for some period, and many in nursing homes. Up to some point, the choice of older adults is most often to remain in their own home. Then, as physical capabilities decline, the older adult begins to think about the various alternatives available and how to achieve the desired alternative. Although living with relatives or in retirement or continuing care communities are all possible choices, each has its limitations as the older adult's physical condition fails. Because nursing homes are home to many older adults and are the setting where most caregivers will be found assisting older adults, these will be discussed in more detail than the other choices.

In planning and obtaining care, the older adult or the family is often interested in continuing care community arrangements, or in private insurance for long-term nursing home care. Caregivers would do their patients a service by always advising them to seek expert assistance in these matters. The contracts for long-term care insurance, for nursing home care, and for continuing care communities are extremely complex and must be interpreted in conjunction with the existing laws concerning the other assistance programs available from the state or federal government. Much overlap often occurs, and the older adult's resources are wasted by having two programs cover the same benefit, because it can only be collected once. These financing arrangements can "offer to the older adult many advantages: independent living, long-term security, and affordable long-term nursing care. The unique financing arrangements, however, present substantial problems and pitfalls for the elderly consumer" (Regan, 1996), and the caregiver should recommend that the older adult obtain professional advice.

Nursing homes

Nursing homes provide care to people who are chronically ill, who are recuperating from an illness, and who need regular nursing care and other health-related services, short of hospitalization, on a long-term basis. For this reason, in addition to providing nursing care and services and basic room and board, nursing homes are also required to provide rehabilitation programs, social programs, and social activities. Because over 200,000 nursing homes are in fact home for over 1.8 million older adults and disabled individuals, nursing homes are also required to recognize and promote the rights of individual residents and to provide care in a homelike environment. A clear understanding of the nursing home's obligations to provide care, and the rights of residents, as established by federal and state laws, is important knowledge for both caregivers and surrogates.

The most far-reaching piece of legislation, known as the Nursing Home Reform Amendments (NHRAs), was passed by the U.S. Congress as part of the Omnibus Budget Reconciliation Act (OBRA) of 1987 and has served as the legal basis for the nursing home regulations published since then.

In enacting the federal NHRAs, Congress sought to strengthen residents' rights. In addition to a substantive expansion of rights, the NHRA mandates that review of compliance with residents' rights be included in the annual standard survey used to determine overall performance and compliance with federal regulations, and that facilities not only protect but also "promote" the rights of each resident. A facility's failure to protect and promote the rights of residents can result in the imposition of intermediate sanctions, such as civil fines, a ban on new admissions, restrictions on the facility's license, or curtailment of federal payments. Where violations of residents' rights are serious and widespread, the facility risks being placed in receivership or being decertified for participation in the Medicare or Medicaid programs. Some states have enacted or are in the process of enacting laws establishing a "private right of action," which allows residents to sue and recover damages for violations of their rights. These laws also often contain provisions that shift the costs of the litigation to the facility in the event that the rights violations are established. For example, in the District of Columbia, Illinois, and New York, if residents sue a facility for violations of their rights and win, the facility must pay the residents' court costs and attorney fees.

In light of the importance of residents' rights as a determinant of quality care and the significant penalties that can attach when rights are not promoted or are violated, it is imperative that caregivers understand the substantive provisions of the residents' bill of rights and recognize that when institutional concerns conflict with the individual right of a resident, the right of the resident must be respected and must supersede the facility's right.

However, what happens when individuals are unable to make decisions or to communicate their choices? Many nursing home residents suffer from cognitive and physical impairments that affect their ability to reason and to communicate effectively. How does the law protect the rights of individuals who, because of these impairments, cannot protect themselves, and how do they manage their affairs? In such cases the laws provide for surrogates to act. As discussed previously, sometimes older adults have established their own surrogates and granted them the powers required. Sometimes there will be no surrogates appointed, nor family consent laws applicable, and at that time the family or caregivers will have to resort to the laws and courts of the appropriate state and have a surrogate appointed. Such surrogates are called "guardians," or, if the powers are less, "conservators." These surrogates, and how they are appointed, are discussed in the section on guardians and conservators.

Reporting laws

In addition to the statewide registry, all 50 states and the District of Columbia have some form of reporting system for monitoring and responding to abuse, neglect, and exploitation of vulnerable adults. Here again, state approaches vary tremendously. In 42 states the reporting system is mandatory. Of these 42 states, 14 impose a mandatory duty to report on any person with knowledge, or reasonable cause to believe, that a person under the statute has been abused, neglected, or exploited. In other states, only certain designated professionals are under such an imposition of mandatory duty. Generally speaking, in states with mandatory reporting laws, physicians, nurses, and other health care professionals are required to report cases of suspected adult abuse, neglect, and exploitation. There may be criminal penalties ranging from fines to imprisonment for failing to do so. In addition, in 17 states the abuse, neglect, or exploitation of a vulnerable adult is punishable as a criminal offense. These criminal sanctions are in addition to and not in lieu of

existing criminal laws dealing with homicide, assault, rape, theft, and fraud. Many state laws protect reporters from liability, provided they have acted in good faith, and most state laws protect the confidentiality of the reporter (American Public Welfare Society and National Association of State Units on Aging, 1986).

In light of the sanctions that may attach, any professional who works with vulnerable adults should become familiar with state law provisions regarding adult protective services. Also, knowledge of how the state's adult protective services program operates may be useful in obtaining needed services for a patient who has been victimized. Many hospitals, nursing homes, and home care agencies provide in-service training to employees regarding these laws. If one of these institutions does not, training should be developed in this area, because ignorance of the law does not excuse a failure to report if indeed a report is required under state law.

Other laws affecting nursing home operation

Two other areas of law that play an important role in defining the rights and obligations of caregivers and residents are the general common law rules of tort law and contract law. They are called "common law" rules because they are court-made rules that have evolved over time through individual case decisions by judges.

Broadly speaking, a "tort" is a civil wrong for which a court will provide a remedy in the form of money damages. A tort may be either intentional or unintentional. An example of an intentional tort is the tort of assault, which occurs when an individual intentionally causes another individual to feel apprehension or fear of bodily injury. Shaking a fist in another person's face would constitute an assault. An unintentional tort occurs when an individual is injured as a result of negligent conduct. Negligence cases constitute the vast majority of lawsuits filed against health care providers.

"Contract law" defines the rights and obligations of institutions and individuals, as established by explicit "bargained-for" agreements between the parties. Generally speaking, a contract is legally enforceable. If one party to a contract fails to perform, the other party can sue to enforce the contract and can obtain money damages to compensate for any loss.

Other laws that relate to the operation of nursing homes, as well as other health care institutions, include certificate-of-need laws and indigent care statutes. These laws are considered tools for health care planning and are considered by some to be necessary to manage scarce resources, to contain costs, and to ensure the availability and accessibility of health care services. Many states have also enacted consumer protection statutes, which can be used to protect consumers from misleading or deceptive advertising. Federal Trade Commission rules concerning misleading trade practices may apply to nursing home chains or other health care providers that operate interstate. In cases where several facilities, a chain, or an association of nursing homes engages in practices that restrict the market in certain ways, such as price fixing, federal antitrust laws may apply. Nursing homes, hospitals, or other health care providers that participate in Medicaid and/or Medicare are also subject to Title VI of the federal Civil Rights Act of 1964, which prohibits discrimination based on race, color, or national origin. Not to be ignored are the numerous state-specific statutes regarding residents' rights, transfer and discharge, and prohibitions barring discrimination against Medicaid recipients.

The long-term care ombudsman program

The long-term care ombudsman plays an important role for residents in long-term care facilities. Under the federal Older Americans Act (1987), every state and the District of Columbia is required to establish and operate a long-term care ombudsman program. The program provides an individual whose full-time job is to investigate and resolve complaints made by or on behalf of residents in long-term care facilities, relating to action or inaction of providers, public agencies,

or social service agencies that may adversely affect the health, safety, welfare, or rights of such residents. Many states have enacted or are in the process of enacting authorizing legislation that defines the powers and duties of the ombudsman in greater detail, and that gives the ombudsman access to residents and their records.

The goal of the long-term care ombudsman program is to promote the highest quality of life and care for residents of nursing homes and board and care homes. The primary function of the ombudsman is to act as an advocate for the residents, but in many jurisdictions the office of the long-term care ombudsman also does the following:

- Acts as a clearinghouse for information on long-term care
- Monitors the implementation of legislation and regulations
- Educates providers, residents, and the public on residents' rights
- Trains and supervises volunteers to advocate in nursing homes on behalf of residents

The long-term care ombudsman programs are also authorized under federal law to pursue legal and administrative remedies on behalf of residents. Some operate toll-free telephone numbers that provide access to ombudsmen.

All programs are obligated to protect the anonymity of any person registering a complaint regarding a particular facility.

The preceding discussions reveal the complexity of the various aspects of the demanding task of caring for older adults in the institutional setting. Many laws and regulations must be followed, institutional policies and procedures must be followed and kept up to date, and the practitioner must attempt to learn about significant changes as they occur. This is an area of great flux as the United States attempts to improve its health care delivery system, and the caregiver has a difficult task in staying knowledgeable about these complexities while attempting to give highest-quality patient care.

■ Guardians and Conservators

The previous discussions were addressed to techniques that can be used by older adults fully able to make their own decisions and for whom knowledge of various techniques will be helpful. By encouraging such people to make their desires known through their plans and their surrogates, the caregiver will be providing valuable support and making the older adult's life more comfortable.

However, many individuals who are in nursing homes today already lack the legal capacity to make health care and financial decisions. For these individuals, family members must look to establishing an appropriate and legally authorized person, a surrogate, for giving consent and direction in many matters affecting the older adult, such as obtaining medical care, refusing such care, or managing financial resources. That person is often, but need not be, a family member. It is important to note that "while the intent of guardianship is benevolent, it can result in substantial deprivation of liberty and property" (Thomas, 1994). Keeping this in mind, caregivers can assist older adults and their families by advocating that the decision authority remain with the older adult as long as feasible and that it be given to a surrogate only to the extent necessary.

There are varied legal steps that a family member might take to manage an older adult's affairs and protect that older adult's rights. These steps include discussions of obtaining surrogates for decision making and of legal actions that will empower a surrogate to make various decisions or plans on behalf of the older adult. The emphasis here is on reacting to an incapacity that has not been adequately planned for.

All states and the District of Columbia have a procedure by which courts can appoint a third party to manage the affairs or to make personal decisions for individuals who are unable to care for themselves. The person appointed is usually called a guardian or conservator, although in some states the term *committee* is used. The terms *guardian* and *conservator* are often used interchangeably. However, some courts may distinguish between a person appointed to manage the financial affairs of the incapacitated person (a conservator) and a person appointed to make decisions, as well, about the incapacitated person's personal care, medical treatment, and/or daily activities (a guardian). The incapacitated person is usually referred to as the "ward."

The process for appointment of a guardian or conservator varies greatly from state to state. Generally speaking, a determination of the need for a guardian or conservator requires that the person bringing the action, sometimes referred to as a "petitioner," show first that the proposed ward has a specified mental or physical impairment and, second, that as a result of the impairment, the proposed ward is unable to manage personal and/or financial affairs. The Uniform Probate Code (1983), which is followed by a number of states, defines an incapacitated person as follows:

Any person who is impaired by reason of mental illness, mental deficiency, physical illness or disability, advanced age, chronic age, chronic use of drugs, chronic intoxication, or other cause (except minority) to the extent [that he or she] lacks sufficient understanding or capacity to make or communicate a responsible decision.

If the court finds that the proposed ward is incapacitated, a guardian or conservator will be appointed. Again, who will be appointed depends on the state law. In some states, preference is given to relatives, whereas in others, the court must give priority consideration to the person chosen by the ward, if that information is known. Many states routinely appoint attorneys, banks, social services agencies, or other disinterested persons or entities. Some states have a public guardian. States following the Uniform Probate Code use priorities such as the following for selecting guardians, and a similar list for selecting conservators (Regan, 1996):

1. The incapacitated person's most recent nomination in a durable power of attorney

2. The person's spouse, or a person nominated by will of a deceased spouse or by other writing signed by the spouse and attested to by at least two witnesses
3. The person's adult child
4. The person's parent, or a nominee by will of a deceased parent or by other writing signed by a parent and attested to by at least two witnesses
5. Any relative of the incapacitated person with whom the person has resided for more than 6 months before the filing of the petition
6. A person nominated by the person who is caring for or paying for the care of the incapacitated person

Once guardians and conservators are appointed, their powers vary greatly, also depending on state law. In many states, guardians and conservators exercise "plenary powers," meaning that they have the power to make decisions affecting virtually every aspect of the ward's life. Increasingly, courts and legislatures are recognizing that persons with mental or physical disabilities do not and should not necessarily lose all their rights to exercise personal autonomy. Thus in some states the guardian's powers, as delineated by the court, must be drawn as narrowly as possible, whereas in other states the courts have broad discretion to structure the guardian's or conservator's authority to fit the needs of the individual ward.

A trend, encouraging to those concerned that the older adult's wishes always be followed, is the increasing application of the doctrine of "substituted judgment" in cases where a guardian has been appointed by a court to make a health care decision for an incapacitated person. Under the doctrine of substituted judgment, a surrogate who has been designated to act for an incapacitated person has a duty to determine what choice the incapacitated person would make with respect to medical treatment if the person were competent to make that decision.

Under the doctrine of substituted judgment the surrogate literally stands in the shoes of the incapacitated person and makes decisions based on the incapacitated person's values, motives, and beliefs.

There are numerous problems with the application of guardianship and conservatorship laws for people who are mentally and physically incapacitated. The proceedings may be very costly and time consuming. The person appointed by the court to make and exercise personal choices on behalf of the ward may in fact be a total stranger to the ward. Although many court-appointed guardians and conservators will make an effort to become familiar with the ward and will make conscientious efforts to fulfill their fiduciary obligations, it is not uncommon to hear complaints about guardians and conservators who fail to establish any personal relationship with the ward, who make personal care decisions in a vacuum, and who even fail to ensure that the ward's bills are paid and that basic needs are met. The ability and willingness of courts to monitor guardianships and conservatorships once established also vary greatly from state to state. Although some states monitor guardianships and conservatorships closely, most only require an annual accounting of financial transactions. Few states have the resources necessary to conduct extensive audits of these accounts or to monitor personal care decisions made under a court appointment.

In spite of these concerns, the use of guardianships is widespread to meet the need for effective management of an incompetent older adult's affairs. Caregivers are in a unique position to observe the older adult's capabilities and to help ensure that the most effective, but least intrusive, type of surrogate power is instituted. Often health care professionals, seeing both the need for, and the effects of, guardianships, are spearheading policy changes to have the process better serve older adults (Coker & Johns, 1994).

■ Conclusion

The information presented here is wide ranging and complex. The delivery of health care in today's environment is challenged by constant changes in personnel, resources, and administrative requirements, and by advances in technology. Education is often narrowed to better serve specified audiences at several nursing levels, sometimes failing to provide a broad view of the complexities of assisting the aging person. Federal and state laws and regulations are changing as attempts are being made to improve care delivery while reducing the costs of health care professionals. There is continuity of concern for the older patient and a growing recognition of the patient's need for control and autonomy. The challenge lies in not reducing the quality of care that will be delivered to our nation's older population, but in assisting this population in as many ways as possible. Encouraging such planning techniques as are presented in this chapter is one way of offering such assistance.

REFERENCES

American Public Welfare Society and National Association of State Units on Aging. (1986). *A comprehensive analysis of state policies and practices related to elder abuse* (Vols. 1-4). Washington, DC: Author.

Black's law dictionary (5th ed. abr.), (1983). St. Paul: West Publishing.

Coker, L.H., & Johns, A.F. (1994). Guardianship for elders: Process and issues. *Journal of Gerontological Nursing, 20*(12), 25-32.

Darr, J. (1995). Guardianship and conservatorship. *Journal of Gerontology Nursing, 21,* 10.

Health Care Financing Administration. (1990). *State operations manual.* Washington, DC: U.S. Government Printing Office.

Huntington, S., & Fry-Revere, S. (1991). Provider responsibilities under the patient self-determination act—Living wills, durable powers of attorney and the law. In *Health law trends.* Washington, DC: Arent, Fox, Kintner, Plotkin, and Kahn.

Mewhinney, K. (1994). Legal aspects of geriatric medicine. In W.R. Hazzard, et al. (Eds.), *Principles of geriatric medicine and gerontology.* New York: McGraw-Hill.

Morris, W. (Ed.). (1979). *The American Heritage dictionary, college edition.* Boston: Houghton Miflin.

Older Americans Act Amendments of 1987, Public Law 100-175 (Vol. 101, Stat. 926) (1987, November).

Omnibus Budget Reconciliation Act of 1987, Public Law 100-203 (1987, December).

Regan, J.J. (1996). *Tax, estate and financial planning for the elderly,* rel 20. New York: Matthew Bender.

Sarrassat v. Sullivan, C.A. No. C 88-20161 RPA (D.C. Cal.) (Stipulation of settlement, May 1, 1989).

Stedman's medical dictionary (25th ed.). (1990). Baltimore: Williams and Wilkins.

Thomas, B.L. (1994). Research considerations: Guardianship and the vulnerable elderly. *Journal of Gerontological Nursing, 20*(5), 10-16.

Uniform Probate Code, S5-108, 8 U.L.A. 437 (West 1983).

Old age has a great sense of calm and freedom; when the passions have relaxed their hold you have escaped, not from one master but from many.

PLATO, *The Republic*

Ethical Perspectives

■ Learning Objectives

On completion of this chapter, the reader will be able to do the following:

1. Compare and contrast four current approaches to studying and applying bioethics: principle-based ethics, virtue theory, communitarianism, and caring.
2. Critique age-based rationing as a means to achieve intergenerational justice.
3. Counsel older adults who seek assistance in making end-of-life treatment decisions.
4. Describe the advocacy responsibilities and related competencies of gerontologic nurses.
5. Identify strategies to prevent and resolve ethical conflict.
6. Use a process of ethical decision making to resolve moral distress and dilemmas.

■ Moral Competency and Gerontologic Nursing

In a now classic article, physician-ethicist Mark Siegler (1984) describes the three ages of medicine as the age of paternalism, the age of autonomy, and the current age of bureaucratic parsimony. Throughout these ages the principal concern of physicians has changed from the good of individual patients, to the good of the patient's freedom and right of self-determination, to the current balancing of the patient's good against the goods of society, health care institutions, and caregivers. The more the standard decision criteria of medical indications and pa-

tient preferences are replaced by quality of life considerations and other external factors, the more vulnerable older adults become. It is no longer unusual to hear intensive care staff (with no knowledge of the patient under consideration) question, "What is this old person doing taking up a critical care bed?" Nor is it out of the ordinary to hear youth complain about being taxed to finance Medicare benefits. Those of us who work with older adults know how difficult it is to attract the "best and brightest" in nursing to choose gerontology as a specialty. The knowledge and experience of gerontologic nurses position us to advocate effectively for older adults. But to do this well, our moral competence

---

BOX 22-1 THE AMERICAN NURSES' ASSOCIATION CODE OF ETHICS

CODE FOR NURSES

1. The nurse provides services with respect for human dignity and the uniqueness of the client, unrestricted by considerations of social or economic status, personal attributes, or the nature of health problems.
2. The nurse safeguards the client's right to privacy by judiciously protecting information of a confidential nature.
3. The nurse acts to safeguard the client and the public when health care and safety are affected by the incompetent, unethical, or illegal practice of any person.
4. The nurse assumes responsibility and accountability for individual nursing judgments and actions.
5. The nurse maintains competence in nursing.
6. The nurse exercises informed judgment and uses individual competence and qualifications as criteria in seeking consultation, accepting responsibilities, and delegating nursing activities to others.
7. The nurse participates in activities that contribute to the ongoing development of the profession's body of knowledge.
8. The nurse participates in the profession's efforts to implement and improve standards of nursing.
9. The nurse participates in the profession's efforts to establish and maintain conditions of employment conducive to high-quality nursing care.
10. The nurse participates in the profession's effort to protect the public from misinformation and misrepresentation and to maintain the integrity of nursing.
11. The nurse collaborates with members of the health professions and other citizens in promoting community and national efforts to meet the health needs of the public.

From American Nurses' Association. (1985). *Code for nurses with interpretive statements.* Kansas City, MO: Author.

---

must be as fine-tuned as other intellectual, technical, and interpersonal competencies.

Moral competence is not an option for nurses—too much is at stake. How (and whether) we choose to nurse can literally determine the human well-being of those entrusted to our care at vulnerable moments of their living and dying. Recognizing this truth, professional nursing organizations such as the American Nurses' Association (1985) have formulated codes of ethics to regulate practice (Box 22-1). More recently the American Nurses' Association (1991) has published standards of clinical nursing

practice and complemented standards of care with a set of professional performance standards, which includes the injunction that "the nurse's decisions and actions on behalf of clients are determined in an ethical manner" (p. 15). See Box 22-2 for related measurement criteria. This chapter describes elements of moral competency that are essential to excellence in gerontologic nursing. A brief examination of popular approaches to "doing bioethics" will provide a theoretic background for later discussions of broad ethical issues and aging, clinical ethics and nursing, and ethical decision making.

BOX 22-2 THE AMERICAN NURSES'
ASSOCIATION STANDARDS OF
PROFESSIONAL PERFORMANCE

Standard v. ethics: The nurse's decisions and
actions on behalf of clients are determined in
an ethical manner.

MEASUREMENT CRITERIA

1. The nurse's practice is guided by the *Code
   for Nurses.*
2. The nurse maintains client confidentiality.
3. The nurse acts as a client advocate.
4. The nurse delivers care in a nonjudgmen-
   tal and nondiscriminatory manner that is
   sensitive to client diversity.
5. The nurse delivers care in a manner that
   preserves and protects client autonomy,
   dignity, and rights.
6. The nurse seeks available resources to
   help formulate ethical decisions.

From American Nurses' Association Task Force on
Nursing Standards Practice. (1991). *Standards of clinical nursing practice.* Kansas City, MO: Author.

■ Approaches to Ethical Inquiry

PRINCIPLE-BASED APPROACH

Ethical theories are systems of reflection that
attempt to explain how we ought to live and
why. These theories may be broadly categorized
as action-guiding theories that answer the question, What ought I to do? or character-guiding
theories that answer the question, What kind of
person ought I to be? In the early days of
bioethics, attention was focused almost exclusively on action-guiding theory of two types:
utilitarian theory, in which the rightness or
wrongness of an action depends on the consequences the action produces, and deontologic
theory, in which an action is right or wrong
independent of the consequences it produces.

From these action-guiding theories, various principles have been derived, such as autonomy
(self-determination), beneficence (doing good),
nonmaleficence (avoiding harm), justice (treating
fairly), veracity (truth telling), confidentiality (respecting privileged information), and fidelity
(keeping promises). All of these are held to
obligate health care professionals in a prima facie
manner (i.e., all things being equal, I am obligated to respect patients, benefit them and cause
them no harm, treat all fairly, be truthful, etc.).

Most applications of bioethics involve the
resolution of dilemmas involving conflicts between two or more of these principles. Unfortunately, there is no agreed upon hierarchy of
principles that specifies which principles may
trump others. Moreover, because many of these
dilemmas highlight dramatic clinical problems—
definitely not of the everyday "to do a terminal
wean or not to do a terminal wean" variety—this
particular type of principle-based ethics, namely,
quandary ethics, has been critiqued as not being
sensitive to the everyday ethical concerns of
practicing nurses and other health care professionals. Beauchamp and Childress (1994) offer a
comprehensive examination of the principle-
based approach to bioethics, and Clouser and
Gert (1994), a strong critique.

VIRTUE THEORY

Dissatisfaction with action-guiding moral theories that ignore the character of the moral agent
has led some ethicists to resurrect virtue theory
and attempt new formulations of virtues or human excellences intrinsic to human flourishing.
Virtue may be defined as a trait of character that
disposes a person habitually to seek excellence
with respect to an end, such as human flourishing. Virtue theorists claim that who health care
professionals are is as important as what they do.
Although many agree with this claim, the harder
task is agreeing upon which virtues and excellen-
cies are intrinsic to the practice of good nursing
or medicine. In a recent text, Pellegrino and
Thomasma (1993) recommend as virtues essen-

tial to the practice of medicine the following: fidelity to trust, compassion, phronesis (prudential judgment), justice, fortitude, temperance, integrity, and self-effacement. Nursing has yet to agree upon its core virtues. Even more elusive is determining how (and if) virtue can be taught and whether virtue should be used as a criterion for admission to and advancement in nursing practice. It may be helpful to reflect on and begin to describe the traits of character that enable gerontologic nurses to secure the outcomes they desire for older patients.

COMMUNITARIANISM

Amitai Etzioni (1993), founder of the communitarian movement, sharply portrays the limitations of the rugged individualism for which Americans are famous and proposes a new balance between our rights as individuals and our social responsibilities. Believing that an allegiance to the shared values and institutions that sustain us is possible, in spite of our pluralism, he directs attention to the common good and calls for a revival of the ideal that small sacrifices by individuals can create large benefits for most all of us. As citizens in the United States struggle to reform health care, the communitarian challenge to set aside individual differences and interests to achieve the laudable goals of access for all, high-quality care, and affordable cost assumes a special urgency and one seemingly compatible with nursing's agenda.

Relevant to the preceding comments about virtue theory, communitarians argue that what youngsters require is to develop the basic personality traits that characterize effective individuals and to acquire core values—in a word, character development.

We mean by *character* the psychological muscles that allow a person to control impulses and defer gratification, which is essential for achievement, performance, and moral conduct. The *core values,* which need to be transmitted from generation to generation, contain moral substances that those with the proper basic personality can learn to appreciate, adapt, and integrate into their lives: hard work pays, even in an unfair world; treat others with the same basic dignity with which you wish to be treated (or face the consequences); you feel better when you do what is right than when you evade your moral precepts (Etzioni, 1994, p. 91).

ETHIC OF CARE

Dissatisfaction with the principle-based approach to nursing ethics, combined with attentiveness to Gilligan's ground-breaking work (1982) in moral development, has led some nurse theorists to begin to articulate an ethic of care (Benner & Wrubel, 1989; Fry, 1989; Watson, 1985). Central to this perspective is the nature of the nurse-patient relationship and attention to the particulars of individual patients viewed within the context of their life's narrative. Rejecting a reductionistic, mechanistic approach to healing, the care perspective calls for a phenomenologic methodology that invites caregivers to empathically enter the patient's world. Characteristics of the care perspective include the following: centrality of the caring relationship, promotion of dignity, respect of patients as people, acceptance of particular patient and health care beliefs, norms of responsiveness and responsibility, and a redefinition of fundamental moral skills (Taylor, 1993). As yet undecided is whether the ethic of care provides sufficient grounding for a distinct theory of nursing ethics.

■ Ethics and Aging

As members of the moral community of health care professionals entrusted with securing the well-being of older adults, gerontologic nurses have a moral obligation to understand and participate in the contemporary moral debate about ethical issues and aging. This chapter highlights four areas of controversy: intergenerational justice, age-based rationing, good dying for older adults, and autonomy and long-term care.

INTERGENERATIONAL JUSTICE

Intergenerational justice is problematic at both the macro and micro levels. When ex–Colorado governor Richard Lamm suggested that older adults have a duty to die to free up resources for younger adults, he sparked a national debate about intergenerational duties. To date there is no consensus about what society as a whole and what individuals owe older adults, nor consensus about what older adults owe society and individuals. For nurses and social workers, the issue often presents itself as a practical question about how much expense and hardship it is reasonable to expect the families of older adults to bear. Can family members refuse to provide care for an older relative who needs assistance with activities of daily living? And conversely, can an older parent refuse to assist an adult child in need of supportive care after discharge? With hospital and long-term care not an option for many older adults because of absent or deficient coverage or finances, home care is becoming a grave problem. Ethicists are beginning to assert the moral relevance of family interests when decisions are being made for individual patients (Blustein, 1993; Hardwig, 1990; Jecker, 1991; Kapp, 1991; Nelson, 1992).

Similar issues present themselves at the policy level as society struggles to distribute the benefits and costs of quality health care. Are older adults entitled to as much health care as they desire, regardless of the costs of this care? To what extent should younger citizens be taxed in order for the government to fund health care for older adults? Are the needs of children being sacrificed to support the entitlements of "greedy geezers"? What degree of sacrifice is reasonable to expect from affluent older adults to provide care for indigent older adults? Philosopher Norman Daniels (1988) offers as one way to avoid intergenerational warfare a "prudential saver" policy of distributive justice. He advocates that we approach the problem of distributing resources between age groups from the perspective of people prudently allocating resources throughout the stages of their own lives, rather than for distinct sets of people. This and other proposals are critiqued by Moody (1992).

Nurses who understand what is at stake for older adults in this dialogue at both the macro and micro levels and who can appreciate the financial and human costs of caregiving have a moral obligation to participate in these debates.

AGE-BASED RATIONING

In a book entitled *Setting Limits,* Dan Callahan (1987), director of the Hastings Center, stimulated public discussion about the future of health care for older adults and shocked many by proposing age as a specific criterion for the allocation and limitation of health care. Urging medicine to give up its relentless drive to extend the lives of older adults and turn its attention instead to the relief of their suffering and an improvement in their physical and mental quality of life, Callahan posits two conditions:

The first condition is that we need, both young and old, to understand that it is possible to live out a meaningful old age that is limited in time, one that does not require a compulsive effort to turn to medicine for more life to make it bearable. The second condition is that as a culture we need a supportive social context for aging and death, one that cherishes and respects the elderly while at the same time recognizing that their primary orientation should be to the young and the generations to come, not to the welfare of their own group (pp. 25-26).

Individuals can agree with Callahan that it is time to rethink the meaning and significance of old age, and yet differ dramatically about what this means for clinical decision making and public policy. Whereas some favor public policy that cites an arbitrary chronologic age as justification for limiting aggressive therapy such as cardiac bypass surgery or dialysis (e.g., no bypass surgery or dialysis for people older than 65 years of age), others prefer to individualize decision making and would only limit treatment for older adults who believe that they have lived their lives and are ready to die. At issue are the questions of who decides when an individual is too old for certain types of care and what criteria are used to make this decision. And whereas attention to the chronic problems of aging is a central theme of Callahan, Battin (1987) has proposed that in an age-based rationing system, direct termination of the lives of older adults more nearly achieves justice than denying them treatment. Two texts deal exclusively with the topic of age-based rationing, examining ethical, legal, medical, and economic consequences (Binstock and Post, 1991; Smeeding et al., 1987).

GOOD DYING FOR OLDER ADULTS

Few today think of death as something totally beyond human control. Some enlist the support of science and technology to rob old age of its infirmities and death itself, whereas others choose to die early, mastering the means and moment of their dying. There is no easy or agreed upon answer for what it means for older adults to die well, but gerontologic nurses must consider the options carefully.

Compassionate palliative care

As the ranks of older adults swell and health care dollars are increasingly targeted to those who represent the best investment risk, keeping compassionate palliative care that is responsive to the particular needs of individual dying patients as an option for older adults will be a real challenge. Gerontologic nurses committed to this type of care do the following:

- Keep all nursing care patient centered
- Clearly articulate the goal of therapy (a comfortable and dignified death) and ensure that the entire team is committed to this goal
- Develop a care system in which it is clearly communicated that comfort and palliation are valued as highly as restoration and cure
- Challenge the dangerous health care professional belief that death is always the enemy and a symbol of failure
- Continue to educate about ethical norms governing the use or nonuse of life-sustaining therapies; respect a patient's right to refuse minimally effective or disproportionately burdensome treatments
- Identify the caregiver competencies that are essential to providing quality compassionate

care and hold caregivers accountable for these competencies
- Value and reward creative care strategies for addressing the fears that underlie requests for voluntary active euthanasia or assisted suicide

Rational suicide

The suicide rate for older people increased steadily and more rapidly than that for any other group during the 1980s. Notably, many of these suicides (one thinks immediately of that of psychologist Bruno Bettelheim) were lauded by the media, who affirmed the ability and willingness to meet death on one's own terms. Interestingly, however, rational suicide in general, and more specifically, rational suicide on grounds of old age, remains a contested concept. Whereas many see it as the last definitive act of one who has always prized independence and being in charge, others question whether one can ever freely choose to end one's life. Harry Moody (1992), deputy director of the Brookdale Center on Aging, writes, "Rational old-age suicide is wrong because it violates deep values of community: relationship, solidarity, and indeed an intergenerational ideal of the human life cycle" (p. 87).

Assisted suicide and voluntary euthanasia

Referenda proposing right-to-die legislation that would legalize physician-assisted suicide and death by lethal injection on humanitarian grounds have been narrowly defeated in Washington and California. However, the measure passed in Oregon, although it was immediately challenged. Furthermore, the initiative continues and is active in several states. As society contemplates the advisability of rescinding the taboo on causing our own or another's death for humane and compassionate reasons, experienced gerontologic nurses must weigh the pro and con arguments on voluntary euthanasia and speak to their potential consequences for older adults. Medical ethicist Edmund Pellegrino (1991) summarizes the major arguments (Box 22-3).

As increasing numbers of older adults request suicide assistance and euthanasia, caregivers

BOX 22-3 ARGUMENTS FOR AND AGAINST VOLUNTARY EUTHANASIA

ARGUMENTS IN FAVOR OF VOLUNTARY EUTHANASIA

1. It is a beneficent and compassionate act.
2. It respects autonomy by preserving the patient's control of the manner, method, and timing of death.
3. It takes the matter outside the reach of "medical power" and scrupulosity.
4. It prevents the injustice that allows some patients to choose death by refusal of life support measures, while denying others the right to do so by active euthanasia.
5. In a pluralistic society, euthanasia must be accepted, whatever its intrinsic morality, since states have no moral justification for intruding into such private decisions.

Proponents of involuntary euthanasia argue that, in addition, it is irrational to afford rights of personhood to anencephalics or patients in a permanent vegetative state and unjust to deny them the right to die to which they are entitled. They argue that beneficence to the patient, family, and health care professionals, as well as conservation of society's resources, makes involuntary euthanasia a positive moral duty of physicians.

ARGUMENTS AGAINST DIRECT VOLUNTARY EUTHANASIA

1. It undermines the value of, and respect for, all human life.
2. Guidelines cannot avoid sliding down the slippery slope to involuntary euthanasia and selective devaluation of the lives of the most vulnerable among us.
3. Euthanasia should be unnecessary since the major reasons for requesting it—intolerable pain and fear of overtreatment—can now be handled by better palliative care, analgesia, and advance directives.
4. A focus on euthanasia will deviate attention from other valuable, palliative techniques.
5. If euthanasia is made legal, it is predicted that patients will feel a subtle pressure to conform so as to relieve the economic and emotional burdens they impose on family and friends.
6. Euthanasia is socially destructive: it undermines trust in physicians and health care professionals, desensitizes society to killing, and imperils the grounds already gained in legitimating passive euthanasia.
7. The religious belief of many Americans is that human life is the gift of the Creator and that humans are its stewards but not its absolute masters.

From Pellegrino, E.D. (1991). Ethics [Contempo issue]. *Journal of the American Medical Association, 265*(23), 3118-3119.

begin to examine factors contributing to these requests. Fear of dying alone, dying in intractable pain, losing control, bankrupting family, and becoming an intolerable burden—these are the most common reasons cited for wanting to choose the time and manner of one's death. Whatever beliefs one holds about the morality of suicide and voluntary euthanasia, it is critical to address and, where possible, to alleviate these fears so that older adults who choose suicide or voluntary euthanasia are doing so freely. Euthanasia should never become the quick fix that relieves us of our obligation to care.

It is no longer farfetched to conceive of euthanasia as society's remedy for the dilemma of how to care for rising numbers of increasingly older adults. Consider Battin's argument for direct termination of the lives of older adults mentioned previously. And should not enough older adults choose to terminate their lives at an appropriate age, voluntary euthanasia can pave the way to involuntary and nonvoluntary euthanasia. This would allow physicians to terminate the lives of older people who lack the capacity to choose this for themselves (involuntary) and for those who aren't wise enough to see that it would really be better for them and all involved if their lives were ended (nonvoluntary). In the Netherlands, where voluntary euthanasia is an accepted, if not legal, option, involuntary euthanasia is already a reality.

At stake in these debates is literally the way in which millions of older adults will spend their last days and moments. Gerontologic nurses who have cared for dying older people have a moral obligation to bring insights gleaned from their experience to the discussion of these options.

AUTONOMY AND LONG-TERM CARE

Among our most prized human abilities is the freedom to choose in light of goods. Individuals are autonomous to the extent that they are self-determining. Much of the bioethics debate in the United States has focused on how we can safeguard the rights of patients to be autonomous. Countering an era of paternalistic medicine in which physicians routinely disregarded the right of patients to be self-determining, bioethicists counseled an ethic of noninterference that left patients free to consent to or to refuse treatment. The growing tendency to not interfere in health care decision making has some physicians reluctant even to offer a recommendation when more than one option exists.

Although older adults today are for the most part free to decide how much and what type of health care they desire, important voices have been raised challenging the adequacy of a noninterference model of autonomy for older adults. Collopy (1988) rejects a negative-rights definition of autonomy, which merely prohibits caregivers

from interfering in older adults' decision making, and calls for a positive-rights approach to autonomy, which obligates caregivers to advocate for, enlarge, and enhance the autonomy of older adults by providing the necessary resources and assistance. He cautions that although many institutionalized older adults have decisional autonomy, that is, the capacity and freedom to make decisions about their lives, they lack executional autonomy—the ability and the freedom to carry out these decisions. Deficient executional autonomy should in no way cause us to ignore an older person's decisional autonomy.

Expanding these themes further, Agich (1993) distinguishes between actual and ideal autonomy, arguing that actual autonomy is better revealed in the everyday experiences of long-term care than in dramatic, conflict-ridden paradigm situations such as decisions to institutionalize, to initiate aggressive treatments, or to withhold or withdraw life-sustaining treatments. Questioning if the choices actually afforded individuals in long-term care are meaningful or worth making, he writes the following:

Respecting the autonomy of persons in long-term care entails a commitment to identifying and establishing conditions that encourage individuals to face adversity and threats to self that are the inevitable result of the illnesses and functional deteriorations that bring elders to long-term care in the first place . . . This means that elders must be treated as individuals, as unique persons with identifiable personal histories and a rich store of experiences and memories (p. 113).

Nurse ethicist Sally Gadow would applaud the work of Collopy and Agich because she advocated a model of existential advocacy for nurses back in 1980. In existential advocacy, individuals are assisted in exercising their freedom of self-determination authentically. An authentic decision is one that is consistent with one's values and interests. Nurses using this model help patients to clarify their values and goals and then assist and support patients as they freely choose in light of these values and goals. The existential advocacy model claims a significant moral role for nurses in patient care. Gerontologic nurses must choose for themselves whether or not to nurse in a way that makes advocacy possible. Nurses can, however, begin to demand ethical competence in advocacy from one another and support one another in attempts to master the advocacy skills that will win respect from colleagues and the credibility and authority to serve patients in this capacity.

■ Clinical Ethics and Nursing

Clinical ethics is an interdisciplinary activity that seeks to identify, analyze, prevent, and resolve ethical problems that arise in the care of particular patients. The major thrust of clinical ethics is to work for outcomes that best serve the interests and welfare of patients and their families. Gerontologic nurses who are sensitive to the ethical dimensions of practice can play a leadership role in preventing and resolving ethical conflict by developing the advocacy competencies highlighted in Box 22-4.

SUPPORTING THE AUTONOMY OF OLDER ADULTS

Individuals with intact decision-making capacity have the right to consent to and to refuse all medically indicated therapy. Nurses who know older patients well need to participate in determinations of capacity. Criteria for decision-making capacity include the following: (1) the ability to comprehend information relevant to the decision at hand, (2) the ability to deliberate in accord with a relatively consistent set of values and goals, and (3) the ability to communicate preferences. In light of the fact that older adults may be reasoning in accord with values and goals that differ from those of the care team, it is important to refute challenges to their capacity arising from differences in values. For example, it is not necessarily unreasonable that an older adult should choose dying with intact limbs over consenting to a life-saving amputation—even if this would not be the health care practitioner's choice.

It is important for nurses working with older adults to support authentically autonomous decision making, that is, to ensure that decisions reflect the identity, decisional history, and moral norms of the patient. A nursing home resident's refusal to eat may reflect an authentic wish to die or may result from a reversible depression or misperception that he or she is too much of a burden to others to continue living. When institutional, caregiver, or family interests interfere with the autonomy of the older adult, nurse advocates will support the older adult and ensure that his or her interests are protected.

Lack of decision-making capacity does not of itself negate the right to be self-determining. So long as the preferences of the incapacitated individual are known, these are to be respected. Nurses advocating for older adults document evidence of capacity carefully and work with the team to elicit and record the preferences of patients with intact decision-making capacity. Advance directives, a living will, and/or a durable power of attorney for health care legally protect an individual's preferences concerning health care.

Finally, nurses may need to assist surrogate decision makers in understanding that their charge is to make the decision that the patient would have made if the patient were able. Valid moral surrogates have intact decision-making capacity, understand the information pertinent to the decision at hand, know the patient's preferences to the extent that this is possible, have no undue conflict of interest, and are not suffering severe emotional problems. Spouses who are legally valid surrogates but who are financially or emotionally dependent on a patient may make treatment decisions based on their own needs rather than the interests of the patient. Nurse advocates can teach such surrogates that their charge is to be a voice for a now incapacitated patient and to decide as the patient would decide.

PROMOTING THE WELL-BEING OF OLDER ADULTS

The first task of the nurse advocate is to work with the patient, family, and health care team to clarify the appropriate goal of therapy: cure and

BOX 22-4 ADVOCACY COMPETENCIES

SUPPORTING AUTONOMY

1. Determining and documenting the patient's decision-making capacity
2. Protecting the right of patients with decision-making capacity to be self-determining
   a. Facilitate communication and documentation of the patient's preferences
   b. Anticipate the types of treatment decisions that are likely to need to be made
   c. Assist in the preparation of advance directives
3. Promoting authentic autonomy; authentic decisions reflect the individual's identity, decisional history, and moral norms
4. Identifying the morally, as well as legally, valid surrogate decision maker
5. Supporting the surrogate decision maker; clarifying the surrogate decision maker's role
6. Identifying limits to patient or surrogate autonomy and limits to caregiver autonomy

PROMOTING PATIENT GOOD

1. Clarifying the goal of therapy: cure and restoration; stabilization of functioning; preparation for a comfortable, dignified death
2. Determining the effectiveness of therapy
3. Weighing the benefits and burdens of therapy
4. Ensuring that all interventions are consistent with the overall goal of therapy
5. Ensuring that the patient's priority needs are addressed (bio-psycho-social-spiritual needs)
6. Ensuring continuity of care as the patient is transferred among services, and intrainstitutionally and interinstitutionally
7. Weighing the moral relevance of third-party interests (family, caregiver, institutional, societal)

PREVENTING AND RESOLVING ETHICAL CONFLICT

1. Establishing that preventing and resolving ethical conflict falls within the authority of all health care professionals engaged in the care of a patient
2. Facilitating timely communication among those involved in decision making: one-on-one meetings; periodic meetings of the patient, family, and interdisciplinary team to clarify goals and plan of care; ethics consult or meeting of the institutional ethics committee
3. Developing awareness of and sensitivity to the conscious and unconscious sources of conflict
4. Documenting pertinent information on the patient record

restoration, stabilization of functioning, or preparation for a comfortable, dignified death. Although the need for clarification would seem to be a given, confusion often exists, making it difficult to ensure that all interventions are consistent with the goal. For example, in the late stages of Alzheimer's disease, whether or not one decides to initiate or continue artificial nutrition and hydration depends upon whether the agreed-upon goal is stabilization of functioning or preparation for a comfortable, dignified death. Obviously, treatment goals may need revision when a patient or resident makes unexpected progress or fails to progress. The families of incapacitated, frail, and debilitated patients may need great support in determining what is in the best interests of the patient, and in deciding when to treat a condition aggressively and when to let nature take its course. Unfortunately, there is no clear line to be drawn between promoting life and needlessly prolonging dying.

Pellegrino (1989) recommends analysis of therapy along two lines: effectiveness and benefit-burden ratio. A treatment is effective to the degree that it reverses or ameliorates the natural progression of the disease. The appropriate antibiotic for an infection is effective therapy. This is an objective medical determination—to the degree that medicine as a science can be objective. Whether or not the antibiotic is beneficial, that is, whether it advances the overall best interests of the patient and outweighs the burdens of therapy, is, however, a subjective determination that can only be made by the patient or by those who know the patient best. Nurses may need to remind physicians that more is at stake in treatment decisions than whether or not the proposed therapy is "medically indicated." Nurses' knowledge is also critical when determining the probability that a particular intervention will contribute to or compromise a goal such as comfort.

Nurses advocating for the patient's interests will also ensure that the patient's priority needs (bio-psycho-social-spiritual needs) are addressed. As health care reform results in increasing fragmentation of services, the likelihood that older adults will be cared for by health care professionals, including nurses, who know them well is decreasing. Nurse managers must critique nursing systems of care that result in no one nurse being responsible for the overall plan of care and identification and resolution of concerns of high priority to patients and families. All too frequently the only patient problems receiving attention today are physical problems. This is of special concern in residential treatment facilities, where older adults may be totally dependent upon caregivers to meet their needs. It is nursing's charge to ensure that wholistic, individualized, prioritized care is a reality for today's older adults.

PREVENTING AND RESOLVING ETHICAL CONFLICT

Gerontologic nurses who wish to prevent ethical conflict will function in care settings where it is established that preventing and resolving ethical conflict falls within the authority of each health care professional engaged in a patient's care. This conviction will facilitate timely communication among all those involved in decision making: one-on-one meetings; periodic meetings of the patient, family, and interdisciplinary team to clarify treatment goals and the plan of care; and ultimately an ethics consult or meeting of the institutional ethics committee if necessary. Sensitivity to, and the ability to communicate about, the factors contributing to ethical conflict are essential to successful mediation of these conflicts. When mediation is not attempted, conflicts tend to escalate and it is not unusual for patients and families to develop hostile, adversarial relationships that all too frequently result in litigation or, at the very least, alienation and a distrust of health care professionals; this, in turn, can color future interactions with caregivers. Gerontologic nurses should be aware of and use wisely the ethics resources available in their institutions and professional community. The National Reference Center for Bioethics Literature offers free bioethics information and computerized literature search assistance (Box 22-5). Mastery of a process of ethical decision making to simplify conflict resolution is also important.

■ Process of Ethical Decision Making

When providing care for older adults, nurses encounter two types of moral problems (Jameton, 1993). *Moral dilemmas* occur when two or more clear moral principles apply but no choice presents itself that preserves both. Caregivers making discharge plans for a frail and debilitated older woman believe that discharge to a nursing home is the only way to ensure the patient's well-being. Competent, the woman insists upon returning to her home and says that somehow

BOX 22-5 NATIONAL REFERENCE CENTER FOR BIOETHICS LITERATURE

Kennedy Institute of Ethics
Georgetown University
Washington, DC 20057
Toll-free phone number: 800-MED-ETHX

A specialized collection of library resources concerned with contemporary biomedical issues in the fields of ethics, philosophy, medicine, nursing, science, law, religion, and the social sciences.

Call for bioethics information; BIOETHICS-LINE searches (computerized data base); search strategies; reference help; publication orders.

she will manage. Respect for her autonomy entails accepting her decision, whereas the strong desire to prevent harm and benefit the patient argues for ignoring her wishes to go home. *Moral distress* arises in situations in which nurses make a moral judgment about a case in which they are involved and the institution or co-workers make it difficult or impossible for the nurse to act on that judgment. When the woman just described develops a strangulated hernia before her discharge and adamantly refuses surgical repair, her nurse ultimately decides that her refusal should be respected. The patient understands that certain death is the consequence of this choice and seems to be freely choosing this outcome. When her physicians order surgery, believing that no one should be allowed to die this way, and close the case to discussion, the nurse finds herself strongly opposed to an order she is powerless to change.

The objective of ethical reasoning when one experiences a moral dilemma is to analyze the ethical dimensions of a clinical problem in hopes of resolving the dilemma or mediating a compromise. The objective of ethical reasoning when experiencing moral distress is to analyze one's moral responsibility to act, given institutional, bureaucratic, or professional constraints. The nursing process provides a sound framework for facilitating ethical reasoning and decision making in both instances. During the diagnosis phase of the process, an ethical problem is identified, not a nursing diagnosis. This framework is highlighted in Box 22-6. What follows is an application of this framework for a dilemma experienced by gerontologic nurses caring for a nursing home resident who begins to refuse food, stating that she wants to die.

ASSESSMENT

The patient is an 82-year-old, widowed resident currently being treated with radiation therapy for a pituitary tumor. Her medical history includes high blood pressure, coronary artery disease, and degenerative joint disease. She moved to this life-care community 6 years ago, and 6 months ago was moved out of her apartment to the skilled nursing floor because of increasing weakness and inability to meet daily needs. She recently reported that she has spent her whole life helping others and now that she can no longer do this she wants to die. She has no children or close family relatives. A devout Methodist, she was actively involved in church work throughout her life. She gets cards and occasional visits from church members she has helped in the past.

The nurse coordinator and aides on this unit are becoming very concerned about her nutritional status because she has returned each meal tray untouched for the last 48 hours. When one aide attempted to spoon food into the patient's mouth, she spit it out. Attempts to reason with her about her need to eat fall on deaf ears. Some aides think that her decision to stop eating should be respected; others say that this is the same thing as watching someone put a gun to his or her head, and that she must be stopped—forcefully if necessary. This is a for-profit, secular life-care community that does not have a policy

BOX 22-6 A PROCESS OF ETHICAL DECISION MAKING

ASSESSMENT

Gather and document pertinent medical and nonmedical facts.

Who: people involved and their relationship to decision needing to be made and authority for decision making and its consequences

What: patient's medical condition, prognosis, therapeutic options, and probable consequences of treatment and nontreatment; patient's beliefs, values, and interests; related family, caregiver, and institutional beliefs, values, and interests; pertinent legal and administrative considerations

When: time parameters

Where: setting

Why: variables creating and fueling conflict

DIAGNOSIS

Identify the ethical issue or issues as clearly as possible. Distinguish ethical problems from communication or general patient care management problems.

PLANNING AND GOAL IDENTIFICATION

1. Identify the objective of doing the ethics workup.
2. List and explore courses of action likely to achieve this goal. Think through the short- and long-term consequences of each.
3. Think of the ethical justification for each course of action and defend it against competing options:
   a. Compatibility with aims of nursing and demands of nurse-patient relationship
   b. Approaches to ethical inquiry: ethical principles, care perspective, virtue theory, and communitarianism
   c. Grounding and source of ethics: philosophic (based in reason), theologic (based in religion), or sociocultural (based in custom)
4. Clearly identify what you take to be the moral obligations of the nurse.
5. Select the course of action you are best able to defend against counter arguments.
6. Seek assistance if unable to work through the above steps independently.

IMPLEMENTATION

Implement the selected course of action and assess consequences.

EVALUATION

Critique your decision, incorporating feedback from involved participants if possible. Decide how you would respond to a similar case in the future. Determine whether or not you need to do something now to optimize future responses. Interventions may be personal (e.g., learn more about advance directives) or institutional (e.g., clarify the hospital's do-not-resuscitate [DNR] policy and reeducate caregivers about the policy).

on force-feeding older adults. The medical director, when called, recommends another day of trying to get the patient to eat but stopping short of force-feeding her. The patient is responding to radiation therapy, and it is very likely that she could live several more years. She states that she has no desire to do this. When she is told that starving herself to death is just like committing suicide, she responds that this doesn't bother her. She believes that God will understand because surely he can't expect her to endure much more. She denies physical pain, which is unrelieved by medication. She has no advance directive and, when asked, is unable to identify anyone she trusts to make health care decisions for her. "I can take care of myself," she says, "and I want you to write down that I'm tired of living and plan to just stop eating."

The nursing coordinator believes that a joint decision must be reached quickly (within 24 hours) that is acceptable to each nurse involved in feeding this resident so that a unified approach will prevail. She understands that among the nursing aides there are very different beliefs about the legitimacy of not intervening if it is decided that the resident is freely choosing to die.

DIAGNOSIS

The ethical dilemma is whether the nurses should respect this woman's decision to end her life by not eating and drinking, or whether they should intervene forcefully, when she is too weak to protest if need be, to ensure an adequate nutritional intake and prevent her death. It will be important to ascertain whether the resident has intact decision-making capacity and is freely deciding on this choice. Should a decision be made to respect the resident's choice, options available to nurses who cannot accept this should be identified.

PLANNING AND GOAL IDENTIFICATION

The objective of doing this ethics workup is to develop a plan of care for this resident that is respectful of her person, promotive of her well-being, and acceptable to those caring for her on an everyday basis.

The first priority is to determine if she possesses the decision-making capacity to freely choose to starve herself to death. If this is the case, options include the following: (1) allowing each nurse to decide for himself or herself how to respond to this dilemma (rejected immediately as unfair to the resident), (2) offering her food and fluid during each mealtime but not pressuring her in any way to eat or drink—accepting that she will die if she does not change her mind, (3) asking her to let someone know if she changes her mind but in the meantime not offering food and drink—accepting that she will die if she does not change her mind, and (4) insisting that she eat and drink and, should she refuse, initiating artificial nutrition and hydration when she is too weak to resist, using restraints if indicated once she becomes stronger.

If the patient lacks decision-making capacity, it is necessary to choose the option that is most consistent with what those who know her best believe she would want (substituted judgment decision-making standard). A legally (and morally) valid surrogate decision maker must be identified. If there are no family members or friends capable and willing to serve in this capacity, in selected situations the physician may assume this role; otherwise, a court-appointed guardian needs to be sought.

Initial discussion revealed that although many caregivers believed that the resident was understandably depressed about moving to the skilled care floor, it was also believed that this depression had not compromised her ability to weigh the consequences of her actions or to make an informed, voluntary choice. Her decision-making capacity was judged to be intact. A decision was made to have the nurse who knew the resident best try to elicit the reasons prompting her refusal to eat, so that these could be addressed to the extent possible (e.g., more discussion about her belief that she no longer had a reason to live because she was not able to care for others and was herself a burden). This was identified to be the priority intervention. Nurses expressed some guilt that they might have failed this resident and contributed to her conviction that her life was no longer worth living, and they discussed constructive ways to address this guilt. This course of action flowed from the ethic of care and the nature of the nurse-patient relationship that obligate nurses to empathically share the resident's world and advocate for her best interests. A model of simple noninterference was rejected. Caring obligated the nurses to intervene positively with the support that would ensure that this was an authentically autonomous decision, that is, consistent with the resident's identity, decisional history, and moral norms.

The nurses also decided that liquids should be available to the resident in her room and that she would be asked before each meal if she would like a tray, but that she would not be pressured to eat or drink. This course of action was made with the acknowledgment that many present believed that a decision to knowingly starve oneself to death is suicide. It was decided that any nurse who expressed moral or religious reasons for not caring for this resident would be assigned to other residents. This course of action was defended as being respectful of the resident's right to be self-determining (autonomy) and respectful of the integrity and moral autonomy of caregivers.

The strongest argument against this course of action was offered by one nurse who expressed the strong conviction that her commitment was to save lives and that she believed their joint duty was to prevent the harm of this resident starving herself to death even if it entailed forcing the resident to eat. The consensus, however, was that a greater harm would be inflicted on the resident if her will was violated in this regard and she was forcibly fed.

IMPLEMENTATION

The above plan of care was implemented. Conversations with the resident, who continued to

refuse to eat but who occasionally took sips of juice or water, revealed that she was quite peaceful with her decision. Attempts to explore with her reasons to reaffirm her commitment to living were gently but persistently refused. An interdisciplinary meeting was held to evaluate ongoing therapies, and once preparation for a comfortable, dignified death was accepted as being the appropriate therapeutic goal, radiation therapy was discontinued and comfort care was made her top priority. The resident became weaker and died 3 weeks later after developing bacterial pneumonia for which antibiotics were declined.

EVALUATION

Nurses caring for this resident generally expressed satisfaction with the team's approach to the resident's refusal to eat and gratitude that a unified approach was adopted. Some concern was expressed about insufficient documentation of the process of decision making, the resultant plan of care, and outcomes. A decision was made to invite the home's ethics consultant and risk manager to address the topic of documentation at the next unit meeting. One nurse volunteered to research the literature to report on how other staffs were dealing with the problem of refusal to eat.

■ Conclusion

Excellence in gerontologic nursing presumes moral competency. Older adults need nurses who are willing and able to challenge care teams and society to be responsive to their needs. Sensitivity to the moral dimensions of practice will foster recognition of the broad human needs of frail older adults and of the creative strategizing required to meet these needs.

REFERENCES

Agich, G.J. (1993). *Autonomy and long-term care.* New York: Oxford University Press.

American Nurses' Association. (1985). *Code for nurses with interpretive statements.* Washington, DC: Author.

American Nurses' Association. (1991). *Standards of clinical nursing practice.* Washington, DC: Author.

Battin, M.P. (1987). Age rationing and the just distribution of health care: Is there a duty to die? *Ethics, 97,* 317-340.

Beauchamp, T.L., & Childress, J.F (1994). *Principles of biomedical ethics* (4th ed.). New York: Oxford University Press.

Benner, P., & Wrubel, J. (1989). *The primacy of caring.* Menlo Park, CA: Addison-Wesley.

Binstock, R.H., & Post, S.G. (Eds.). (1991). *Too old for health care? Controversies in medicine, law, economics, and ethics.* Baltimore: Johns Hopkins University Press.

Blustein, J. (1993). The family in medical decision making. *Hastings Center Report, 23*(3), 6-13.

Callahan, D. (1987). *Setting limits: Medical goals in an aging society.* New York: Simon and Schuster.

Clouser, K.D., & Gert, B. (1994). Morality vs. principlism. In R. Gillon (Ed.), *Principles of health care ethics.* New York: John Wiley and Sons.

Daniels, N. (1988). *Am I my parents' keeper?* New York: Oxford University Press.

Etzioni, A. (1994). *The spirit of community: Rights, responsibilities, and the communitarian agenda.* New York: Crown.

Fry, S. (1989). The role of caring in a theory of nursing ethics. *Hypatia, 4,* 88-103.

Gadow, S. (1980). Existential advocacy: Philosophical foundations of nursing. In S.F. Spicker & S. Gadow (Eds.), *Nursing: Images and ideals—Opening dialogue with the humanities* (pp. 79-101). New York: Springer.

Gilligan, C. (1982). *In a different voice: Psychological theory and women's development.* Cambridge, MA: Harvard University Press.

Hardwig, J. (1990). What about the family? *Hastings Center Report, 20*(2), 5-10.

Jameton, A. (1993). Dilemmas of moral distress: Moral responsibility and nursing practice. *AWHONN's Clinical Issues in Perinatal and Women's Health Nursing, 4,* 542-551.

Jecker, N.S. (1991). *Aging and ethics: Philosophical problems in gerontology.* Clifton, NJ: Human Press.

Kapp, M.B. (1991). Health care decision making by the elderly: I get by with a little help from my family. *Gerontologist, 11,* 619-622.

Moody, H.R. (1992). *Ethics in an aging society.* Baltimore: Johns Hopkins University Press.

Nelson, J.L. (1992). Taking families seriously. *Hastings Center Report, 22*(4), 6-12.

Pellegrino, E.D. (1989). Withholding and withdrawing treatments: Ethics at the bedside. *Clinical Neurosurgery 35,* 164-184.

Pellegrino, E.D. (1991). Ethics [Contempo issue]. *Journal of the American Medical Association, 265*(23), 3118-3119.

Pellegrino, E.D., & Thomasma, D.C. (1993). *The virtues in medical practice.* New York: Oxford University Press.

Siegler, M. (1984). Should age be a criterion in health care? *Hastings Center Report, 14*(5), 24-27.

Smeeding, T.M., Battin, M.P., Francis, L.P., & Landesman, B.M. (Eds.). (1987). *Should medical care be rationed by age?* Totowa, NJ: Rowman and Littlefield.

Taylor, C. (1993). Nursing ethics: The role of caring. *AWHONN's Clinical Issues in Perinatal and Women's Health Nursing, 4*(4), 552-560.

Watson, J. (1985). *Nursing: The philosophy and science of caring.* Boulder: Colorado Associated University Press.

BIBLIOGRAPHY

American Association of Retired Persons. (1989). *A matter of choice: Planning ahead for health care decisions.* Washington, DC: Author.

American Hospital Association. (1991). *Put it in writing: A guide to promoting advance directives.* Chicago: Author.

Berlowitz, D.R., Wilking, S.V.B., & Moskowitz, M.A. (1991). Do-not-resuscitate orders at a chronic care hospital. *Journal of the American Geriatric Society, 8,* 472-476.

Buchanan, A.E., & Brock, D.W. (1989). *Deciding for others: The ethics of surrogate decision making.* New York: Cambridge University Press.

Callahan, D. (1990). *What kind of life: The limits of medical progress.* New York: Simon and Schuster.

Callahan, D. (1993). *The troubled dream of life.* New York: Simon and Schuster.

Collopy, B. (1988). Autonomy and long-term care: Some crucial distinctions. *Gerontologist, 28*(Suppl.), 10-17.

Concern for Dying. (1991). *Advance directive protocols and the Patient Self-Determination Act: A resource manual for the development of institutional protocols.* New York: Author.

Gadow, S. (1984, March 29). Gov. Lamm asserts elderly, if very ill, have "duty to die." *New York Times,* p. A16.

Hastings Center. (1987). *Guidelines on the termination of life-sustaining treatment and the care of the dying.* Bloomington and Indianapolis: Indiana University Press.

President's Commission for the Study of Ethical Problems in Medicine and Biomedical and Behavioral Research. (1982). *Making health care decisions* (Vols. 1-3). Washington, DC: U.S. Government Printing Office.

President's Commission for the Study of Ethical Problems in Medicine and Biomedical and Behavioral Research. (1983). *Deciding to forego life-sustaining treatment: Ethical, medical, and legal issues in treatment decisions.* Washington, DC: U.S. Government Printing Office.

Weir, R.F., & Gostin, L. (1990). Decisions to abate life-sustaining treatment for nonautonomous patients: Ethical standards and legal liability for physicians after Cruzan. *Journal of the American Medical Association, 264,* 1846-1853.

C H A P T E R   23

*The quality of a life's experience cannot
be measured in the same way as its quantity;
numbers of years may have little to do with
satisfactions in living.*

M.B. WEINER, A.J. BROK, AND A.M. SNADOWSKY,
Working with the Aged

The Future

■ Learning Objectives

On completion of this chapter, the reader will be able to do the following:

1. Appreciate the importance of stating ideas and contributing suggestions in public policy discussions to advance professional nursing.
2. Contribute to the refinement of nursing language, including nursing diagnoses, that will improve the understanding of nursing and encourage clear and frequent communication.
3. Emulate models of care that enable improved practice, research, and education to be understood and applied in patient care.
4. Prepare for and be prepared to cope with the adjustments that are anticipated to be imposed in the twenty-first century.

Only if a person were denied access to electronic or print media would that person be unaware of the prevalence of older adults in today's population. No matter the subject for discussion in the current media, it is difficult to ignore the ever-increasing numbers of older adults in social, civic, economic, or other gatherings of people. Awareness of one's surroundings and consciousness of one's associates present a clear message: there are increased numbers of older people in the population today. An examination of the status and the activities of these people—at this, the end of the twentieth century—leads to the question, What will be the status of older adults in the twenty-first century?

There is no magic wand to create situations for the future, nor is there a seer to portray what the future will hold in terms of the numbers of older adults or the status of older adults. The best we can do is to look at some of the events that are occurring today and project *what might be the future* for older adults in the years ahead. This chapter presents some of the ideas that have been suggested by people who have worked with older adults in the recent past and by our discussions and collaborations with others who are equally interested in and concerned about what will happen to older adults in the future. Some of the trends that can now be identified point to the directions that one can expect to be taken in the future.

The availability of educational opportunities and of various and diverse experiences—both personal and professional—and the opening of windows of opportunity around the globe have all contributed to the development of the professional nurse's expertise. As numbers of older people increase in the world, the nurse observes people in various states of health, residing in various settings that are more or less conducive to maintaining health, with full recognition of the responsibility for assisting and/or supporting a few or many of the people who are amenable to the benefits the nurse can offer.

■ Future Roles of Nursing

Few people debate the issues that are ahead in the world of professional nursing. Rather, debate revolves around the "how" of coping with the challenges that will be faced. This chapter considers the debatable issues of coping with the challenges that will occur.

The following statements summarize the present state of affairs and suggest what lies ahead:

Throughout the world, health care is undergoing dramatic transition, perhaps better described as a quiet revolution. And clearly, the health profession most affected by these changes is nursing. The intensely technological components, physician-driven components of health care, will remain in hospitals, while the care, comfort, rehabilitation, education and counseling—the nursing piece—has shifted to community settings along with the nurses who provide it (Dreher, 1995).

The nurses of this latter part of the twentieth century are much more savvy than were the nurses of pre–World War II. They are an articulate group of professionals, and they are knowledgeable about the issues that are critical to their survival and the welfare of the people who will be dependent on their expertise in the twenty-first century. This group of caregivers will be able to use their abilities to speak, analyze situations, and establish priorities that will ultimately benefit the health care givers, as well as the health

care consumers. Recognition of the influence of the political system in the United States will thrust the nurses into that arena to state their cases and to plead for justice in the workplace, as well as justice in the care system for the consumers of health care. A recent report from an attorney and policy analyst suggests five challenges as the new century approaches; it will be important to do the following:

1. Demonstrate that nurses provide cost-effective, high-quality care that can be measured. Good and valid data are needed to illustrate the cost of care, as well as patient outcomes.
2. Adopt uniform licensure and educational requirements for the nursing profession and establish fewer and simpler titles.
3. Overcome the mentality of an oppressed minority. Develop the self-confidence necessary to provide leadership in clinical situations, as well as in positions of administration and government.
4. Accept the reality of job insecurity; other health care givers, besides nurses, will be faced with the same downsizing.
5. Sustain a commitment to lifelong professional learning. This is one of the defining characteristics of professionals (Hadley, 1996).

To emphasize the significance that nursing will achieve in the twenty-first century, Hadley (1996) pays tribute to Florence Nightingale, who used her intellect and her compassion to shape the nursing profession. Nightingale recognized, more than 100 years ago, that nursing outcomes must be measured with good data. The quality of good nursing care must be measured and documented to be valued. The following quotation accompanies a portrait of Florence Nightingale: "To understand God's thoughts we must study statistics, for these are the measure of His purpose." Careful reading of this quote suggests that it expresses the relationship among epidemiology, biostatistics, and the health of populations that is at the heart of public health and managed care. Hadley pleads with nurses to combine this intellectual legacy with the well-known compassion of nursing to master both the political and economic marketplaces (Hadley, 1996).

■ Changes and Transitions in Aging

As one ponders the thought of aging, whether it be the aging of self or of others, it is the optimist's view of aging that is most appealing. A review of all the benefits of aging and careful reflection on the "good life" can produce happy thoughts and good feelings about self and those nearby. Although it is the pessimist's tendency to think negatively, to think of all the wrong things that will occur as "age creeps up," observation of aging people reveals that there are often many more positives than there are negatives about the process of aging.

For example, one of the prevalent fears among older adults is that brain function will be impaired as they age. This fear is especially strong if the aging person has been mentally active and very much involved in multiple cerebral activities. A recent study confirms what some scientists have long believed: brain power decreases very little in healthy people as they age. As a result of a study conducted by Dr. John Morris, it was concluded that impairment of brain function is a result of disease, not age (Crowley, 1996). Reports of studies such as this one are important to share with people who are concerned about what the future might hold.

Literature and conversations about the fears that are faced by older adults often revolve around concern about change; they are fears about the changes that will, or might, occur as people grow older. Some of the concerns are very real—based on factual data that are available now. Some of the concerns are not reality based—they have no basis in fact. One of the approaches to helping the older person cope with these fears is to distinguish between "transition" and "change"; it is helpful in adjusting the perspective of the older person and the caregiver, especially if there is an undue focus on change. A dictionary definition of *change* suggests that this term means to substitute one thing for another, to adopt one thing in place of another; change tends to be abrupt. The idea of transition, however, suggests a process that occurs over time; there is a sense of flow and movement. For example, a brief, self-limiting illness usually creates some necessary changes. Few people have not experienced an upper respiratory tract infection, and no one looks forward to such an experience. Various changes must be made in work schedules, in activities of daily living, in eating schedules, and in sleeping routines, and these changes usually continue for a number of days. All who experience this type of illness know that an adjustment in living is necessary, but they also know that these changes are not prolonged. Very soon the ill person will be able to return to the usual schedule. At the same time, a chronic illness has been viewed as requiring a process of transition that goes beyond the realm of change. An illness that requires major adjustments in life patterns is viewed as creating a major transition in one's lifestyle. For instance, an occurrence of cancer, bronchiectasis, diabetes, or other major interruption in life pattern will be considered in a different manner than a head cold. A period of change can occur, but most likely, the chronic ailment will require major transitions in living patterns. Internal processes usually make up the process of transition, whereas external processes tend to characterize change (Bridges, 1991; Meleis & Trangenstein, 1994).

■ Changes in Nursing Frameworks

Whether concerned with change or with transition, caregivers need a framework or a structure within which care can be planned and given. To enable universal acceptance of what is the caregiver's responsibility, a clear statement is needed to define the responsibility of the nurse to the patients for whom the nurse cares. Since 1992, the Congress of Nursing Practice has been revising the social policy statement for nursing.

This 3- to 4-year effort on the part of many nurses in the United States has resulted in the acceptance and publication of a social policy statement that represents nursing's commitment to society and to the people who are served by the professionals. It is a document that nurses can use as a framework for understanding "nursing's obligation to those who receive nursing care" (American Nurses' Association [ANA], 1995). With this as a basis for planning the directions for the twenty-first century, nurses can proceed with a sound framework for setting directions for the future.

Significant strides have been made in nursing since midcentury; the twentieth century will be noted for defining the historical development of nursing theory and nursing diagnosis, as well as for providing a clear definition of nursing. In 1980 the ANA defined nursing as "the diagnosis and treatment of human response to actual or potential health problems" (p. 9). At the North American Nursing Diagnosis Association (NANDA) conference inclusive in 1990, a more inclusive definition of nursing was accepted that is more inclusive of the full range of nursing thought and that reflects a wholistic approach to the patient. The following definition was found quite acceptable: Nursing diagnosis is a clinical judgment about an individual, family, or community response to actual or potential health problems or life processes. Nursing diagnosis provides the basis for selection of nursing interventions to achieve outcomes for which the nurse is accountable (NANDA, 1992).

After many years of work and much energy expenditure by many nurses, the NANDA Foundation will be incorporated by the end of 1996. This will enable NANDA to continue the development of a nursing language for the international classification of nursing practice.

Having defined the framework for nursing via *Nursing's Social Policy Statement* (American Nurses Publishing, 1995), the next logical step in defining nursing's responsibility was to accept the *Scope and Standards of Gerontological Clinical Nursing Practice* (ANA, 1995). Once these revised data were discussed and promulgated, they were accepted and the directions were clear for examining and analyzing the essence of nursing in a more profound way than had been done in the past.

It can be predicted that multiple efforts will continue to be pursued to clarify the definition of nursing. One of the more profound discussions that have recently been addressed is that of *data bases.* An appointed group became the ANA steering committee on data bases to support clinical nursing practice. Topics for discussion included the following: electronic information activities; the ways, means, and rationales for linking nursing research language with the clinical language of nursing; and the progress of the International Council of Nurses (ICN) project on an international classification of nursing practice (ICNP). With multiple efforts such as these, coming from multiple sources, the involvement of nurses will be encouraged for many of these data base projects. The National Library of Medicine (NLM) has been examining linkages between the NLM staff nomenclatures and ANA-recognized nursing nomenclatures. One of the major goals is to incorporate the nursing interventions classification (NIC) and the OMAHA system into the metathesaurus. This linkage will assist in the development of a unified nursing language, as well as examining the implications for staff nurses. This is a strategic goal that will bear watching in the immediate future ("Steering Committee," 1995).

Another role for which nurses will be responsible in the not-too-distant future is that of advocacy. Traditionally, nurses have perceived themselves as being the patient's advocate, although this has been more difficult in some places than in others. The ANA position statement on ethics and human rights calls for nurses to value the differences among persons. British epidemiologist Sir Richard Doll considered the greatest threats to health to be poverty, pollution, and population. A member of the ANA board of directors, Thomas Stenvig, added prejudice, suggesting that in today's practice we must be concerned about threats of economic or political prejudice that pose a threat to human rights (Burtt, 1995).

■ The Changing Face of Health Care

In the 1990s the system of health care is quite different than it was in the past. Whether the differences can be labeled "transitions" or "changes," the fact is that the face of health care is hardly recognizable from what it was in the past. The regulation of health professions and occupations is being questioned, and a major overhaul of the licensure systems throughout the country is being debated. Some of this initiative is the result of efforts to protect the consumers; other causes are directed at removing government and insurance interference. As a result of this increased visibility of the health care system, several foundations with ample financial resources are becoming interested in extending their finances to the health care arena. The Pew Charitable Trust is one such foundation. One of their many projects is the Pew Health Professions Commission, which is looking at approaches to reforming state educational, workforce planning, and licensure systems of health professionals so that they can better cope with the demands of the present health care system. A task force was convened to explore "health professions education, governance, credentialing and regulation and recommend improvements to the regulatory system" (Whittaker and Minich, 1995).

The recommendations of the Pew task force are being reviewed by professional leaders in nursing, and stress is being placed on pursuing interdisciplinary collaboration and assurance of continued competency of health care personnel. ANA has been and is resisting a "consolidated board of Medicine/Nursing care." The concern regarding this idea is that such a board would lead to renewed efforts by medicine to control nursing practice and to limit its scope.

Among the Pew recommendations are the closing of 20% of the nation's medical schools and reducing the number of new professionals, including nurses, by 10% to 25% to prepare for the massive hospital closings that are predicted by the year 2000. Hadley (1996) cautions that nurses need to prepare for the inevitable dislocation that will result from hospital downsizing, as well as other dramatic changes that are apt to occur in the health delivery system. (A full copy of the Pew task force report can be obtained by writing to Pew Health Professions Commission Task Force on Health Care Workforce Regulation, UCSF Center for the Health Professions, 1388 Sutter Street, Suite 805, San Francisco, CA 94109.)

Even as the focus is upon change and there are attempts to envision what will be the changes of tomorrow, there are certain messages that are evident now. It is possible to visualize many more older people in the United States in the years ahead than are encountered today. Barring a major catastrophe, it is unlikely that the population of this country will decrease. The message that health care givers and providers can count on is this: get ready for increased numbers of patients of all ages, especially older patients. Related to this message, it seems that predictions can include struggles with establishing a system that will enable health care problems to be cared for, and along with that, there will be struggles to provide for the economic problems that will accompany the health care challenges. Three factors seem to be critical in this regard:

- There is concern over the number of people who will need care in the future.
- There is an expected dilemma in regard to defining and establishing the system that will enable care of older adults.

• There is concern about the economic factors that will be faced in resolving this dilemma.

Changes that will be seen, undoubtedly, as a result of advances today are the following: increased methods of treatment (new medications, new technologies, and new approaches to care); different approaches to therapies, whether new or traditional; and changes in assigned responsibilities for personal care.

■ Educational Issues in the Future of Nursing

Most people, especially educators, would agree that a major influence in setting directions for the future involves education. Not only is it possible to influence learners by word and by action, but it is also possible to influence observers by role-modeling what are desirable and recommended ways of performing selected professional functions. When considering health care responsibilities, the education of health care givers becomes critical to preparing those who will care for people who are in need of attention and care.

A review of literature will reveal a number of models of care that can be duplicated and emulated by those who are in clinical practice, in administration, doing clinical research, and performing as educators. In addition to reading the reports of experiences that can act as models, a productive way of acquiring knowledge about improving practice in the care of older adults is attending the meetings of people who have acted as pioneers in the planning and implementation of care models. One such meeting was held in December 1995. The dialogue among this group was historic in nature, and the written reports to follow will contain critical information that will help others in the care of older adults.

This meeting of well-known gerontologic nursing leaders underscores the significance and importance of considering the future of gerontologic nursing. It was at this invitational conference in New York City that these influential professionals met under an "umbrella" of *Gerontological Nursing Partnerships between Practice and Education: Learning from the Past—Designing for the Future.* This conference presented the opportunity to review several projects that were funded by well-known organizations with the hope that the care of older adults would be improved. The outcomes of the meeting included the following: recognition of the changing demography of older adults in America; opportunity to describe the salient characteristics of the nursing home projects that were conducted during a 10-year period; analysis of the good and not-so-good outcomes of the projects; recognition of the implications of fiscal and other factors that relate to the success of any project; and identification of opportunities for student learning and for interdisciplinary training in the various projects.

Each of the projects can be considered a model for functioning with older adults and for the ultimate goal of realizing positive benefits in gerontologic nursing.

■ Projects Aimed at Improving Care of Older Adults

The Community College Nursing Home Partnership Project modeled situations in which partnerships were built between two community-based organizations—the community college and the nursing home. The partnerships resulted in improved care of older adults, as well as stimulating curricular changes in associate degree education.

The Robert Wood Johnson Teaching Nursing Home Projects were located in 11 different sites with the ultimate goal of expanding the clinical, educational, and research initiatives in gerontologic nursing. A close linkage between schools of nursing and nursing homes was perceived as the means by which this might be done. Currently a 1-year grant awarded to New York University will be used to do a follow-up on these participants to identify the salient features of the project.

Nurses Improving Care to the Hospitalized Elderly (NICHE): Outcomes in Four Hospitals was an 18-month collaborative effort to develop, test, and disseminate two key features of the NICHE project: (1) the institutional assessment profile and (2) the clinical protocols. A process evaluation of the NICHE project will be conducted to facilitate replication in hospitals nationwide.

Another project involved geriatric education centers and their contribution to practice and education. This project focused on the training needs of the health professionals who serve older adults. Most of the geriatric education centers aim to improve and expand geriatric health care, particularly for minority, multiethnic, low-income, and underserved older adults. The means by which these centers hope to achieve their goals include providing knowledge and training for health professionals, providing for leadership by academic faculty, encouraging interdisciplinary linkages among gerontologic health care professions and provider agencies, and providing tuition-free training programs.

Another project was called Interdisciplinary Team Training in Geriatrics (ITTG): The Contribution of the Team to the Practice and Education of Healthcare Professionals. This project focused on creating partnerships between health care providers and graduate health professionals' education programs so that there will be preparation for the service imperatives of the next century—geriatrics and interdisciplinary care.

Work groups and discussions were held at the completion of the project presentations. Based on these activities, the group "developed a vision for future development of gerontological nursing" (Woodside, 1996).

Continuing with the opportunity to talk about and to plan for the future of older adults in America, for the first time since 1981 a White House Conference on Aging was held in May 1995. Some 2200 delegates proceeded through a variety of preconference events where multiple and diverse topics were addressed. The theme of the conference was America Now and Into the Twenty-First Century: Generations Aging Together with Independence, Opportunities, and Dignity. The purpose of the conference was to address issues pertinent to older Americans and to make public policy recommendations. Four goals were defined to achieve this purpose:

1. To ensure comprehensive health care, including long-term care
2. To promote economic security
3. To maximize housing and support service options
4. To maximize options for a quality life

One of those who spoke during the preconference activities was Dr. Robert Butler, a powerful and influential friend of older adults. His plea was to put research high on the agenda for planning the future for older citizens. If adequate consideration is given now to systematic study of the issues and problems faced by older adults, the positive outcomes will be cost containment and improved services for those over age 65, as well as a higher quality of life for those who will pass the half-century mark in 1996 (Butler, 1995).

PREDICTIONS FOR THE FUTURE

As noted earlier, it is impossible for anyone who is living today to predict with any sense of accuracy what the coming century will present in terms of older adults, or the older generation. How many people will there be who are over 65 years of age? What will the designation of age (over 65) mean? How healthy will this group of people be? Who will be available to provide health care for these people who are in need of care? Within what type of system will health care be provided? Posing the questions is much easier than providing the answers; however, if the trends of today are any indication, a few predictions can be suggested.

The number of older people will continue to grow, and there will be increased numbers of older adults as compared to the number who are alive today. This will pose challenges for a variety of systems, especially the health care system. A greater variety of health services to provide for the multiple types of needs, and creativity in devising and implementing novel ways of providing service will be given priority. There will be fewer examples of the "same old things" offered as assistance for the needy.

The older people in society will be given freedom to choose. Systems of care will be optional and no one system will be mandated. Probably the "over 65" group will be happier and more comfortable with the selections they make for health care, for living, for recreation, for socializing, and for other activities of living. Rather than being forced into one pattern or mold, they will have the option to choose in which direction they wish to go and how they wish to be treated; there will be much more satisfaction among those who are growing older, and there will be more compliance in those areas that are not rigidly mandated. The beliefs of those who are providing care or who are supporting and assisting the older people will be guided by the conviction that each person has a right to decide his or her own destiny. Respect for the decision-making capability of each individual will be paramount.

There will be increased numbers of group homes, homes for assisted living, or retirement facilities. New and different residences will appear with a variety of options for payment, as well as a variety of services available. There will be multiple choices offered to older adults in this area, and given the variety of choices, once the decision has been made by the individual in need, there will be noticeable satisfaction derived from having been able to make one's own choice. It is possible that nursing home beds will be reduced in number. Even though the number of older people may increase, it is also possible that the people in the older age group will be healthier than is the group of older adults today.

The educational level of older adults will be higher than it is today. Opportunities for formal education will be greater than ever, and contin-

ued education will be opted for by all people. With more time available to pursue interests in various specialties, older individuals will be able to become a more learned group of people.

With many of the older adults having purchased their own homes, most will have satisfied their home mortgages; hence they will have the option of moving elsewhere to a spot of equal value, or they will be able to opt for staying where they are. Many will take the option of "aging in place." There will be a certain amount of security in knowing the neighborhood, knowing what resources (such as churches, grocery stores, banks, barbers, beauty shops, and clinics) are nearby, and knowing the means of transportation available to get there. Increased numbers of support services are becoming available to older people in many neighborhoods, making it reasonable and possible to age in place.

Nurse-managed centers are a recent and growing trend in health care for older adults. These centers can take on one of the following emphases: they can function as a community clinic, as a center associated with another institution such as a hospital or a health maintenance organization; as an academic center; or as a private nursing practice operated by nurse entrepreneurs. These centers are organizations that enable the patient to contract directly with the professional nurses who diagnose and treat responses to health problems, as well as offering wholistic, patient-centered health services. Acute care and illness management are provided in these centers by nurse practitioners; community health nursing care is the focus, with emphasis on education, health promotion, health-related research, and case management (Yoder, 1996).

This review of selected activities in which nurses are involved and some of the topics that are being addressed by nurses provides a preview of what will be the concerns of the profession as the twentieth century comes to a close and the twenty-first century arrives.

REFERENCES

American Nurses' Association. (1980). *Nursing: A social policy statement.* Kansas City, MO: Author.

American Nurses' Association. (1995). *Scope and standards of gerontological clinical nursing practice.* Washington, DC: Author.

American Nurses Publishing. (1995). *Nursing's social policy statement.* Washington, DC: Author.

Bridges, W. (1991). *Managing transitions: Making the most of change.* Reading, MA: Addison-Wesley.

Burtt, K. (1995). Nurses advocate for human rights. *American Nurse, 27*(8), 21.

Butler, R.N. (1995). Put research on the nation's agenda [Editorial]. *Geriatrics, 50*(4), 8.

Crowley, S.L. (1996, April). Aging brain's staying power. *AARP Bulletin, 37*(4), 1ff.

Dreher, M. (1995, Winter). Standing on honor with diverse spirit. *Reflections, 21*(4), 4-5.

Hadley, E.H. (1996, January-February). Nursing in the political and economic marketplace: Challenges for the twenty-first century. *Nursing Outlook, 44*(1), 6-10.

Meleis, A.I., & Trangenstein, P.A. (1994). Facilitating transitions: Redefinition of the nursing mission. *Nursing Outlook, 42*(6), 255-259.

North American Nursing Diagnosis Association. (1992). *NANDA nursing diagnosis: Definitions and classification.* Philadelphia: Author.

Steering committee on databases. (1995). *The American Nurse, 27*(5), 27.

Webster's New Collegiate Dictionary. (1961). Springfield, MA: G. and C. Merriam.

Weiner, M.B., Brok, A.J., & Snadowsky, A.M. (1987). *Working with the aged* (2nd ed.). Norwalk, CT: Appleton-Century-Crofts.

The White House conference—and NCOA pre-events. (1995, July-September). *NCOA Perspective on Aging, 24*(3), 30-31.

Whittaker, S., & Minich, L. (1995, October). Pew efforts seek to change how health professions are regulated. *American Nurse, 27*(7), 1.

Woodside, K.J. (1996, February). NLN conference explores the future of gerontological nursing. *NLN Update, 2*(1), 1, 3.

Yoder, M.K. (1996, January-February). Starting a nurse-managed center for older adults: The needs assessment process. *Geriatric Nursing, 17*(1), 14-19.

BIBLIOGRAPHY

Gallagher, R.M. (1995). *Community-based long term care: Agenda for the twenty-first century.* Washington, DC: American Nurse.

Knollmueller, R.N. (Ed). (1994). *Prevention across the life span: Healthy people for the twenty-first century.* Waldorf, MD: American Nurses Publishing.

Minimum Data Set (MDS) Federal Requirement for Assessment of Nursing Home Residents for Medicare

Numeric Identifier_____

MINIMUM DATA SET (MDS) - VERSION 2.0
FOR NURSING HOME RESIDENT ASSESSMENT AND CARE SCREENING

BASIC ASSESSMENT TRACKING FORM

SECTION AA. IDENTIFICATION INFORMATION

1.	**RESIDENT NAME**	**a.** (First) **b.** (Middle Initial) **c.** (Last) **d.** (Jr/Sr)
2.	**GENDER**	1. Male 2. Female
3.	**BIRTHDATE**	Month — Day — Year
4.	**RACE/ETHNICITY**	1. American Indian/Alaskan Native 4. Hispanic 2. Asian/Pacific Islander 5. White, not of 3. Black, not of Hispanic origin Hispanic origin
5.	**SOCIAL SECURITY AND MEDICARE NUMBERS** [C in 1st box if non med. no.]	**a.** Social Security Number **b.** Medicare number (or comparable railroad insurance number)
6.	**FACILITY PROVIDER NO.**	**a.** State No. **b.** Federal No.
7.	**MEDICAID NO.** ["+" if pending, "N" if not a Medicaid recipient]	
8.	**REASONS FOR ASSESS-MENT**	[Note-Other codes do not apply to this form] **a.** Primary reason for assessment 1. Admission assessment (required by day 14) 2. Annual assessment 3. Significant change in status assessment 4. Significant correction of prior assessment 5. Quarterly review assessment 0. *NONE OF ABOVE* **b.** *Special codes for use with supplemental assessment types in Case Mix demonstration states or other states where required* 1. 5 day assessment 2. 30 day assessment 3. 60 day assessment 4. Quarterly assessment using full MDS form 5. Readmission/return assessment 6. Other state required assessment
9.	**SIGNATURES OF PERSONS COMPLETING THESE ITEMS:**	

a. Signatures   Title   Date

b.   Date

GENERAL INSTRUCTIONS

Complete this information for submission with all full and quarterly assessments (Admission, Annual, Significant Change, State or Medicare required assessments, or Quarterly Reviews, etc.)

MDS 2.0 10/18/94N

Numeric Identifier_____

MINIMUM DATA SET (MDS) - VERSION 2.0
FOR NURSING HOME RESIDENT ASSESSMENT AND CARE SCREENING

DISCHARGE TRACKING FORM [do not use for temporary visits home]

SECTION AA. IDENTIFICATION INFORMATION

1.	RESIDENT NAME				
		a. (First)	b. (Middle Initial)	c. (Last)	d. (Jr/Sr)

2.	GENDER	1. Male 2. Female

3.	BIRTHDATE			
		Month	Day	Year

4.	RACE/ ETHNICITY	1. American Indian/Alaskan Native 4. Hispanic 2. Asian/Pacific Islander 5. White, not of 3. Black, not of Hispanic origin Hispanic origin

5.	SOCIAL SECURITY AND MEDICARE NUMBERS [C in 1st box if non med. no.]	a. Social Security Number
		b. Medicare number (or comparable railroad insurance number)

6.	FACILITY PROVIDER NO.	a. State No.
		b. Federal No.

7.	MEDICAID NO.[*+* if pending, *N* if not a Medicaid recipient]	

8.	REASONS FOR ASSESS- MENT	[Note-Other codes do not apply to this form] a. Primary reason for assessment 6. Discharged - return not anticipated 7. Discharged - return anticipated 8. Discharged prior to completing initial assessment

9. SIGNATURES OF STAFF COMPLETING FORM:

a. Signatures	Title	Sections	Date
b.			Date
c.			Date

SECTION R. ASSESSMENT/DISCHARGE INFORMATION

3.	DISCHARGE STATUS	*Skip if not discharged* a. *Code for resident disposition upon discharge* 1. Private home/apartment with no home health services 2. Private home/apartment with home health services 3. Board and care/assisted living 4. Another nursing facility 5. Acute care hospital 6. Psychiatric hospital, MR/DD facility 7. Rehabilitation hospital 8. Deceased 9. Other b. *Optional State Code*

4.	DISCHARGE DATE	*Date of death or discharge*		
		Month	Day	Year

SECTION AB. DEMOGRAPHIC INFORMATION
[Complete only for stays less than 14 days] (AA8a=8)

1.	DATE OF ENTRY	*Date the stay began. Note - Does not include readmission if record was closed at the time of temporary discharge to hospital, etc. In such cases, use prior admission date*		
		Month	Day	Year

2.	ADMITTED FROM (AT ENTRY)	1. Private home/apt. with no home health services 2. Private home/apt. with home health services 3. Board and care/assisted living/group home 4. Nursing home 5. Acute care hospital 6. Psychiatric hospital, MR/DD facility 7. Rehabilitation hospital 8. Other

SECTION A. IDENTIFICATION AND BACKGROUND INFORMATION

6.	MEDICAL RECORD NO.	

Numeric Identifier_____

MINIMUM DATA SET (MDS) - VERSION 2.0
FOR NURSING HOME RESIDENT ASSESSMENT AND CARE SCREENING

REENTRY TRACKING FORM

SECTION AA. IDENTIFICATION INFORMATION

1.	RESIDENT NAME				
		a. (First)	b. (Middle Initial)	c. (Last)	d. (Jr/Sr)
2.	GENDER	1. Male	2. Female		
3.	BIRTHDATE	Month — Day — Year			
4.	RACE/ ETHNICITY	1. American Indian/Alaskan Native 4. Hispanic 2. Asian/Pacific Islander 5. White, not of 3. Black, not of Hispanic origin Hispanic origin			
5.	SOCIAL SECURITY AND MEDICARE NUMBERS [C in 1st box if non med. no.]	a. Social Security Number b. Medicare number (or comparable railroad insurance number)			
6.	FACILITY PROVIDER NO.	a. State No. b. Federal No.			
7.	MEDICAID NO. ["+" if pending, "N" if not a Medicaid recipient]				
8.	REASONS FOR ASSESS- MENT	[Note-Other codes do not apply to this form] a. Primary reason for assessment 9. Reentry			

9. SIGNATURES OF STAFF COMPLETING FORM:

a. Signatures	Title	Sections	Date
b.			Date
c.			Date

SECTION A. IDENTIFICATION AND BACKGROUND INFORMATION

4a.	DATE OF REENTRY	Date of reentry Month — Day — Year
4b.	ADMITTED FROM (AT REENTRY)	1. Private home/apt. with no home health services 2. Private home/apt. with home health services 3. Board and care/assisted living/group home 4. Nursing home 5. Acute care hospital 6. Psychiatric hospital, MR/DD facility 7. Rehabilitation hospital 8. Other
6.	MEDICAL RECORD NO.	

Resident_____   Numeric Identifier_____

MINIMUM DATA SET (MDS) - VERSION 2.0
FOR NURSING HOME RESIDENT ASSESSMENT AND CARE SCREENING

BACKGROUND (FACE SHEET) INFORMATION AT ADMISSION

SECTION AB. DEMOGRAPHIC INFORMATION

1.	DATE OF ENTRY	Date the stay began. Note - Does not include readmission if record was closed at the time of temporary discharge to hospital, etc. In such cases, use prior admission date

☐☐ – ☐☐ – ☐☐☐☐
Month   Day   Year

2.	ADMITTED FROM (AT ENTRY)	1. Private home/apt. with no home health services 2. Private home/apt. with home health services 3. Board and care/assisted living/group home 4. Nursing home 5. Acute care hospital 6. Psychiatric hospital, MR/DD facility 7. Rehabilitation hospital 8. Other
3.	LIVED ALONE (PRIOR TO ENTRY)	0. No 1. Yes 2. In other facility
4.	ZIP CODE OF PRIOR PRIMARY RESIDENCE	☐☐☐☐☐
5.	RESIDEN-TIAL HISTORY 5 YEARS PRIOR TO ENTRY	(Check all settings resident lived in during 5 years prior to date of entry given in time AB1 above) Prior stay at this nursing home — a. Stay in other nursing home — b. Other residential facility-board and care home, assisted living, group home — c. MH/psychiatric setting — d. MR/DD setting — e. NONE OF THE ABOVE — f.
6.	LIFETIME OCCUPA-TION(S) [Put "/" between two occupations]	☐☐☐☐☐☐☐☐☐☐☐☐☐☐☐
7.	EDUCATION (Highest Level Completed)	1. No schooling 5. Technical or trade school 2. 8th grade/less 6. Some college 3. 9-11 grades 7. Bachelor's degree 4. High School 8. Graduate degree
8.	LANGUAGE	(Code for correct response) **a.** Primary Language 0. English 1. Spanish 2. French 3. Other **b. if other, specify**
9.	MENTAL HEALTH HISTORY	Does resident's RECORD indicate any history of mental retardation, mental illness, or developmental disability problem? 0. No 1. Yes
10.	CONDITIONS RELATED TO MR/DD STATUS	(Check all conditions that are related to MR/DD status that were manifested before age 22, and are likely to continue indefinitely) Not applicable - no MR/DD (Skip to AB11) — a. MR/DD with organic condition Down's syndrome — b. Autism — c. Epilepsy — d. Other organic condition related to MR/DD — e. MR/DD with no organic condition — f.
11.	DATE BACK-GROUND INFORMA-TION COMPLETED	☐☐ – ☐☐ – ☐☐☐☐ Month Day Year

SECTION AC. CUSTOMARY ROUTINE

1.	CUSTOMARY ROUTINE	(Check all that apply. If all information UNKNOWN, check last box only.)

(In year prior to DATE OF ENTRY to this nursing home, or year last in community if now being admitted from another nursing home)

CYCLE OF DAILY EVENTS

Stays up late at night (e.g., after 9 pm)	a.
Naps regularly during day (at least 1 hour)	b.
Goes out 1+ days a week	c.
Stays busy with hobbies, reading, or fixed daily routine	d.
Spends most of time alone or watching TV	e.
Moves independently indoors (with appliances, if used)	f.
Use of tobacco products at least daily	g.
NONE OF ABOVE	h.

EATING PATTERNS

Distinct food preferences	i.
Eats between meals all or most days	j.
Use of alcoholic beverage(s) at least weekly	k.
NONE OF ABOVE	l.

ADL PATTERNS

In bedclothes much of day	m.
Wakens to toilet all or most nights	n.
Has irregular bowel movement pattern	o.
Showers for bathing	p.
Bathing in PM	q.
NONE OF ABOVE	r.

INVOLVEMENT PATTERNS

Daily contact with relatives/close friends	s.
Usually attends church, temple, synagogue (etc.)	t.
Finds strength in faith	u.
Daily animal companion/presence	v.
Involved in group activities	w.
NONE OF ABOVE	x.
UNKNOWN - Resident/family unable to provide information	y.

☐ END

SECTION AD. FACE SHEET SIGNATURES

SIGNATURES OF PERSONS COMPLETING FACE SHEET:

a. Signature of RN Assessment Coordinator			Date
b. Signatures	Title	Sections	Date
c.			Date
d.			Date
e.			Date
f.			Date
g.			Date

Resident_____   Numeric Identifier_____

MINIMUM DATA SET (MDS) - VERSION 2.0
FOR NURSING HOME RESIDENT ASSESSMENT AND CARE SCREENING
FULL ASSESSMENT FORM
(Status in last 7 days, unless other time frame indicated)

SECTION A. IDENTIFICATION AND BACKGROUND INFORMATION

1. RESIDENT NAME
a.(First)   b.(Middle Initial)   c.(Last)   d.(Jr/Sr)

2. ROOM NUMBER

3. ASSESSMENT REFERENCE DATE
a. Last day of MDS observation period
Month — Day — Year
b. Original (0) or corrected copy of form (enter number of correction)

4a. DATE OF REENTRY
Date of reentry from most recent temporary discharge to a hospital in last 90 days (or since last assessment or admission if less than 90 days)
Month — Day — Year

5. MARITAL STATUS
1. Never Married
2. Married
3. Widowed
4. Separated
5. Divorced

6. MEDICAL RECORD NO.

7. CURRENT PAYMENT SOURCES FOR N.H. STAY
(Billing Office to indicate; check all that apply in last 30 days)
Medicaid per diem — a.
Medicare per diem — b.
Medicare ancillary part A — c.
Medicare ancillary part B — d.
CHAMPUS per diem — e.
VA per diem — f.
Self or family pays for full per diem — g.
Medicaid resident liability or Medicare co-payment — h.
Private insurance per diem (including co-payment) — i.
Other per diem — j.

8. REASONS FOR ASSESSMENT
[Note - If this is a discharge or reentry assessment, only a limited subset of MDS items need be completed]
a. Primary reason for assessment
1. Admission assessment (required by day 14)
2. Annual assessment
3. Significant change in status assessment
4. Significant correction of prior assessment
5. Quarterly review assessment
6. Discharged - return not anticipated
7. Discharged - return anticipated
8. Discharged prior to completing initial assessment
9. Reentry
0. NONE OF ABOVE
b. Special codes for use with supplemental assessment types in Case Mix demonstration states or other states where required
1. 5 day assessment
2. 30 day assessment
3. 60 day assessment
4. Quarterly assessment using full MDS form
5. Readmission/return assessment
6. Other state required assessment

9. RESPONSIBILITY/ LEGAL GUARDIAN
(Check all that apply)
Legal guardian — a.
Other legal oversight — b.
Durable power of attorney/health care — c.
Durable power attorney/financial — d.
Family member responsible — e.
Patient responsible for self — f.
NONE OF ABOVE — g.

10. ADVANCED DIRECTIVES
(For those items with supporting documentation in the medical record, check all that apply)
Living will — a.
Do not resuscitate — b.
Do not hospitalize — c.
Organ donation — d.
Autopsy request — e.
Feeding restrictions — f.
Medication restrictions — g.
Other treatment restrictions — h.
NONE OF ABOVE — i.

SECTION B. COGNITIVE PATTERNS

1. COMATOSE
(Persistent vegetative state/no discernible consciousness)
0. No   1. Yes   (If yes, skip to section G)

2. MEMORY
(Recall of what was learned or known)
a. Short-term memory OK - seems/appears to recall after 5 minutes
0. Memory OK   1. Memory problem
b. Long-term memory OK - seems/appears to recall long past
0. Memory OK   1. Memory problem

3. MEMORY/ RECALL ABILITY
(Check all that resident was normally able to recall during last 7 days)
Current Season — a.
Location of own room — b.
Staff names/faces — c.
That he/she is in a nursing home — d.
NONE OF ABOVE are recalled — e.

4. COGNITIVE SKILLS FOR DAILY DECISION-MAKING
(Made decisions regarding tasks of daily life)
0. INDEPENDENT - decisions consistent/reasonable
1. MODIFIED INDEPENDENCE - some difficulty in new situations only
2. MODERATELY IMPAIRED - decisions poor; cues/supervision required
3. SEVERELY IMPAIRED - never/rarely made decisions

5. INDICATORS OF DELIRIUM - PERIODIC DISORDERED THINKING/ AWARENESS
(Code for behavior in the last 7 days.) [Note: Accurate assessment requires conversations with staff and family who have direct knowledge of resident's behavior over this time].
0. Behavior not present
1. Behavior present, not of recent onset
2. Behavior present over last 7 days appears different from resident's usual functioning (e.g., new onset or worsening)
a. EASILY DISTRACTED - (e.g., difficulty paying attention; gets sidetracked)
b. PERIODS OF ALTERED PERCEPTION OR AWARENESS OF SURROUNDINGS - (e.g., moves lips or talks to someone not present; believes he/she is somewhere else; confuses night and day)
c. EPISODES OF DISORGANIZED SPEECH - (e.g., speech is incoherent, nonsensical, irrelevant, or rambling from subject to subject; loses train of thought)
d. PERIODS OF RESTLESSNESS - (e.g., fidgeting or picking at skin, clothing, napkins, etc; frequent position changes; repetitive physical movements or calling out)
e. PERIODS OF LETHARGY - (e.g., sluggishness; staring into space; difficult to arouse; little body movement)
f. MENTAL FUNCTION VARIES OVER THE COURSE OF THE DAY - (e.g., sometimes better, sometimes worse; behaviors sometimes present, sometimes not)

6. CHANGE IN COGNITIVE STATUS
Resident's cognitive status, skills, or abilities have changed as compared to status of 90 days ago (or since last assessment if less than 90 days)
0. No change   1. Improved   2. Deteriorated

SECTION C. COMMUNICATION/HEARING PATTERNS

1. HEARING
(With hearing appliance, if used)
0. HEARS ADEQUATELY - normal talk, TV, phone
1. MINIMAL DIFFICULTY when not in quiet setting
2. HEARS IN SPECIAL SITUATIONS ONLY - speaker has to adjust tonal quality and speak distinctly
3. HIGHLY IMPAIRED/absence of useful hearing

2. COMMUNICATION DEVICES/ TECHNIQUES
(Check all that apply during last 7 days)
Hearing aid, present and used — a.
Hearing aid, present and not used regularly — b.
Other receptive comm. techniques used (e.g., lip reading) — c.
NONE OF ABOVE — d.

3. MODES OF EXPRESSION
(Check all used by resident to make needs known)
Speech — a.
Writing messages to express or clarify needs — b.
American sign language or Braille — c.
Signs/gestures/sounds — d.
Communication board — e.
Other — f.
NONE OF ABOVE — g.

4. MAKING SELF UNDERSTOOD
(Expressing information content - however able)
0. UNDERSTOOD
1. USUALLY UNDERSTOOD - difficulty finding words or finishing thoughts
2. SOMETIMES UNDERSTOOD - ability is limited to making concrete requests
3. RARELY/NEVER UNDERSTOOD

5. SPEECH CLARITY
(Code for speech in the last 7 days)
0. CLEAR SPEECH - distinct, intelligible words
1. UNCLEAR SPEECH - slurred, mumbled words
2. NO SPEECH - absence of spoken words

6. ABILITY TO UNDERSTAND OTHERS
(Understanding verbal information content - however able)
0. UNDERSTANDS
1. USUALLY UNDERSTANDS - may miss some part/intent of message
2. SOMETIMES UNDERSTANDS - responds adequately to simple, direct communication
3. RARELY/NEVER UNDERSTANDS

7. CHANGE IN COMMUNICATION/ HEARING
Resident's ability to express, understand, or hear information has changed as compared to status of 90 days ago (or since last assessment if less than 90 days)
0. No change   1. Improved   2. Deteriorated

Resident_____   Numeric Identifier_____

SECTION D. VISION PATTERNS

1.	**VISION**	*(Ability to see in adequate light and with glasses if used)* 0. *ADEQUATE* - sees fine detail, including regular print in newspapers/books 1. *IMPAIRED* - sees large print, but not regular print in newspapers/books 2. *MODERATELY IMPAIRED* - limited vision; not able to see newspaper headlines, but can identify objects 3. *HIGHLY IMPAIRED* - object identification in question, but eyes appear to follow objects 4. *SEVERELY IMPAIRED* - no vision or sees only light, colors, or shapes; eyes do not appear to follow objects
2.	**VISUAL LIMITATIONS/ DIFFICULTIES**	Side vision problems - decreased peripheral vision (e.g., leaves food on side of tray, difficulty traveling, bumps into people and objects, misjudges placement of chair when seating self) a. Experiences any of following: sees halos or rings around lights; sees flashes of light; sees "curtains" over eyes b. NONE OF ABOVE c.
3.	**VISUAL APPLIANCES**	Glasses; contact lenses; magnifying glass 0. No 1. Yes

SECTION E. MOOD AND BEHAVIOR PATTERNS

1.	**INDICATORS OF DEPRES-SION, ANXIETY, SAD MOOD**	*(Code for indicators observed in last 30 days, irrespective of the assumed cause)* 0. Indicator not exhibited in last 30 days 1. Indicator of this type exhibited up to five days a week 2. Indicator of this type exhibited daily or almost daily (6, 7 days a week)

VERBAL EXPRESSIONS OF DISTRESS	h. Repetitive health complaints - e.g., persistently seeks medical attention, obsessive concern with body functions
a. Resident made negative statements - e.g., "Nothing matters; Would rather be dead; What's the use; Regrets having lived so long; Let me die"	
b. Repetitive questions - e.g., "Where do I go; What do I do?"	i. Repetitive anxious complaints/concerns (non-health related) e.g., persistently seeks attention/reassurance regarding schedules, meals, laundry, clothing, relationship issues
c. Repetitive verbalizations - e.g., calling out for help, ("God help me")	**SLEEP-CYCLE ISSUES**
d. Persistent anger with self or others - e.g., easily annoyed, anger at placement in nursing home; anger at care received	j. Unpleasant mood in morning k. Insomnia/change in usual sleep pattern **SAD, APATHEIC, ANXIOUS APPEARANCE**
e. Self deprecation - e.g., "I am nothing; I am of no use to anyone"	l. Sad, pained, worried facial expressions - e.g., furrowed brows
f. Expressions of what appear to be unrealistic fears - e.g., fear of being abandoned, left lone, being with others	m. Crying, tearfulness n. Repetitive physical movements - e.g., pacing, hand wringing, restlessness, fidgeting, picking
g. Recurrent statements that something terrible is about to happen - e.g., believes he or she is about to die, have a heart attack	**LOSS OF INTEREST** o. Withdrawal from activities of interest - e.g., no interest in long standing activities or being with family/friends p. Reduced social interaction

2.	**MOOD PERSIS-TENCE**	One or more indicators of depressed, sad or anxious mood were not easily altered by attempts to "cheer up", console, or reassure the resident over the last 7 days 0. No mood indicators 1. Indicators present, easily altered 2. Indicators present, not easily altered
3.	**CHANGE IN MOOD**	Resident's mood status has changed as compared to status of 90 days ago (or since last assessment if less then 90 days) 0. No change 1. Improved 2. Deteriorated
4.	**BEHAVIORAL SYMPTOMS**	**(A)** *Behavioral symptom frequency in last 7 days* 0. Behavior not exhibited in last 7 days 1. Behavior of this type occurred 1 to 3 days in last 7 days 2. Behavior of this type occurred 4 to 6 days, but less than daily 3. Behavior of this type occurred daily **(B)** *Behavioral symptom alterability in last 7 days* 0. Behavior not present OR behavior was easily altered 1. Behavior was not easily altered (A) (B)

a. WANDERING (moved with no rational purpose, seemingly oblivious to needs or safety)	
b. VERBALLY ABUSIVE BEHAVIORAL SYMPTOMS (others were threatened, screamed at, cursed at)	
c. PHYSICALLY ABUSIVE BEHAVIORAL SYMPTOMS (others were hit, shoved, scratched, sexually abused)	
d. SOCIALLY INAPPROPRIATE/DISRUPTIVE BEHAVIORAL SYMPTOMS (made disruptive sounds, noisiness, screaming, self-abusive acts, sexual behavior or disrobing in public, smeared/threw food/feces, hoarding, rummaged through others' belongings)	
e. RESISTS CARE (resisted taking medications/injections, ADL assistance, or eating)	

5.	**CHANGE IN BEHAVIORAL SYMPTOMS**	Resident's behavior status has changed as compared to status of 90 days ago (or since last assessment if less than 90 days) 0. No change 1. Improved 2. Deteriorated

SECTION F. PSYCHOSOCIAL WELL-BEING

1.	**SENSE OF INITIATIVE/ INVOLVE-MENT**	At ease interacting with others	a.
		At ease doing planned or structured activities	b.
		At ease doing self-initiated activities	c.
		Establishes own goals	d.
		Pursues involvement in life of facility (e.g., makes/keeps friends; involved in group activities; responds positively to new activities; assists at religious services)	e.
		Accepts invitations into most group activities	f.
		NONE OF ABOVE	g.
2.	**UNSETTLED RELATION-SHIPS**	Covert/open conflict with or repeated criticism of staff	a.
		Unhappy with roommate	b.
		Unhappy with residents other than roommate	c.
		Openly expresses conflict/anger with family/friends	d.
		Absence of personal contact with family/friends	e.
		Recent loss of close family member/friend	f.
		Does not adjust easily to change in routines	g.
		NONE OF ABOVE	h.
3.	**PAST ROLES**	Strong identification with past roles and life status	a.
		Expresses sadness/anger/empty feeling over lost roles/status	b.
		Resident perceives that daily routine (customary routine, activities) is very different from prior pattern in the community	c.
		NONE OF ABOVE	d.

SECTION G. PHYSICAL FUNCTIONING AND STRUCTURAL PROBLEMS

1.	**(A)** ADL SELF-PERFORMANCE (Code for resident's *PERFORMANCE OVER ALL SHIFTS during last 7 days - Not including setup*)
	0. *INDEPENDENT* - No help or oversight -OR- Help/oversight provided only 1 or 2 times during last 7 days
	1. *SUPERVISION* - Oversight, encouragement or cueing provided 3 or more times during last 7 days -OR- Supervision (3 or more times) plus physical assistance provided only 1 or 2 times during last 7 days
	2. *LIMITED ASSISTANCE* - Resident highly involved in activity; received physical help in guided maneuvering of limbs or other nonweight bearing assistance 3 or more times - OR- More help provided only 1 or 2 times during last 7 days
	3. *EXTENSIVE ASSISTANCE* - While resident performed part of activity, over last 7-day period, help of following type(s) provided 3 or more times:
	   - Weight-bearing support
	   - Full staff performance during part (but not all) of last 7 days
	4. *TOTAL DEPENDENCE* - Full staff performance of activity during entire 7 days
	8. *ACTIVITY DID NOT OCCUR* during entire 7 days

(B) ADL SUPPORT PROVIDED - *(Code for MOST SUPPORT PROVIDED OVER ALL SHIFTS during last 7 days; code regardless of resident's self-performance classification)* 0. No setup or physical help from staff 1. Setup help only 2. One person physical assist 8. ADL activity itself did not occur during entire 7 days 3. Two+ persons physical assist	(A) Self-Perf	(B) Support
a. **BED MOBILITY** How resident moves to and from lying position, turns side to side, and positions body while in bed		
b. **TRANSFER** How resident moves between surfaces - to/from: bed, chair, wheelchair, standing position (EXCLUDE to/from bath/toilet)		
c. **WALK IN ROOM** How resident walks between locations in his/her room		
d. **WALK IN CORRIDOR** How resident walks in corridor on unit		
e. **LOCOMO-TION ON UNIT** How resident moves between locations in his/her room and adjacent corridor on same floor. If in wheelchair, self-sufficiency once in chair		
f. **LOCOMO-TION OFF UNIT** How resident moves to and returns from off unit locations (e.g., areas set aside for dining, activities, or treatments). If facility has only one floor, how resident moves to and from distant areas on the floor. If in wheelchair, self-sufficiency once in chair		
g. **DRESSING** How resident puts on, fastens, and takes off all items of street clothing, including donning/removing prosthesis		
h. **EATING** How resident eats and drinks (regardless of skill). Includes intake of nourishment by other means (e.g., tube feeding, total parenteral nutrition)		
i. **TOILET USE** How resident uses the toilet room (or commode, bedpan, urinal): transfer on/off toilet, cleanses, changes pad, manages ostomy or catheter, adjusts clothes		
j. **PERSONAL HYGIENE** How resident maintains personal hygiene, including combing hair, brushing teeth, shaving, applying makeup, washing/drying face hands, and perineum (EXCLUDE baths and showers)		

Resident_____

2.	BATHING	How resident takes full-body bath/shower, sponge bath, and transfers in/out of tub/shower (EXCLUDE washing of back and hair.) Code for most dependent in self-performance and support (A) BATHING SELF-PERFORMANCE codes appear below	(A)	(B)
		0. Independent - No help provided		
		1. Supervision - Oversight help only		
		2. Physical help limited to transfer only		
		3. Physical help in part of bathing activity		
		4. Total dependence		
		8. Activity itself did not occur during entire 7 days (Bathing support codes are as defined in Item 1, code B above)		
3.	TEST FOR BALANCE (see training manual)	(Code for ability during test in last 7 days) 0. Maintained position as required in test 1. Unsteady, but able to rebalance self without physical support 2. Partial physical support during test; or stands (sits) but does not follow directions for test 3. Not able to attempt test without physical help		
		a. Balance while standing		
		b. Balance while sitting - position, trunk control		
4.	FUNCTIONAL LIMITATION IN RANGE OF MOTION (see training manual)	(Code for limitations during last 7 days that interfered with daily functions or placed resident at risk of injury) (A) RANGE OF MOTION (B) VOLUNTARY MOVEMENT 0. No limitation 0. No loss 1. Limitation on one side 1. Partial loss 2. Limitation on both sides 2. Full loss	(A)	(B)
		a. Neck		
		b. Arm - Including shoulder or elbow		
		c. Hand - Including wrist or fingers		
		d. Leg - Including hip or knee		
		e. Foot - Including ankle or toes		
		f. Other limitation or loss		
5.	MODES OF LOCOMO-TION	(Check all that apply during last 7 days)		
		Cane/walker/crutch	a.	Wheelchair primary mode of locomotion	d.
		Wheeled self	b.	
		Other person wheeled	c.	NONE OF ABOVE	e.
6.	MODES OF TRANSFER	(Check all that apply during last 7 days)		
		Bedfast all or most of time	a.	Lifted mechanically	d.
		Bed rails used for bed mobility or transfer	b.	Transfer aid (e.g., slide board, trapeze, cane, walker, brace)	e.
		Lifted manually	c.	NONE OF ABOVE	f.
7.	TASK SEGMENTA-TION	Some or all of ADL activities were broken into subtasks during last 7 days so that resident could perform them 0. No 1. Yes		
8.	ADL FUNCTIONAL REHABILITA-TION POTENTIAL	Resident believes he/she is capable of increased independence in at least some ADLs	a.	
		Direct care staff believe resident is capable of increased independence in at least some ADLs	b.	
		Resident able to perform tasks/activity but is very slow	c.	
		Difference in ADL Self-Performance or ADL Support, comparing mornings to evenings	d.	
		NONE OF ABOVE	e.	
9.	CHANGE IN ADL FUNCTION	Resident's ADL self-performance status has changed as compared to status of 90 days ago (or since last assessment if less than 90 days) 0. No change 1. Improved 2. Deteriorated		

SECTION H. CONTINENCE IN LAST 14 DAYS

1.	CONTINENCE SELF-CONTROL CATEGORIES (Code for resident's PERFORMANCE OVER ALL SHIFTS)
	0. CONTINENT - Complete control [includes use of indwelling urinary catheter or ostomy device that does not leak urine or stool]
	1. USUALLY CONTINENT - BLADDER, incontinent episodes once a week or less; BOWEL, less than weekly
	2. OCCASIONALLY INCONTINENT - BLADDER, 2 or more times a week but not daily; BOWEL, once a week
	3. FREQUENTLY INCONTINENT - BLADDER, tended to be incontinent daily, but some control present (e.g., on day shift); BOWEL, 2-3 times a week
	4. INCONTINENT - Had inadequate control BLADDER, multiple daily episodes; BOWEL, all (or almost all) of the time

a.	BOWEL CONTI-NENCE	Control of bowel movement, with appliance or bowel continence programs, if employed	
b.	BLADDER CONTI-NENCE	Control of urinary bladder function (if dribbles, volume insufficient to soak through underpants), with appliances (e.g., foley) or continence programs, if employed	
2.	BOWEL ELIMINATION PATTERN	Bowel elimination pattern regular - at least one movement every three days	a.	Diarrhea	c.
				Fecal impaction	d.
		Constipation	b.	NONE OF ABOVE	e.

Numeric Identifier_____

3.	APPLIANCES AND PROGRAMS	Any scheduled toileting plan	a.	Did not use toilet room/commode/urinal	f.
		Bladder retraining program	b.	Pads/briefs used	g.
		External (condom) catheter	c.	Enemas/irrigation	h.
		Indwelling catheter	d.	Ostomy present	i.
		Intermittent catheter	e.	NONE OF ABOVE	j.
4.	CHANGE IN URINARY CONTI-NENCE	Resident's urinary continence has changed as compared to status of 90 days ago (or since last assessment if less than 90 days) 0. No change 1. Improved 2. Deteriorated			

SECTION I. DISEASE DIAGNOSES

Check only those diseases that have a relationship to current ADL status, cognitive status, mood and behavior status, medical treatments, nursing monitoring, or risk of death. (Do not list inactive diagnoses)

1.	DISEASES	(If none apply, CHECK the NONE OF ABOVE box)			
		ENDOCRINE/METABOLIC/NUTRITIONAL		Hemiplegia/Hemiparesis	v.
				Multiple sclerosis	w.
		Diabetes mellitus	a.	Paraplegia	x.
		Hyperthyroidism	b.	Parkinson's disease	y.
		Hypothyroidism	c.	Quadriplegia	z.
		HEART/CIRCULATION		Seizure disorder	aa.
		Ateriosclerotic heart disease (ASHD)	d.	Transient ischemic attack (TIA)	bb.
		Cardiac dysrhythmias	e.	Traumatic brain injury	cc.
		Congestive heart failure	f.	**PSYCHIATRIC/MOOD**	
		Deep vein thrombosis'	g.	Anxiety disorder	dd.
		Hypertension	h.	Depression	ee.
		Hypotension	i.	Manic depression (bipolar disease)	ff.
		Peripheral vascular disease	j.	Schizophrenia	gg.
		Other cardiovascular disease	k.	**PULMONARY**	
		MUSCULOSKELETAL		Asthma	hh.
		Arthritis	l.	Emphysema/COPD	ii.
		Hip fracture	m.	**SENSORY**	
		Missing limb (eg, amputation)	n.	Cataracts	jj.
		Osteoporosis	o.	Diabetic retinopathy	kk.
		Pathological bone fracture	p.	Glaucoma	ll.
		NEUROLOGICAL		Macular degeneration	mm.
		Alzheimer's disease	q.	**OTHER**	
		Aphasia	r.	Allergies	nn.
		Cerebral palsy	s.	Anemia	oo.
		Cerebrovascular accident (stroke)	t.	Cancer	pp.
		Dementia other than Alzheimer's disease	u.	Renal failure	qq.
				NONE OF ABOVE	rr.
2.	INFECTIONS	(If none apply, CHECK the NONE OF ABOVE box)			
		Antibiotic resistant infection (e.g., Methicillin resistant staph)	a.	Septicemia	g.
				Sexually transmitted diseases	h.
		Clostridium difficile (c.diff.)	b.	Tuberculosis	i.
		Conjunctivitis	c.	Urinary tract infection in last 30 days	j.
		HIV infection	d.	Viral hepatitis	k.
		Pneumonia	e.	Wound infection	l.
		Respiratory infection	f.	NONE OF ABOVE	m.
3.	OTHER CURRENT OR MORE DETAILED DIAGNOSES AND ICD-9 CODES	a._____			
		b._____			
		c._____			
		d._____			
		e._____			

SECTION J. HEALTH CONDITIONS

1.	PROBLEM CONDITIONS	(Check all problems present in last 7 days unless other time frame is indicated)			
		INDICATORS OF FLUID STATUS		Dizziness/Vertigo	f.
				Edema	g.
		Weight gain or loss of 3 or more pounds within a 7 day period	a.	Fever	h.
				Hallucinations	i.
				Internal bleeding	j.
		Inability to lie flat due to shortness of breath	b.	Recurrent lung aspirations in last 90 days	k.
		Dehydrated; output exceeds input	c.	Shortness of breath	l.
				Syncope (fainting)	m.
		Insufficient fluid; did NOT consume all/almost all liquids provided during last 3 days	d.	Unsteady gait	n.
				Vomiting	o.
		OTHER		NONE OF ABOVE	p.
		Delusions	e.		

Resident_____   Numeric Identifier_____

2.	PAIN SYMPTOMS	(Code the highest level of pain present in the last 7 days)			
		a. FREQUENCY with which resident complains or shows evidence of pain 0. No pain (skip to J4) 1. Pain less than daily 2. Pain daily		**b. INTENSITY** of pain 1. Mild pain 2. Moderate pain 3. Times when pain is horrible or excruciating	
3.	PAIN SITE	(If pain present, check all sites that apply in last 7 days)			
		Back pain	a.	Incisional pain	f.
		Bone pain	b.	Joint pain (other than hip)	g.
		Chest pain while doing usual activities	c.	Soft tissue pain (e.g., lesion, muscle)	h.
		Headache	d.	Stomach pain	i.
		Hip pain	e.	Other	j.
4.	ACCIDENTS	(Check all that apply)			
		Fell in past 30 days	a.	Hip fracture in last 180 days	c.
		Fell in past 31-180 days	b.	Other fracture in last 180 days	d.
				NONE OF ABOVE	e.
5.	STABILITY OF CONDITIONS	Conditions/diseases make resident's cognitive, ADL, mood or behavior patterns unstable - (fluctuating, precarious, or deteriorating)			a.
		Resident experiencing an acute episode or a flare-up of a recurrent or chronic-problem			b.
		End-stage disease, 6 or fewer months to live			c.
		NONE OF ABOVE			d.

SECTION K. ORAL/NUTRITIONAL STATUS

1.	ORAL PROBLEMS	Chewing problem			a.
		Swallowing problem			b.
		Mouth pain			c.
		NONE OF ABOVE			d.
2.	HEIGHT AND WEIGHT	Record (a.) height in inches and (b.) the weight in pounds. Base weight on most recent measure in last 30 days; measure weight consistently in accord with standard facility practice - e.g., in a.m. after voiding, before meal, with shoes off, and in nightclothes			
		a. HT (in.)		**b. WT (lb.)**	
3.	WEIGHT CHANGE	**a. Weight loss** - 5% or more in **last 30 days**; or 10% or more in **last 180 days** 0. No 1. Yes			
		b. Weight gain - 5% or more in **last 30 days**; or 10% or more in **last 180 days** 0. No 1. Yes			
4.	NUTRITIONAL PROBLEMS	Complains about taste of many foods	a.	Leaves 25% or more of food uneaten at most meals	c.
		Regular or repetitive complaints of hunger	b.	NONE OF ABOVE	d.
5.	NUTRITIONAL APPROACHES	(Check all that apply in last 7 days)			
		Parenteral/IV	a.	Dietary supplement between meals	f.
		Feeding tube	b.	Plate guard, stabilized built-up utensil, etc.	g.
		Mechanically altered diet	c.		
		Syringe (oral feeding)	d.	On a planned weight change program	h.
		Therapeutic diet	e.	NONE OF ABOVE	i.
6.	PARENTERAL OR ENTERAL INTAKE	(Skip to Section L if neither 5a nor 5b is checked)			
		a. Code the proportion of total calories the resident received through parenteral or tube feedings in the last 7 days 0. None 3. 51% to 75% 1. 1% to 25% 4. 76% to 100% 2. 26% to 50%			
		b. Code the average fluid intake per day by IV or tube in last 7 days 0. None 3. 1001 to 1500 cc/day 1. 1 to 500 cc/day 4. 1501 to 2000 cc/day 2. 501 to 1000 cc/day 5. 2001 or more cc/day			

SECTION L. ORAL/DENTAL STATUS

1.	ORAL STATUS AND DISEASE PREVENTION	Debris (soft, easily movable substances) present in mouth prior to going to bed at night	a.
		Has dentures or removable bridge	b.
		Some/all natural teeth lost - does not have or does not use dentures (or partial plates)	c.
		Broken, loose, or carious teeth	d.
		Inflamed gums (gingiva); swollen or bleeding gums; oral abscesses; ulcers or rashes	e.
		Daily cleaning of teeth/dentures or daily mouth care - by resident staff	f.
		NONE OF ABOVE	g.

SECTION M. SKIN CONDITION

1.	ULCERS (Due to any cause)	(Record the number of ulcers at each ulcer stage - regardless of cause. If none present at a stage, record *0* (zero). Code all that apply during last 7 days. Code 9 = 9 or more.) [Requires full body exam.]	Num. at Stage
		a. Stage 1. A persistent area of skin redness (without a break in the skin) that does not disappear when pressure is relieved.	
		b. Stage 2. A partial thickness loss of skin layers that presents clinically as an abrasion, blister, or shallow crater.	
		c. Stage 3. A full thickness of skin is lost, exposing the subcutaneous tissues - presents as a deep crater with or without undermining adjacent tissue.	
		d. Stage 4. A full thickness of skin and subcutaneous tissue is lost, exposing muscle or bone.	
2.	TYPE OF ULCER	(For each type of ulcer, code for the highest stage in the last 7 days using scale in item M1 - i.e., 0=none; stages 1, 2, 3, 4)	
		a. Pressure ulcer - any lesion caused by pressure resulting in damage of underlying tissue	
		b. Stasis ulcer - open lesion caused by poor circulation in the lower extremities	
3.	HISTORY OF RESOLVED ULCERS	Resident had an ulcer that was resolved or cured in LAST 90 DAYS	
		0. No 1. Yes	
4.	OTHER SKIN PROBLEMS OR LESIONS PRESENT	(Check all that apply during last 7 days)	
		Abrasions, bruises	a.
		Burns (second or third degree)	b.
		Open lesions other than ulcers, rashes, cuts (e.g., cancer lesions)	c.
		Rashes - e.g., intertrigo, eczema, drug rash, heat rash, herpes zoster	d.
		Skin desensitized to pain or pressure	e.
		Skin tears or cuts (other than surgery)	f.
		Surgical wounds	g.
		NONE OF ABOVE	h.
5.	SKIN TREATMENTS	(Check all that apply during last 7 days)	
		Pressure relieving device(s) for chair	a.
		Pressure relieving device(s) for bed	b.
		Turning/repositioning program	c.
		Nutrition or hydration intervention to manage skin problems	d.
		Ulcer care	e.
		Surgical wound care	f.
		Application of dressings (with or without topical medications) other than to feet	g.
		Application of ointments/medications (other than to feet)	h.
		Other preventative or protective skin care (other than to feet)	i.
		NONE OF ABOVE	j.
6.	FOOT PROBLEMS AND CARE	(Check all that apply during last 7 days)	
		Resident has one or more foot problems - e.g., corns, calloures, bunions, hammer toes, overlapping toes, pain, structural problems	a.
		Infection of the foot - e.g., cellulitis, purulent drainage	b.
		Open lesions on the foot	c.
		Nails/calloures trimmed during last 90 days	d.
		Received preventative or protective foot care (e.g., used special shoes, inserts, pads, toe separators)	e.
		Application of dressings (with or without topical medications)	f.
		NONE OF ABOVE	g.

SECTION N. ACTIVITY PURSUIT PATTERNS

1.	TIME AWAKE	(Check appropriate time periods over last 7 days) Resident awake all or most of time (i.e., naps no more than one hour per time period) in the:			
		Morning	a.	Evening	c.
		Afternoon	b.	NONE OF ABOVE	d.

(If resident is comatose, skip to **Section O**)

2.	AVERAGE TIME INVOLVED IN ACTIVITIES	(When awake and not receiving treatments or ADL care)			
		0. Most - more than 2/3 of time 2. Little - less than 1/3 of time 1. Some - from 1/3 to 2/3 of time 3. None			
3.	PREFERRED ACTIVITY SETTINGS	(Check all settings in which activities are preferred)			
		Own room	a.	Outside facility	d.
		Day/activity room	b.		
		Inside NH/off unit	c.	NONE OF ABOVE	e.
4.	GENERAL ACTIVITY PREFERENCES (adapted to resident's current abilities)	(Check all PREFERENCES whether or not activity is currently available to resident)			
		Cards/other games	a.	Trips/shopping	g.
		Crafts/arts	b.	Walking/wheeling outdoors	h.
		Exercise/sports	c.	Watching TV	i.
		Music	d.	Gardening or plants	j.
		Reading/writing	e.	Talking or conversing	k.
		Spiritual/religious activities	f.	Helping others	l.
				NONE OF ABOVE	m.

Resident _____   Numeric Identifier _____

5.	PREFERS CHANGE IN DAILY ROUTINE	*(Code for resident preferences in daily routines)*
		0. No change 1. Slight change 2. Major change
		a. Type of activities in which resident is currently involved
		b. Extent of resident involvement in activities

SECTION O. MEDICATIONS

1.	NUMBER OF MEDICA-TIONS	*(Record the number of different medications used in the last 7 days; enter "0" if none used)*	
2.	NEW MEDICA-TIONS	*(Resident currently receiving medications that were initiated during the last 90 days)* 0. No 1. Yes	
3.	INJECTIONS	*(Record the number of DAYS injections of any type received during the last 7 days; enter "0" if none used)*	
4.	DAYS RECEIVED THE FOLLOWING MEDICATION	*(Record the number of DAYS during last 7 days; enter "0" if not used. Note - enter "1" for long-acting meds used less than weekly)*	
		a. Antipsychotic d. Hypnotic	
		b. Antianxiety	
		c. Antidepressant e. Diuretic	

SECTION P. SPECIAL TREATMENTS AND PROCEDURES

1.	SPECIAL TREAT-MENTS PROCE-DURES, AND PROGRAMS	**a. SPECIAL CARE** - *Check treatments or programs received during the last 14 days [Note - count only post admission treatments]*		
		TREATMENTS		Ventilator or respirator	l.
		Chemotherapy	a.	**PROGRAMS**	
		Dialysis	b.	Alcohol/drug treatment program	m.
		IV medication	c.		
		Intake/output	d.	Alzheimer's/dementia special care unit	n.
		Monitoring acute medical condition	e.	Hospice care	o.
		Ostomy care	f.	Pediatric unit	p.
		Oxygen therapy	g.	Respite care	q.
		Radiation	h.	Training in skills required to return to the community (e.g., taking medications, house work, shopping, transportation, ADLs)	r.
		Suctioning	i.		
		Tracheostomy care	j.		
		Transfusions	k.	*NONE OF ABOVE*	s.

b. THERAPIES - *Record the number of days and total minutes each of the following therapies was administered (for at least 15 minutes a day) in the last 7 calendar days (Enter 0 if none or less then 15 min. daily)* **[Note-count only post admission therapies]**
(A) = # of days administered for 15 minutes or more
(B) = total # of minutes provided in last 7 days

	DAYS (A)	MIN (B)
a. Speech - language pathology and audiology services		
b. Occupational therapy		
c. Physical therapy		
d. Respiratory therapy		
e. Psychological therapy (by any licensed mental health professional)		

2.	INTERVEN-TION PROGRAMS FOR MOOD BEHAVIOR, COGNITIVE LOSS	*(Check all interventions or strategies used in last 7 days - no matter where received)*	
		Special behavior symptom evaluation program	a.
		Evaluation by a licensed mental health specialist in last 90 days	b.
		Group therapy	c.
		Resident-specific deliberate changes in the environment to address mood/behavior patterns - e.g., providing bureau in which to rummage	d.
		Reorientation - e.g., cueing	e.
		NONE OF ABOVE	f.

3.	NURSING REHABILITA-TION/ RESTOR-ATIVE CARE	*Record the NUMBER OF DAYS each of the following rehabilitation or restorative techniques or practices was provided to the resident for more than or equal to 15 minutes per day in the last 7 days (Enter 0 if none or less than 15 min. daily.)*	
		a. Range of motion (passive)	**f.** Walking
		b. Range of motion (active)	**g.** Dressing or grooming
		c. Splint or brace assistance	**h.** Eating or swallowing
		TRAINING AND SKILL PRACTICE IN:	**i.** Amputation/prosthesis care
			j. Communication
		d. Bed mobility	**k.** Other
		e. Transfer	

4.	DEVICES AND RESTRAINTS	*(Use the following codes for last 7 days:)* 0. Not used 1. Used less than daily 2. Used daily	
		Bed rails	
		a. - Full bed rails on all open sides of bed	
		b. - Other types of side rails used (e.g., half rail, one side)	
		c. Trunk restraint	
		d. Limb restraint	
		e. Chair prevents rising	
5.	HOSPITAL STAY(S)	Record number of times resident was admitted to hospital with an overnight stay in last 90 days (or since last assessment if less than 90 days). *(Enter 0 if no hospital admissions)*	
6.	EMERGENCY ROOM (ER) VISIT(S)	Record number of times resident visited ER without an overnight stay in last 90 days (or since last assessment if less than 90 days). *(Enter 0 if no ER visits)*	
7.	PHYSICIAN VISITS	In the LAST 14 DAYS (or since admission if less than 14 days in facility) how many days has the physician (or authorized assistant or practioner) examined the resident? *(Enter 0 if none)*	
8.	PHYSICIAN ORDERS	In the LAST 14 DAYS (or since admission if less than 14 days in facility) how many days has the physician (or authorized assistant or practioner) changed the resident's orders? *Do not include order renewals without change. (Enter 0 if none.)*	
9.	ABNORMAL LAB VALUES	Has the resident had any abnormal lab values during the last 90 days (or since admission)? 0. No 1. Yes	

SECTION Q. DISCHARGE POTENTIAL AND OVERALL STATUS

1.	DISCHARGE POTENTIAL	a. Resident expresses/indicates preference to return to the community	
		0. No 1. Yes	
		b. Resident has a support person who is positive towards discharge	
		0. No 1. Yes	
		c. Stay projected to be of a short duration - discharge projected within 90 days (do not include expected discharge due to death)	
		0. No 2. Within 31-90 days	
		1. Within 30 days 3. Discharge status uncertain	
2.	OVERALL CHANGE IN CARE NEEDS	Resident's overall self sufficiency has changed significantly as compared to status of 90 days ago (or since last assessment if less than 90 days).	
		0. No change 1. Improved - receives fewer supports, needs less restrictive level of care 2. Deteriorated - receives more support	

SECTION R. ASSESSMENT INFORMATION

1.	PARTICIPA-TION IN ASSESS-MENT	a. Resident: 0. No 1. Yes	
		b. Family: 0. No 1. Yes 2. No family	
		c. Significant other: 0. No 1. Yes 2. None	

2. SIGNATURES OF PERSONS COMPLETING THE ASSESSMENT:

a. Signature of RN Assessment Coordinator (sign on above line)

b. Date RN Assessment Coordinator signed as complete

	Month	Day	Year

c. Other signatures	Title	Sections	Date
d.			Date
e.			Date
f.			Date
g.			Date
h.			Date

A P P E N D I X B

Functional Assessment Tools

BARTHEL INDEX

Action	With help	Independently
1. Feeding (if food needs to be cut up = help)	5	10
2. Moving from wheelchair to bed and return (includes sitting up in bed)	5-10	15
3. Personal toilet (washing face, combing hair, shaving, cleaning teeth)	0	5
4. Getting on and off toilet (handling clothes, wiping, flushing)	5	10
5. Bathing self	0	5
6. Walking on level surface (or if unable to walk, propelling wheelchair)	0*	5*
7. Ascending and descending stairs	5	10
8. Dressing (includes tying shoes, fastening fasteners)	5	10
9. Controlling bowels	5	10
10. Controlling bladder	5	10

A patient scoring 100 BDI is continent, feeds himself, dresses himself, gets up out of bed and chairs, bathes himself, walks at least a block, and can ascend and descend stairs. This does not mean that he is able to live alone—he may not be able to cook, keep house, and meet the public—but he is able to get along without attendant care.

DEFINITION AND DISCUSSION OF SCORING

1. Feeding
   - 10 = Independent. The patient can feed himself a meal from a tray or table when someone puts the food within his reach. He must put on an assistive device if this is needed, cut up the food, use salt and pepper, spread butter, etc. He must accomplish this in a reasonable time.
   - 5 = Some help is necessary (with cutting up food, etc., as listed previously).

BARTHEL INDEX—cont'd

2. Moving from wheelchair to bed and return

   15 = Independent in all phases of this activity. Patient can safely approach the bed in his wheelchair, lock brakes, lift footrests, move safely to bed, lie down, come to a sitting position on the side of the bed, and change the position of the wheelchair, if necessary, to transfer back into it safely and return to the wheelchair.

   10 = Either some minimal help is needed in some step of this activity or the patient needs to be reminded or supervised for safety of one or more parts of this activity.

   5 = Patient can come to a sitting position without the help of a second person but needs to be lifted out of bed, or he transfers with a great deal of help.

3. Doing personal toilet

   5 = Patient can wash hands and face, comb hair, clean teeth, and shave. He may use any kind of razor, but he must put in blade or plug in razor without help, as well as getting it from the drawer or cabinet. Female patients must put on own makeup, if used, but need not braid or style hair.

4. Getting on and off toilet

   10 = Patient is able to get on and off toilet, fasten and unfasten clothes, prevent soiling of clothes, and use toilet paper without help. He may use a wall bar or other stable object for support if needed. If it is necessary to use a bed pan instead of toilet, he must be able to place it on a chair, empty it, and clean it.

   5 = Patient needs help because of imbalance or in handling clothes or in using toilet paper.

5. Bathing self

   5 = Patient may use a bathtub, shower, or take a complete sponge bath. He must be able to do all the steps involved in whichever method is employed without another person being present.

6. Walking on a level surface

   15 = Patient can walk at least 50 yards without help or supervision. He may wear braces or prostheses and use crutches, canes, or a walkerette, but not a rolling walker. He must be able to lock and unlock braces if used, assume the standing position and sit down, get the necessary mechanical aids into position for use, and dispose of them when he sits. (Putting on and taking off braces is scored under dressing.)

6a. Propelling a wheelchair

   5 = Patient cannot ambulate but can propel a wheelchair independently. He must be able to go around corners, turn around, maneuver the chair to a table, toilet, etc. He must be able to push a chair at least 50 yards. Do not score this item if the patient gets a score for walking.

7. Ascending and descending stairs

   10 = Patient is able to go up and down a flight of stairs safely without help or supervision. He may and should use handrails, canes, or crutches when needed. He must be able to carry canes or crutches as he ascends or descends stairs.

   5 = Patient needs help with or supervision of any one of the above items.

8. Dressing and undressing

   10 = Patient is able to put on and remove and fasten all clothing, and tie shoelaces (unless it is necessary to use adaptations for this). This activity includes putting on and removing and fastening corset or braces when these are prescribed. Such special clothing as suspenders, loafer shoes, or dresses that open down the front may be used when necessary.

Continued

BARTHEL INDEX—cont'd

    5 = Patient needs help in putting on and removing or fastening any clothing. He must do at least half the work himself. He must accomplish this in a reasonable time. Women need not be scored on use of a brassiere or girdle unless these are prescribed garments.

9. Continence of bowels

    10 = Patient is able to control his bowels and have no accidents. He can use a suppository or take an enema when necessary (as for spinal cord injury patients who have had bowel training).

    5 = Patient needs help in using a suppository or taking an enema or has occasional accidents.

10. Controlling bladder

    10 = Patient is able to control his bladder day and night. Spinal cord injury patients who wear an external device and leg bag must put them on independently, clean and empty bag, and stay dry day and night.

    5 = Patient has occasional accidents or cannot wait for the bed pan or get to the toilet in time or needs help with an external device.

The total score is not as significant or meaningful as the breakdown into individual items, since these indicate where the deficiencies are.

Any applicant to a chronic hospital who scores 100 BDI should be evaluated carefully before admission to see whether such hospitalization is indicated. Discharged patients with 100 BDI should not require further physical therapy but may benefit from a home visit to see whether any environmental adjustments are indicated.

From Mahoney, F.I., & Barthel, D.W. (1965). Functional evaluation: The Barthel Index. *Maryland State Medical Journal, 14,* 62. Reprinted with permission.
*Score only if unable to walk.

INSTRUMENTAL ACTIVITIES OF DAILY LIVING SCALE

Action	Score
A. Ability to use telephone	
1. Operates telephone on own initiative—looks up and dials numbers, etc.	1
2. Dials a few well-known numbers	1
3. Answers telephone but does not dial	1
4. Does not use telephone at all	0
B. Shopping	
1. Takes care of all shopping needs independently	1
2. Shops independently for small purchases	0
3. Needs to be accompanied on any shopping trip	0
4. Completely unable to shop	0
C. Food preparation	
1. Plans, prepares, and serves adequate meals independently	1
2. Prepares adequate meals if supplied with ingredients	0
3. Heats and serves prepared meals, or prepares meals but does not maintain adequate diet	0
4. Needs to have meals prepared and served	0
D. Housekeeping	
1. Maintains house alone or with occasional assistance (e.g., "heavy work—domestic help")	1
2. Performs light daily tasks such as dishwashing, bed making	1
3. Performs light daily tasks but cannot maintain acceptable level of cleanliness	1
4. Needs help with all home maintenance tasks	1
5. Does not participate in any housekeeping tasks	0
E. Laundry	
1. Does personal laundry completely	1
2. Launders small items—rinses socks, stockings, etc.	1
3. All laundry must be done by others	0
F. Mode of transportation	
1. Travels independently on public transportation or drives own car	1
2. Arranges own travel via taxi, but does not otherwise use public transportation	1
3. Travels on public transportation when assisted or accompanied by another	1
4. Travel limited to taxi or automobile with assistance of another	0
5. Does not travel at all	0
G. Responsibility for own medications	
1. Is responsible for taking medication in correct dosages at correct times	1
2. Takes responsibility if medication is prepared in advance in separate dosages	0
3. Is not capable of dispensing own medication	0
H. Ability to handle finances	
1. Manages financial matters independently (budgets, writes checks, pays rent and bills, goes to bank), collects and keeps track of income	1
2. Manages day-to-day purchases, but needs help with banking, major purchases, etc.	1
3. Incapable of handling money	0

From Lawton, M.P., & Brody, F. (1969). Assessment of older people: Self-maintaining and instrumental activities of daily living. *Gerontologist,* 9:181. Reprinted with permission.

Organizations Providing Resources and Information for and about Older Adults

Administration on Aging
330 Independence Avenue S.W.
Washington, DC 20201
(202) 619-0556

Age and Aging
Bailliere Tindall
7-8 Henrietta Street
Covent Garden
London, England WCZE 8QE

Alzheimer's Association
919 N. Michigan Avenue, Suite 1000
Chicago, IL 60611-1676
(800) 272-3900

American Academy of Physical Medicine and Rehabilitation
122 S. Michigan Avenue, Suite 1300
Chicago, IL 60603-6107
(312) 922-9366

American Association for Continuity of Care
1730 N. Lynn Street, Suite 520
Arlington, VA 22209
(703) 525-1191

American Association for Geriatric Psychiatry
P.O. Box 376-A
Greenbelt, MD 20768
(301) 220-0952

American Association for International Aging
1133 20th Street N.W., Suite 333
Washington, DC 20036
(202) 822-8893

American Association of Homes and Services for the Aging
901 E. Street N.W., Suite 500
Washington, DC 20004-2037
(202) 783-2242

American Association of Retired Persons (AARP)
601 E. Street N.W.
Washington, DC 20049
(202) 434-2277

American Bar Association
Commission on Legal Problems of the Elderly
1800 M Street N.W.
Washington, DC 20036
(202) 331-2297

*American College of Nursing Home
Administrators*
4650 East-West Freeway
Washington, DC 20014

American Council of the Blind
1155 15th Street N.W., Suite 720
Washington, DC 20005
(202) 467-5081

American Diabetes Association
Diabetes Information Service Center
1660 Duke Street
Alexandria, VA 22314
(800) ADA-DISC

*American Federation for Aging Research
(AFAR)*
1414 Avenue of the Americas, 18th Floor
New York, NY 10019
(212) 752-AFAR
(212) 832-2298 (fax)

American Foundation for the Blind, Inc.
National Office
15 W. 16th Street
New York, NY 10011
(212) 620-2000

American Geriatrics Society
770 Lexington Avenue, Suite 300
New York, NY 10021
(212) 308-1414

American Health Care Association
1201 L Street N.W.
Washington, DC 20005-4014
(202) 842-4444

American Heart Association
7320 Greenville Avenue
Dallas, TX 75231
(214) 373-6300

American Lung Association
1740 Broadway
New York, NY 10019-4373
(212) 315-8700

American Medical Association (AMA)
515 N. State Street
Chicago, IL 60610
(312) 464-5000

*American Medical Directors Association
(AMDA)*
10480 Little Patuxeny Parkway, Suite 760
Columbia, MD 21044
(800) 876-2632

American Nurses' Association
600 Maryland Avenue S.W.
Washington, DC 20024-2571
(202) 544-4444

American Parkinson's Disease Association
60 Bay Street, Suite 401
Staten Island, NY 10301
(800) 825-2732

American Public Health Association
1015 15th Street N.W.
Washington, DC 20005
(202) 789-5600

American Red Cross
National Headquarters
430 17th Street N.W.
Washington, DC 20006
(202) 737-8300

American Society for Geriatric Dentistry
211 E. Chicago Avenue, 17th Floor
Chicago, IL 60611
(312) 440-2500, x 2660

*American Society for Parenteral and Enteral
Nutrition*
8630 Fenton Street, Suite 412
Silver Spring, MD 20910-3805
(301) 587-6315

American Society on Aging
833 Market Street, Suite 512
San Francisco, CA 94103-1824
(415) 882-2910

*American Speech-Language-Hearing
Association*
10801 Rockville Pike
Rockville, MD 20852
(301) 897-5700
(800) 638-8255

Arthritis Foundation
1330 West Peachtree Street
Atlanta, GA 30309
(800) 283-7800

*Association for Gerontology in Higher
Education*
1001 Connecticut Avenue N.W., Suite 410
Washington, DC 20036-5504
(202) 429-9277

Catholic Charities U.S.A.
1731 King Street
Alexandria, VA 22314
(703) 549-1390

Catholic Health Association of the U.S.
4455 Woodson
St. Louis, MO 63134-3797
(314) 427-2500

Center for Social Gerontology
2307 Shelby Avenue
Ann Arbor, MI 48103-3895
(313) 665-1126

Children of Aging Parents
1609 Woodbourne Road, Suite 302-A
Levittown, PA 19057
(215) 945-6900

Department of Veteran's Affairs
Veterans Health Administration
Nursing Service Programs (118c)
810 Vermont Avenue N.W.
Washington, DC 20420
(202) 299-4000

Federal Council on Aging
330 Independence Avenue S.W.
Room 4280 HHS-N
Washington, DC 20201

Food and Drug Administration (FDA)
Professional and Consumer Programs
5600 Fishers Lane, Suite 1685
Parklawn Building
Rockville, MD 20857
(301) 443-5006

Foundation for Hospice and Home Care
519 C Street N.E.
Washington, DC 20002
(202) 547-6586

Gerontological Nutritionists
4103 44th Street
Sacramento, CA 95820
(916) 451-7149

Gerontological Society of America
1275 K Street N.W., Suite 350
Washington, DC 20005-4006
(202) 842-1275

Gray Panthers
1424 16th Street N.W., Suite 602
Washington, DC 20036
(202) 387-3111

House Select Committee on Aging
House Office Building
Annex 1, Room 712
Washington, DC 20515

*Lighthouse National Center for Vision
and Aging*
800 Second Avenue
New York, NY 10017
(212) 808-0077

*Mountain States (Human Services
Organization)*
950 N. Cole Road
P.O. Box 6756
Boise, ID 83704
(208) 322-4880

National Association for Hispanic Elderly
3325 Wilshire Boulevard, Suite 800
Los Angeles, CA 90010-1724
(213) 487-1922

National Association for Home Care
519 C Street N.W.
Washington, DC 20002-5809
(202) 547-7424

National Association of Directors of Nursing
Administration in Long-term Care
(NADONA-LTC)
10999 Reed Hartman Highway, Suite 229
Cincinnati, OH 45242
(800) 222-0539

National Association of the Deaf
814 Thayer Avenue
Silver Spring, MD 20910-4500
(301) 587-1788
(301) 587-1789 (TTY)

National Cancer Institute
Office of Communications
Room 10A24
9000 Rockville Pike
Rockville, MD 20892
(800) 4-CANCER

National Caucus and Center on the
Black Aged, Inc.
1424 K Street N.W., Suite 500
Washington, DC 20005
(202) 637-8400

National Citizens Coalition for Nursing Home
Reform
1224 M Street N.W., Suite 301
Washington, DC 20005
(202) 393-2018

National Conference on Geriatric Nurse
Practitioners
P.O. Box 270101
Fort Collins, CO 80527-0101
(303) 493-7793

National Council of Senior Citizens, Inc.
1331 F Street N.W.
Washington, DC 20004-1171
(202) 347-8800
(202) 624-9595 (fax)

National Council on the Aging
(Includes National Institute of Senior Citizens
and National Institute on Adult Day Care)
409 3rd Street S.W., Suite 200
Washington, DC 20024
(202) 479-1200

National Gerontological Nursing Association
c/o Mosby, Inc.
7250 Parkway Drive, Suite 510
Hanover, MD 21076
(800) 723-0560

National Hospice Organization (NHO)
1901 N. Moore Street, Suite 901
Arlington, VA 22202
(703) 243-5900

National Indian Council on Aging
6400 Uptown Boulevard N.E., Suite 510W
Albuquerque, NM 87110
(505) 242-9505

National Institute on Aging
31 Center Drive, MSC 2292
9000 Rockville Pike
Bethesda, MD 20892-2292
(301) 496-1752

National League for Nursing
350 Hudson Street
New York, NY 10014
(212) 989-9393

National Meals on Wheels Foundation
1133 20th Street N.W., Suite 321
Washington, DC 20036
(202) 463-6039

National Osteoporosis Foundation
1150 17th Street N.W., Suite 500
Washington, DC 20036
(202) 223-2226

National Policy Center on Housing and Living
Arrangements for the Older Americans
University of Michigan
2000 Bonisteel Boulevard
Ann Arbor, MI 48109

National Rehabilitation Association
633 S. Washington Street
Alexandria, VA 22314
(703) 836-0850

National Senior Citizens Law Center
1815 H Street N.W., Suite 700
Washington, DC 20006
(202) 887-5280

National Stroke Association
8480 E. Orchard Road, Suite 1000
Englewood, CO 80111-5015
(303) 771-1700

Older Women's League (OWL)
666 11th Street N.W., Suite 700
Washington, DC 20001
(202) 783-6686

Oncology Nursing Society
501 Holiday Drive
Pittsburgh, PA 15220-2749
(412) 921-7373

Senate Special Committee on Aging
Dirksen Senate Office Building
Room 623
Washington, DC 20510
(202) 224-5364

Social Security Administration
6401 Security Boulevard
Baltimore, MD 21235
(800) 772-1213

INDEX